Dimensions of

Community Health

9

Dimensions of

Community Health

Fourth Edition

Dean F. Miller

University of Toledo

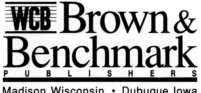

WCB Brown &
Benchmark
PUBLISHERS

Madison, Wisconsin • Dubuque, Iowa

Book Team

Editor *Ed Bartell*
Developmental Editor *Megan Rundel*
Production Editor *Kristine McQuigg*
Designer *Anna Manhart*
Art Editor *Tina Flanagan*
Photo Editor *Laura Fuller*
Visuals/Design Developmental Consultant *Marilyn A. Phelps*
Visuals/Design Freelance Specialist *Mary L. Christianson*
Marketing Manager *Pamela S. Cooper*
Advertising Coordinator *Susan J. Butler*
Production Manager *Beth Kundert*

Brown & Benchmark

A Division of Wm. C. Brown Communications, Inc.

Executive Vice President/General Manager *Thomas E. Doran*
Vice President/Editor in Chief *Edgar J. Laube*
Vice President/Marketing and Sales Systems *Eric Ziegler*
Director of Production *Vickie Putman Caughron*
Director of Custom and Electronic Publishing *Chris Rogers*

Wm. C. Brown Communications, Inc.

President and Chief Executive Officer *G. Franklin Lewis*
Senior Vice President, Operations *James H. Higby*
Corporate Senior Vice President and Chief Financial Officer *Robert Chesterman*
Corporate Senior Vice President and President of Manufacturing *Roger Meyer*

The credits section for this book begins on page 489 and is considered an extension of the copyright page.

Copyedited by Nikki Herbst

A Times Mirror Company

Library of Congress Catalog Card Number: 94–70177

ISBN 0–697–15262–6

Printed in the United States of America by Wm. C. Brown Communications, Inc., 2460 Kerper Boulevard, Dubuque, IA 52001

10 9 8 7 6 5 4 3 2 1

BRIEF CONTENTS

CONTENTS

This fourth edition of *Dimensions of Community Health* has been written for individuals who have had little experience with community health programs. It also is directed toward those people with minimal knowledge about community health. The book provides an overview of the field of community health and focuses on a variety of community health problems and issues.

This text is most timely, since it discusses many significant changes occurring in the mid-1990's that have a direct impact on community health. Some of these changes involve philosophical and financial foundations of community health.

The various problems and issues discussed in *Dimensions of Community Health* focus upon three different dimensions: political, social (cultural), and economic. Each dimension is independently discussed in the first portion of the book, but integrated with other facets of community health in the remainder of the text.

This edition of *Dimensions of Community Health* is organized into four units. The first unit introduces the reader to the various organizational structures of community health: international, national, state, and local along with an examination of the role played by the private sector.

In unit two the emphasis is on the provision of health care in the United States. Increased escalation of health care costs and the many problems associated with the lack of accessibility to health care for many individuals, particularly the economically disadvantaged, has led to major concern about what kind of health care system should be in place by the latter part of the 1990s. This section has been revised and a new chapter on economic factors relating to health care added in this edition for the purpose of keeping as current as possible in the national debate over health care reform.

In unit three the reader will find discussion of nine different areas of community health programming that usually can be found in most localities throughout the nation. In unit four, several specific target groups or program activities are examined for which community health programming is of particular concern, both locally and nationally.

The first unit, "Organization of Community Health," includes presentations concerning the basic concept of "community" and an overview of federal, state and local, and international organizations, activities, and programming. The reader is also exposed to a broader interpretation of community, with international health problems being emphasized.

Many important, and necessary, activities of health and social programming are carried out by the private sector. Chapter 5 analyzes this sector and its importance in community health. The private sector includes the philanthropic foundations, the religious agencies and organizations, and the voluntary health organizations.

No discussion of community health can be complete without an understanding of issues concerning the provision of health care. Unit two, "Health Care and Community Health," has been revised in this fourth edition to include as much as is currently possible about the country-wide discussion and debate over national health care reform. Health care costs have risen dramatically during the past decade. Chapter 6 examines various issues impacting this escalation of health care costs, with particular focus upon the problems faced by the economically disadvantaged, the medically uninsured, and the homeless.

Payment for health care services is a concern of every American. A major new section is presented in chapter 7 that examines state and national initiatives aimed at health care reform. The importance of health care reform has been "front page news" since the beginning of the national presidential election campaign in 1992. The issues associated with this debate and current developments are a part of this chapter.

The third chapter in this unit, chapter 8, discusses various issues involving health care facilities and the medical work force in the latter part of this century.

The third unit, "Programming for Community Health," presents nine different areas of community health programming that have traditionally been found in most local and state health departments. In any kind of health program planning, the various skills and knowledge of epidemiology are important. These factors are presented in brief overview in chapter 9.

Since the early days of community health in the United States, health programming has included activities designed to control and prevent diseases and to provide a clean sanitary environmental setting. For this reason, disease prevention and control measures are presented in chapters 10 and 11 and environmental health in chapter 12. Information is included about both communicable and chronic diseases.

Possibly the most feared communicable disease confronting the world in the mid-1990s is acquired immunodeficiency syndrome (AIDS). Information about HIV/AIDS is presented in several different sections of this edition, with special focus in the chapter on disease control.

Thousands of fatalities and injuries occur each year due to various kinds of traumatic occurrences. These factors have a major impact on the health care services and agencies of every community. Chapter 13 presents updated information about injury prevention and control.

The next four chapters present information concerning community nutrition, community mental health, school health, and health promotion/health education. In each chapter, selected problems and programs germane to the topic are noted. The impact of political, social, and economic factors are interwoven throughout these chapters.

In the last unit, "Community Health for Special Target Groups," discussions are presented that focus upon special groups of concern in communities throughout the country. Any student of community health or any health care worker cannot long escape realizing the cultural dimensions of community health. Many community health activities and programs are designed to meet the needs of minorities throughout the nation. The health status of three minority populations is presented in chapter 18: African-Americans, Native Americans, and Hispanics. The text also includes information about community health concerns of an expanding minority in the United States—refugees who have left their homelands in an attempt to find peace, stability, and economic opportunity. This influx of refugees in recent years has introduced a variety of unique community health problems.

A review of the health status of women and infants tells much about the health status of any community. Chapter 19 presents information on maternal-child health (MCH) issues. Important matters such as infant mortality, immunization, and contraception are presented. A matter of specific concern in communities across America in recent years is the epidemic of teenage pregnancies. Probably the most controversial health and social issue confronting the American society in the 1990s is the matter of abortion. Unfortunately, resolution to this conflict is not to be found in the foreseeable future. The issue is presented in this chapter.

At the opposite end of the life cycle from birth and infancy is old age. Senior citizens are the most rapidly increasing demographic population in America today. With this in mind, the need for increased thinking about care and life-style of the elderly is presented in chapter 20.

Chapters 21 and 22 present information about abuse of drugs, alcohol, and tobacco, and occupational health and safety. Factors concerning these matters that affect everyone in some way are analyzed and discussed.

The last chapter (chapter 23) presents discussions on the subject of violence and its impact on community health. This is a problem that seems to have escalated to tragic proportions in the past several years. Initially, child abuse and neglect, spouse abuse, and elder abuse are discussed. Then concerns relating to rape are introduced. The chapter ends with material about homicide and suicide.

A short epilogue is included at the end of the book. The author hopes this material will challenge the reader to consider what responsibilities and challenges await each of us in the field of community health during the remainder of the twentieth century.

To assist the reader in the use of this text, each chapter contains a chapter outline, a summary, discussion questions, suggested relevant readings, and endnotes. Most chapters also contain a short story, a case study, an inventory, or other "boxed" information that illustrates the actual workings of community health programs and workers. The charts and photographs also elaborate on textual information. Several new case studies and discussion questions have been added to this edition to assist the reader.

The dynamic, ever changing nature of community health makes it very difficult to maintain total currentness of information. During the period of time that this revision has been taking place, almost daily some news release, news report, or journal article either changes, adds to, or increases information about some concept or fact that is presented. The reader will need to keep abreast of developments in the news as this edition serves as a foundation. Community health and health care are ever developing dynamics in the American society.

Many individuals with whom I have had the opportunity to interact professionally have provided assistance in the development of this book. I appreciate the efforts of all who have answered my questions, sent information when requested, or just had the time to talk with me about the issues found in the book. It has been particularly refreshing to obtain important insights that keep one current by working with students in internships and field experiences. Through these contacts, I have acquired an expanded view of community health and an appreciation of this dynamic, challenging field of activity.

In addition to the many opportunities I have had in this country, my global consciousness has been expanded by working in community health projects in several countries of the world. I hope this consciousness will be extended to the users of *Dimensions of Community Health*.

D.F.M.

ACKNOWLEDGEMENTS

Thanks are extended to the many reviewers who critically appraised this edition of the text:

Vivien C. Carver
University of Southern Mississippi

Marietta Deming
Eastern Illinois University

Janet B. Douglass
University of Massachusetts–Lowell

William C. Gross
Western Michigan University

Jacquie Rainey
Ball State University

Patricia A. Tyra
University of Massachusetts–Lowell

Sydney C. Walston
Central Michigan University

Lynn D. Woodhouse
East Stroudsburg University

Thanks are also extended to the many respondents to a written questionnaire regarding how this edition of *Dimensions of Community Health* could be improved. These respondents include:

G. Robert Bowers
Tallahassee Community College

Denise Depalma
Montclair State College

Robert I. Fisher
Baldwin Wallace College

Mary L. Gress
Lorain County Community College

Laurie Jossey
Brewton-Parker College

Frances Makowski
University of Portland

Kelli McCormack-Brown
Western Illinois University

Arthur J. Rubens
Northern Illinois University

Junella Silvey
Tallahassee Community College

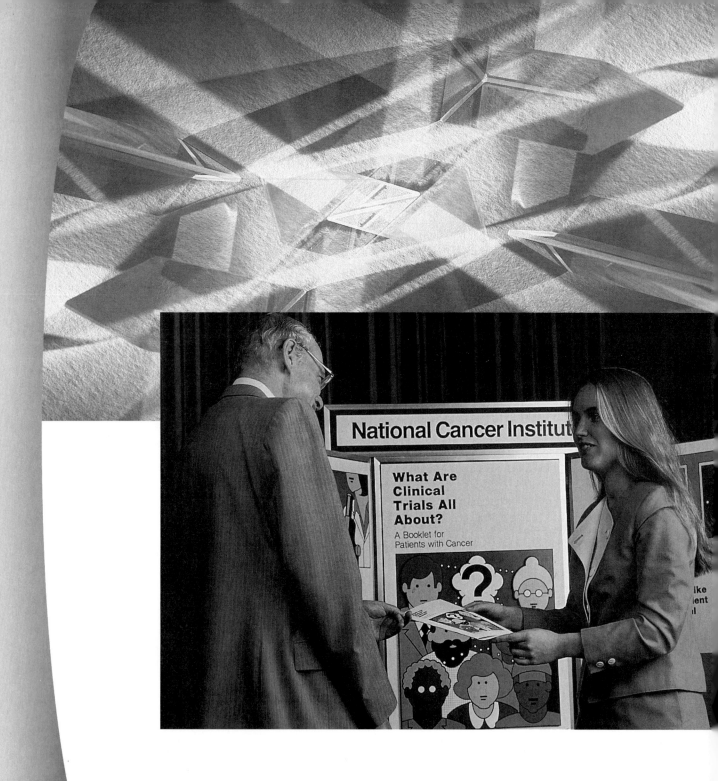

UNIT **ONE**

Organization of Community Health

CHAPTER **ONE**

Health

Involvement of the Community

Angela graduated from college last term with a major in community health. She has been employed for the past several months by the community hospital as a program coordinator in health promotion. During these past months Angela has learned more about community health than she did in all of her college course work. Reflecting upon the many experiences she has had so far, Angela considers the many people she has met and the many challenging and interesting activities and responsibilities involved in their work.

Last week she had the opportunity to meet a sanitarian with nearly thirty years of experience in the city health department. This individual possessed a wealth of knowledge about water and sewage sanitation in the community. It was fascinating for Angela to learn of the many responsibilities that a sanitarian is required to carry out.

Angela's exposure was further expanded when she was asked to become part of a community coalition on health promotion for mothers of preschool-age children. She learned that the funding for much of this coalition project came through something called a "block grant." Since the grant was being prepared just at the time that Angela became involved with the coalition, she found opportunity to work on the writing team involved with the grant proposal.

One day Angela received a telephone call asking if she could present a three hour seminar on stress management. This request was made by the owner of a small company in town, who felt a need to provide this seminar for the employees of his company.

On a recent weekend there was a health fair at the major shopping mall in the community. Since the hospital health promotion department was the principal sponsor of the fair, Angela came to know a variety of people from several different agencies. She worked very closely with a team from the local school system who have been involved in developing a drug-free program for the junior high school students. A family-planning counselor and a health department public health nurse have also worked closely with Angela on this health fair. In addition, a staff person from the regional safety council has developed an interesting display on alcohol and driving.

Knowledge about the work and activities of all these professionals has helped Angela to understand that the efforts to improve the health and well-being of the community involve more than just the medically oriented activities of health care providers. Numerous organizations, agencies, and personnel are a part of community health activities.

4

Traditionally, community health programs were principally directed toward the control of communicable diseases and the improvement of the sanitary conditions of the community. The current scope of community health has broadened considerably. It includes not only these goals but also activities directed at provision of mental health services, drug and alcohol control and rehabilitation, improved nutrition, fitness, and general wellness, control of chronic diseases such as heart disease and cancer, and many other concerns related to the provision of health care. Community health used to be the principal responsibility of the state and/or local departments of health. Today numerous programs are conducted in hospitals, by nongovernmental private agencies, in schools, and in a variety of other settings. Since the health of each person has a collective effect upon the health of the community, health and well-being necessitate community involvement.

Historical Perspective

As the early explorers and colonists came to North America during the sixteenth and seventeenth centuries, they brought along numerous communicable diseases and the need for health care. Epidemics of smallpox, yellow fever, cholera, typhoid, measles, and other contagious diseases caused the death of thousands of Native Americans as well as settlers. Many of the early colonists witnessed the near destruction of entire populations from these epidemics.

At that time nothing was known of the "germ theory" of disease causation, and it was difficult to establish disease prevention programs when the exact etiology was unknown. There was widespread belief that many of the diseases were caused by decaying animal and vegetable substances. Noxious odors in the air were another suspected source of contagious diseases. Because of these beliefs, most of the colonies prior to the American Revolution took measures designed to improve poor environmental sanitation. There was concern about pollution along many of the waterways of the East Coast where settlement was occurring.

To reduce the presence of communicable diseases, quarantine measures often became law. For example, in the Massachusetts Bay Colony individuals with smallpox were placed in isolation so as not to come in contact with other residents and in turn spread this highly contagious disease. Houses and buildings where an individual with a contagious disease resided were placed under quarantine. Ships docked at ports often were quarantined when diseases were present among the passengers. People were not permitted to come and go to and from these locations and facilities.

After the Declaration of Independence and the American Revolution, the newly formed states became responsible for the health of their citizens. By 1800, legislation in such states as New York and Massachusetts had provided for the establishment of state health departments. At this same time most major cities—Boston, New York, Philadelphia, Baltimore, and others—established health departments to provide services related to environmental sanitation and disease control.

The federal government established a public health service in 1798. It was known as the Marine Hospital Service and was the forerunner of today's Public Health Service. This agency was created by action of President John Adams to care for sick and disabled merchant seamen and to prevent the spread of disease epidemics. The first Marine Hospital was established in an abandoned barracks on Castle Island in Boston Harbor. The health of seamen and their families was a major concern at this time because the merchant fleet was the principal economic lifeline for the nation. Transportation, economic growth, and prosperity, as well as national defense, were closely intertwined with a strong merchant marine fleet.

Throughout the nineteenth century as the nation grew in population and expanded geographically, there was minimal growth of public health initiatives. The provision of health services was considered to be a private matter. Physicians and other health care providers practiced independently, with care being rendered on a fee-for-service basis. The education and training of health care workers during this time lacked strong controls and regulations, and so skills and abilities varied greatly.

Hospitals and other health care facilities were not considered to be important by most Americans. Many believed that hospitals were only for the poor and the aged. Those with incurable communicable diseases and those who were insane went to the hospitals. Most people identified admission to a hospital as evidence there was little hope for rehabilitation and recovery. The hospital was a place to go to die.

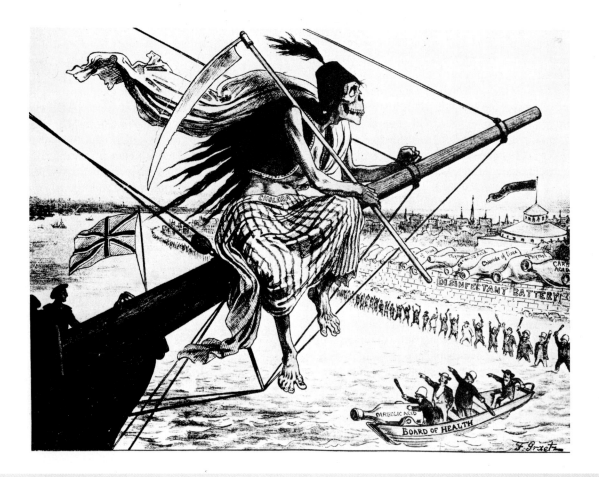

The United States tightened quarantine and sanitation laws after the cholera pandemic. Cartoon 1883.

During the 1800s many European immigrants came to America to escape famine, poverty, and difficult living conditions. As these large numbers of people began to settle in seaport cities such as New York City, Boston, and Baltimore, many problems arose. Sanitation and housing problems became very acute. The need for dealing with poorly ventilated, filthy tenement houses, inadequate sewage disposal and drainage, a poor water supply, and poor food distribution services put increasing pressure on communities to develop some type of public health program. It became obvious that these conditions were taking their toll in lives and illnesses.

By the latter part of the nineteenth century, a number of states had established state health departments. Many programs were developed during these years, including state hospitals for the care of the mentally ill. State and local health departments also had responsibility for improving the sanitation of food and dairy products, and for sewage removal and disposal.

As America changed from a rural, agricultural society to an urban, industrialized nation, hygiene and safety in the workplace became an issue. There was little regulatory control over workplace conditions. However, by the early twentieth century workers' compensation

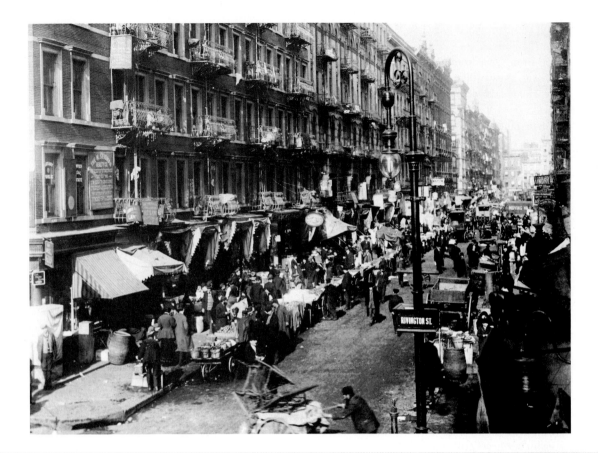

Crowding and poor sanitary conditions were seen in New York City in the 1800s.

laws were providing some assistance to employees who were injured or disabled while at work.

Increased federal legislation led to expanded public health initiatives in programming and research in the latter part of the 1800s and the early 1900s. Contagious disease control measures were the responsibility of state and local government. Nevertheless, recognizing that many of these governments had ineffective plans for coping with these problems, Congress passed a Federal Quarantine Act in 1878. This legislation authorized investigations into the origin and causes of epidemic diseases, especially yellow fever and cholera. The Marine Hospital Service developed quarantine laws for ports along the coasts and rivers of the nation where there were no state or local regulations.

Medical research being carried out throughout the 1800s by Louis Pasteur, Edward Jenner, Robert Koch, and other notable scientists expanded the knowledge of microorganisms and the etiology of disease. These new concepts led to the development of a number of vaccines and serums to protect against contagious diseases. By 1887 the new science of bacteriology was being practiced in a one-room building at the Marine Hospital on Staten Island to study cholera and other contagious diseases.

By the latter part of the nineteenth century, an increasing number of Americans were purchasing food that was produced by factories, shipped over long distances, and sold in commercial grocery stores. Prior to this most food was made or purchased locally from neighbors and surrounding farmers. Because of these changes, a greater amount of food being provided to consumers was not safe for human consumption. The need to transport food over long distances from farm to market led to the development of chemical preservatives. Used without controls, some of these chemicals were found to be dangerous to human health.

More instances of food adulteration began to occur. In some cases the adulteration was accidental, but in others it was due to carelessness in food handling. A number of state and national laws were passed to protect all people from poor quality, contaminated food. Eventually this led to the establishment of the federal Food and Drug Administration from passage of the first Federal Food and Drug Act in 1906.

During the early twentieth century medical research was making discoveries that were to have an impact on broadening the responsibilities of public health organizations. An evolution in health care and a shift in attention to different health problems helped to bring about this broadened concept. Though communicable diseases still received emphasis, a different set of problems including chronic diseases was now a greater cause of morbidity and mortality. They began to receive wider public health organization concern and attention. Other debilitating conditions have led to a greater involvement of many agencies, organizations, and programs in our communities, all related to the health of the general population.

The roles and responsibilities of a public health agency are no longer clearly delineated, although public health law and sanitary codes are quite specific in identifying many tasks. Previously clear distinctions between the functions of public health departments, hospitals, ambulatory care facilities, and other community health agencies are now somewhat blurred. For example, primary health tasks that were formerly conducted by public health departments, voluntary health agencies, schools, and universities are now often performed by hospitals. In fact, an expanding hospital activity is the development of wellness programs that focus upon a healthier life-style and improved well-being. These community outreach programs may involve fitness measurement and screening followed by prescribed personal exercise and nutrition programs.

Many community agencies, funded by federal or private grant monies, provide a broad range of health care services once fulfilled principally by public health departments. These new programs are not designed by, nor are they responsible to, health departments. In many communities, family-planning services, mental health care, maternal and child health activities, and other services are obtainable in settings apart from private medicine and official public health structures.

Local and state health departments are involved both directly and indirectly in health care functions. For example, they often license various health care institutions, are responsible for issuing credentials for allied health personnel, and have responsibilities in the administration of Medicare and Medicaid. Some public health departments and public hospitals have combined their resources to provide a full range of health care in both metropolitan and rural areas.

Concept of Community

The concept of community has traditionally been limited to a political or geographical region and its respective subdivisions. In its report, the National Commission on Community Health Services referred to a "community of solution."[1] The commission suggested that such a community was established ". . . by the boundaries within which a problem can be defined, dealt with, and solved."[2] Each health problem must be considered in light of the population involved.

Several factors must be considered in dealing with health problems in a community. Physical considerations including geography, topography, and climate play important roles in health concerns. In addition, social and cultural factors involving socioeconomic status, and political and religious influences, along with tradition and social norms, will have significant impact on the community. Organizational factors can also be important in coping with health problems. Numerous agencies and individuals influence health both directly and indirectly. All these must be considered in developing community health programs.

This concept of "community" leads to a functional definition relating to specifically identified problems. Such a notion may find some health problems very geographically limited, while others take on global dimensions. Yet each, regardless of its magnitude, is of vital importance in attaining the goal of creating a healthy society.

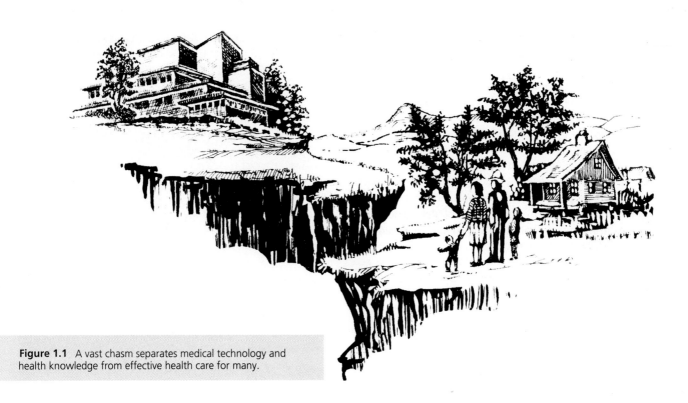

Figure 1.1 A vast chasm separates medical technology and health knowledge from effective health care for many.

This community concept is illustrated by two health problems. The first example is a common occurrence—an outbreak of a childhood disease in a local section of a metropolitan area. This type of problem is limited geographically, and the local health agency is usually able to solve the problem, since the outbreak probably occurred only in a given age group of children within a single school building. The second example is the problem of acid rain, which necessitates the efforts and services of a number of different agencies and political jurisdictions for its resolution. This problem may affect a "community" of several hundred square miles, including several different states, as well as having international ramifications, as in the conflict between the United States and Canada over damage being done to forests and fish in the Canadian northeast.

As the structure of community health has expanded from the traditional political and geographical entities to the concept of "communities of solution," its scope has broadened. Today, whenever a problem that relates to the health and well-being of people must be resolved, it becomes a concern of community health. Community health closely relates to the provision of health care in the nation, since each community health program, activity, organization, and agency, though unique in some manner, contributes to the overall goal of wellness and positive health for all humanity.

The Great Chasm

Most persons are well aware of the spectacular advances in medical science that have taken place in the twentieth century—new drugs, the control of numerous communicable diseases, body organ transplants, and highly sophisticated technological procedures. The advancement of medical and health knowledge (research and technology) improves the quality of life and has a profound effect upon millions of people throughout the world.

In spite of these developments, the provision of needed health services to multitudes of persons is far from adequate. A vast chasm separates medical technology and knowledge from effective health care for many individuals (figure 1.1). Too often efforts to bridge this chasm have been limited by inaccessible health care, the high cost of obtaining adequate health provisions, and the failure of many people to comprehend the complex system of health and medicine.

Not only is there a notable disparity between health care services in the United States and in less-developed countries, but in this country many persons are unable to obtain even minimal health care. Although many reasons can be suggested why this situation exists, the limitations usually belong to one of three categories. These categories relate to the chasm separating what is known about medical and health care from the provision of health services and proper effective health care. They are (1) *political considerations,* (2) *economic concerns,* and (3) *sociological* or *cultural ramifications.* Each of these dimensions, though important in and of itself, interacts with others and gives substance to community health.

Health for All by 2000

The importance of projecting long-range goals in the field of health care was highlighted by action taken in 1977 by the World Health Assembly of the World Health Organization. Recognizing the need for mobilizing various aspects of government as well as the health care field, the assembly called for "Health for All by the Year 2000."

Implied in this declaration is that major program goals that will permit all people throughout the world to lead socially and economically productive lives must be encouraged. It means that new and creative approaches to meeting the health needs of all people have to be introduced. Emphasis on curative medicine must give way to an emphasis on primary health care and preventive measures. A consideration of social problems relating to hunger, poverty, and overpopulation is needed in addition to traditional efforts at communicable disease control. It does not mean that all disease will be eliminated. However, the concept implies that the resources for health will be evenly distributed and that essential health care will be accessible for everyone.

Governments must be willing to allocate or reallocate adequate resources for health care needs. One of the goals of the World Health Organization was that nations would spend five percent of their national income on health care. This goal has not been realized. There is little likelihood that it will be attained in many nations by the year 2000.

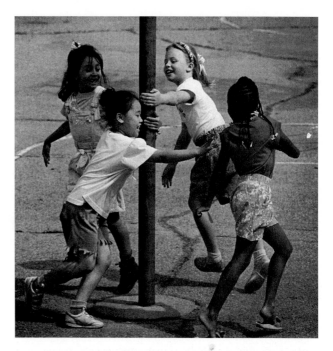

Children in the United States and throughout the world will be the major beneficiaries of programs designed to provide "Health for All by the Year 2000."

Though most governments have been less than supportive of moving their national resources to the health sectors, some positive measures have occurred. Many governments have reexamined their national health policies and have identified specific health problems needing attention. Reorientation of national health systems toward primary health care has taken place.[3] There have been reported reductions in many countries of maternal mortality rates. Also, life expectancy has improved in various nations of the world. The percentage of children receiving immunizations for basic diseases of childhood has increased in many localities.

Regardless of some improvements, the gap between the developed, industrial nations and the less developed, Third World nations continues to widen. The need now is for a greater will to provide the needed resources, in terms of economy and personnel, to achieve "health for all." Such an international goal is attainable only if individual nations identify goals and establish plans within their countries. "Health for All by the Year 2000" will not be achieved if economic resources, political will, and cultural differences are not addressed by those involved in community health. The chasm separating optimal health care and the present health status of millions in the world must be narrowed if the World Health Assembly goal is ever to be reached.

Year 2000 National Health Objectives

If a major commitment is made to the goal of health for all, it is reasonable to suggest that such a goal is attainable. It is hoped that new directions in community health will be charted leading to "Health for All by the Year 2000" in the United States. This commitment and planning began in 1979. After examining data concerning the leading causes of death and/or morbidity, the federal government—through the Surgeon General's Report on Health Promotion and Disease Prevention—issued a publication entitled *Healthy People*.[4] Specific risk factors for the leading causes of death were identified, and national goals were then established for five different age groups.

To reach these goals, extensive professional review and discussion involving individuals and organizations from both the public (governmental) and private sectors took place for the purpose of setting specific, measurable objectives for the nation. These objectives—encompassing such concerns as premature death, diseases, and other disabling conditions—were the focus of community health programming and resource allocation for the 1980s.

Fifteen areas were identified that, with planned and appropriate action, would meet these health promotion and disease prevention objectives and so lead to improved health for all Americans. The fifteen health problem areas were: control of hypertension; family planning; pregnancy and infant health; immunization; sexually transmitted diseases; toxic agent control; occupational health and safety; injury control; fluoridation of drinking water supplies; control of infectious diseases; smoking; alcohol and drug abuse; nutrition; physical fitness; and stress management. These problem areas were grouped into three categories: health services, health protection, and life-style change. In all, two hundred and twenty-six measurable objectives were identified and published.[5] It was felt that if these objectives could be achieved, the health status of Americans would be greatly improved.

These "National Health Goals for 1990" served as major guidelines for state and local health departments, private health agencies, corporations, schools, and other health-related organizations in program development and planning. Many states established their own state health goals.

The development of this initiative was the first time that the United States had established a set of measurable health objectives. By 1990 success in meeting the objectives was mixed: some were met, others surpassed, and about one-fourth not met.[6] A problem of this initiative was that baseline data for a number of the objectives were not available in 1979. Therefore, it was impossible to ascertain whether the individual objective had been reached during the 1980s.

Looking to the turn of the century, the government announced a new health objective program for the year 2000 in 1990. After a number of hearings, and review and comment by hundreds of health agencies, state and local health departments, and thousands of health professionals, new goals and objectives were established.

Goals for the Nation, Year 2000

1. Increase the span of a healthy life.
2. Reduce disparities in health status among different populations.
3. Provide access to preventive health care services for all people.

Three broad goals have been identified for the year 2000. Two hundred ninety-eight specific objectives have been detailed. These objectives have been spread over twenty-two subject priority areas as compared with fifteen in the 1979 plan. The objectives within each subject priority area are classified according to health status, risk reduction, public awareness, professional education and awareness, and services and protection.

Each objective area has been assigned to one of the agencies of the Public Health Service for administration, monitoring, and oversight. These objectives were developed after two years of information gathering in an effort coordinated by the Office of Disease Prevention and Health Promotion of the Public Health Service. Specific activities include working with national, state, and local agencies in program development and the dissemination of scientific and technical information as well as public information on health promotion and disease prevention.

Year 2000 National Health Objectives

Category	Number of Objectives	Lead Agency
Health Promotion		
Nutrition	21	Food and Drug Administration
		National Institutes of Health
Physical Activity and Fitness	12	President's Council on Physical Fitness and Sports
Tobacco	16	Centers for Disease Control and Prevention
Alcohol and Other Drugs	19	Alcohol, Drug Abuse, and Mental Health Administration
Family Planning	11	Office of Population Affairs
Violent and Abusive Behavior	18	Centers for Disease Control and Prevention
Mental Health and Mental Disorders	14	Alcohol, Drug Abuse, and Mental Health Administration
Educational and Community-Based Programs	14	Health Resources and Services Administration
Health Protection		
Environmental Health	16	National Institutes of Health
		Centers for Disease Control and Prevention
Occupational Safety and Health	15	Centers for Disease Control and Prevention
Unintentional Injuries	22	Centers for Disease Control and Prevention
Food and Drug Safety	6	Food and Drug Administration
Oral Health	16	National Institutes of Health
		Centers for Disease Control and Prevention
Preventive Services		
Maternal and Infant Health	16	Health Resources and Services Administration
Immunization and Infectious Diseases	19	Centers for Disease Control and Prevention
Human Immunodeficiency Virus Infection (AIDS)	14	National AIDS Program Office
Sexually Transmitted Diseases	15	Centers for Disease Control and Prevention
Heart Disease and Stroke	17	National Institutes of Health
Cancer	16	National Institutes of Health
Diabetes and Chronic Disabling Conditions	20	National Institutes of Health
		Centers for Disease Control and Prevention
Clinical Preventive Services	8	Health Resources and Services Administration
		Centers for Disease Control and Prevention
Surveillance		
Surveillance and Data Systems	7	Centers for Disease Control and Prevention

Source: Public Health Service. *Healthy People 2000: National Health Promotion and Disease Prevention Objectives for the Year 2000.* Washington, D.C.: U.S. Department of Health and Human Services. DHHS Publication no. (PHS) 91-50212 (1991).

The office's activities are also conducted in cooperation with business and industry, and professional and voluntary organizations.

In the year 2000 initiative, greater emphasis has been placed on target populations at risk for premature death, disease, and disability than in the earlier program. Three particular population groups that are at especially high risk have been identified. These include individuals of low socioeconomic status, certain minorities, and people having either physical and/or mental disabilities. Health education, statistical analysis, and prevention of disability and morbidity have been given more attention.[7] In setting specific measurable objectives, baseline data have been identified for most of the objectives.

Health through Health Promotion and Disease Prevention

As mentioned earlier, medicine has historically been oriented to *curative* measures. Throughout the United States and most of the industrial world, emphasis in health care has focused on the treatment and cure of disease. Medical

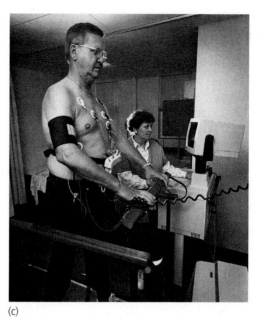

(a)

(b)

(c)

(a) The United States public is becoming aware of the values to be found in physical fitness activities. Fitness classes are conducted in schools, at worksites, and in YMCAs, churches, and other community centers. (b) Fitness programming includes aerobic exercise. Many such activities can be done alone at little cost. (c) It is wise to have a physical fitness evaluation before beginning a regular, planned exercise program. Fitness evaluations check the cardiovascular and respiratory systems.

education has prepared the physician to provide service that will cure, resolve, or reduce a maladaptation, and millions of dollars are spent on facilities and equipment to provide such medical care.

In recent years, increasing emphasis is being directed toward the *prevention* of illness and disease and to the promotion of positive health and wellness. Maintaining a high level of wellness is important to a larger segment of the American population. Individuals who are overweight are concerned about their weight and are looking for ways to reduce. In a society filled with stress-producing situations, the need and desire to find appropriate and effective ways to cope with stress are being examined. Physical fitness activities, such as jogging, walking, bicycling, and participating in active individual sports, are yet other measures being undertaken by millions to contribute to a more positive level of wellness.

Disease prevention is primarily a personal matter. However, there are community dynamics involved in health promotion. Many environmental activities such as pollution control, provision of a pure water supply, and sewage and toxic waste disposal have preventive values for both the individual and the community. Immunization of children for common childhood diseases also provides a preventive dimension for a community.

The Surgeon General's Report on Health Promotion and Disease Prevention noted that only 4 percent of federal expenditures for health were spent for prevention-related activities. This report pointed out three reasons for the importance of an increased emphasis on disease prevention and health promotion: (1) prevention saves lives; (2) prevention improves the quality of life; and (3) prevention is cost effective.[8]

An important focus of preventive health care is early intervention. This may involve personal evaluation of one's life-style. It means making decisions concerning factors that contribute to illness or to poor health—nutritional patterns, smoking behavior, stress dynamics, or drinking. In addition to personal life-style, a number of environmental factors affect health. Early intervention in environmental health hazard recognition and control is equally important in disease prevention.

A basic premise of preventive health care is that it will decrease the incidence, duration, and severity of disease. Theoretically, then, the cost of health care will be reduced and the well-being of people enhanced.

First, though, health promotion strategies must become cost beneficial for individuals, industry, and the community. Some economic incentive must be developed for health care providers to keep people well. With this in mind, hospitals are developing wellness centers or clinics where people in the community receive a variety of preventive services. These services include education, health counseling, screening for hypertension and other chronic disorders, fitness activities, and nutrition awareness.

Health insurance programs have not provided coverage for preventive health services to any great extent. So entrenched is the health insurance payment system in curative medicine that only rarely are routine physical examinations and health-counseling services covered. Increased interest in group prepaid health programs, known as health maintenance organizations, that provide an emphasis on preventive measures occurred in the 1980s. These organizations have economic motivators built into their programs to encourage people to maintain health and wellness.

In several states, efforts have been made to provide special tax funds to promote nonuse or better use of certain health-threatening substances. In one midwestern state, a penny state tax was added to all cigarette sales to finance the development of anti-smoking education programs in schools and community settings. The more cigarettes that are purchased, the more money that is made available for health promotion activities. With a reduction in cigarette purchases, less monies would be available, but it is hypothesized that the need for such activities would also be reduced. In another state, funds from the state alcohol tax revenues are appropriated for various alcohol programs, including detoxification programs and halfway houses.[9]

Emphasis on prevention creates some interesting dilemmas. Antismoking programs have been somewhat effective. Many state and local governments have passed laws and ordinances restricting smoking in public places as well as at public and private worksites. However, the political and economic power of the tobacco-producing industry has been opposed to these initiatives. They argue that tobacco is a legally manufactured product and as such should not have governmental restrictions placed on it.

Increased emphasis on prevention leads to improved health status. This means less need for curative medicine and the services of the medical care system. The medical profession is then forced to seek revenues for physicians and other health care providers from preventive activities. This has resulted in the development of a variety of health promotion programs by health care provider organizations.

A very important question has been raised concerning health promotion programming. Should prevention be mandated? In the view of many Americans, any disease prevention activity is a private matter. A person should have a choice of whether or not to smoke, of what to eat, of whether or not to wear a seat belt when driving an automobile, or of his or her individual drinking patterns.

Establishing rules that require certain behavioral patterns, though preventive in nature, is considered by many an infringement of individual rights. A clear example of this is the controversy over the helmet requirement for motorcycle riders. In the early 1970s all but three states had laws mandating that all motorcyclists wear helmets. But public opposition to these regulations has led many states to rescind this requirement. Today less than half the states require all motorcyclists to wear helmets. Because of this, motorcycle injuries and fatalities have increased, a fact which evidently has had little impact since the issue remains controversial.

Another controversial issue centers on the fluoridation of public drinking water. It is a widely accepted fact that the fluoridation of drinking water prevents tooth decay. Fluoridation, then, is a common procedure in many communities throughout the United States. But there are many people who are opposed to such a practice, claiming that this is an infringement of their individual rights and is in fact forced medication.

On the other hand, states require children to be immunized prior to enrolling in school. Though an occasional parent may object to this immunization requirement,

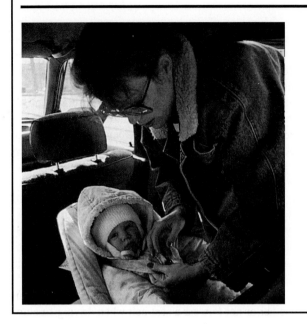
most comply with little complaint. This issue, however, is somewhat different from the fluoridation and helmet controversies because it relates to the health of the general public. Others can contract communicable diseases from nonimmunized individuals, so immunization is considered by many to not be a matter of individual rights.

Obviously then, in some preventive activities public policy and mandate are viewed as appropriate; in others they are not. When and in which situations preventive health requirements and provisions are an infringement of individual rights is an ongoing debate having no easy resolution.

Competition or Regulation?

The structure and form of community health programming and of health care provision within a nation are dependent upon that nation's position in an economic and political debate. Some individuals view the provision of health care and health services as part of the free market economy. As such, the health care system operates on the fee-for-service concept, with costs determined by the economic principle of supply and demand and by competition in the marketplace. Government involvement in the form of regulatory measures is minimal.

This economic and political view suggests that broad-based geographical planning is not needed. Those health providers—clinics, hospitals, physicians, and pharmacists—that can operate in the competitive economic marketplace will survive. Those who cannot will go out of business. Therefore, overexpansion of hospitals and a surplus of health personnel and equipment do not need to be regulated by government. As in all American private industry, health care costs "find" a level commensurate with the level of the basic national economy. Free market enterprise principles, it is held, dictate the percent of the gross national product (GNP) spent on health. Highly inflationary governmental controls and regulations do not result, and the increases in health care costs should be minimal.

Supporters of this marketplace competition concept of health care argue that competition improves the quality of health care. It also makes the consumer more cost conscious. With governmental regulatory programs, there is no incentive to cut costs. If a hospital, through conscious effort, is able to reduce costs to a patient, it does not receive any financial benefit. (See table 1.1.)

Those supporters also suggest that there should be increased patient cost-sharing measures, more copayments, and greater deductibles in payment for the health care services rendered. It is argued that these measures would reduce the demands for minor health care now covered by third-party payment.

Another competitive measure is to provide employee health insurance options. The worker can then choose the type and amount of coverage, and so dictate personal cost. The employer's cost is the same regardless of the coverage selected, but the employee pays a greater premium for more inclusive coverage. It is believed that with this measure, only the most creative underwriters of health insurance plans will survive and prosper.

Some proponents of this free enterprise position have suggested that the government withdraw from the health provider business completely with the exception of providing health care for military personnel. Support for community health centers, health facilities for the needy and for medically underserved areas, and even some provisions for governmental health care in Public Health Service facilities should be eliminated and provided in the private health care sector. The government would then be removed from the provision of as many direct health care services as possible.

On the opposite end of the political, economic, and philosophical spectrum are those who hold that access to health care services is a *right* and not a privilege. This is based on the assumption that all people, regardless of race, religion, or economic status, have a right to adequate health services and freedom from sickness. When this premise is accepted, provisions must be made available for all to receive the benefits and services they need for healthy lives. As an outgrowth of this belief, the government is forced to play an extensive role in providing these health services.

Supporters of this position suggest that the free enterprise, open market system of health care provision fails to meet the needs of many, particularly the economically disadvantaged. There is less accessibility to health care for the poor, the elderly and those living in medically underserved locations. Price competition often results in health care for only those who can afford to make the payments.

Because of these concerns, many argue that the government must intervene. The specific intervention measures vary: some nations have a national health care system wherein all health facilities and personnel are controlled and employed by the government; others have national health insurance schemes that provide payment for comprehensive health services at little or no direct cost to the consumer (patient). Though the United States does not have a national health insurance program, the needs of the elderly and the poor are partially met through federally funded insurance and assistance programs.

This approach to health care involves the government in extensive planning and regulatory procedures. Many aspects of health care are regulated, based upon decisions arrived at through a systematic legislative planning process. Thus, health provision independence is often overruled by government direction.

During the 1960s and 1970s the predominant political view in the United States was one of increasing federal support and governmental regulation of health care services. Numerous federal laws were passed resulting in the widespread regulation of the health scene. Emphasis on curbing environmental pollution, improving industrial health and safety, and reducing the number of automobile accidents resulted in the government establishing many mandatory regulatory procedures. Every consumer was affected by governmental regulations of health and safety matters.

A dramatic reversal of this process came about in 1980. The administration of President Ronald Reagan, with its commitment to a free market approach in the health field, brought about diverse changes in the budgeting and structure of health care provision.

The escalating costs of health care by the early 1990s led many to reexamine their views in this debate. This is particularly true regarding the need for some type of federally supported health insurance. For the first time in U.S. history, increasing numbers of leaders in the business and industrial community are suggesting that government must help control the continuing rise in health care costs. Concerns about the despoiling of the environment have also led to a demand for more governmental regulation.

Table 1.1 Philosophical View of Health Care

GOVERNMENT CONTROLLED AND REGULATED HEALTH CARE SYSTEM		PRO-COMPETITIVE HEALTH CARE SYSTEM
├───┤		
	PAYMENT	
National health insurance system—provide coverage for everyone		Fee-for-service through private funds and third-party pay (health insurance)
	COST CONTROLS	
Federal regulations through national planning		Free enterprise principles of supply and demand determine and control costs
Cost controls put in place by government		
	PERSONNEL/FACILITIES	
Government controlled and operated		All physicians, dentists, nurses, and other health care providers operate on a fee-for-service basis
Medical personnel employed on salary basis		
Health facilities nationally owned and operated		Minimal or no support for professional education, training, or facility construction
	PUBLIC HEALTH	
Increased involvement in regulatory enforcement of environmental issues		Minimal provision of health care services through public clinics
Provision of care for the poor through public health department clinics		Major focus on local and state health initiatives and concerns

Where on the continuum do you place yourself with regard to your philosophical beliefs?

Those involved in community health and in the provision of health care have had to readjust planning priorities and program directions to adapt to these philosophical and political policy changes. Many accept certain concepts of both the free enterprise and government intervention views and find themselves philosophically somewhere between the two positions. This creates a dynamic community health atmosphere that incorporates much more than simple medical answers to health problems.

Your position on this issue will play a major role in determining your understanding of many of the issues presented throughout this book. As the many issues facing community health in the 1990s are examined and better understood, it is likely that one's placement on the continuum will change. This can be analyzed by using table 1.1.

Summary

Health and personal well-being are more than an individual matter. Humankind does not live in isolation, unaffected by others. As a result, health must be seen as a dynamic of community.

In the past, collective efforts for communicable disease control, environmental sanitation, and health protection were the domain of public health officials. With expanded programs designed to provide a greater level of wellness, however, community health has evolved into dynamic issues with varying program emphases. The concept of "community of solution" sets a pattern for focusing upon each specific health-related problem in program development and planning.

In bringing needed health care personnel and services to a broader range of citizens, three different—but interrelated—dimensions can be noted: (1) political considerations, (2) economic concerns, and (3) sociological and cultural ramifications.

The World Health Organization goal of "Health for All by the Year 2000" necessitates a reexamination of traditional community health programming. New and creative approaches are needed if this goal is to be achieved. It means moving away from the curative medical model of solving health problems to a greater emphasis upon disease prevention and health maintenance.

The federal government has identified three specific, measurable health goals to be achieved by the year 2000. More than three hundred specific objectives have been detailed. These goals will be the focus of program planning, implementation, and evaluation by federal, state, and local health agencies; private sector organizations; and professional and voluntary health organizations during the 1990s.

Underlying all community health discussions is your philosophical view of the role of government. Is health to be managed on the free enterprise economic system, determined by the law of supply and demand, or is governmental regulation and control necessary? Your position on this issue determines the extent and types of community health programming, funding, and activities that are supported. Regardless of your view of this issue, the government has and will continue to have some influence on community health.

Discussion Questions

1. During colonial times, what were the basic beliefs underlying community efforts in health?

2. What role did the Marine Hospital Service play after its creation in 1798?

3. Describe the kinds of health problems the nation was faced with during the 1800s.

4. Compare the community health concerns and initiatives of the latter part of the 1800s with those of the 1990s.

5. What is your understanding of the concept of a "community of solution"?

6. Identify some specific matters in your community that relate to the following dimensions mentioned in this chapter:
   a. political considerations
   b. economic concerns
   c. sociological and cultural ramifications

7. What is meant by the concept of the goal of "Health for All by the Year 2000"?

8. Is it reasonable to expect that the goal of "Health for All" can be achieved in the United States by the year 2000? Explain your answer.

9. What are the Year 2000 Health Objectives for the Nation?

10. Discuss the identified goals to be achieved by the year 2000 by the federal government.

11. How does preventive health differ from curative medicine?

12. Do you believe that preventive health programming should be mandated? Why do you take this position?

13. Explain the pro-competitive position of health care provision.

14. Do you support increased federal regulation of the health care industry? Explain your response to this question.

Suggested Readings

Able-Smith, Brian. "Financing Health for All." *World Health Forum* 12, no. 2 (1991): 191–200.

Agich, George J., and Charles E. Begley. "Some Problems with Pro-Competition Reforms." *Social Science Medicine* 21, no. 6 (1985): 623–30.

Centers for Disease Control and Prevention. "Health Objectives for the Nation." *Morbidity and Mortality Weekly Report* 38, no. 37 (September 22, 1989): 629–33.

Cunningham, Robert M. "Competition and Regulation: We Need Them Both." *Hospitals* 54, no. 19 (October 1, 1980): 63–64.

Friedman, Emily. "Does Market Competition Belong in Health Care?" *Hospitals* 54, no. 13 (July 1, 1980): 47–50.

Goldbeck, Willis. "Health Is Not a Free Market Commodity." *Business and Health* 7, no. 7 (July 1989): 48.

Institute of Medicine. *The Future of Public Health.* Washington, D.C.: National Academy Press, 1988.

Little, Craig. "Health for All by the Year 2000: Where Is It Now?" *Nursing and Health Care* 13, no. 4 (April 1992): 198–201.

Pollard, Michael R. "Competition or Regulation: A Critical Choice for Organized Medicine." *Journal of the American Medical Association* 249, no. 14 (April 8, 1983): 1860–63.

Public Health Service, U.S. Department of Health and Human Services. *Healthy People 2000: National Health Promotion and Disease Prevention Objectives.* Washington, D.C.: U.S. Government Printing Office, DHHS Publication No. (PHS) 91–50212 (1991).

Quelch, John A. "Marketing Principles and the Future of Preventive Health Care." *Milbank Memorial Fund Quarterly, Health and Society* 58, no. 2 (1980): 310–47.

Endnotes

1. Report of the National Commission on Community Health Services. *Health Is A Community Affair.* Cambridge, Mass.: Harvard University Press, 1967.

2. *Ibid.,* 20.

3. World Health Organization. *The Work of WHO, 1984–1985.* Geneva: WHO, 1986, p. 49.

4. Surgeon General's Report on Health Promotion and Disease Prevention. *Healthy People.* Washington, D.C.: U.S. Government Printing Office, 1979.

5. Department of Health, Education, and Welfare (HEW). *Promoting Health, Preventing Disease: Objectives for the Nation.* Washington, D.C.: U.S. Government Printing Office, 1979.

6. "Progress Toward Achieving the National 1990 Objectives for Fluoridation and Dental Health." *Morbidity and Mortality Weekly Report* 37, no. 37 (September 23, 1988): 578–83. "Progress Toward Achieving the National 1990 Objectives for Injury Prevention and Control." *Morbidity and Mortality Weekly Report* 37, no. 9 (March 11, 1988): 138–49. "Progress Toward Achieving the National 1990 Objectives for Sexually Transmitted Diseases." *Morbidity and Mortality Weekly Report* 36, no. 12 (April 3, 1987): 173–76.

7. "Health Objectives for the Nation." *Morbidity and Mortality Weekly Report* 38, no. 37 (September 22, 1989): 630.

8. Surgeon General's Report on Health Promotion and Disease Prevention. *Healthy People.* Washington, D.C.: U.S. Government Printing Office, 1979.

9. Fielding, J. E. "Health Promotion—Some Notions in Search of a Constituency." *Journal of the American Medical Association* 67, no. 11 (November 1977): 1083.

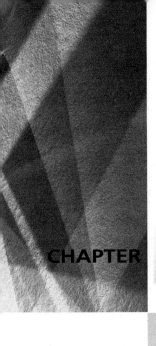

CHAPTER **TWO**

Official Health Organization

Federal Government's Role

Official health agencies are those administrative bodies of government involved in programs that are designed to improve people's health. These are found at the local, state, and national levels of government. These agencies are financially supported by public monies (taxes) and are established for the purpose of implementing health laws, informing the people about health matters, providing various health services, and conducting research.

Federal Involvement in Health Care

The preamble to the United States Constitution states that one of the purposes of the federal government is to "promote the general welfare" of the people. From a broad interpretation of this, the federal government derives its powers to become involved in health-related activities. Yet there is no specific constitutional basis requiring federal control of the nation's health programs.

    A number of health activities are supervised by different federal agencies, but most of the responsibility for health belongs to the **Department of Health and Human Services (HHS)**, and in particular, the Public Health Service. There are also health programs that fall under other government departments, though these programs are usually specific to the responsibilities of that department.

    The following are examples of specific health concerns of several departments of the federal government.

Department of Defense—health of military personnel and their dependents and operation of several veterans' hospitals throughout the nation

Department of Interior—a number of environmental pollution control activities

Department of Labor—health concerns of the working person and environmental conditions of the work location

Treasury Department—control over the importation of drugs of abuse

Health Services for Governmental Employees

The provision of health services for the general population has historically been the concern of private enterprise. The individual physician provided medical care on a fee-for-service basis, a concept that has been the cornerstone of medical care provision in this country. Philosophically and constitutionally, health care was outside the realm of government.

At first, the federal government became involved in the health care field on a specialized basis, for example, when health services were needed by governmental employees. As early as 1798 the Marine Hospital Service was established to provide health care to sick and disabled American seamen. In 1852, St. Elizabeth's Hospital in Washington, D.C., was established for the purpose of providing health care for federal employees.

The federal government makes provisions for the health and medical care of all federal civilian employees. Usually, the health needs of each federal employee are covered by government-paid health insurance. However, the federal government also operates a system of direct medical services for civilian employees. The Federal Bureau of Medical Services Division of Hospitals and Clinics operates the oldest continuous hospital system in the United States, consisting of eight general hospitals and a hospital for patients with Hansen's disease (leprosy). In addition to hospitals, outpatient clinics make available a number of ambulatory services to governmental employees.

Military hospitals treat military and selected governmental personnel. Any active duty or retired military person, as well as their dependents, may receive treatment at a medical facility administered by the Department of Defense. When, however, these facilities are incapable of treating a particular ailment, the costs incurred by military personnel and their dependents in a civilian hospital are also covered.

The Veterans Administration (VA) operates an extensive network of medical centers and clinics. It is the largest health care system in the United States. Currently, VA medical centers number more than 170, with 226 outpatient clinics, over 100 nursing homes, and nearly 50 VA satellite clinics. Many different health and rehabilitative services are available in these VA facilities, with over one million patients receiving inpatient hospital care annually. More than twenty-two million outpatient visits

were reported in 1990.[1] These facilities are open to any person who has actively served in the military and who has received an honorable discharge, with priority being given to individuals who have a problem that is service related. The individual's dependents also qualify for care through the Veterans Administration medical system.

The VA health programs encompass all aspects of medicine. Mental health services are part of the VA system as are physical rehabilitation services. The goal of these services is to return handicapped veterans to their communities as functioning and productive citizens. In addition, ambulatory and dental care are available on an outpatient basis.

The Veterans Administration also sponsors a health professions education program and research activities. The medical education program provides academic and clinical experience for students in medicine, dentistry, nursing, pharmacy, social work, and other allied health professions. Research efforts cover a broad range of health problems. Loss of limbs and spinal cord injury research have been given high priority, but recent programs have focused upon alcoholism and delayed stress disorders in Vietnam-era veterans. Following the Vietnam War readjustment counseling services were established.

Health Services for the General Population

It was not until after World War II that the federal government increased its participation in health care and community health programs for the general population. In 1946, the Hill-Burton Act was passed by Congress. This act provided funds for the building of badly needed hospital facilities in many communities. In the years since the passage of this legislation, several thousand projects for the construction and modernization of various health facilities have been financed.

Government funding of actual treatment for illnesses was not an actuality until the 1960s. Prior to that, government involvement in health care was limited to the support of programs for the economically disadvantaged and minority populations. The increase in social welfare programs during the 1960s brought about the establishment of numerous plans, projects, and programs, many of which were attempts to make available adequate medical care to citizens who otherwise could not afford or receive such services.

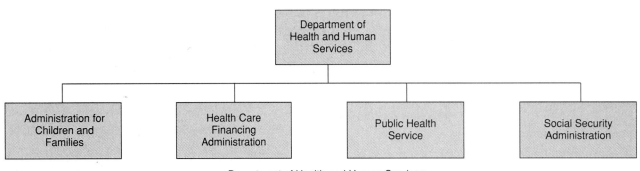

Department of Health and Human Services

The establishment of Medicare in 1965 inaugurated the first government payments for health services to a certain segment of citizens other than federal government employees. The basic purpose of Medicare has been to make available quality health care for the elderly. Senior citizens who are entitled to Social Security or railroad retirement benefits receive health insurance coverage in the Medicare program.

Another federal medical insurance program established in 1965 was the Medicaid program for low-income individuals. Three population groups were identified for participation in this program: (1) the needy, including all federally aided public assistance recipients— the aged, blind, disabled, or those families with dependent children; (2) the medically needy (as identified in number one) who have the income to meet daily needs but not medical expenses; and (3) children under twenty-one whose parents cannot afford to provide medical care for them.

A major change in political philosophy occurred during the 1980s regarding government involvement in the provision of health care and public health programming. Philosophically, the political leadership of this time advocated less federal government involvement in the field of health. Associated with this philosophical view were the concepts that health care should remain part of the private enterprise system and that federal government involvement in public health programming and funding should be reduced. Greater emphasis was placed on development and support of programs at the state and local levels of government. This meant that federal funds were to be provided to the individual states as block grants. The state was required to implement and manage the specific programs. A more detailed look at the block grant approach to health programming is presented later in this chapter.

Department of Health and Human Services

The Department of Health and Human Services (HHS) was established in May 1980. Prior to this, federal health administration and programming were part of the Department of Health, Education, and Welfare (HEW), which was organized as a cabinet-level department of government in 1952. As the result of expanded legislative mandate, federal programming, and national needs, HEW became the largest department of the federal government. Social legislation passed by Congress during the 1960s and 1970s led to such tremendous growth of HEW that many felt it should be reorganized. Educators in particular were desirous of the separation of education from HEW. As a result, the Department of Education was organized in 1980, and health concerns were made a part of the new Department of Health and Human Services.

The Department of Health and Human Services is composed of four operating divisions: the Administration for Children and Families, the Health Care Financing Administration, the Social Security Administration, and the Public Health Service. Each division is assigned special roles that contribute to the health of the American people.

The *Administration for Children and Families,* organized in 1991, is the federal agency that oversees programs for children and families. Program priorities are focused upon children considered to be at risk for health and development. The Head Start Program for economically disadvantaged preschool children is administered by this agency. Also, the Aid to Families with Dependent Children (ADC) Program is administered within this agency. The National Center on Child Abuse and Neglect provides a broad range of programming designed to protect and

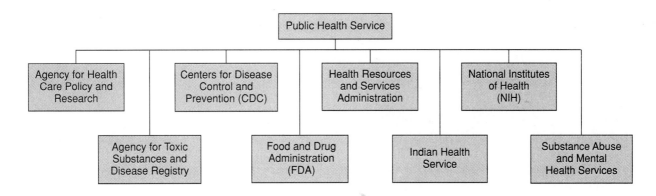

treat at-risk children. Support is provided to states for child abuse prevention and treatment initiatives. This agency also provides support to states to help refugees become employed and self-sufficient. The National Youth Sports Program, a recreational activities and counseling program for low income youth, is supported by this federal agency.

The main task of the *Health Care Financing Administration* is to manage the Medicare and Medicaid programs. Medicare provides health insurance coverage for the elderly through Social Security. Medicaid is a jointly funded state and federal health insurance program for the economically disadvantaged. Both of these federal health insurance programs were legislated by Congress in the mid-1960s.[2]

The *Social Security Administration* directs the various programs of the Social Security system. Americans pay into this system with payroll deductions. Social Security benefits are given to an individual at the time of retirement or disability, or to one's dependents in the event of death. The Social Security Administration also administers benefits for disabled coal miners suffering from black lung disease, pneumoconiosis.

The *Public Health Service* plays the most direct role in maintaining the health of the nation's general population.

Public Health Service

The Public Health Service is the governmental agency principally responsible for maintaining and protecting the health of the American people. The Public Health Service presently consists of the following eight agencies:

Centers for Disease Control and Prevention

Food and Drug Administration

Health Resources and Services Administration

National Institutes of Health

Substance Abuse and Mental Health Services

Indian Health Service

Agency for Toxic Substances and Disease Registry

Agency for Health Care Policy and Research

Centers for Disease Control and Prevention

The Centers for Disease Control and Prevention (CDC) is the part of the Public Health Service that has responsibility for controlling and preventing disease, injury, and disability. The CDC, headquartered in Atlanta, Georgia, was established in 1946 and was known at that time as the Communicable Disease Center. The primary program emphasis at that time was to study and combat various communicable diseases. The original disease surveillance activities included study of malaria, typhus, smallpox, psittacosis, diphtheria, leprosy, and plague.[3] As communicable diseases became less of a health threat in the United States and as other health problems came into prominence, the program emphasis of the Communicable Disease Center expanded. This led to the establishment of the Center for Disease Control in 1970.

Throughout the 1970s prevention of infectious and chronic diseases became an increasingly important aspect of the CDC. This meant putting more emphasis on examining health problems as they related to environmental hazards. Industrial safety and prevention of occupational diseases became important parts of the CDC's mission. The promotion of health and wellness through health education and health promotion efforts was also emphasized.

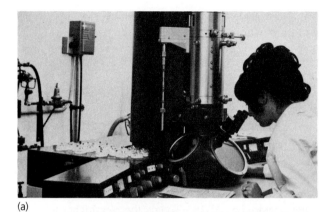

(a)

The various programs of the Centers for Disease Control and Prevention include such research activities as (a) electronmicroscopy pathological studies of pesticides in animals, (b) removing fluid from cell cultures in the Maximum Containment Lab, and (c) examining plates with the first environmental isolates of *Legionella pneumophilia.*

(b)

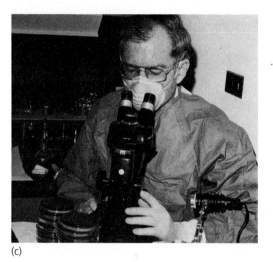

(c)

This expanded focus has led to the realignment of the CDC, renaming it the Centers for Disease Control and Prevention.

Center for Infectious Diseases

Efforts to control infectious diseases include investigations, diagnosis, surveillance, and immunization. Close working relationships between state and local health departments in disease prevention programs are established. In addition, the CDC works with other nations and with the World Health Organization to control diseases throughout the world. Currently of concern are such diseases as HIV/AIDS, toxic shock syndrome, and Reye's syndrome, and the elimination of tuberculosis.

Center for Environmental Health and Injury Control

Efforts designed to control environmentally related diseases, particularly through research of environmental matters and their effects on health, are the focus of the Center for Environmental Health and Injury Control.

Lead poisoning is the major environmental threat to children, causing developmental and learning disabilities, retardation of intellectual development, and in some cases death. The federal government has established a program designed to eliminate childhood lead poisoning. In addition to research initiatives, lead screening and public education efforts are a part of this program.

This center has added programming related to injuries from motor vehicle and household accidents. The importance of this is realized when it is learned that nonintentional injuries are the leading cause of death between the ages of one and forty-four.

Another concern being addressed is prevention of violence. Funding has been made available to support demonstration projects that will result in violence prevention.

National Institute for Occupational Safety and Health

Activities designed to encourage a safe and healthful work environment are a primary responsibility of the National Institute for Occupational Safety and Health (NIOSH). Both laboratory research and epidemiological studies are carried out by NIOSH to ascertain the hazard levels of substances found in the work environment. For example, standards have been recommended for work-related exposure to a broad range of disease-causing substances.

NIOSH assists OSHA, which conducts on-site health and safety inspections at the request of both employees and employers and offers assistance for the prevention and control of occupational health hazards to both groups. Most of the authorization for this type of programming comes from the Occupational Safety and Health Act (OSHA). NIOSH also provides medical, technical, and consultative assistance to state and local agencies.

Center for Prevention Services

This agency funds, conducts, and oversees a variety of service programs that have a preventive focus. Several programs specifically identified by the government are the concern of this center: immunizable diseases, sexually transmitted diseases, dental disease, kidney disease, diabetes, AIDS, and tuberculosis. Special coordination with state and local health departments is designed to provide appropriate services to all citizens.

Center for Chronic Disease Prevention and Health Promotion

Increased awareness that health preventive measures and health promotion are effective in reducing chronic and communicable diseases has resulted in increased activity of the Center for Chronic Disease Prevention and Health Promotion. This activity includes the designing, piloting, evaluating, and disseminating of health education and health promotion programs, which take place in schools, in work environments, in health care facilities, and throughout many community settings.[4]

The National AIDS Information Clearinghouse

The National AIDS Information Clearinghouse is part of the National AIDS Information and Education Program of the Centers for Disease Control and Prevention. The clearinghouse was established in 1987 as an information service to health professionals about the human immunodeficiency virus (HIV) and Acquired Immunodeficiency Syndrome (AIDS). Today, the clearinghouse provides service to all Americans about HIV infection and AIDS. A major focus of the clearinghouse is to increase public awareness of the cause and prevention of AIDS.

The National AIDS Hotline is an information center available on a twenty-four-hour-a-day basis for anyone in the country. All that one needs to do is call an 800 telephone number (800–342–AIDS) and they can obtain any information they request. This service is staffed with bilingual speakers of English and Spanish.

There is also a communications section to the clearinghouse. This unit prepares and conducts media-based information campaigns using the mass media, particularly television and radio. Posters and free educational materials are prepared and made available on any factor relating to HIV/AIDS.

The clearinghouse works with state and local agencies working with AIDS patients, conducting AIDS education programs, and building community coalitions to impact the AIDS epidemic.

Food and Drug Administration

How sure are you that the foods you purchase are safe? When you purchase a prescribed drug, can you be confident that it will be effective in combating the illness you have had for several days? Should health products have labels indicating possible dangers to your health? These and many other questions are seldom considered by most American consumers.

This assurance of safety is the primary responsibility of the Food and Drug Administration (FDA). The FDA is charged with ensuring that foods are safe and wholesome, that all medicines and medical devices are safe and effective, that cosmetics are harmless, and that radiation emitted from consumer products is not injurious to the health of the consumer. In an effort to make sure that governmental standards are met, FDA personnel inspect factories, warehouses, and stores, collecting samples for testing.

The initial legislative mandate for the Food and Drug Administration occurred in 1906 when Congress passed the Pure Food and Drug Act. In 1938 a much changed Food, Drug, and Cosmetic Act became law. Whereas the previous legislation focused on adulterated and misbranded foods and drugs, the 1938 legislation extended coverage to cosmetics, required predistribution clearance for safety of new drugs, and authorized factory inspections.

For the first time a manufacturer was required to have an effective application for a new drug before it could be introduced for interstate commerce. To obtain the application the manufacturer had to present clear evidence from chemical, pharmacological, and human testing that the drug was safe. However, it was not necessary to prove that the drug was effective. As a result, many new drugs appeared on the market that were safe, but showed no evidence that they could cure diseases for which they were advertised. Not until passage of an amendment (the Kefauver-Harris Amendment) in 1962 did drug manufacturers have to prove to the FDA the effectiveness of the drug before it could be marketed.

Through the years several other amendments to the Federal Food, Drug, and Cosmetic Act have been passed. Such amendments prohibit new food additives from being marketed until proved safe (1958), limit the amount of color additives in foods (1960), outline procedures for new drug applications (1979), and require that food labeling be honest and informative (1966).

Four principal areas within the jurisdiction of the Food and Drug Administration have received major emphasis in recent years: (1) food labeling, (2) food safety, (3) human drugs, and (4) radiological health. Any product that does not meet established federal standards in any of these areas is confiscated. The Food and Drug Administration can remove a product from the marketplace and prosecute either the manufacturer or vendor if it can be shown that the food, drug, or cosmetic is unsafe or contaminated, or if the labeling or advertising can be proved false or misleading.

An important responsibility of the FDA is to make certain that all labeling is truthful, informative, and correctly stated. Consumer interest in the past decade has led to more informative labeling of health products, and especially of food. The FDA had the responsibility of rewriting regulations governing both food labeling and medical devices as mandated in the Nutrition Labeling and Education Act and the Safe Medical Devices Act of 1990. Nutrition labeling is now required on virtually all foods.

Food safety is another major concern of the Food and Drug Administration. FDA scientists carry out more than 70,000 inspections a year to test foods and food additives to ensure their safety and purity.[5] For instance, food served in interstate carriers, such as planes and trains, must be inspected periodically. Also the FDA ensures that milk has been properly processed and is safe for human consumption. If food is found to be contaminated, the FDA takes appropriate corrective action.

The FDA also has responsibility for assuring that food entering the United States is safe for human consumption. For example, in 1991 six million pounds of peanuts were refused entry from several countries. Many of these peanuts had been in storage for two or more years and had become contaminated with rodent and insect filth. These nuts were reexported. Under law, refused shipments can be reexported or destroyed.[6]

The Food and Drug Administration certifies the safety and effectiveness of prescription and over-the-counter drugs. The FDA does not conduct research, but examines the results of studies carried out by the manufacturer. Before a drug can be marketed, it must pass certain research standards established by the Food and Drug Administration. It is the responsibility of the drug manufacturer to have all newly manufactured drugs tested and approved. This procedure, from the time of development of the drug until final FDA approval is given and the drug is marketed, often takes several years.

Once a drug is approved by the Food and Drug Administration, it is tested on a random basis to ensure purity and potency. All insulin and antibiotics marketed for human use, for example, must be certified for purity and effectiveness. In addition, the FDA is responsible for monitoring the proper labeling of prescription drugs.

An example of a drug that has received FDA approval is Cladribine, which was approved in 1993 for treatment of a rare, often fatal cancer of the blood and bone marrow. Treatment with this drug is a one-time, intravenous procedure. In 1992 the FDA approved three biological products for use in the prevention and control of excessive bleeding from hemophilia. The FDA has also approved the drug selegiline for use in the treatment of Parkinson's disease. This drug has been shown to be useful in controlling the symptoms of this disorder.

In 1992 the FDA gave approval to Depo Provera for use as an effective preventive of pregnancy. Depo Provera is a form of the hormone progesterone that is used in birth control pills. It contains no estrogen. This hormone has been available in many countries for some time as a treatment for cancer. Approval had been delayed for several years due to fear that the drug might increase the risk of some cancers. However, after reviewing several studies the FDA decided there was no increase in overall risk of cancer and gave its approval.

The Food and Drug Administration has responsibility for assuring the safety of the nation's blood supply. FDA investigators examine on a routine basis the various blood bank operations, testing for contaminants.

The FDA is also involved in the protection of consumers from unnecessary exposure to radiation. Of particular concern are such sources of radiation as color television sets and microwave ovens. Electric blankets, like many home appliances, produce low-intensity electric and magnetic fields. The FDA conducted research to determine if there was any association between electric blanket use and cancer and in 1989 reported finding no conclusive evidence that electric blankets are a health hazard.

Also, the FDA maintains constant surveillance of medical devices and equipment to ensure the safety of the medical patient. For example, all pacemakers must receive FDA approval before they can be marketed, and caution has been advised with silicone breast implants.

Health Resources and Services Administration

The function of the Health Resources and Services Administration is to assist various agencies throughout the nation in improving health resources and in administering the activities of specific organizations that deliver health services. This administration's programs work with health care providers in an effort to provide excellent health care to medically underserved individuals such as residents of rural communities, migrant workers, and the homeless, as well as mothers and children.

The programs administered by this agency fall under one of three bureaus: (1) the Bureau of Maternal and Child Health and Resources Development, (2) the Bureau of Health Professions, and (3) the Bureau of Health Care Delivery and Assistance.

The *Bureau of Maternal and Child Health and Resources Development* supports a broad range of activities, with a particular focus on programs designed to improve the health of mothers and infants and children. The maternal-child health block-grant program is administered by this bureau, and research and service programs relating to genetic diseases, hemophilia, pediatric emergency medical services, and pediatric AIDS are also major activities.

Activities to improve the procurement of organs for transplant are supported. A scientific registry of all transplantation recipients is maintained, thus facilitating collection and analysis of data on organ transplantation.

The *Bureau of Health Professions* manages a variety of programs designed to enhance the development, distribution, and quality of professional training of health personnel. These activities include the financial support of medical, nursing, and allied health care training and efforts to improve this training with in-service programs. A particular emphasis is providing greater access to health careers for minorities and the economically disadvantaged. The goal of other recent program activities is to increase the supply of medical doctors trained in primary care and to improve the knowledge and skills of those who serve the elderly.

The *Bureau of Health Care Delivery and Assistance* conducts several programs designed to meet the needs of people not adequately served by the normal private health care system. Some programs are directed at specific health problems and others at certain population groups.

A number of community health centers have provided a wide range of health services in rural and inner-city settings, including primary health care, mental health services, health education, and other health and social services for the residents of these medically underserved areas.

Since many rural and inner-city localities lacked adequate medical personnel, the National Health Service Corps was established for the purpose of recruiting personnel to serve in such settings. Physicians, nurses, and other health-related personnel are appointed to an underserved locality for a given time. Upon completion of this federal service, it is hoped that the health providers will continue serving this same area in a private practice.

Many initiatives focusing on specific health problems have been supported by the Health Resources and Services Administration. Infant mortality and low infant birthweight have been concerns, and making available effective prenatal care for economically disadvantaged women has been an initiative of support.

The Health Resources and Services Administration (HRSA) HIV/AIDS initiative has supported a variety of programs authorized by the Ryan White Comprehensive AIDS Resources Act of 1990. The basic purpose of funding under authorization of this program is to help HIV patients who are not eligible for public or private reimbursement programs. Support has been given to demonstration projects that are developing coalitions of health service providers and community organizations working with AIDS patients and their families. These coalitions are needed to ensure continuity of services and to identify and resolve any gaps.

Pediatric AIDS has been an increasing concern of HRSA. Programs have been supported which seek effective ways to prevent HIV infection, particularly through perinatal transmission. Also initiatives designed to provide service to families with AIDS infected infants have been supported.

National Institutes of Health

The National Institutes of Health (NIH), one of the largest medical research centers in the world, conducts and supports extensive biomedical research for the benefit of Americans. In addition to this research, conducted in NIH laboratories and in various institutions throughout the nation, the National Institutes of Health trains young researchers and disseminates research-related information.

The National Institutes of Health began in 1887 in a one-room facility at the Marine Hospital on Staten Island. From that time until 1930 it was known as the Hygienic Laboratory. In 1930 the name was changed to the National Institutes of Health.

From 1953 to 1979, the NIH was a part of the Department of Health, Education, and Welfare (HEW). Today NIH is one of the health agencies that make up the Public Health Service of the Department of Health and Human Services.

The National Institutes of Health is organized into seventeen research institutes plus a research hospital, the National Library of Medicine, and the Fogarty International Center. Each of these institutes is assigned a specific focus. Research activities are supported and conducted in programs designed to solve the specific health problem.

The research hospital, known as the Warren G. Magnusen Clinical Center, houses five hundred beds. It is the world's largest medical research hospital. Admission to this facility is limited to individuals with illnesses and diseases that are institute study topics and who are referred by their personal physicians. Annually about 9,000 patients receive treatment in clinical studies at NIH.

The National Library of Medicine houses over three-and-a-half million volumes, the world's largest single-subject medical reference center. In addition to housing medical works, the library publishes numerous periodicals. The other component of the NIH, the Fogarty International Center, conducts research into international health concerns and problems and holds conferences and seminars involving international collaboration.

Most of the National Institutes of Health departments are now located outside Washington, D.C., in Bethesda, Maryland. The National Institute of Environmental Health Sciences, however, is housed in North Carolina, and several other smaller field stations and facilities are located outside the Bethesda headquarters.

National Institute on Aging

The senior citizen population is rapidly increasing in the United States. As a result, recent years have seen an increased interest in the aging process and in the problems of senior citizens. Research supported by the National Institute on Aging (NIA) has investigated several of these problems.

Research has focused on the interaction of aging and diseases and disorders associated with aging, such as Alzheimer's disease, osteoporosis, osteoarthritis, injuries caused by falls, and urinary incontinence. Biomedical and

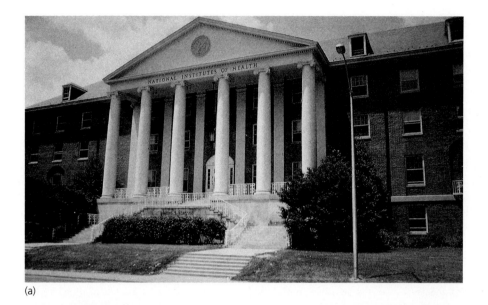

(a)

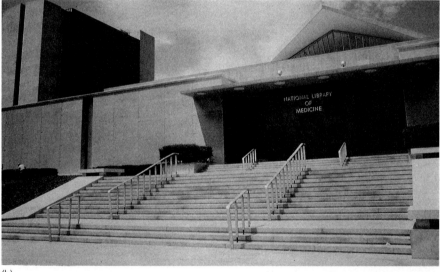

(b)

(a) In 1938, government officials broke ground for the National Institutes of Health in Bethesda, Maryland. These institutes, staffed by scientific personnel, conduct research on a variety of different health problems and diseases. (b) The National Library of Medicine is a part of the National Institutes of Health in Bethesda, Maryland. This is the largest medical reference center in the world, containing over 3.5 million items. The medical reference journal *Index Medicus,* an index to articles in about twenty-five hundred medical journals, is published by the National Library. The Lister Hill National Center for Biomedical Communications and the National Medical Audiovisual Center are a part of the National Library of Medicine.

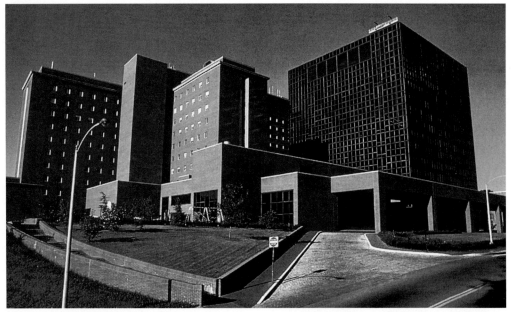

(a)

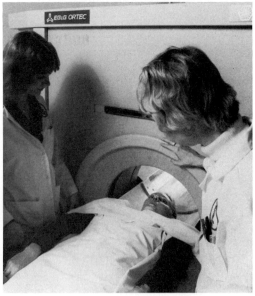

(b)

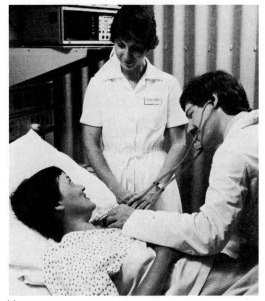

(c)

(a) The principal clinical facility for the National Institutes of Health is this building, the Warren G. Magnusen Clinical Center, in Bethesda, Maryland. (b) There are many laboratories throughout the Center where study and research are carried out. Such instruments as the Positron Scanner are used. The scanners can locate minute pieces of tissue in the brain, deeply embedded tumors, and metabolic changes in the body that other noninvasive techniques are unable to detect. (c) About nine thousand patients are admitted annually to this facility, with another 120,000 outpatient visits taking place.

psychosocial factors in maintaining health and effective functioning in the middle and later years are another emphasis of research in this institute. The institute also has responsibility for research concerned with the biological, social, psychological, cultural, and economic factors that affect both the process of growing old and the status and roles of older people in society.

The NIA supports research on the structure and function of the aging nervous system and behavioral manifestations of the brain among the elderly. Specific focus is on the cause, treatment, and prevalence of Alzheimer's disease. Fifteen Alzheimer's disease research centers have been established throughout the nation where basic, clinical, and behavioral aspects of this chronic disease of the elderly are being studied.

Another research finding reported by the NIA is that the mechanisms for exercise-stimulated muscle building are slowed or turned off in adults. Therefore, exercise does lead to fat reduction and weight loss in the elderly, but an increase in muscle mass is not achieved in these exercisers as it is in younger athletes. This is not to suggest that the senior citizen cannot benefit from exercise, but that muscle growth will not be a major outcome.

The NIA has funded research relating to aging and cancer. These research projects have examined the epidemiology of cancer in the elderly, with an emphasis on changes in the immune system. In the behavioral sciences, projects have sought the development of effective psychosocial support systems for elderly cancer patients.

Concern about nutritional disorders of the elderly has resulted in NIA support of research initiatives on malnutrition. Studies have been conducted to ascertain the prevalence of and preventive measures for malnutrition among senior citizens.

National Institute of Allergy and Infectious Diseases

The basic focus of the National Institute of Allergy and Infectious Diseases (NIAID) is discovering why the body's immune system defenses are disrupted and learning how these disruptions can be corrected and prevented. Research efforts at the molecular level expand scientists' knowledge of microorganisms responsible for infectious diseases. Studying immunologic defects, enhancing immunization procedures, and correcting malfunction as in asthma and other allergic disorders are important activities of this institute.

Its research programs are directed at acquiring knowledge that will lead to the treatment and prevention of infectious diseases. This involves research in microbiology looking at the isolation, characterization, and biology of disease-causing microorganisms. It also includes the development of successful and safe antimicrobial compounds, particularly for viruses and parasites. The institute oversees investigations into the nature of infectious diseases. Although these diseases no longer pose the health threat that they did half a century ago, they are still a major cause of acute illnesses in the United States today.

Because allergies are one of the most difficult problems to diagnose and treat, the institute is conducting research into their cause, pathogenesis (origination and development), prevention, and treatment. Reactions to insect bites, foods, chemicals, and a variety of airborne allergens are being studied by institute scientists in the hope that some relief for those suffering from allergies will be found.

In recent years NIAID has established a network of centers throughout the nation where scientists are studying the molecular causes of allergy symptoms. The use of several drugs for treating allergies has been developed under institute-sponsored research. The biochemical basis of the emotional reactions that occur during an asthma attack is also being investigated.

Other research programs have been directed toward the development of new vaccines for pertussis, hepatitis B, and rabies. The National Institute of Allergy and Infectious Diseases is the principal agency supporting research in parasitology and tropical medicine. This has been accomplished through bilateral projects with other nations as well as through the World Health Organization. Six tropical diseases—filariasis, leishmaniasis, leprosy, malaria, schistosomiasis, and trypanosomiasis—have been given priority.

The institute's research efforts have also increased in the area of sexually transmitted diseases (STDs). Attempts have been made to learn more about the biology and physiology of such diseases as herpes, chlamydia, and trichomoniasis. The researchers' efforts are proving effective. Experimental vaccines have been developed and tested for preventing genital herpes, syphilis, and gonorrhea, and new drug treatments have been investigated for most STDs. A test that allows diagnosis of chlamydial infection within thirty minutes has been developed, as well as a technique to detect chlamydia from a Pap smear.

Along with several other of the National Institutes of Health, this institute has placed major emphasis on AIDS in the past few years. Researchers have been working on antiviral drugs, the use of bone marrow transplants, and basic understanding of the immune system in attempting to bring about a cure for AIDS.

A major goal of NIAID research is to find procedures for treating diseases caused by the HIV virus that may lead to AIDS. Currently three types of drug studies are being carried out: (1) testing of drugs that may control the HIV virus—these drugs may prevent or delay the onset of AIDS; (2) development of drugs that may strengthen the immune system; and (3) identification and development of drugs that treat diseases that attack AIDS patients.

National Institute of Diabetes, and Digestive and Kidney Diseases

This institute focuses its research efforts on a variety of problems related to diabetes and the kidneys.

Research efforts relating to the kidneys are concentrating on developing new methods of preventive therapy, early diagnosis, and more effective treatment. As a result of research work, long-term results of kidney transplants have been successful in recent years, and long-term rehabilitation is now possible.

Kidney stones often present a very painful disorder of the urinary tract. Research has focused on procedures to dissolve these stones and to develop means for medical interventions. One procedure uses a urine sample to warn of the likelihood of kidney stones formation.

Improved forms of kidney dialysis therapy continue to be a goal of the institute. A measure known as continuous ambulatory peritoneal dialysis (CAPD) has been an important research topic in recent years. This procedure, portable and possibly less expensive than other traditional kidney dialysis measures, frees the patient from daily dialysis treatment. Research continues in an effort to make CAPD more efficient and safe.

Diabetes is a metabolic disorder that affects an estimated eleven million Americans. The National Institute of Diabetes, and Digestive and Kidney Diseases conducts a variety of programs attempting to reduce the problems

related to diabetes and to increase early risk identification. Studies of the role of diet and obesity in the development of diabetes among populations at high risk are being undertaken. Interesting research directed at the transplantation of pancreatic tissue for treatment of diabetes has been a new area of work. New procedures for screening the retina of the eye may identify a blood factor found in patients at risk for vision loss from diabetes.

Not all research is conducted in the NIH laboratories in Bethesda. Researchers at the Mayo Clinic in Rochester, Minnesota, are also supported by institute funds. They have been trying to develop better therapy regimens for diabetics. Their goal is to design a more efficient system of determining individual insulin doses and a better alarm system to warn that the regimen is malfunctioning.

National Institute of Arthritis and Musculoskeletal and Skin Diseases

The National Institute of Arthritis and Musculoskeletal and Skin Diseases supports research, education, and prevention activities related to arthritic conditions and diseases and problems of the musculoskeletal system.

Studies of arthritic conditions are concentrated on learning more about the causes of rheumatic diseases, connective tissue diseases, and associated musculoskeletal disorders. Twenty multipurpose arthritis centers have been established throughout the country, with research conducted at each center. In addition, medical and community educational programs, and community and health services research programs, occur in these centers.

This institute supports research on sports medicine and spinal injuries. Also, it has encouraged research into the role of exercise as a preventive of arthritic conditions.

There has been an increase in the number of artificial joint replacements among arthritics in the United States in recent years. It is estimated that 150,000 total joint replacements are performed annually, particularly of the hip and knee.[7] Research is being supported looking for more effective substances that can be used in replacement.

National Cancer Institute

Since cancer is the second leading cause of death in the nation (cardiovascular disease is number one), the importance of the institute's research into the cause, prevention, diagnosis, and treatment of cancer is obvious.

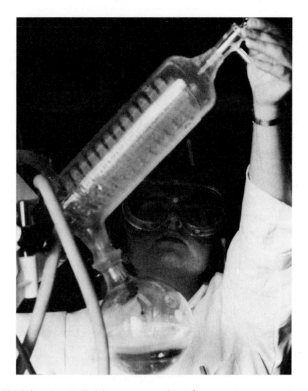

This laboratory technician removes solvent from a rotary evaporator, used to concentrate a chemical solution, while performing an experiment to synthesize an anticancer drug. The National Cancer Institute has been instrumental in the development of several such drugs.

National Cancer Institute (NCI) grants have promoted cancer prevention, detection, treatment, and rehabilitation activities. Programs about these aspects of cancer have been set up for the education of health professionals and the public. Future directions, however, will emphasize prevention of and screening for this disease, as well as cancer control surveillance activities.

The NCI has established the goal of reducing cancer mortality by 50 percent by the year 2000. To achieve this goal, the institute has specified several areas for emphasis: reduction in cigarette smoking, dietary changes involving reduction of fat consumption and increase of fiber consumption, increase in breast and cervical examinations, and application of research findings into improved cancer treatment modalities. The NCI estimates that achieving a 50 percent reduction would mean saving 250,000 lives a year.[8]

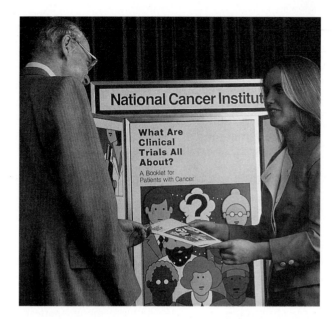

Not all the initiatives of the National Cancer Institute involve biomedical research. Public information is an important component of the mission of this Institute.

Basic biomedical research has led to a better comprehension of the carcinogenic process at the cellular level. The genetic and biochemical changes that cause a normal cell to become cancerous and the cancer to metastasize and spread are now better understood. As more is learned about the origin and progression of cancer, better diagnosis, treatment, and preventive measures should follow. For example, NCI-funded research has recently centered on biological therapies in the treatment of cancer, as well as refinement of chemotherapy and radiotherapy techniques.

Specific cancer research takes a variety of directions. Leukemia is one of the least treatable cancers, but recent research has developed an antileukemic therapy program that has had positive results. Some patients have remained disease free for up to four years. The objective of this particular research is to lengthen the duration of remission and to prevent a relapse.

Epidemiological research has shown a low incidence of colon cancer among populations with high-fiber diets. Other epidemiological studies have established a relationship between use of smokeless tobacco, particularly oral snuff, and excessive rates of oral cancer.

Improvements in cancer patient survival are related to better knowledge of chemotherapy. New drugs that are more effective but less toxic for patients have been developed. For example, the percentage of patients with Hodgkin's disease who are cured with chemotherapy has increased in recent years.

An interesting anticancer research program involves the study of herbal medicine to discover new anticancer drugs. Thousands of plant samples from throughout the world have been collected and studied. There is great value in such research. Two major cancer drugs used today—vinblastine, used to treat Hodgkin's disease, and vincristine, an effective drug in the treatment of childhood leukemia—come from Madagascar periwinkle. This herb has been used for generations in folk medicine to treat many health problems.[9]

Another National Cancer Institute program is the diet, nutrition, and cancer program, which includes research into the relationship between dietary patterns and cancer incidence. This program also helps the cancer patient to cope with dietary problems provoked by the disease.

A number of research initiatives concerning AIDS have been undertaken by the NCI. Investigators isolated HIV, a retrovirus, which is now understood to be the primary cause of AIDS. Researchers of this institute also developed and successfully tested the drug azidothymidine (AZT), an antiretroviral agent used against AIDS. Other anticancer drugs have been examined for potential use in the battle against AIDS.

National Institute of Child Health and Human Development

The program activities of this institute do not focus upon any one disease, but upon a wide variety of health problems related to maternal health, child health, and human development. Such concerns as fertility regulation, pregnancy, and labor have been recent emphases of this institute. Prenatal development has also received much attention.

Research designed to reduce abnormalities resulting from factors associated with pregnancy has been an important emphasis in both the biomedical and the behavioral sciences. The nutritional needs of the pregnant woman, the fetus, and the newborn infant are determining factors in the early life development of the child. The more that is known about the relationship between nutrition and development, the better the chance of having healthy young children. The impact of malnutrition during pregnancy and early childhood on physiological development and personal behavior has also been explored.

Realizing that injuries are the major cause of death after the first year of life, the National Institute of Child Health and Human Development (NICHHD) has supported more research seeking to identify factors linked to injuries, such as behavioral and developmental patterns and the role of family and parents.

A center for population research is also part of this institute. Here programs are conducted to find better ways of regulating fertility. The development of more effective contraceptive methods is one area of study. Under investigation are new drugs, devices, and techniques, including hormones for male use. In addition, research on the social and personal behavioral patterns related to family life and child care have been important.

National Institute of Deafness and Other Communication Disorders

The National Institute of Deafness and Other Communication Disorders carries out support of research and training on disorders of hearing and communication processes. Biomedical and behavioral problems that affect individuals with communication impairment and disorder are the primary focus of this institute. The diagnosis, treatment, and prevention of several communicative disorders have also been investigated. Specific emphasis has been placed on hearing, language, and speech disorders related to abnormalities of the brain, including measures to assess hearing loss in infants and young children. Disorders of taste and smell in adults have also been project topics.

Hearing impairment in children has been one major area of research emphasis. Research has been conducted to learn more about hereditary factors related to deafness.

Language disorders are another concern of this institute. Stuttering is little understood and in need of research. Adult aphasia is a language disorder which results from damage to the part of the brain dominant for speech. This condition often results in conjunction with stroke. Research is being directed at learning more about this disorder.

Eight Research Areas of the National Institute of Child Health and Human Development

Category	Sample Research
1. Pregnancy, birth, and the infant	Genetic and environmental factors related to abnormal pregnancies
2. Congenital abnormalities	Inherited defects with emphasis on birth defects that are major causes of infant mortality and long-term morbidity
3. Sudden infant death syndrome	Ways to identify infants at risk for sudden infant death syndrome
4. Nutrition	Nutritional and health benefits of human milk for young infants
5. Contraceptive development	Safe contraceptives for both men and women
6. Contraceptive evaluation	Long-range safety of currently marketed contraceptives such as oral contraceptives, spermacides, and IUDs
7. Fertility and infertility	Biology, chemistry, and endocrinology as they affect fertility
8. Population dynamics	Population change in terms of fertility, mortality, and migration

Source: Department of Health and Human Services, Public Health Service, National Institutes of Health, National Institute of Child Health and Human Development—synthesis of various documents published by this institute.

In order to provide information about deafness and communication disorders to health professionals, patients, and the public, the NIDCD National Information Clearinghouse has been established.

National Institute of Dental Research

The research at the National Institute of Dental Research (NIDR) has focused on the identification of microorganisms that cause oral diseases. Oral bacteria, the biochemistry of plaque, and the physiochemistry of the caries process have been investigated. Research has increasingly concentrated on oral health promotion with initiatives on adoption of preventive measures. Other oral health programs emphasizing such problems as malocclusion, dental caries, viral diseases of the mouth, mineralization, and periodontal disease are also supported by this institute. These programs continue to provide a wealth of new information on dental health.

Since the ultimate goal of the National Institute of Dental Research is the elimination of tooth decay as a major health problem, there is interest in identifying a vaccine that would accomplish this. The problem with obtaining such a vaccine, though, is that antibody levels decrease after a time, rendering the vaccine ineffective. It is hoped this problem will soon be resolved and an effective vaccine made available to the public.

One area of study is examining the effects of lasers on hard dental tissues. There is some evidence that early tooth decay can be stopped by laser treatment.

It appears that application of lasers makes teeth resistant to acid attack and decay.

A current area of research concern is whether female dental assistants, dental hygienists, and dentists are at risk for reduced fertility. Nitrous oxide is an anesthetic gas used in dentistry, and female employees are exposed to this gas. There is question as to whether nitrous oxide has any effect on reducing fertility of females exposed in dental offices over periods of time.

Other research activities involve such areas as salivary glands and secretions, mineralization and fluorides, tooth pulp biology, nutrition, and research related to dental implants, replants, and transplants. Developing and improving materials and techniques used in restorative fillings, bonding agents, and cements and in rebuilding and restoring tooth attachments are research topics supported by this institute.

Canker sores, lesions that form inside the mouth, are yet another facet of dental health in which the institute is involved. Research now suggests that the tendency to develop these mouth ulcers may be genetic. NIDR-funded projects are investigating this possibility.

Research supported by NIDR grants has concluded that cleft lip may be linked to a gene that puts a fetus at risk for this condition. Efforts to identify the specific gene are now under way. At the other end of the life cycle, the NIDR is interested in problems of oral health among senior citizens, specifically the aging of oral tissues.

Oral health research of the National Institute of Dental Research covers work in fourteen different areas:

Dental caries
Periodontal diseases
Congenital craniofacial malformations
Acquired craniofacial defects
Dentofacial malrelations
Soft tissue disease
Craniofacial pain and sensory-motor dysfunction
Salivary glands and secretions
Mineralized tissues and fluoride studies
Pulp biology
Nutrition research
Behavioral studies
Implants, replants, and transplants
Restorative materials

Source: National Institute of Dental Research, NIH, Bethesda, Md., 20205.

The oral health of economically disadvantaged minorities is poor. In 1992 the NIDR announced a program to create research and service centers focusing on the oral health of minorities. These centers are established to provide regional coverage within major metropolitan localities.

NIDR researchers have conducted studies of the oral manifestations of AIDS, particularly the presence of the HIV virus in saliva. One rather interesting preliminary finding is that the salivary glands secrete a factor that blocks the HIV virus from infecting cells. This may explain why AIDS is not transmitted orally.[10] Much more research needs to be undertaken concerning this factor.

National Institute of Environmental Health Sciences

This institute focuses on the chemical, physical, and biological components of the environment that adversely affect health. Researchers are concerned about the effect of long-term exposure to low concentrations of these dangerous components.

Institute scientists, for example, have discovered that anticonvulsant drugs used to manage human epilepsy cause birth defects in animals. Such adverse reactions are unknown in humans, but these findings are cause for concern among women of childbearing age who use these drugs.

Under authorization of the Superfund legislation, the institute is responsible for health and safety training of workers involved in hazardous waste removal. Research is conducted that can provide information about how various toxic agents can harm the environment and humans. Also, diseases that are caused or aggravated by these environmental toxic agents are studied by scientific investigators.

Every year new synthetic chemicals are introduced in the form of food additives, drugs, cosmetics, insecticides, and herbicides. Many of these chemicals have not been tested to ascertain their negative effects on humans. Some, previously thought to be safe, have now been shown to cause genetic mutations in animals. This mutation process and other dangerous side effects of synthetic chemicals are yet another concern of the National Institute of Environmental Health Sciences.

National Eye Institute

A number of eye problems result in blindness or limited vision for millions of people throughout the world. The National Eye Institute conducts research to learn more about visual disorders and diseases of the eye such as cataracts, strabismus, amblyopia, and retinal and choroidal diseases. Related research is aimed at the rehabilitation of the visually handicapped.

Research programs have made it possible to detect glaucoma in the early stages and to determine whether the use of laser surgery is more useful than treatment with medications alone. Scientists have also been studying different types of lasers to determine their effectiveness. Investigators are attempting to identify factors that contribute to a much higher incidence of glaucoma among the African-American population than the non-African-American.

The National Eye Institute is supporting research to ascertain how and why cataracts develop so that procedures can be recommended for preventing cataracts and more effective treatment modalities developed.

The institute has supported training programs aimed at improving the prevention, diagnosis, and treatment of visual disorders. It has also supported research on the epidemiology, treatment, and cell biology of ocular tumors. The two most frequent ocular tumors are choroidal melanoma and retinoblastoma—conditions that can not only cause loss of sight but may also be fatal. Of particular interest has been the hereditary relationship of retinoblastoma. Close to 40 percent of these cases are hereditary.

The elderly often suffer from loss of vision. A leading cause of this loss is age-related macular degeneration (AMD). This disease affects a part of the retina, the

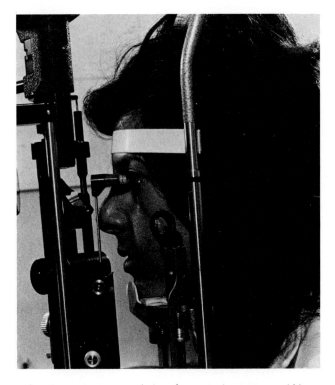

Aplanation tonometry, a technique for measuring pressure within the eye, is used for glaucoma testing at the National Eye Institute. A flat disc is placed on the eye and pressure is exerted until the cornea is flattened. The amount of pressure needed to flatten the cornea is equal to the pressure inside the eye.

macula. Researchers are trying to identify the underlying causes of AMD. Success in this endeavor will lead to effective means of prevention and treatment. Several different kinds of laser treatment have been developed or are being experimented with.

National Institute of General Medical Sciences

A broad spectrum of health concerns is covered in the research subjects of the National Institute of General Medical Sciences. This institute supports research into genetics, biomedical engineering, pharmacology, and the cellular and molecular basis of disease. The institute supports research on pain and the actions and side effects of anesthetics, including metabolic and respiratory changes.

Researchers at the National Institute of General Medical Sciences are also studying the structure and function of human cells in order to help the medical world better understand the body's response to trauma. Special attention is given to the care and treatment of posttraumatic infections and the rehabilitation of injured individuals.

Genetic research initiatives focus on understanding the basic genetic processes and the role of heredity in health and disease. Scientists have been determining the location of particular genes on the chromosomes. Such research efforts help in understanding more precisely the cause of genetic defects.

National Heart, Lung, and Blood Institute

Research into heart and lung diseases and circulatory system problems is conducted by this institute. Coronary heart disease, hypertension, congenital heart disease, atherosclerosis, cerebral vascular disease, and heart failure are some of the cardiovascular diseases of concern to this institute.

Chronic obstructive lung disease, respiratory failure, pediatric pulmonary disease, and other respiratory system problems are subjects of research. In 1989 a National Asthma Education Program was started by the National Heart, Lung, and Blood Institute in cooperation with a number of professional and voluntary organizations. The purpose of this initiative is to increase public awareness of asthma, particularly among children.

The NHLBI has established programs that focus upon cardiovascular and respiratory disease among employees in the workplace. The special focus in this program is upon worksite conditions that contribute to these diseases.

Research into bleeding and clotting disorders is another area of support. Sickle cell disease is one disorder of the red blood cells that has received particular notice.

Recognizing that it is important to get information from the results of heart, lung, and blood research to health care professionals, patients, and the public, the NHLBI has established five major prevention and education programs. These programs are the National Asthma Education and Smoking Education Program, National High Blood Pressure Education Program, National Cholesterol Education Program, and National Blood Resource Education Program.

National Institute of Neurological Disorders and Stroke

This institute conducts research into a wide range of health problems related to the brain and to nervous system disorders.

The causes and early detection of stroke, especially, have received much attention from this institute. For instance, new monitoring devices and techniques have been developed to identify transient ischemic attack (TIA), which is often a forerunner of a major stroke. Studies of tumors of the brain, the spinal cord, and the peripheral nerves are current research activities. These studies often lead to the development of surgical techniques.

Many neurological disorders have been studied. Cerebral palsy, autism, and dyslexia are childhood problems that have been of interest to institute research teams. A wide range of other neurological conditions such as Parkinson's disease, Huntington's disease, muscular dystrophy, myasthenia gravis, and narcolepsy have also been studied. New methods of preventing, diagnosing, and treating epilepsy are being sought, and new antiepileptic drugs have been developed.

Injury of the central and peripheral nervous systems in cases of trauma has been a research initiative of this institute. Special focus has been on head and spinal cord injuries caused by accidents. New medical technologies, such as magnetic resonance imaging and positron emission tomography for the diagnosis and management of diseases, have been another major area of institute activity.

Other research programs have been directed at studying the causes of headaches, particularly migraine, and seeking effective treatment measures. Biological research with emphasis on the neurology of pain is also an emphasis of this institute.

National Institute of Nursing Research

The National Institute of Nursing Research supports research related to nursing. Seven priority areas for research efforts have been identified: low infant birthweight, long-term care, symptom management, information systems, health promotion, technology dependence, and AIDS-positive patients and families.

Investigators have tested methods to help patients in nursing homes deal with depression. Behavioral and environmental factors that contribute to illness and disability have been the focus of other programs. Women's health

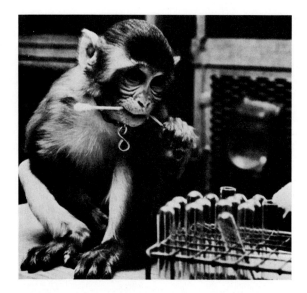

Researchers use animals—like this monkey at an NIH laboratory—for much of their experimental work. Guidelines protect the animals under investigation, and routine daily treatment of animals includes medical care.

concerns have been another area of interest, including mood disorders associated with premenstrual syndrome (PMS) as well as different aspects of menopause.

In addition to research, the institute has conducted conferences exploring the issue of widespread nursing staff shortages in the United States. Other conferences have provided information about the care of AIDS patients and their families to health care practitioners.

Methods of managing diseases of the elderly, including programs for prevention of osteoporosis, procedures for supporting recovery from hip fracture, and development of techniques to control urinary incontinence, are also of interest.

A number of AIDS-related research initiatives have been carried out with the support of this institute. Studies of infants born to mothers carrying the AIDS virus have been conducted, and the physical, environmental, and behavioral nursing needs of AIDS patients have been examined.

National Institute on Alcohol Abuse and Alcoholism

This institute conducts biomedical, clinical, epidemiological, and behavioral research on alcohol abuse and associated problems. For example, extensive study of the neurochemistry and neurophysiology of the action of alcohol on the body is one area of medical research being carried out by this institute. Biological factors underlying the development of alcoholism have been another research focus.

Increasing concern is being expressed concerning fetal alcohol syndrome. It is unknown exactly how much exposure of the fetus to alcohol is necessary to cause physiological damage. NIAAA research is looking at underlying mechanisms that result in this syndrome. Of particular concern is at what points during the pregnancy does alcohol exposure result in problems.

Epidemiologic research is seeking to find clues to the underlying causes and consequences of alcohol abuse. There is interest in identifying individual characteristics and environmental factors associated with the development of alcohol problems.

It is interesting to note that prevention research is a priority of this institute's research programs. Studies have been designed to learn more of the effectiveness of alcohol advertising and alcohol warning labels on alcohol consumption. Also, the NIAAA has conducted studies to learn more about effective interventions to reduce driving while under the influence of alcohol.

National Institute on Drug Abuse

The principal governmental agency for conducting research on drug abuse is the National Institute on Drug Abuse (NIDA). Research has been undertaken to ascertain underlying biological and biochemical factors associated with drug abuse and the effects of specific drugs on the human body.

Also, research has been conducted attempting to learn more about the many causes of drug use. For example, studies of brain chemical sites responsible for the compulsive use of cocaine and buprenorphine treatment for heroin have been conducted.[11] Not only are physiological factors being considered, but also social, environmental, and behavioral causes have been investigated.

NIDA researchers have developed initiatives designed to develop new treatment medications for drug abuse. In addition, as with most of the other institutes, prevention and educational initiatives have been implemented. For several years the institute has conducted surveys of high school seniors, attempting to measure the prevalence of current drug use. The same type of survey has also been conducted among the general household population to measure the prevalence of drug use.

National Institute of Mental Health

The National Institute of Mental Health is the largest scientific institute in the world to focus on mental disorders.[12] It conducts biological, psychological, clinical, epidemiological, and behavioral investigations into the various factors associated with mental health. Specific institute programs are discussed in a later chapter.[13]

Substance Abuse and Mental Health Services Administration

The Substance Abuse and Mental Health Services Administration was created as an agency of the Public Health Service in 1992. This agency replaced the former Alcohol, Drug Abuse, and Mental Health Administration. Creation of the new agency brought together several federal departments involved in administering governmental substance abuse and mental health treatment and prevention programs. It was decided that preventive and treatment services for alcohol, drug abuse, and mental health problems could be improved under the new agency format. Three centers were established: the Center for Substance Abuse Prevention, the Center for Mental Health Services, and the Center for Substance Abuse Treatment.

The *Center for Substance Abuse Prevention* administers a variety of programs designed to reduce the use of alcohol, tobacco, and illicit drugs. For example, a grant program for high-risk youth has been designed to provide support to communities establishing initiatives to help young people at risk for using substances of abuse. Also, initiatives have been supported to help small businesses who cannot afford to establish Employee Assistance Programs (EAPs). Another center activity has been providing grant monies to communities for the purpose of establishing coalitions. These coalitions, consisting of a variety of organizations within the community, will plan to use their funds to establish model comprehensive substance abuse prevention activities.

The *Center for Mental Health Services* works with state and local governmental agencies to provide access for treatment, prevention, and rehabilitation services for individuals with mental illness. One program administered by this center is designed to support community

Women's Health Initiative

In 1993 the National Institutes of Health announced a long-term project—possibly as long as fourteen years—designed to provide information on women's health. The focus of this study will be on the three most common causes of death and disability of females: cardiovascular disease, cancer, and osteoporosis.

The controlled clinical component of the project is to be carried out at about forty-five clinical centers throughout the country. Three factors will be studied in postmenopausal women between the ages of 50 and 79. The effect of low-fat dietary eating patterns on the prevention of breast cancer, cancer of the colon, and coronary heart disease will be one study. Another study will examine the effect of hormonal replacement therapy on the prevention of coronary heart disease and osteoporosis. The effect of calcium and vitamin D supplementation on the prevention of cancer of the colon and osteoporosis will be a third focus of this initiative. It is anticipated that more than 150,000 women will participate in this study.

Another component of the project will examine various community approaches designed to develop healthful behaviors. It is anticipated that through education and improvement of social support within communities, procedures to enhance the adoption of healthful behaviors by women will become standard community practices. Special focus for this component of the initiative will be upon minorities and the medically underserved.

It is anticipated that funding for this decade and a half long project will exceed $600 million. However, it is hoped that a significant amount of information about women's health will be obtained. From this data should come the impetus for establishment of effective health promotion and disease prevention initiatives that will enhance the health of all women.

Source: Personal memorandum provided by the National Institutes of Health, March 1993.

centers providing services for children and adolescents with severe emotional, behavioral, or mental disorders. Also, demonstration grants have been funded for communities establishing model housing, treatment programs, and support services for adults with severe mental illness. The community mental health services block grant program is administered by this center.

Grants have been provided to individuals seeking careers in providing mental health services in community agencies. Persons receiving this support are trained to deliver mental health services to minorities, the homeless, and AIDS patients.

The *Center for Substance Abuse Treatment* provides support for state and local agencies that provide treatment and recovery services for persons with alcohol and drug problems. For example, support has been provided for establishing comprehensive residential treatment programs for pregnant women and new mothers who are using illicit drugs. In these residential programs they will be provided primary health care. Another program provided outpatient drug treatment programs for pregnant women and infants. The National Capitol Area Demonstration Program in Washington, D.C., was funded as a model substance abuse prevention and treatment program.

Several programs designed to help illicit drug users get diagnostic assistance and counseling for HIV/AIDS have been funded by this center. The substance abuse block grant program is also administered by this center.

Agency for Health Care Policy and Research

The purpose of this agency of the Public Health Service is to enhance the quality of patient care. This is designed to result from promoting improvements in clinical practice and in the financing, organization, and delivery of the health care service system. One other goal of the agency is to increase access to quality medical care.

Several research initiatives are being undertaken to learn more about finding new ways to finance and direct health care. Also, the agency carries out research on medical treatment effectiveness of diagnostic and therapeutic medical procedures. For example, research has suggested that elimination of unnecessary, routine kidney x-rays prior to prostate surgery could save $50–$60 million annually.

There have been a number of initiatives introduced that give increased attention to issues important to the health and well-being of women and children.

Agency for Toxic Substances and Disease Registry

The mission of this agency of the Public Health Service is protecting the public from hazardous wastes and from spills of these substances in the environment. Information concerning the effects of toxic substances on people's health is made available to the public as well as health care providers. A registry of the diseases and illnesses of all those who have been exposed to toxic substances is maintained. The agency also aids communities in times of emergencies involving exposure to hazardous substances.

Indian Health Service

The Indian Health Service (IHS) is the principal federal agency that provides health care to Native Americans living throughout the United States. More than one million American Indians and Alaska Natives are eligible to use the preventive, curative, and rehabilitative services of the IHS. The Indian Health Service provides medical inpatient care in hospitals as well as operating outpatient facilities. A more complete examination of the Indian Health Service and health problems of Native Americans receiving care provided by this federal health care system are presented in chapter 8.

Health Block-Grant Program

Beginning in 1980 a change in political thinking led to a change in philosophy concerning federal and state government programming. The states were to assume responsibility for most programs that had previously been federally legislated and funded. This change stemmed from the desire of the president, Congress, and many citizens to reduce the role of the federal government in the lives of the people of the United States.

A major vehicle to effect these transferrals of responsibility was the 1981 Omnibus Budget Reconciliation Act. This legislation created a block-grant program for federal funding to consolidate federal support programs.

Congress felt that each state could best determine its own health needs and priorities. Thus, it was argued, the individual states should play the major role in developing and administering the health programs for the citizens of the state. Instead of appropriating money for specific programs, the federal government would deliver funds to each state in the form of block grants. The

individual states could then select the specific areas in which these "health" dollars would be of greatest benefit. This has resulted in increased responsibilities in program planning, management, and evaluation at the state and local health departments.

Most health programs and services have been lumped together under several health block grants: (1) preventive health services, (2) substance abuse services, (3) community mental health services, and (4) maternal and child health services. Another block grant, the Child Care and Development Block Grant, does not provide primarily health support. It provides assistance to low-income families for child care, child development, and also for preschool programs and after-school activities. Some of these initiatives have impact on the health of children.

The *preventive health services block* includes eight formerly categorical programs:

1. Home health
2. Rodent control
3. Water fluoridation
4. Health education/risk reduction
5. Health incentive grants
6. Emergency medical services
7. Rape crisis centers
8. Hypertension

Since the implementation of the block-grant program in the early 1980s, several modifications and additions have been made to the preventive health and health services block. Today dental health, tuberculosis control, and environmental health initiatives are also supported. In 1987 the program began to include projects designed to reduce chronic diseases, to control serum cholesterol, and to provide immunizations against hepatitis B, as well as projects relating to breast and uterine cancer. Injury control and diabetes control demonstration programs were added in 1990.

The largest individual amount of funding support in this block is for hypertension control programming and health education/risk reduction activities. Every state is required to spend a portion of this block-grant allocation on sexual assault services to provide support for the victims.

A new law implemented in 1989 required states to supply more information about how they were using their preventive health services block-grant monies.

Applicants for funding under this program must show how their requests will help to achieve specific health objectives and priorities as identified by the state health department. They must be consistent with the national health promotion and disease prevention year 2000 objectives.

The *substance abuse block grant* provides support to states for alcohol and drug abuse prevention initiatives. States must use at least thirty-five percent of allocated funds from this block grant each for alcohol and drug abuse services, twenty percent for primary prevention services, and five percent to increase services for pregnant women and women with dependent children. In order to qualify for funds under this block grant, states must ensure that intravenous drug abusers receive drug treatment within fourteen days of requesting it. Also, in order to qualify for substance abuse block-grant money, a state must have a law prohibiting the distribution and sale of tobacco to children under the age of eighteen. States may also use these block-grant funds for data collection and for program evaluations.

The *community mental health services block grant* provides the state with funds to provide mental health services to adults with serious mental illnesses and to children with emotional disturbances.

The *maternal and child health block grant* involves several programs for maternal and child health care. Adolescent pregnancy services and several childhood disease research programs are part of this block grant. In addition, genetic disease, sudden infant death syndrome, and hemophilia research are included.

Since the establishment of this block-grant program, other initiatives have been added. Support for well-child clinics, child health assessments, immunizations, and neonatal screening activities is now included. Family planning, genetic testing and counseling, and lead-poisoning prevention are funded by maternal and child health block grants. These funds are also used to diagnose and treat children with handicapping conditions.

Each block grant has certain regulations stipulating the percentage of money the state can spend on administrative costs, the percentage that can be transferred to other programs, and whether state matching funds are required to receive the federal money.

To its proponents, the health block-grant concept is a good idea. Allowing states to decide health priorities and to administer these programs at the state level seems meritorious. The federal block-grant program has given state health departments more responsibility and greater authority than they had in the past.

Those who question the block-grant approach point out that federal services were developed primarily because the health needs of certain individual groups were not met in the past by individual states' services. Opponents also argue that politics may affect the distribution of grant monies, with groups wielding less political clout left wanting.

The effectiveness of this concept of community health funding continues to need to be evaluated and reviewed.

Summary

Official government agencies at the federal level play important roles in community health programming. These agencies are supported financially by public tax monies. Many health programs are administered by the Department of Health and Human Services (HHS). The Public Health Service (within the Department of HHS) is the governmental agency primarily responsible for maintaining and protecting the health of the American citizens.

The Public Health Service is composed of eight different agencies: (1) the Centers for Disease Control and Prevention, (2) the Food and Drug Administration, (3) the Health Resources and Services Administration, (4) the National Institutes of Health, (5) the Substance Abuse and Mental Health Services Administration, (6) the Indian Health Service, (7) the Agency for Toxic Substances and Disease Registry, and (8) the Agency for Health Care Policy and Research.

Since the early 1980s, the prevailing political attitude has been to reduce federal programming in all areas. Health programs, it is believed, should be the responsibility of state and local governments. Thus, funding for federal programs has been reduced and a renewed and redirected emphasis, in the form of block grants, has led to a broader program concept by state and local health departments.

Discussion Questions

1. In what ways can political changes in government affect a nation's health program?
2. To what groups has the federal government historically provided health care?
3. What is the basic organizational structure and what are the responsibilities of the Department of Health and Human Services?
4. What are some of the programs administered by the Administration for Children and Families?
5. What is the function of the Public Health Service?
6. Explain some of the program activities of the Centers for Disease Control and Prevention (CDC).
7. Identify several of the activities carried out by the National AIDS Information Clearinghouse.
8. Trace the legislative mandate for program activities of the Food and Drug Administration.
9. What role does the Food and Drug Administration play in the approval of prescription drugs?
10. Discuss some of the issues involved in food labeling.
11. How does the Health Resources and Services Administration differ from other agencies of the Public Health Service?
12. Describe some of the research efforts of the National Institutes of Health.
13. Explain the program components of the Women's Health Initiative of the National Institutes of Health.
14. Discuss the various program support activities of the Substance Abuse and Mental Health Services Administration.
15. What kinds of initiatives are the responsibility of the Agency for Health Care Policy and Research?
16. Do you believe that there should be an increased or decreased involvement by the federal government in health programming? Explain your answer.
17. What is the health block-grant program?
18. What is the preventive health services block?
19. Discuss some of the initiatives that are funded by the substance abuse block grant.
20. Explain the various relationships that exist between the Department of Health and Human Services and state and local health departments.

Suggested Readings

Specific publications explaining the various federal agencies are available from the specific agencies. Most governmental documents are also available from the United States Government Printing Office, Washington, D.C.

Centers for Disease Control and Prevention. "Public Health Service Report on Fluoride Benefits and Risks." *Morbidity and Mortality Weekly Report* 40, RR–7 (June 14, 1991): 14 pp.

Farley, Dixie. "The ELF in Your Electronic Blanket." *FDA Consumer* 26, no. 10 (December 1992): 22–27.

National Institutes of Health. *NIDR at 40.* NIH Publ 88–1868.

Endnotes

1. Department of Health and Human Services. *Health: United States, 1991.* DHHS Pub. No. (PHS) 92–1232 (1992): 300.
2. An expanded discussion of Medicare and Medicaid is found in chapter 6.
3. Centers for Disease Control. *Morbidity and Mortality Weekly Report. Surveillance Summaries, 1985,* Vol. 34, no. 255, p. 3SS.
4. These activities are discussed in greater detail in chapter 17.

5. Department of Health and Human Services. *Public Health Service Fact Sheet.*

6. *Ibid.*

7. Department of Health and Human Services. *1992 Research Highlights: Arthritis, Rheumatic Diseases, and Related Disorders.* NIH Publication No. 92–3413 (1992): 9.

8. National Cancer Institute. *Directors Report and Annual Plan FY 1986–1990,* p. 1.

9. *News and Features from NIH* (June 1981): 12.

10. Department of Health and Human Services. *NIDR at 40.* NIH Publication No. 88–1868: 39.

11. Department of Health and Human Services. *National Institute on Drug Abuse Fact Sheet.*

12. Department of Health and Human Services. *National Institute of Mental Health Fact Sheet.*

13. Specific program activities of the National Institute of Mental Health are presented in chapter 15.

CHAPTER

THREE

State and Local Health

Expanded Importance

State and local public health departments have always played important roles in the health of American society. In 1940 the American Public Health Association defined public health as having six basic functions: (1) communicable disease control, (2) health education, (3) laboratory services, (4) maternal and child health care, (5) sanitation, and (6) vital statistics.

Historically, the responsibility for the general health and well-being of America's communities has not been federal but rather state and local. Increased federal legislation and budget appropriations, beginning with the "Great Society" legislation in the 1960s, resulted in a reduction of program responsibility for state and local health departments. Federally funded programs either replaced state and local efforts or provided controls that effectively reduced the program identity at the community level. Since the development of the New Federalism concepts of the 1980s, where responsibility for social and health programs were returned to the local communities, state and local health departments have assumed an increased and expanded importance.

State Health Department

Article X of the United States Constitution states that "the powers not delegated to the United States by the Constitution, nor prohibited by it to the States, are reserved to the States respectively, or to the people." Since there is no direct mention of health in the Constitution, under a broad interpretation of the tenth amendment the responsibility for the health and well-being of the people rests with the individual states. States are expected to develop the rules, regulations, and laws that are necessary for the positive health status of their citizens.

Each of the fifty states has a state health department, headed by a state health commissioner. Half, twenty five, of these are independent, cabinet-level public health agencies. Thirteen of the state health departments are combined with another state agency such as social services, welfare services, and environmental health. Other departmental structures are integrated with the human resources department of the state.[1] The health commissioner is usually a physician who is either selected by the state governor or is appointed by the state board of health.

The policy-making decisions, overall planning and budgeting, and program development and evaluation rest with the particular state board of health. Selection to the state board of health is usually by appointment of the governor or by legislative confirmation. Health professionals serve in a majority of health department board positions, while consumers occupy only a minority of the memberships.[2]

Funding for the operation of the state health departments is obtained from several sources. The major funding comes from state tax revenues. Other major sources of state funding include bonds and fees for license permits and various types of registrations, laboratory fees, and fees for clinical services. Less than 5 percent of state health department budgets come from fee payments. Several states channel fees back into program services. One state uses monies collected for marriage licenses and divorce decrees to fund the state health department family-planning and domestic violence programs. In another state fines from traffic violations support the state emergency medical service program.

Federal funds are provided for some state health department activities through the block-grant program. The federal government provides money to state agencies for the operation of previously federal categorical-grant support programs. This concept of funding through the "block-grant" program gives the state health department greater responsibility in the programming and management of a range of health activities. The state health department is able to make more accurate determination as to specific needs within the state.

More than half of the federal monies that go to state health departments are for the Special Supplemental Food Program for Women, Infants, and Children (WIC). This is the third largest provider of food assistance in the United States after the food stamp and the school lunch programs.

Private foundations also support many programs developed and managed by state departments of health. These are usually programs specific to a given activity.

The operational organization and administrative structures of the state health departments are not the same for any two states. In most states, district or regional offices throughout the state provide the direct health department services. For instance, in Texas and Florida there are eleven public health districts, in Minnesota and Illinois there are eight, and in the state of Ohio there are four. The number of districts or regional offices and the specific services rendered are determined by the needs and geographical distribution of the state's population.

There are many similarities in the health services provided by the different state health departments. Each department's services are provided by physicians, dentists, public health nurses, nutritionists, dietitians, educators, sanitarians, researchers, environmentalists, and other related health professionals. State health departments also employ economists, engineers, attorneys, computer programmers, and a variety of other professional staff members.

Vital statistics are maintained by each state health department. These data are sent to the state health department from the local health departments. Vital records include data concerning births, deaths, marriages, and divorces. This information is useful in determining the prevalence and incidence of various diseases, for analyzing trends for program planning, and for research purposes.

The role of environmental sanitarians is important in every state health department. These personnel work to ensure a healthful environment in the state. Their tasks include developing standards, conducting regular inspections, regulating licensure and certification, and enforcing sanitary codes and public health laws. They also monitor the health and safety regulations in mobile home parks, in migrant labor camps, and at recreational areas and youth camps. Food and water sanitation is yet another very necessary responsibility of the sanitarian. The state health department must ensure that water supplies and food are safe for human use.

The state health department is also responsible for the prevention and control of communicable diseases. Epidemiology and immunization programs enable the department to successfully accomplish this task. State health departments are becoming more involved in chronic disease control with cancer, hypertension, and diabetes control programs.

Another important state health department facility is the public health laboratory. A state health department public health laboratory provides a number of essential services. In addition to the testing necessary for the prevention and control of communicable diseases, these laboratories provide specialized services unavailable in many private facilities to diagnose and treat a broad range of health problems.

Most state health departments have zoonosis control programs. These activities are designed to detect and control animal diseases that can be transmitted to humans. Control of rabies, a disease that can be fatal to humans, is a principal concern. Other zoonotic diseases of concern to state health departments include several types of encephalitis, ornithosis (a poultry disease), and psittacosis (parrot fever).

In many states the state health department administers various hospital, nursing home, and health professional licensing laws. Hospital and nursing home licensing activities ensure that these facilities are meeting state and local codes for providing a safe environment. They also assure that high standards of patient care are occurring. Professional licensing includes dietitians, audiologists, and medical technicians. In Texas the licensing of athletic trainers is a responsibility of the Texas Department of Health.

All state health departments are responsible for their individual state Medicaid programs, including the administration of the Medicaid program and the establishment of specific regulations.

A primary function of most state public health programs is to support the local health department. State public health care institutions, with some exceptions, are not direct service providers. A direct service institution that is found in all states is the mental health establishment. Generally, mental health facilities are operated by state departments of mental health. Occasionally hospitals for crippled children and cancer institutions are state operated.

Local Health Department

The local health departments were created because of local sanitation and disease control needs. These health departments were originally established to serve limited political and geographical jurisdictions, such as townships, counties, or cities. The early local public health departments included a physician, a public health nurse, and a sanitary inspector.

Actual person-to-person public health services are most often provided at the local level. The local health department is the official governmental agency having legal responsibility for the health and well-being of the citizens within its jurisdiction. This jurisdiction may encompass any of the geographical divisions of a region. Today the county health department is the most common

department jurisdiction in the United States. Other local health department jurisdictions include city and town departments, units combining city with county, or other multiple jurisdictional arrangements.

There are more than 2,900 local health departments throughout the nation. The importance of the local health department is noted by the health promotion and disease promotion objectives for the nation. One objective calls for increasing the services of local health departments to include at least 90 percent of the nation's population by the year 2000.[3]

Though a wide range of services is offered, those most commonly provided by the local health department include immunization, environmental surveillance, tuberculosis control, maternal and child health care, nursing, sexually transmitted disease control, chronic disease programs, dental care, home care, family planning, education, and ambulatory care.

Some public health clinics have scheduled appointments. However, most health department services are available on a first-come, first-served basis. Fees for these services vary—some services are provided free of charge; others require a small charge based on a sliding scale of fees determined by family size and income. Follow-up visits are not made unless the problem is severe, and preventive care visits are rare.

The services of the local health department are often targeted at the poor. Because many citizens view the local department of health as public funding of health services for the economically disadvantaged, its acceptance in the community is not widespread. It is important, though, that the local health department be seen as a health care provider for the entire community, not just for a limited sector.

The Health Department Commissioner

The organization and structure of most local health departments are patterned after the state health departments. As at the state level, there is a local health commissioner (historically a physician) as well as a board of health. Today one-third of all local health directors and an increasing number of local health officers (administrators) are not members of the medical profession.

There are a number of reasons for this development. The shortage of qualified physicians who are interested in public health is one. Economics have also contributed to this change. The salary of a physician serving as the public health commissioner is much greater than that of a nonmedical person. Most physicians can make a greater income from private medical practice than they can from work in public health. Finally, the nature of the administrative position favors employment of a person who is not medically trained. Many of the abilities necessary for administering a public health department include budgeting, public relations, management, and other business-related skills. The chief administrator of a public health department need not have earned a medical degree if he or she possesses these skills.

However, before the nonmedical health officer is accepted in many jurisdictions, the laws must be modified to permit such officials. In nearly one-half of the states, a nonmedical health officer is not permitted by law.[4] But nonmedical public health directors have been received very positively by the community in states allowing it. A nonmedical director does need the services of a medical advisor or a medical advisory committee, however, to compensate for the lack of medical training. Medically related decisions are then the responsibility of this individual or committee.

The health commissioner is usually appointed by the board of health. In some large cities the appointment is made by the mayor with city council confirmation.

Programming

Local community health problems need to be identified, dealt with, and solved at the local level.[5] Local health department activities are determined by state and local laws and other governing codes. Forty-four services that are commonly authorized by state statute have been identified.[6] Included among these are controlling communicable diseases and keeping vital statistics. Tuberculosis and sexually transmitted disease control and the establishment of quarantine are mandated by 90 percent of the states' health laws.[7]

In order to be most effective, a local health department should serve a population of at least fifty thousand residents. Because larger agencies are more efficient, the trend in recent years has been to merge small health departments into larger units and to consolidate the services of other social services with the public health department. Such mergers have economic benefits, too.

Administrative costs are reduced, and funds can be reallocated to better serve the needs of the community.

Today local health department programming must identify and assess the health status and needs of the citizens it serves. Part of this identification process includes an evaluation of the effectiveness in meeting specific needs of current programs. Those areas that are found lacking then become the focus of future planning and programming.

The local health department must become more of an advocate for improved health within the community. This requires the setting of priorities. In too many instances local health departments basically respond to current identified health problems. There is little long-range planning, a major need for development in local health department programming.

Upon setting priorities, plans must be made to confront each identified issue. This usually requires building constituencies and coalitions within the community. Coalition building requires the involvement of resources from the medical community and the private community, as well as the public agencies.

Budgetary Problems

More than one-half of the local health department budget comes from local and state tax revenues. In recent years reduction in both state and local tax revenues in some communities due to economic recession, combined with greater demand for health department services, has caused serious program constraints. Many localities have experienced program cutbacks. This lack of funds has led to a reduction in local health department staffing, which in turn has resulted in the inability to perform seriously needed and at times legislatively mandated services. Usually the first programs eliminated are those with a health promotion focus such as nutrition services, health education, and visiting nurses' services. Only those programs that are mandated by legislation are retained, and these are often operated at a bare minimum.

With the increased demand for funding made by various state and local agencies and organizations, the health department will continue to have to "fight" for a necessary share of the tax dollar. When the cost of health care increases, so do the operational costs of an effective local health department. If funding is unavailable, it then

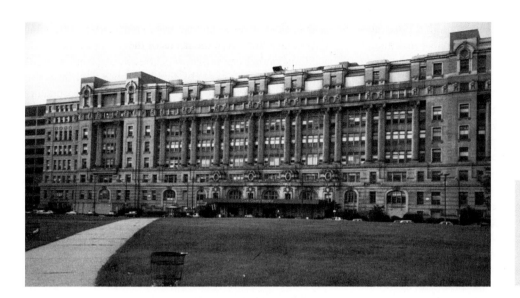

Health care is provided for thousands of people at Cook County Hospital in Chicago. Many of these people do not have access to any other source for meeting their health care needs.

becomes necessary for the local health department board and staff to make difficult decisions about the programs that can be continued and those that must be eliminated.

State expenditures for the Medicaid program have risen sharply in recent years. Dwindling state revenues accompanied by increased Medicaid costs have led to serious state budgetary deficits. Some states have been forced to roll back coverage to their citizens under Medicaid. One reason for this is that during years of prosperity some states added or increased health benefits beyond the minimums required by federal guidelines. Now they are reducing benefits to the original minimums. Eligibility standards have been reduced, as have the type and amount of coverage for eligible persons. Limitations on inpatient hospital coverage as well as physician and outpatient services have been instituted in many states. These budgetary problems have resulted in serious problems for state and local health departments, as well as other state governmental agencies.

Provision of Health Care Services

The Public Health Clinic

For many people the clinical facilities and health centers of the local health department are the main source of health care. In many large cities, the health department clinic is the only place that the economically disadvantaged, the homeless, and a large segment of the minority community can go when in need of emergency or primary care. For example, the Chicago Department of Health is the largest provider of outpatient care in that city: more than half a million patient visits a year occur in the health centers, health clinics, and outreach centers.[8]

Many services differ from one location to another. Whereas large urban health departments employ thousands of employees and have budgets exceeding $80 million, departments in small communities may employ only a couple of nurses in their clinic. Obviously, the extent of services available will be quite different.

Maternal-child health services are found in many local health departments. Well-baby or well-child clinics are available. Here infants are given regular examinations and check-ups to make sure proper growth and development are taking place. Health problems and risk factors can be identified early in the life of the newborn, and appropriate follow-up care obtained. The parents can be given help and advice. These clinics also provide immunizations and screening for vision, height and weight, and anemia. Information about diet, child rearing, safety, and other matters of importance to child development are often provided.

Prenatal and postpartum care are available in many local health department clinics. Here pregnant women receive physical examinations, counseling, and other assistance. For most of these individuals there would be no other source of prenatal care. An important part of postpartum services is family-planning instruction designed to assist in child spacing.

Dental clinics can be found in many local health departments. For many citizens without a family dentist, this clinic is the only place they can go when having tooth pain or problems associated with the oral cavity. The Chicago Department of Health provides basic dental services for children at some public elementary schools.

Most health departments provide clinics for diagnosing and treating sexually transmitted diseases. These are still referred to in some localities as VD clinics. For thousands of economically disadvantaged teenagers in large cities, this clinic is the only place where treatment is available.

Some local health departments provide services to the elderly. Because many of the problems of the elderly are related to long-term, chronic diseases, however, follow-up and continuation of care is often sporadic and noneffective.

Though the environment in a local health clinic is made as attractive as possible, there are problems. Individuals must often wait since most clinics do not take appointments. Because of this long waiting time, many people do not go unless in serious need of care. This is particularly a problem for working people, students having to miss school, and mothers with infants or small children.

Also, patients cannot usually select their health care providers. Physicians, dentists, and other personnel are assigned at random so that the patient who returns for several visits usually will be seen by a variety of different health professionals. This can mean a lack of continuity of care.

Budgetary considerations have an impact on the extent of care available at the clinic facility of the local health department since it is chiefly funded by taxes. In times of budgetary constraints, health departments find it necessary to close or curtail their services. The number of hours the clinic is open and the number of health care professionals available to serve clients are often determined by the level of funding. Unfortunately, in times of budgetary constraints the people in the greatest need of health care are often without the only services available to them.

Payment for services at the health department clinic takes many different forms. Direct payment may be required, with the rate often based on the economic status of the patient. Many people are covered under Medicare and Medicaid. Some services are funded by governmental and foundation grant programs. For example, some screening clinics provide services in conjunction with migrant programs supported by the state or federal government, others with nutrition programs like WIC and Head Start.

Public Health Laboratories

Over last weekend, fifteen students living in the north wing of Smith Dormitory became ill with diarrhea, vomiting, and stomach cramps. Some type of food poisoning was thought to be responsible. Food samples were sent to the state health department for laboratory analysis. It is hoped that this analysis will identify the actual cause of the students' illness.

The services and information obtained from a health department laboratory are very important to a community health agency. The World Health Organization (WHO) has suggested that any health administrator must have available the information that a health laboratory can provide. To achieve maximum efficiency and usefulness, each laboratory must be adapted to the specific needs of the population it serves. Therefore, the functions of a health laboratory vary from one locality to another.

Numerous services are performed in a health laboratory. Lab work is performed by different agencies. Much laboratory work takes place at the Centers for Disease Control and Prevention in Atlanta, Georgia. Some laboratory services are conducted by the state health department and others by the local health department; sometimes they are fulfilled under contract with a private laboratory.

Microbiology and serology laboratories are important in any communicable disease control program. The bacteriology laboratory does blood tests and cultures to help diagnose such communicable diseases as syphilis and gonorrhea. In addition, microbiological examinations of throat cultures for streptococcal infections, tuberculosis, and parasites are performed.

The health laboratory also conducts tests for viruses to prevent any outbreak of a viral epidemic. For example, animals suspected of having rabies are often examined in a health laboratory. This laboratory service is networked with communicable disease departments so that outbreaks are quickly and efficiently controlled.

Before a new well can be used, the water must be tested by the health department and certified as safe for use. Existing water sources, such as private wells, public drinking water, and water in parks, camps, and schools, are also tested periodically to ensure safety. These laboratory tests determine the presence of toxic materials and pesticides as well as the level of bacteria present in the water. If any one of these tests indicates a contaminated water supply, the health department will not certify it for use.

The various sanitary program activities of a health department must be supplemented by a laboratory facility. Water, milk, and many foodstuffs are tested to ensure that they are free of disease-causing organisms. This laboratory testing can also help identify the specific cause of food poisoning.

Blood samples of newborn infants are analyzed for hereditary and metabolic diseases. Screening for sickle-cell anemia, phenylketonuria, hypothyroidism, galactosemia, and homocystinurea is a regular function of a public health laboratory. Early detection and treatment of these diseases are important.

Laboratory testing relating to environmental concerns is another important activity of the health department laboratories. Tests are conducted for such hazards as air pollution contaminants, radioactivity, and solid waste contaminants. These tests ensure compliance with pollution control laws.

Many public health laboratories have provided services free of charge. However, because of greater need for laboratory services, it is becoming increasingly necessary to limit public health laboratory work to problems that are clearly of a public health nature. Personal laboratory testing would then be performed by the many private health laboratories throughout our communities.

Health Department Personnel

State and local health departments employ a broad range of individuals to carry out their mandates. For the direct provision of health care there are physicians, dentists, and a variety of technicians and therapists. Administrators are employed to direct department activities and to manage the budget, facilities, and personnel. A number of different social service professionals can be found in these departments. Statisticians are responsible for recording and analyzing the many vital statistics that are filed and recorded by health departments. Many types of public health engineers play important roles in sanitation and pollution control as well as in occupational health and safety initiatives.

Of the many personnel employed by state and local health departments, two categories have a long tradition of service and importance: (1) the community health nurse and (2) the environmental sanitarian. Every health department has such individuals in its employment. Public (community) health nursing has a long and storied history in state and local health departments. In the early years of public health in the United States, public health nurses often played important roles as social reformers.[9] Since those early years the scope of responsibilities of the community health nurse has expanded. Environmental sanitarians have also played important roles in the health of communities since the early days of state and local health departments in this country. Their tasks and opportunities, like those of community health nurses, have expanded and changed with the passage of time.

Community Health Nursing

Many times the most visible public health person in the community is the public (community) health nurse. As public health has expanded from a traditional official agency to a broader community-based health service, so the role of the community health nurse has expanded. Community health nursing provides services to a variety of people. These services are offered in industrial settings, in schools, in homes, or through community health screening programs. The community health nurse also performs services in clinical settings, in community mental health centers, with visiting nurses associations, and in nursing homes. Health education and maternal-child health programming are major components of the work of community health nursing today.[10] Most commonly, however, the community health nurse operates in schools, in homes, or in community clinics.

Schools

The community health nurse provides many services in the local schools. The roles and responsibilities in the schools vary, but a common activity of the community health nurse is conducting various health screening and appraisal activities. Oftentimes, such screening programs as those for vision and hearing are required in many

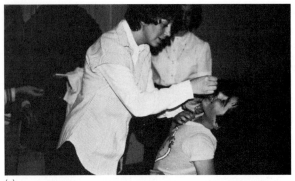
(a)

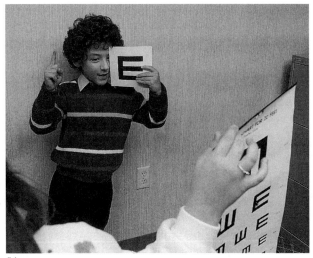
(b)

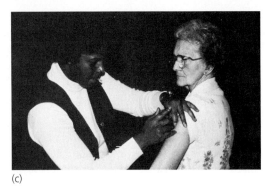
(c)

The public health nurse serves people of all ages. For youngsters, the nurse (a) administers oral polio vaccine and (b) performs visual testing. (c) The senior citizen is given influenza shots by the local public health nurse.

states. Also, evaluation for scoliosis and screening for communicable diseases commonly are conducted in the schools by the community health nurse.

The community health nurse may make periodic visits to the classroom. He or she observes the children and notes those who seem to deviate from normal well-being. The children who appear to have a health-related problem are referred to the appropriate school authorities. Their parents, too, are notified of a potential problem. The nurse's responsibilities also include follow-up of these referrals, since no school screening program is effective if the recommended medical care is not obtained.

If the child's parents are not familiar with the appropriate community medical resources for treating the problem, the public health nurse will assist them. This may mean recommending the social services available in the community. The role of the nurse, then, includes not only the education of the parents about appropriate care but also the actual follow-up treatment for the child.

The community health nurse is often called upon by health education instructors to help in the planning of a health lesson or to serve as a content resource person. Though the community health nurse usually does not teach regularly scheduled health classes, she or he may talk to the children about special topics. Not only are presentations made for the children, but classes and presentations for parents on specific health concerns are often given.

Home Health Care Service

Many community health nurses provide health care services with visits to the home. Historically, such visits investigated cases of chronic and communicable diseases. But today home visitation has expanded so that a very large portion of the nurse's time is now directed toward maternal and child health concerns.

In some communities, health department services are provided to any new mother and her infant. The nurse visits the home and evaluates the health status of the mother and the baby. He or she advises the mother on the care and feeding of the infant and counsels her on an appropriate immunization schedule for the child. The nurse attempts to direct the mother to a medical care service if there is no family physician.

The community health nurse also becomes involved with families having multiple health problems. Most of the people who seek the health department services are economically disadvantaged. This population group all too often has a number of compounded health problems. Their needs are made known to the health department by many sources including direct visitation and referral by the school, the court, or a community social service. In all instances, the nurse enters the home and attempts to work with the family as a unit.

The demand for more community health nurses providing home visitations has increased as a result of the aging of the American population, the HIV/AIDS epidemic, and the early discharge of most patients from hospitals who are in need of additional care at home. As people live longer they will experience health conditions resulting in the need for long-term care. Many of these people will be able to remain in their homes, needing regular nursing care. Also, many people with AIDS are not in hospitals, yet they have the need for regular health care. Nurses are the primary providers of care to these individuals. The need for community health nurses who will work in home care will increase significantly during the remaining years of this century.[11]

Clinics

Most local health departments operate a variety of clinics. In these clinics the community health nurse provides a number of basic nursing services. Here the nurse assists the physician in conducting medical examinations, in taking health histories, in maintaining records, and in a host of other services. For example, many people come to the health department clinic for immunizations. Children frequently require the nurse's services for inoculations, but many adults (those considering international travel or work in a specific environment) also seek these immunizations. Another important role played by the public health nurse in the clinical setting is that of patient counselor. This counseling may involve informing the patient of the health condition, helping the patient to cope or adjust to the situation, or recommending additional measures.

The Environmental Sanitarian

Within most state and local health departments are programs that contribute to the improvement of environmental conditions. These programs include monitoring the water supply, restaurant sanitation, housing and swimming pool inspection, milk sanitation, pest and rodent control, and a variety of other activities. They are often mandated by state or local laws, codes, and ordinances. These laws, codes, and ordinances are in the public domain and are designed to protect the general public from sickness, disease, and disability. The public health sanitarian is important to the functioning of an environmental sanitation program.

The public health environmental sanitarian plays an important role in maintaining an environment that is conducive to good health. In the past, this individual was instrumental in the control of communicable diseases. In recent years, as a result of the greater awareness of environmental problems, the responsibilities of the environmental sanitarian have expanded.[12]

Air and water pollution have always been a challenge to the sanitarian. State and federal legislation in both these areas have transferred power and responsibility to the environmentalist. The environmental sanitarian is concerned—in addition to the problems of air and water pollution, noise abatement, and radiation—with food sanitation, housing, rodent control, and many other environmental conditions and their effects upon individual health and the quality of community life.

The sanitarian performs the tasks that are mandated by law at the local, state, and federal levels. These actions may include inspection of food service establishments, mobile home parks, public housing centers, or public schools. A sanitarian may also respond to a complaint and conduct a search to ascertain if a given condition is in violation of the law.

The sanitarian conducts inspections to make sure that public facilities meet appropriate laws and regulations. For example, a food service establishment must be inspected and approved before it can open its doors to public customers. On a periodic basis the sanitarian will conduct additional inspections to ensure that the restaurant is still in compliance with appropriate regulations. Where conditions do not meet standards, the sanitarian must inform the owner and then take action to make sure the defect is corrected or to close down the facility.

Searches occur in response to specific complaints and are not conducted on a regular basis. The sanitarian, upon receiving the complaint, must visit the facility and determine if any violations of laws and regulations exist. If evidence of wrongdoing is noted, the sanitarian files an appropriate report, and correction must be made or a penalty paid.

An inspection can be viewed as a preventive health measure since compliance with certain laws and regulations is checked. On the other hand, a search is more corrective in nature, looking specifically for wrongdoing as reported by another party. Most sanitarians prefer to conduct inspections, where they can teach the public about a sanitary environment, rather than searches, where they act as enforcers.

Community Sanitation and Environmental Services

Food Sanitation

The prevention of foodborne disease and illness is the basic objective of public health food sanitation programs. The most widely known cause of foodborne disease in the United States is salmonella. This usually results from insufficient cooking and improper holding temperatures. The usual signs of food poisoning are vomiting, abdominal cramps, and diarrhea. The public health sanitarian inspects restaurants and other food services to identify unsafe and unclean conditions and to prevent food poisoning and contamination.

Though there are many causes of salmonella outbreaks, eating of contaminated eggs is the leading cause.[13] When eggs are undercooked and left at room temperature for a short period of time, salmonella may develop. Outbreaks occur when eggs have been taken to picnics. Infants and the elderly are particularly at risk for salmonella. Concern about the increasing rise in outbreaks of salmonella during the 1980s was noted when the federal government set as a goal the reduction of salmonella outbreaks by the year 2000.[14]

Eating at public food establishments has increased dramatically in recent years. Fast-food franchises operate in nearly every city of the country. Because so many people eat out on a regular basis at such establishments, maintaining environments that meet food service codes is of greater importance today than in the past.

The responsibilities of the sanitarian include checking the quality of the food served. Thus, sanitarians are specially trained in food, meat, and milk sanitation measures. These procedures call for meat and milk inspection. In addition, the sanitarian must certify that the food establishment meets all regulations for the general sanitation of the food preparation and eating areas.

There are several factors that contribute to foodborne diseases. The food itself may be contaminated with microorganisms that cause disease in humans. Often the cause of this contamination may be mishandling in the food-processing plants or contact with a contaminated employee. For this reason, it is not only important to make sure that food service facilities meet regulations, but that the food-processing procedures are sanitary as well.

Inadequate heat processing of food can also result in foodborne disease. If foods are not heat processed, people may ingest toxins and disease follows. Toxins vary in heat stability, but most are destroyed after a few seconds in temperatures reaching 165 degrees F. Bacteria in foods can be killed at lower temperatures if exposed for longer periods of time. Cooking food at too low a temperature or for too short a time will not destroy toxins, and thus disease results.

In late 1992 and the early part of 1993 there was an outbreak of infection with *Escherichia coli* (*E. coli*) which resulted in four fatalities and more than 500 laboratory-confirmed infections.[15] These infections occurred in four western states and were found to principally occur among people who had eaten hamburgers in the same fast-food chain restaurant.

E. coli is a pathogenic bacterium which when injested has been shown to cause severe bloody diarrhea. It resides in the intestines of healthy cattle. In this situation the meat became contaminated during the slaughtering process. The ground beef was then delivered to several different restaurant locations in the far west. The Centers for Disease Control and Prevention (CDC) identified six slaughter plants as the likely sources of carcasses which were used in the preparation of the ground beef that was in turn transported to the specific restaurants, all of the same fast-food chain.

During preparation it was likely that the meat was not cooked properly. When cooked thoroughly to temperatures of 155 degrees F. or greater, the *E. coli* organisms are destroyed. The Food and Drug Administration

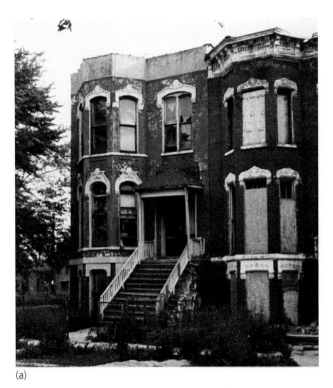

(a)

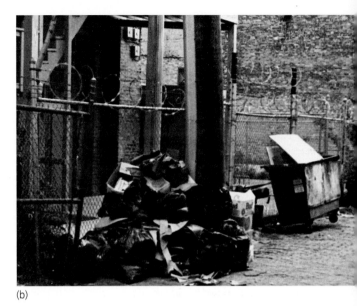

(b)

Unhealthy living conditions are manifest in a variety of ways in urban localities. (a) Old abandoned structures and (b) poor sanitation are major contributors to rodents.

recommends that ground beef be cooked until the interior is no longer pink, and the juices are clear.[16]

In addition to improper cooking of food, disease can be caused by improper storage of certain foods. Foods that should be refrigerated but are left in warm surroundings are likely to become contaminated and so cause illness.

Disease can be spread with the use of inadequately cleaned cooking equipment. Also, the cleanliness of personnel handling food is a contributing factor. There are numerous items that must be inspected to ensure that cleanliness and sanitary procedures are maintained.

Some organisms cause food poisoning, or more accurately, intoxication, because the organisms release a toxin on the food. *Clostridium perfringens* and staphylococcal infections are capable of causing such food intoxication.

Housing

In many cities throughout the United States, there is a shortage of adequate low-income housing, and problems of overcrowding and substandard buildings exist. These problems have grown in recent years as the cost of housing has risen. Lower-income families cannot afford the price of houses, when perhaps a decade ago they could have purchased a home. Thus, these families establish their households in older buildings, apartments, or housing that is only marginally standard.

Most communities have regulations that ensure a safe and healthy living environment. These regulations have to do with water supply, waste removal, and pest control. Usually, local public health departments are responsible for upholding these regulations.

Since inspectors usually do not conduct regular inspections and are too few in number in most large cities, housing often becomes substandard or even a threat to human well-being. In most instances, the building inspectors approve the construction of new buildings. After this initial approval, they are likely to return only to deal with occupants' complaints or if social workers or public health personnel consider that conditions warrant an inspection.

Inadequate housing has both direct and indirect effects upon the health of people. Unintentional injuries in the home are a cause of many deaths and disabilities each year. Over nineteen thousand deaths occur each year in the home as the result of accidents.[17] More than half of these fatalities involve children under five years of age and the elderly over the age of sixty-five. The National Safety Council has estimated that in a recent year there were more than 6 million disabling injuries from home accidents, costing at least 85 billion dollars.[18] Not all of these accidents occurred in substandard housing, but many times improperly maintained structures were responsible for accidents and related fatalities or injuries.

Inadequate housing is also responsible for the high incidence of lead poisoning among children living in older homes and apartments. Lead poisoning is a problem particularly among preschool children living in old, dilapidated houses where lead-based paint has peeled from walls, floors, doorways, and other parts of the building. The young children chip at the peeling lead-based paint, then eat the pieces that fall off the wall. Lead is a toxic element that causes a number of health problems: anemia, headaches, weakness, and impaired kidney function. If untreated, the nervous system may be affected, resulting in blindness, paralysis, and eventually coma and death.

A number of gastrointestinal diseases are caused by poor sanitation, inappropriate water supply, and lack of adequate waste disposal. In many localities, particularly in rural settings, septic systems do not meet required standards. As a result, leaching from the septic system contaminates the water table. In many communities private contractors remove wastes. Some poor, rural families cannot pay for such service, so solid waste accumulates and leads to problems with insects, rodents, and other disease-causing agents.

In an indirect manner, overcrowding contributes to a lower level of health and well-being. When people are forced to live in overcrowded housing, respiratory diseases are likely to spread. Also, crowding over a long period of time has detrimental effects on the mental health of individuals.

There is a need to establish and support programs that rehabilitate existing housing, both in urban communities and in rural settings. It is important that housing improvement is considered a public health concern because

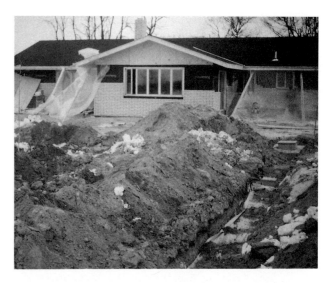

Septic disposal systems must be provided whenever new homes are built in areas not having access to a municipal sewage system—usually in rural and suburban localities. Before a new home can be occupied the septic disposal system must be inspected by the local health department and a usage permit issued.

poor, substandard, unsanitary living conditions have a major effect on the health of a community.

Pest Control

Insects and rodents are a public health concern throughout the United States. Flies, especially, constitute a serious public health problem. The household fly feeds upon human waste, garbage, and other filth and debris. It then travels into the home or restaurant and feeds upon food prepared for human consumption. By carrying the pathogens on parts of its body, the fly is carrying disease. Many different diseases are spread by domestic flies, including typhoid, cholera, dysentery, hookworm, and pinworm. Mosquitoes, too, are a reservoir of infection and a mode of microorganism transmission. They are particularly a problem in the transmission of malaria, the most widespread disease in the world. Cockroaches also carry various disease organisms.

Pesticides are helpful in controlling insects. Nevertheless, the importance of maintaining a clean, sanitary environment cannot be overlooked. Garbage must be covered and kept where insects cannot invade it.

Possibly the most widespread pest problem is rodent control. Rats have caused extensive sickness and death throughout the history of humanity. Bubonic plague, or the "black death," is transmitted to humans chiefly by fleas from infected rats. This plague killed millions of people in Europe during the Middle Ages. In India, as many as ten million people died from bubonic plague at the turn of this century. Today the plague is controlled somewhat by medicine and public sanitation.

Another disease caused by fleas that live on rats is typhus. This disease is symptomatically similar to bubonic plague, but is usually less severe.

Several thousand cases of diseases caused by organisms that live on rats are reported in the United States each year. The rat carries fleas and a number of internal parasites that can affect humans.

Because of a weak bladder, the rat urinates often and spoils food and grain. Public health authorities speculate that many cases of indigestion and "flu" in people living in poor inner-city neighborhoods where there is a rodent population are caused by eating food contaminated by rodents.

Rodents are indigenous to the entire United States. But they are particularly populous in urban communities among the lower socioeconomic populations and in cities located on international waterways. There is always the danger that infected rodents are aboard incoming ocean vessels.

Fear spread throughout the Native American population in the southwest during the spring of 1993 when about twelve individuals died from "unknown causes." Extensive investigations by CDC, the state health departments of the affected states, and the Indian Health Service identified a viral infection, *hantavirus*, as the etiological agent of this outbreak. It was concluded that rodents were the likely primary source of transmission of this infectious disease.[19] Measures were initiated to learn more about the problem, to find ways to disrupt the rodent burrows, and to encourage people to avoid exposure to rodents.[20]

Numerous rodent bites are reported each year. Children are the most common victims of rat bites. Most of these bites occur in the home, not out-of-doors. All too often a small child is bitten while asleep in the crib. In such cases, rabies transmission is feared.

The rodent population has increased in recent years because of several circumstances. The natural predators of rodents in the wild are foxes, hawks, and owls. As society has become more urbanized, it has encroached upon the natural habitat of these predators, thus decreasing their population.

Rat poisons have been used widely to control rodents but are only moderately effective. Unfortunately, rodents have developed a resistance and immunity to certain of the more effective rodenticides. It has thus become necessary to develop a more effective poison. The problem with this, however, is that such poisons kill domestic animals and humans as well as rats.

Improved sanitation and cleanliness have been emphasized as the most positive public health measures in rodent control. Preventive procedures include the cleanup of environments that attract rodents: picking up garbage and other waste materials, covering garbage cans, repairing cracks and holes in walls of buildings, and cleaning areas where rats may be living. If a rodent cannot find a place to burrow and live and cannot obtain food, it will not remain in the area.

Rodent control programs emphasize prevention, cleanliness, and education. The environment should be as unattractive for rats as possible. Some communities have mobilized citizens in efforts to clean city lots and old, dilapidated structures, and to mow long grass. As people learn rodent control procedures and the importance of cleanliness, this public health problem can be reduced.

Community Dental Health

The most prevalent of human diseases are dental caries (tooth decay). In the past it was estimated that nearly 95 percent of the population in the United States had at least one dental cary. However, there have been declines reported in the amount of dental caries during the past decade. This may be attributed to better oral hygiene and greater emphasis on prevention by the dental profession.

Dental caries and periodontal diseases are the most common causes of tooth loss. Malocclusion, or misalignment of the teeth, is another dental concern that can also lead to tooth loss and cause numerous social and emotional difficulties as well.

Dental caries are the result of decalcification of the enamel or cementum by bacteria-produced organic acids. Dental caries develop under a bacterial mass on the tooth structure referred to as dental plaque. They will not heal without treatment. Also, visible scarring is left where decay has been repaired. Regular visits to the dentist for diagnosis and practicing of preventive measures play significant roles in reducing dental caries. The principle preventive procedure to protect against both tooth decay and periodontal disease is the removal of dental plaque through brushing, flossing, and regular visits to the dentist.

The objective of dental health services is the prevention of dental disease of all kinds, as well as the treatment of dental disorders. Most Americans receive this preventive and curative treatment from a dentist in a private practice on a fee-for-service basis. In addition, public dental health services are available through local health department clinics and health dispensaries in many communities. Usually, charges for services rendered in these settings vary with the ability to pay.

Fluoridation

Possibly the most effective public health preventive measure against dental caries and related problems is fluoridation. Historically, the dental profession has played a major role in encouraging the fluoridation of public drinking water and other measures designed to result in better dental hygiene.

As early as the 1930s, epidemiological studies indicated that dental caries were reduced in localities having fluoride naturally present in the drinking water. These observations increased the interest in the role of fluoride as a preventive to tooth decay. It was not until the 1940s, though, that fluoride was purposefully added, in controlled amounts, to the public drinking water. In 1945 Grand Rapids, Michigan, became one of the first large communities to have fluoride added to its water.[21]

This practice verified the 1930s studies: where fluoride had been added to the community water supply, the amount of tooth decay had decreased significantly. Through the years, a significant body of data has only added weight to the argument that fluoridation of public water is not only safe, but contributes to better dental health. It has been estimated that for every one dollar spent on fluoridation, fifty dollars can be saved on dental treatment.[22]

The American Medical Association Council on Foods and Nutrition, after carefully reviewing the clinical effectiveness of fluoride in public drinking water supplies, concluded that this measure is safe and desirable in the reduction of dental decay. This council also noted that fluoride may be helpful in preventing or alleviating osteoporosis (a condition where the bones become weakened) in the aged.[23] The concept of fluoridation of public drinking water is endorsed by seventy-five national science and health organizations.

By the early 1990s some one hundred thirty-five million people residing in 9,800 communities had access to a fluoridated public water supply.[24] Nine states had mandatory fluoridation laws. In two of these states, Maryland and Illinois, about 99 percent of the people have fluoridated public water supplies.[25] The other seven states require fluoridation in communities of certain population sizes. The federal goal for the nation is that 75 percent of the population with public water systems will have fluoridation by the year 2000. Should this goal be achieved, an additional thirty million individuals would have access to fluoridated public drinking water.[26]

The recommended concentration of fluoride in the water supply is 0.7 to 1.2 parts of fluoride per million parts of water. Not until rather large amounts of fluoride (eight to twenty milligrams/day) are ingested for several years have adverse effects been noted.

In spite of the fact that the benefits of fluoridation have been known for years, many Americans still do not have access to fluoridated drinking water because they have individual water systems, a well, or are on a community water system that is deficient in natural fluoride. Another important reason why many people have no access to fluoridated water is the strong opposition to such programs by small but vocal groups.

Antifluoridation

The reasons for the opposition to fluoridation of public drinking water vary from an ignorance of the value of fluoridation in the prevention of tooth decay, to concern over forced medication, to religious beliefs. Often the rejection of fluoridation has been expressed in emotional terms, unsubstantiated by facts.

Opponents have publicized their opinions using a number of approaches. Most commonly, these people take their concern to the voters of the community. Another recent approach involved local groups attempting to pass statewide legislation to prohibit any community from fluoridating its water supply.[27] In the 1980s nearly two out of every three public referendums on fluoridation of public drinking water were defeated.[28]

Several reasons for opposing fluoridation are given. Some believe fluoride causes cancer, although the American Cancer Society has found no evidence that this is the case. A study from the National Toxicology Program in 1990 reported an increased incidence of osteosarcoma, a rare bone cancer, in laboratory rats that had been given high levels of fluoridated water; none of the rats fed nonfluoridated water developed this condition. Again, as in the past, opponents of public fluoridation of water supplies had new scientific research to support their positions. However, the National Institute for Dental Research issued a statement indicating that the evidence present in this report was insignificant.

Others suggest that fluoridation of the public water supply is a violation of federal clean water statutes. Adding fluoride to the water supply, they argue, is polluting or contaminating the water with a foreign substance, which is illegal and an environmental hazard.

Another antifluoridation argument is that this action is an infringement upon the Constitutional guarantee of freedom of choice. Their view is that this addition constitutes forced medication. A citizen has no choice but to drink the fluoridated, or "medicated," water.

Opponents of fluoridation have used AIDS as a reason for opposition. They remind people that a majority of AIDS victims come from urban communities with fluoridation, hence suggesting that fluoridated water fosters AIDS. No medical and/or scientific evidence in any way links fluoridation with AIDS.

Opponents also claim that fluoride can be obtained in other ways, without affecting the community water supply. Fluoride mouth rinses are effective but must be used continually and regularly. Dietary fluoride supplements have been used quite successfully but these, too, must be given on a daily basis from infancy through adulthood. Another approach has been the application of fluoride directly to the teeth, particularly to children's teeth. This procedure usually is necessary twice a year throughout the growing years if it is to be effective.

The dental profession has proved to be fluoridation's greatest advocate. Members have played a major role in supporting community fluoridation programs, primarily with programs in preventive dental care. Public health dentists and dental hygienists continue to educate the general public on good dental health practices, including fluoride treatment, a very important aspect of the public dental health service program.

Coalition Building

Resolving specific community health problems and concerns is not always the responsibility of one given agency or organization. Often several different agencies or organizations, some in the official governmental sector and others in the private sector, have interest in and program resources for work on an identified issue. Sometimes the concern is broad and will involve state, national, and/or international interests. Other times the focus will be limited to a small geographical area. Regardless, the formation of coalitions has become a recent trend in community health programming.

Coalition building is working together to mobilize community resources in technical, programmatic, and advocacy roles. Constituent groups with similar interests come together. Each has its own agenda, resources, and goals, but these organizational goals and activities must be transcended. There can be power in cooperating and working together.

It is not always easy to build community coalitions. Some agencies have a specific limited focus and will not become involved in coalition efforts. Often these are larger, more powerful governmental organizations with specific program priorities. Coalitions bring together agencies and organizations that otherwise might compete with one another. In joining a coalition, an agency usually must relinquish something.

While building the coalition, all the agencies and organizations must listen to each other. They need to ask what is already happening in their community relating to the problem under consideration. It is important to learn from and to help each other. Overlapping activities and program duplications must be identified and eliminated, and any existing gaps must be filled.

In recent years there has been an increasing interest in coalition building for community health concerns. Many communities have developed areawide coalitions to deal with the problem of substance abuse. These coalitions usually involve community health and social service agencies, local hospitals, and educational organizations. The media and religious, civic, and economic communities are often included. Other local coalitions concentrate on nutritional problems, violence and abuse, teen pregnancy, school health legislation, and safety initiatives. Some coalitions have been developed on a national scale. For example, in 1988 a National Coalition for Adult Immunization was formed consisting of some forty public and private health organizations.

In a number of states coalitions have been formed to improve the comprehensive school health program.[29] For example, in Maine state agencies, the Department of Education and Department of Human Services along with a variety of voluntary health agencies, and universities have formed a coalition to develop and carry out a number of school health initiatives. This coalition has sought and received funding for many of its activities. In Michigan a coalition of seven state agencies working with a number of voluntary and professional health groups have developed the Michigan Model for Comprehensive School Health Education.[30]

Whether at the national, state, or community level, effective coalition formation and programming will be necessary in the 1990s. Duplication of services and individual efforts will not be acceptable in times of economic constraints. Networking to solve community health concerns will be an increasing pattern of action.

Summary

The official health organization at the state and local level is the health department. Each of the fifty states has a state department of health, with local health departments serving the states' many communities. Funding for these departments comes principally from tax revenues.

State and local health departments provide a range of services, the most common being immunization, environmental surveillance, tuberculosis control, communicable and chronic disease programs, school health services, maternal and child health, and family planning. Legal mandate and budgetary constraint affect the number of services provided. The activities of the local and state health departments are often conducted in cooperation with each other.

Many people rely on the clinical facilities of local health departments for much of their health care. Several different kinds of services are provided in these facilities, for example, maternal-child health services, prenatal and postpartum care, dental clinics, sexually transmitted disease clinics, and services for the elderly. The majority of those using the clinics of the health department are people from minority and lower socioeconomic groups.

Health departments rely on the services of public health laboratories. The functions of a health laboratory vary from one locality to another. Microbiology and serology laboratories are important for communicable disease control activities. Chemical analysis, blood analysis, and laboratory testing of environmental factors are also part of the health department laboratory activities.

A broad range of professionals are employed to carry out the activities of state and local health departments. Two of the most visible state or local health department personnel are the community health nurse and the sanitarian. The community health nurse provides nursing, education, counseling, and social service skills in a variety of settings. Most commonly, the community health nurse is found working in health department clinics, schools, or private homes providing home health care.

Health department sanitarians perform a broad range of services. They conduct food and food establishment inspections to ensure that proper sanitation measures are being met and that the food being served is safe for consumption. Other health concerns of the sanitarian are housing inspections and the control of insects, rodents, and other pests. Rodent control programs have involved cleaning up wastes, garbage, and other materials that attract rodents. Such problems and related programs are more commonly found in poor, urban neighborhoods.

Dental health is more than a personal matter, especially in terms of one issue. Possibly the most effective public health preventive measure against dental caries is the fluoridation of public drinking water. Though a proven measure in reducing the incidence of dental problems, fluoridation of public drinking water has been very controversial. Some people see it as mandated health care, social medicine, or environmental pollution of the drinking water and have fought for its prohibition. These matters have placed the state and local health departments in the middle of a continuing controversy.

Increasingly, state and local health departments are working with coalitions within their communities and states to solve health problems. Coalition building is working together to draw on the unique resources of all organizations in the region that have focused programming on a common concern.

Discussion Questions

1. Review the annual report of the state health department program in your state and discuss the various programs conducted.

2. In what ways are state and local health departments funded?

3. What are the most common services provided by local health departments?

4. Do you believe that the local health department commissioner should be a physician? Defend your answer.

5. What types of medical services are provided in health department clinics?

6. What laboratory services are usually found in health departments?

7. Identify some of the responsibilities of a community health nurse.

8. What does the public health nurse do in the school setting?

9. What are some health problems that continue to place greater demand on the need for community health nurses in provision of home health care?

10. Discuss some of the responsibilities of the environmental sanitarian employed by local health departments.

11. If you were a public health department sanitarian, what would you look for during food inspections?

12. Explain the difference between a sanitarian's inspection and a sanitarian's search.

13. Discuss some of the reasons why housing concerns are a public health program activity.

14. What procedures for rodent control should a community implement?

15. Identify several reasons why fluoridation of public drinking water is beneficial?

16. Discuss some of the reasons given for opposing fluoridation of public drinking water.

17. How has the dental profession effectively educated the public on dental hygiene?

18. Discuss the concept of coalition building for use in community health.

19. What are some coalitions that are currently working in your community to improve the health of the community?

Suggested Readings

Materials, data, and assorted information concerning state and local health departments is available from: Association of State and Territorial Health Officials, 1311A Dolley Madison Blvd., Suite 3A, McLean, Virginia 22101

Berkseth, Janet Kempf. "Public Health Nursing for America's Children." *Public Health Nursing* 2, no. 4 (December 1985): 221–31.

Browne, Sanford M. "A Comparison of Inspection and Search." *Journal of Environmental Health* 44, no. 5 (March/April 1982): 245–48.

Buhler-Wilkerson, Karen. "Public Health Nursing: In Sickness or in Health?" *American Journal of Public Health* 75, no. 10 (October 1985): 1155–61.

Cameron, Charles M., and Anthony Kobylarz. "Nonphysician Directors of Local Health Departments: Results of a National Survey." *Public Health Reports* 95, no. 4 (July/August 1980): 386–97.

Centers for Disease Control and Prevention. "Knowledge of the Purpose of Community Water Fluoridation—United States, 1990." *Morbidity and Mortality Weekly Report* 41, no. 49 (December 11, 1992): 919, 925–27.

Centers for Disease Control and Prevention. "Public Health Focus: Fluoridation of Community Water Systems." *Morbidity and Mortality Weekly Report* 41, no. 21 (May 29, 1992): 372–81.

Corbin, Stephen B. "Fluoridation Then and Now." *American Journal of Public Health* 79, no. 5 (May 1989): 561–63.

Liang, Arthur P. "Survey of Leadership Skills Needed for State and Territorial Health Officers, United States, 1988." *Public Health Reports* 108, no. 1 (January/February 1993): 116–20.

Lindsay, Gordon B., and Gary Edwards "Creating Effective Health Coalitions." *Health Education* 19, no. 4 (August/September 1988): 35–36.

Loe, Harold. "The Fluoridation Status of U.S. Public Water Supplies." *Public Health Reports* 101, no. 2 (March/April 1986): 159–62.

Roberts, Doris E., and Janet Heinrich. "Public Health Nursing Comes of Age." *American Journal of Public Health* 75, no. 10 (October 1985): 1162–72.

Roper, William D., and others. "Strengthening the Public Health System." *Public Health Reports* 107, no. 6 (November/December 1992): 609–15.

Endnotes

1. Institute of Medicine. *The Future of Public Health.* Washington, D.C.: National Academy Press, 1988.

2. Gossert, Daniel J., and C. Ardon Miller. "State Boards of Health, Their Members and Commitments." *American Journal of Public Health* 65 (1973).

3. Department of Health and Human Services. *Healthy People 2000: National Health Promotion and Disease Prevention Objectives.* Washington, D.C.: U.S. Government Printing Office, 1991, p. 264.

4. Cameron, Charles M., and Anthony Kobylarz. "Nonphysician Directors of Local Health Departments: Results of a National Survey." *Public Health Reports* 95, no 4 (July/August 1980): 386–97.

5. Roper, William D., and others. "Strengthening the Public Health System." *Public Health Reports* 107, no. 6 (November/December 1992): 615.

6. Miller, C. Ardon, and others. "A Survey of Local Public Health Departments and Their Directors." *American Journal of Public Health* 67, no. 10 (October 1977): 932.

7. *Ibid.,* 943.

8. Personal communication with the Chicago Department of Health, January 1990.

9. Combs-Orme, Terri. "Effectiveness of Home Visits by Public Health Nurses in Maternal and Child Health: An Empirical Review." *Public Health Reports* 100, no. 5 (September/October 1985): 490.

10. *Ibid.,* 491.

11. Public Health Service. *Seventh Report to the President and Congress on the Status of Health Personnel in the United States.* DHHS Publication No. HRS-P-09-90-1 (1990).

12. Vandusen, Karen. "The Challenge of Chronic Physical and Mental Disease to Environmental Sanitarians." *Public Health Reports* 95, no. 3 (May/June 1980): 223–38.

13. Department of Health and Human Services, *Healthy People 2000,* 342.

14. *Ibid.,* 342.

15. Centers for Disease Control and Prevention. "Update: Multistate Outbreak of Escherichia coli O157:H7 Infections from Hamburgers—Western United States, 1992–1993." *Morbidity and Mortality Weekly Report* 42, no. 14 (April 16, 1993): 258.

16. *Ibid.,* 262.

17. National Safety Council. *Accident Facts, 1993.* Chicago, Ill.: National Safety Council, 1992, p. 98.

18. *Ibid.,* 98.

19. Centers for Disease Control and Prevention. "Update: Outbreak of Hantavirus Infection—Southwestern United States, 1993." *Morbidity and Mortality Weekly Report* 42, no. 24 (June 25, 1993): 478.

20. *Ibid.,* 478.

21. Arnold, F. A., Jr. "Grand Rapids Fluoridation Study: Results Pertaining to the 11th Year of Fluoridation." *American Journal of Public Health* 47 (1957): 539.

22. Loe, Harold. "The Fluoridation Status of United States Public Water Supplies." *Public Health Reports* 101, no. 2 (March/April 1986): 157.

23. "Revised Statement of Fluoridation." *Journal of the American Medical Association* 231, no. 11 (March 17, 1985): 1167.

24. Centers for Disease Control and Prevention. "Public Health Focus: Fluoridation of Community Water Systems." *Morbidity and Mortality Weekly Report* 41, no. 21 (May 29, 1992): 372–81.

25. Centers for Disease Control and Prevention. "Dental Caries and Community Water Fluoridation Trends—United States." *Morbidity and Mortality Weekly Report* 34, no. 6 (February 15, 1985): 78.

26. Department of Health and Human Services, *Healthy People 2000*, 357.

27. Rosenstein, David I., and others. "Fighting the Latest Challenge to Fluoridation in Oregon." *Public Health Reports* 93, no. 1 (January/February 1978): 69–72.

28. Loe, Harold. "The Fluoridation Status of United States Public Water Supplies." *Public Health Reports* 101, no. 2 (March/April 1986): 159.

29. Association for the Advancement of Health Education. *Healthy Networks: Models for Success.* Metropolitan Life Foundation (1992).

30. *Ibid.,* 53–60.

CHAPTER **FOUR**

International Health

The Need for Cooperation in Problem Solving

umanity has rarely made a concerted effort to solve international health problems. Through the years attempts have been made to develop global cooperation in solving the problems of disease, sickness, and starvation. Yet warfare, natural disaster, poverty, and illiteracy continue to thwart these efforts at international cooperation.

In the past, this cooperation may not have been as necessary as it is today. Peoples of the world were isolated from one another by space, time, and culture. Contact between nations and between cultural groups within nations was limited, so disease was slow to move from place to place. But with the advent of increased mobility and communication, world exploration, industrial development, and growth in population, health problems can no longer be contained by national boundaries or tribal geography. In the latter part of the twentieth century the need for cooperation and improvement of health programs on an international scale is vital. Quality of life is much more likely to be affected by conditions half the world away than was ever the case before.

International Agencies

World Health Organization

In 1946 an International Health Conference was held in San Francisco. At this conference representatives of sixty-one different governments agreed on the need for an international health organization. As a result, the constitution of the World Health Organization (WHO) was written. Not until April 1948, however, did ratification of the constitution take place, creating the World Health Organization. It was founded as an agency of the United Nations, with central headquarters located in Geneva, Switzerland. Since its founding, this international agency has met with varied degrees of success in improving health and well-being throughout the world.

The basic objective of WHO is to "help nations to help themselves" in dealing with specific health problems and concerns. One of WHO's earliest contributions to the health professions was the development of a definition for health: "Health is a state of complete physical,

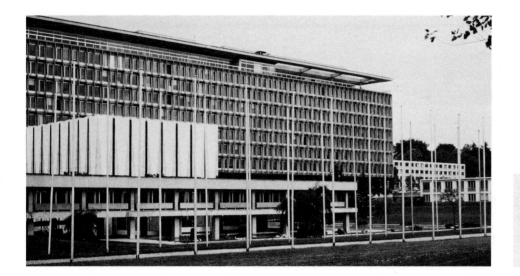

The World Health Assembly, the governing body of the World Health Organization, meets annually at WHO headquarters in Geneva, Switzerland.

mental, and social well-being, and not merely the absence of disease or infirmity." This definition has received worldwide recognition and acceptance and has served as a foundation for program planning, development, and implementation.

The World Health Organization consists of two official bodies: a governing body and an executive body. The governing body, the World Health Assembly, meets annually to establish policy, program, and budget. A nation does not have to belong to the United Nations to belong to the World Health Organization. Each member nation is represented by three official delegates in the World Health Assembly. However, each nation has only one vote. The executive arm of the World Health Organization is the Executive Board. Representatives of thirty-one nations, selected on a rotating basis, constitute this board, whose responsibility is to conduct and guide the routine activities initiated by the World Health Assembly.

Six regional offices for WHO have been established. (See table 4.1.) Personnel from these offices supervise and coordinate the actual fieldwork in their respective regions. Specific program focus varies from one region to another, depending on the principal health problems.

Table 4.1 Regional Offices of the World Health Organization

Area	Office Location
Africa	Brazzaville, Zaire
Americas	Washington, D.C.
Europe	Copenhagen, Denmark
Eastern Mediterranean	Alexandria, Egypt
Southeast Asia	New Delhi, India
Western Pacific	Manila, Philippines

The World Health Organization helps nations in planning and providing health services. Projects are conducted for the most part in the developing nations, with professional expertise provided by scientists, educators, engineers, nurses, physicians, dentists, administrators, and other staff personnel. These personnel from developed nations are made available to the developing nations on a short-term consultant basis. In addition, programs for the education and training of Third World inhabitants are established so that they can eventually assume the duties of the consultants.

Programs tend to be extensive, depending on the need. Wide-scale activities that the World Health Organization has undertaken include development of an international disease classification system; control of communicable diseases worldwide; establishment of international standards for foods, drugs, and vaccines; standardization of statistics on disease and mortality; health work force development programs; and development of modern laboratory facilities for comprehensive diagnostic purposes. WHO activities in health work force development have included the training of health science personnel and specialists; the design, production, and distribution of teaching materials; plus the promotion of health development centers. Other activities include maternal-child health activities and aggressive immunization programs.[1]

The sanitation and improvement of water supplies are examples of specific needs that the World Health Organization believes are vitally important objectives in its overall programming. For example, potable water—water that is suitable for drinking—is unavailable for 75 to 80 percent of citizens living in rural areas of some developing nations. One person out of every four in the world suffers from some type of waterborne disease. As a result, 1980 to 1989 was designated the International Drinking Water Supply and Sanitation Decade. WHO's objective was that nations provide a clean water supply for their inhabitants.

Since 1948, WHO priorities have been expanded, revised, shifted, and redirected according to changes in the needs of a particular period of time and geographic location. Original WHO priorities included eradication of malaria and tuberculosis and control of venereal disease. Starvation and malnutrition, also serious health problems, have been the focus of various World Health Organization programs, too.

An example of the modification in priorities is the smallpox eradication program. In 1967 the World Health Organization decided to inaugurate a program designed to eradicate smallpox. At that time smallpox was endemic in forty-four nations of the world.[2] Through surveillance, vaccination, and education, this long-feared disease, which had killed millions throughout history, has been eradicated. The last known case of smallpox was diagnosed in a resident of Somalia, East Africa, in 1977.[3] In December 1979 the World Health Organization declared the world free from smallpox, and an official certificate of

eradication was issued. This program has been without question one of the most successful carried out by the World Health Organization. It demonstrates that international cooperation and program efforts can solve health problems.

Hansen's disease (leprosy) is another example of a health problem that WHO has worked to eliminate. Assisted by the World Health Organization, a number of nations today have control programs for Hansen's disease. Not only are case finding and treatment important, but research is also conducted in a number of localities.

In 1988 the World Health Assembly approved a resolution to establish a polio eradication initiative. The goal is to eradicate polio by the year 2000. Each year two hundred thousand children worldwide are paralyzed by this disease. In many of the Third World countries crippled children have little opportunity for rehabilitation because services are inadequate. In any case, most families cannot afford the services that are available. Specific programs of the WHO initiative will focus on worldwide polio immunization, case surveillance, and rehabilitation services, as well as research. Advancement toward this goal seems to be occurring. In 1991 WHO reported that more than one hundred countries reported having no cases of polio, and fewer than twenty countries reported having more than ten cases of polio.

Not all WHO disease prevention and eradication programs have been successful. In the early 1950s malaria was identified as a "priority disease" for eradication. Malaria control programs (where all buildings were sprayed with DDT) were developed in some ninety-five different countries. The largest program was in India, where over 150,000 people were employed in the project. But although the program was the largest disease eradication effort in history, malaria continues to be one of the most widespread international diseases. It is still considered to be a very serious problem in many parts of Africa, Asia, and Latin America.

The primary reason for the malaria control failure was the international ban on DDT because of biological magnification in the food chain. This action required the use of alternative insecticides with shorter residual times and higher costs. Another reason for the failure of malaria eradication programs has been that the mosquitoes that transmit the microorganisms of malaria have become increasingly resistant to insecticides and drugs used to combat the disease. In addition, efforts to educate people to remove standing water, a breeding source for mosquitoes, have not been successful.

The World Health Organization, in conjunction with many nations of the world, continues to study ways to control malaria. It is felt that an effective program must include more than just the spraying of insecticides. A more comprehensive program that includes removal of standing water and effective education as well as regular primary health care is required.

The World Health Organization has opened an emergency preparedness center in Ethiopia. This center is designed to provide information on droughts, floods, earthquakes, hurricanes, and other natural disasters. With this information, nations in affected regions should be able to provide services, food, and protection for their citizens more effectively.

The incidence of cardiovascular disease is increasing in many Third World nations. Many health care workers in these nations have little skill and experience in dealing with heart attack, stroke, or other cardiovascular problems. In particular, these health providers often do not have the training or equipment to carry out preventive screenings. Therefore, the World Health Organization has recommended that health workers in Third World nations be given stethoscopes and sphygmomanometers for checking the hearts and measuring the blood pressures of people in their villages. These health care providers must be instructed about how to care for and use these instruments.

The worldwide concern regarding AIDS (acquired immunodeficiency syndrome) has led WHO to initiate a number of programs and to assist nations in AIDS activities. WHO has established a surveillance system for worldwide identification and epidemiological study of AIDS. Increasing the awareness of the world's population regarding AIDS has also been a major activity. Funding of AIDS control programs, especially those designed to provide facilities for AIDS victims, has been provided by WHO.

Joint Agency Programs

The World Health Organization has joint programs with other international agencies such as the United Nations Children's Fund (UNICEF)—formerly the United Nations International Children's Emergency Fund—the Food and Agricultural Organization (FAO), and the International Fund for Agriculture Development. In addition to jointly sponsored programs conducted with WHO, these agencies conduct a variety of health-related programs with a special focus on nutrition.

UNICEF conducts programs to help children, particularly those in the developing nations. Numerous programs have been implemented to control communicable diseases and to improve nutrition. Funding for this agency comes from voluntary contributions from governments and private citizens.

The Food and Agriculture Organization oversees programs designed to relieve hunger and malnutrition throughout the world. Research, school lunch programs, education, and direct services to those in need are vital parts of FAO involvement.

An example of an interagency program is the Onchocerciasis Control Program, which has been implemented in eleven countries of West Africa.[4] Onchocerciasis is a debilitating disease that has caused blindness in several million people worldwide. The Onchocerciasis Control Program has brought together the resources of the United Nations Development Program, FAO, the World Bank, and the World Health Organization. Research has been conducted to find effective drugs to counter the filariae in the human body that cause this disease. The drug ivermectin has been developed as an effective treatment. Field personnel have been trained in ways to assist people with onchocerciasis.

In a joint venture between WHO, UNESCO (the United Nations Educational, Scientific, and Cultural Organization), and UNICEF, a document was released in 1989 entitled *Facts for Life*. This initiative identified ten areas of emphasis for primary health care programs concentrating on maternal and child health. Strategies for implementing activities and concepts that should be understood by those conducting the activity were presented for each of the ten areas. The *Facts for Life* initiative has been designed to assist any agency, organization, or individual conducting primary health activities anywhere in the world.

Many other agencies and organizations throughout the world have programs designed to meet the health needs of people. Some are government sponsored, such as the United States Agency for International Development (AID). AID provides funds for health and nutrition programs to Third World countries. Other medical- and

Facts for Life—Ten Areas of Emphasis

1. Timing of births. Spacing of births is an important way of improving the health of women and children.
2. Safe motherhood. Prenatal care and assistance at birth by a trained person greatly reduces the dangers of childbearing.
3. Breast-feeding. Babies that are breast-fed have fewer illnesses and less malnutrition than those fed on other foods.
4. Child growth. Physical and mental development is retarded by malnutrition and infectious diseases.
5. Immunization. Affordable vaccines that can give protection against the major childhood diseases are available.
6. Diarrhea. Poor hygiene and lack of clean drinking water are the major causes of diarrhea, which result in death and malnutrition among children.
7. Coughs and colds. Much childhood debilitation can be prevented if coughs and colds are adequately cared for by parents and health care providers.
8. Hygiene. Much illness can be prevented by practicing personal and community hygiene.
9. Malaria. Much death and illness is associated with this disease.
10. AIDS. Preventing the spread of this disease is a paramount goal in all nations of the world.

Source: UNICEF, WHO, and UNESCO. *Facts for Life.* Oxfordshire, U.K.: P&LA, 1989.

health-related activities are conducted by nonprofit, volunteer organizations, referred to as nongovernmental organizations (NGOs). NGOs include many religious agencies, such as Catholic Relief Services, Compassion International, and World Vision. Other nonprofit groups that are active in many health, nutrition, and population projects include Save the Children and Helen Keller International. In 1980 the World Bank announced that funds would be directly available for these health projects.[5] The purpose of supporting health projects is to strengthen a nation's primary health care system. It is hoped that such actions will improve access to basic health care, particularly for the poor of the world.

Primary Health Care

Changing concepts have led the World Health Organization and other agencies involved in international health to place more emphasis upon primary health care, not just disease control. Primary health care is now considered a major program objective in the Third World nations.

In 1978, an international conference on primary health care was held in Alma-Ata, USSR. This conference was organized and sponsored by the World Health Organization and the United Nations Children's Fund (UNICEF) following worldwide national and regional meetings on primary health care. A major objective of the conference was to promote the concept and development of primary health care in all nations of the world.

The most important outcome of this conference was the Declaration of Alma-Ata. This document has provided significant direction for World Health Organization programming as well as for other international health agencies and organizations, both governmental and voluntary.

The concept of primary health care varies from one location to another. However, there are certain health problems that most agree fall into the category of primary health care. As stated in the recommendations of the Alma-Ata conference, primary health care should include at least: ". . . education concerning prevailing health problems and the methods of identifying, preventing, and controlling them; promotion of food supply and proper nutrition, an adequate supply of safe water, and basic sanitation; maternal and child health care, including family planning; immunization against the major infectious diseases; prevention and control of locally endemic diseases; appropriate treatment of common diseases and injuries; promotion of mental health; and the provision of essential drugs."[6]

Primary health care focuses attention on principal health problems and so must be a part of the health policy planning of any government. The government may have to reevaluate its health priorities, however, in incorporating primary health care into its policy planning. This may mean developing different types of health personnel and reducing emphasis on curative facilities, particularly in the Third World. Or it may mean integrating the traditional methods of healing with the modern concepts of medicine in many nations.

The Declaration of Alma-Ata has served as an impetus for the World Health Organization, other international agencies, and the governments of the world to set specific, practical goals in their health planning. The declaration called for all governments to formulate national policies and action plans and to include primary health care as a part of their national health systems. It also called for the cooperation and commitment of governmental bodies in striving for "an acceptable level of health for all people . . . by the year 2000."

Whereas Alma-Ata emphasized primary health care, previous international conferences had focused on curative health provisions emphasizing facilities, research, technological development, and increasing health care personnel. The emphasis on primary health care should result in lower costs and be much more effective in attaining the long-range goal of improving people's lives.

UNICEF: State of the World's Children

In a statement issued in 1982, UNICEF suggested that developments in social and biological sciences make it possible to significantly improve the health of children throughout the world at very low cost.[7] UNICEF stated that a serious commitment by nations' governments and international health organizations could reduce disability and death among children by as much as one half within a decade. This could be accomplished by simple oral rehydration, universal child immunization, promotion of breast-feeding, and mass distribution and use of simple cardboard weight charts for coping with malnutrition.

In a follow-up report issued in 1993 it was noted that significant improvements had been made in the health of children of the world since the early 1980s.[8] It was projected that within a decade it should be possible to end child malnutrition, preventable disease, and widespread illiteracy throughout the world. UNICEF projected a cost of $25 billion a year to accomplish these goals.

Oral Rehydration Therapy

In the early 1980s, at the start of the UNICEF initiative, diarrhea was the major cause of death of children throughout the Third World. At that time it was estimated that five million children a year died from dehydration caused by diarrhea. By 1993 deaths from diarrhea had been replaced by respiratory infections as the leading cause of death of children in the world. It is now estimated that three million deaths occur annually resulting from diarrhea, while there are 3.5 million deaths a year from respiratory infections.[9]

The principle factor that has brought about this reduction in deaths from dehydration/diarrhea has been the use of oral rehydration therapy (ORT). As recently as fifteen years ago the standard treatment for dehydration was intravenous infusion of fluids. This was not only costly but necessitated the presence of trained medical personnel and sterile equipment. However, a procedure of rehydrating patients by oral administration of a solution of water, sugar, and salts has become widely used. This procedure, known as oral rehydration therapy, or ORT, is inexpensive, can be done by the patient's parents, and has been shown to be very successful. Through the use of oral rehydration therapy, it is projected that one million fewer children in the world now die each year from dehydration/diarrhea.[10]

UNIVERSAL CHILDHOOD IMMUNIZATION INITIATIVES

Bangladesh—has raised child immunization coverage from about zero in 1980 to 62 percent in 1990.
Latin America—polio has nearly been eradicated.
People's Republic of China—immunization levels have risen from around 20 percent in 1980 to about 90 percent in 1990.
Mexico—more than 90 percent of the eleven million children under five years of age have been immunized.

Source: UNICEF, *The State of the World's Children, 1993*. Oxfordshire, UK: Oxford University Press, 1993, pp. 16, 24.

Universal Child Immunization

Millions of children die each year throughout the world from common childhood diseases for which protection is available in the form of immunization. Measles, diphtheria, tetanus, whooping cough, polio, and tuberculosis account for about one-third of all childhood deaths. The development of more heat stable, effective, and inexpensive vaccines has made it possible to immunize children in the remotest of Third World nations. For agencies conducting child survival programs, immunization must be a top priority.

A typical **ROAD TO HEALTH CHART SHOWING A CHILD'S PROGRESS:**

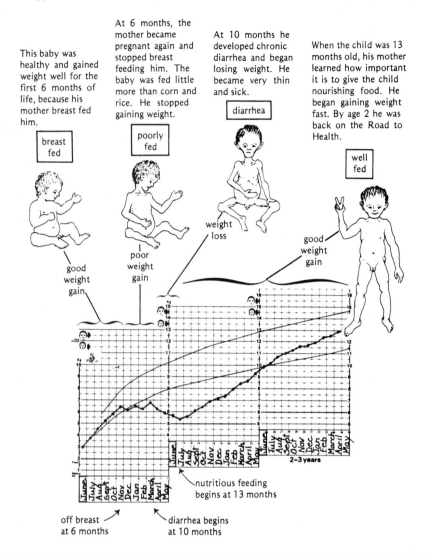

This baby was healthy and gained weight well for the first 6 months of life, because his mother breast fed him.

breast fed

good weight gain

At 6 months, the mother became pregnant again and stopped breast feeding him. The baby was fed little more than corn and rice. He stopped gaining weight.

poorly fed

poor weight gain

At 10 months he developed chronic diarrhea and began losing weight. He became very thin and sick.

diarrhea

weight loss

When the child was 13 months old, his mother learned how important it is to give the child nourishing food. He began gaining weight fast. By age 2 he was back on the Road to Health.

well fed

good weight gain

nutritious feeding begins at 13 months

off breast at 6 months

diarrhea begins at 10 months

2-3 years

Simple, cardboard growth charts can be helpful to the mother in identifying deviations from normal health related to proper growth and development. This chart and instructional information have been used by thousands of village health workers throughout the world.

The World Health Organization reported to the United Nations in 1991 that 80 percent of the world's children had been immunized against these six diseases. It was estimated that three million child deaths a year can be prevented as a result of this achievement.

Breast-Feeding

Children who are breast-fed are healthier and obtain all the necessary nutrients needed for early childhood growth and development. Breast milk alone is adequate until most infants are four to six months of age, yet mothers in many Third World nations are choosing to stop breast-feeding and use bottle-feeding.[11] At the time of weaning, the child is at high risk for infection, diarrheal diseases, and malnutrition. This is the result of such factors as illiteracy, in which mothers are unable to read the instructions on the infant formula labels; the use of impure, polluted water to dilute the formula; and basic poverty. It is important that women be educated regarding the advantages of breast-feeding and the disadvantages of switching to the use of infant formula and bottle-feeding.

Malnutrition

Millions of children worldwide suffer from malnutrition. Protein and vitamin A deficiencies are often present, but malnutrition may not be noticed by mothers until the problem has become serious and life-threatening. Using rather simple, inexpensive cardboard growth charts, mothers can be taught to enter the weight of the child each month. Over time they can see abnormal changes in growth and can be taught to seek help when these abnormal growth patterns develop.

Health Care Needs

The lack of medical care in many countries is related to the inadequate health care facilities and work force. In most Third World nations whatever health care provisions are available are usually found in the urban areas. Since these health providers usually practice fee-for-service medicine, the poor and the disadvantaged often do not receive appropriate care.

Those living in rural areas are denied access to health care because of geography, just as the urban poor are denied because of economics. Even though there is a pattern of movement to urban centers from rural areas, millions of people still reside in the small towns, villages, and hamlets of the world. Health care facilities are seldom located in these outposts, and the small-town inhabitants rarely venture to larger cities for treatment.

Numerous strategies have been introduced to meet the needs of these people. Some nations require all physicians, nurses, and other health care providers to serve in these rural settings for a specific period upon completion of their education. This measure helps meet some health needs, but the health personnel seldom

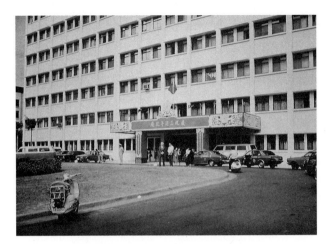

The China Medical College in Taichung, Taiwan, R.O.C., includes education for both traditional Chinese doctors and modern medicine. This medical college provides a setting for the integration of both medical care systems.

remain in the rural areas once the required service is fulfilled. The urban centers, with their modern health care facilities, specialized medicine, and greater income potential, are far more attractive to the physicians, nurses, and other health care personnel than the impoverished rural areas of their nation.

There are other reasons, too, for the health care providers to immediately return to the city after their required service is completed. They sometimes see their roles as medical administrators in a clinical setting where direct clinical services are not priorities. Personnel seldom venture from the clinic to administer medicine directly to the people in the small villages. Many times there are cultural and linguistic differences between the health care providers and the rural people. This creates a feeling of distance and of distrust and sometimes results in failure to provide optimum health care.

Thus, in spite of governmental efforts to provide adequate health care in rural areas, most rural Third World residents do not have access to needed health provisions. For many people, the principal health care provider is still the traditional village healer who has learned his or her skills and techniques from long apprenticeship with an older healer, quite often a parent or other relative.

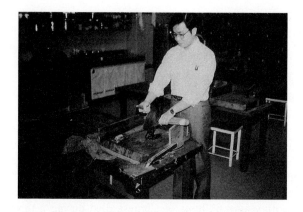

At the China Medical College, traditional Chinese herbal medicines are prepared, studied, and used. The students enrolled in the traditional medical curriculum learn what herbal preparations are effective for specific health problems. Research is conducted to ascertain in what ways the herbs have healing properties.

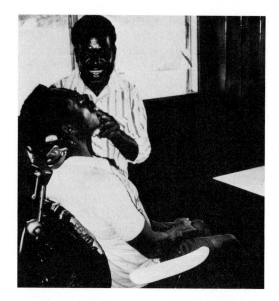

These village dental workers, known as dental montris, in Irian Jaya, Indonesia, are trained to perform extractions and to do simple fillings. They provide the only dental care to thousands of people living in the rural communities of Irian Jaya.

Traditional medicine makes use of different herbs, spices, and procedures in the healing process. Many times the healing concepts are rooted in religious beliefs and practices. Traditional medicine has been looked upon by many modern medical practitioners as basically unacceptable. Modern medicine has tended to ignore and to reject these traditional health systems and procedures. Therefore, when modern medicine is introduced into a locality, the people are often urged to turn from the traditional ways of healing.

In recent years it has been suggested that traditional healing systems have much to offer in providing health care to many of the world's population. One important reason for traditional medicine's effectiveness is that many rural, Third World citizens trust, understand, and can afford this form of medicine, whereas modern medicine is mistrusted and the facilities and work force are too costly. Also, people do not have to be educated to seek the healer's help; she or he is a visible presence in the community. For these reasons, with the support of governments and the World Health Organization, practitioners of modern medicine are being encouraged to cooperate with and to integrate traditional healers into health care programs. Measures have been taken in many countries to use the best of traditional medicine along with basic concepts of more modern medical care. In fact, some traditional healers have even been given training in the rudiments of modern medical practice.

Another development, which has gained widespread interest, is the use of village health workers as providers of primary health care among the poor, particularly the rural people, of the Third World. Primary medical care skills are taught to a person selected from a village. This individual continues to live in his or her village and acts as the basic health care provider. This concept, popularized during the 1970s, is based on the barefoot doctor programs of the People's Republic of China.

The village health workers—*promotores del salud* as they are known in many parts of Latin America, or medical *montris* as they are called in Indonesia—are able to give basic first aid, diagnose certain diseases and provide some medicines, deliver babies, and often help in elementary preventive health strategies. More advanced skills may include nursing and midwifery.

These health workers play an important part in many integrated rural health, agriculture, and economic development projects.[12] Such programs make available a broader base of health personnel for primary health care than a program employing only physicians and nurses.

In an attempt to meet the health needs of rural people, community development has also become a goal in many Third World nations. The community development concept is based on two premises: (1) there are not enough health care providers in rural settings, so village people should be trained to help meet certain needs, and (2) health problems relate to agriculture, education, and economics, as well as to medicine.

World Health Problems in the 1990s

If you were asked the following hypothetical question, "What one world health problem would you solve to help the greatest number of people?" how would you respond? Before you can consider such a question, however, you must be aware of some of the major world health problems. Initially, world hunger comes to mind. Millions in the world today are starving to death or are seriously malnourished. Population growth is another concern, particularly in parts of South America, Africa, and the Orient. Overpopulation in these areas is an obvious reality. Communicable diseases, though not as extensive a problem as in the past, still cause debilitation and death. The lack of a pure water supply in some 70 to 80 percent of the world causes many of these diseases. Illiteracy, urbanization, pollution, and political and economic systems are yet other obstacles to the health of the world's people.

Compounding these individual problems is the fact that most of them are interrelated. World hunger is often the result of political upheaval and warfare, which creates a flood of poor, homeless, and hungry refugees. Increased population growth leads to greater pollution problems as well as to urban sprawl. Impure water results in various communicable diseases. Illiteracy is interwoven into nearly all of these problems.

Each of these concerns demands thorough and intensive examination. Here, however, we will explore three problems that are paramount in the twentieth-century world: (1) hunger, (2) population growth, and (3) lack of a pure water supply.

World Hunger Crisis

The pictures of starving children in Somalia and Mozambique, of hungry refugee families throughout Africa and parts of Asia, or of young children with bloated stomachs suffering from kwashiorkor and other protein deficiency diseases in Central America are not pleasant reminders to those who live in North America. Not only are they displeasing to view, but they can, and should, make us feel guilty about our own excessive food consumption. Even more unsettling is the knowledge that such pictures can be multiplied millions of times throughout the world. Malnutrition, hunger, starvation, and resultant death are increasing problems in the world. Estimates suggest that five hundred million people (one in eight) in the world today are hungry or malnourished.

Famine is not new to our world; records tell of many such occurrences throughout history. Food shortages have been recorded as far back in history as ancient Egypt, Rome, Greece, and biblical times. In India in 1837 famine took some eight hundred thousand lives. And only a century ago, millions of Chinese died during a three-year famine.

Today the world food crisis is more significant because there are many other related problems. Population growth makes movement to new lands impossible when agricultural fields become too impoverished for food production. Mass migration to urban areas from rural localities to search for jobs and economic security compounds the problem. The lack of adequate fresh water in many parts of the world is also related to malnutrition and hunger.

The present world hunger crisis has evolved over a period of time. The conditions that have led to the present lack of adequate food supplies and related worldwide hunger have been developing for years. However, several human-made and natural occurrences have accelerated the crisis. At the beginning of the 1970s, there was a surplus of grain in the world. Many developed nations had enough to feed their own populations, help nations with serious food-related problems, and still retain a measure of reserves. But in the past two decades this surplus of world grain has been seriously depleted.

For example, in southern Africa eleven countries have historically been grain exporting nations. More than enough food was grown to adequately feed the population and in turn be able to sell agricultural commodities to other nations. However, since 1991 drought in this region has caused serious food depletion. Cereal production has fallen to half the normal production.[13] Acute water shortages have led to the death of thousands of cattle. Food is having to be brought to hungry and starving people in these nations. Major causes of these developments are the lack of rain and the effects of civil war that has taken place in several of these nations.

Worldwide economic inflation has contributed to the food crisis. In many poor nations of the world, people spend as much as 80 percent of their income on food. With the escalating costs of importation, fertilizer, and fuel, food costs have more than doubled in the past decade. Thus, the poor cannot afford to pay for adequate food.

The price of oil has been particularly disastrous to people living in poor, underdeveloped nations. Since the Middle East boycott of oil production in the early 1970s and the companion rise in crude oil costs, nations that must import oil have had to pay exceedingly high prices for food production. Many of the Third World nations must import oil to operate irrigation pumps, cultivation machinery, and produce-transport vehicles and for heating and cooking. Fertilizers and pesticides, which are oil based, have also risen in price. As a result, the quality of planted grains has decreased and insect loss increased.

Weather patterns have also played a part in the grain shortage and thus the world food crisis. Throughout the past decade, several regions of the world suffered serious drought. The Sahel region of Africa was especially hard hit. Thousands of acres of marginal farming land were destroyed through desertification. Many people in these areas, previously able to raise enough food for survival, became dependent upon food supplied by external sources.

Another contributing factor to the present world food shortage is the food consumption pattern of developed nations. Meat products, particularly beef, are widely consumed in the United States, and cattle are usually fed grain to fatten them before they are butchered. It has been estimated that beef cattle in the United States eat forty million tons of grain per year—enough grain to feed two hundred million people for a year at the basic level of four hundred pounds of grain per person per year.

Fertilizers are very important for farmers in the Third World, as their use can increase production. For example, one pound of fertilizer stimulates production of five to ten additional pounds of grain. Yet each year millions of pounds of fertilizer are used in North America on lawns, flower gardens, and golf courses. If even this amount of fertilizer were allocated to impoverished nations, food production would improve significantly.

Population growth has clearly contributed to the world food crisis. Each year there are as many as ninety-five million more people in the world than the previous year. This means more mouths to feed but less available land on which to raise adequate food supplies. This relationship of population increase to food production has been discussed for years. As long ago as 1798, Thomas R. Malthus wrote a classic essay on this topic entitled *Essay on the Principle of Population, 1798.* Malthus's basic thesis was that population increases more rapidly than resources do. He held that food production would not keep up with the ability of the human race to reproduce. Malthus hypothesized that population, if unchecked, increases in a geometric ratio, while food production increases only arithmetically. In spite of opposition to Malthus's ideas and continuing research efforts to increase food production, population growth is still outstripping the available food supplies in many nations of the world.

As nations become more industrialized, the citizens desire eating patterns similar to those in developed countries. Their diets change from vegetable to animal protein, increasing the demand for meat products. As consumption patterns of the developing world follow those of the more affluent societies, the food shortage will become even more pronounced.

Landownership patterns in many Third World nations also contribute to the world food crisis. Poor, landless farmers are often forced to pay much of their food production profit to the landowner. Many tenant farmers owe the landowner money for seed, fertilizer, and other items needed to plant and grow the crops. There is little motivation for landless peasants to increase food productivity when the landowner absorbs the profits. In many countries, landowners constitute only a fraction of the entire population but are usually wealthy and well fed, and have the political clout to continue the manipulation of landless peasants and food products prices.

In Central America, as in other parts of the world, the problems of hunger and malnutrition are worsening. One important factor in this situation is that agricultural products are exported to developed nations rather than used to feed the local population. This process has been termed *export cropping* and has been an important basis of Central American economy for years. Coffee, cotton, sugar, beef, and bananas account for the majority of Central American exports. Unfortunately, export economy has not benefited the majority of people in these countries. The large landowners and the rich have benefited, and the peasants are faced with higher food prices.

Beef exportation from Central America to the United States shows how American eating patterns can affect malnutrition and hunger in another part of the world. Since the 1950s beef exporting from Central American ranches has increased. The beef usually is cut-rate because of the low production costs. However, in the years since 1960, beef consumption by Central Americans has actually fallen by 20 percent because less beef is available for them. As the majority of the meat is exported to the United States, there is often an inadequate supply in the shops and markets of many towns and villages.

The cost of beef in Latin America has risen dramatically because the ranchers would prefer to sell to markets in the United States where they can get a higher price. The poor peasant in Central America cannot afford the inflated prices, and the local landowner will not lower the price if there are greater profits in exporting. Therefore meat consumption drops, an important source of protein is lost, and malnutrition increases. In the meantime, the poor workers and their families, without an adequate amount of protein, spend their days working to supply the tables of the overfed in the United States.

The problem of hunger is cyclical. The human body needs food for physiological growth and repair and for energy to keep the body systems functioning. The necessary minerals, vitamins, fats, carbohydrates, and calories can only be obtained from eating a balanced diet. The inability to obtain food leads to limited functioning—or malfunctioning—of the human body and mind. When the body systems do not function properly, disease invades the body, muscles become thinner, and every organ focuses its efforts on simply keeping alive. As starvation sets in, the mind is dominated by a desire for food; other matters have little importance. Obviously, then, as social and environmental conditions reduce food sources, people are unable to work or to function optimally, and greater debilitation occurs.

Food Assistance Programs

A broad range of activities focused upon the world's hungry and starving are carried out by different organizations and agencies, both governmental and private. Many television specials conducted by different private volunteer organizations (PVOs) have been used to raise funds to provide food for world hunger. The work of an American group of recording artists known as USA for Africa has

been instrumental in providing grants to organizations and agencies to combat famine and to provide direct food supplies to many hungry and starving people in the world since the mid-1980s.

Numerous international agencies have made food available to help those in need. Food assistance programs take a variety of forms. The food aid program of the United Nations is the World Food Programme based in Rome. The primary priority of this program is to provide food to victims of natural and human-made disasters. For example, millions of tons of emergency food aid have been provided for people who are most seriously affected by recent droughts in Africa by this United Nations agency. Other program work occurs through the provision of grants to private organizations as well as to international agencies working in areas of severe hunger.

Many problems must be overcome in channeling food to people in need. (1) Logistics is one problem that is very difficult to solve. Often roadways are poor, making it nearly impossible to transport food and grain from the docks and the cities to rural isolated villages. As a result thousands of people have flocked to the cities in the hope that food might be obtained. This has resulted in hundreds of thousands of poor people living in slum conditions within urban areas. Numerous health, social, and environmental problems occur associated with the influx to the cities. (2) Many localities do not have adequate food storage facilities. All too often food rots or is infested with rodents or is stolen and sold at greatly inflated prices before it gets to those in the most need. Obviously adequate storage facilities must be planned and constructed as part of any food aid program. (3) The food that is "imported" is often not compatible with the traditional food habits of the people for whom it is intended. Foods should be provided that are local staples rather than surpluses from the sending nations.

In 1992 the U.S. military was used to assist the people of Somalia. The purpose of this military intervention was to secure the ports where food was delivered and stored. Then the military moved the food out to towns and communities in the countryside that had not been able to get food because of warfare between various factions within the country. In most instances the actual feeding of the people was carried out by relief personnel with the necessary infrastructure already in place to assist people in need.

Food aid is more than raising funds and "sending" the hungry something to eat. It involves all the dimensions relevant to community health.

Population

Is there a problem of overcrowding in the world? Do you consider population growth to be an issue in need of resolution during the latter part of the twentieth century? Most Americans would respond to these two questions with a very emphatic yes. Indeed, population growth is viewed as a very serious concern by most informed Americans.

The population explosion is evident in the crowded streets of many of the world's major cities. The stress created by population problems in such localities as Hong Kong, Mexico City, and Calcutta, India, plus literally thousands of other cities throughout the world, convinces most westerners of the seriousness of this problem. But it hits closer to home as American farmlands, woods, and natural beauty spots give way to expanding cities, suburbs, factories, and shopping centers.

Despite our concern about population growth, literally millions of people throughout the world do not see it as a problem. At a worldwide conference on population sponsored by the United Nations and held in Bucharest, Romania, in 1974, there was disagreement about whether or not the world is actually experiencing a population problem. As a matter of fact, some nations, including those of Eastern Europe, expressed a desire for *increased* population in their countries.[14]

Other nations suggested that the population problems identified by many of the developed nations are really economic matters. They felt that the unequal distribution of the world's resources and wealth significantly contributes to population problems and that economic equality must be achieved by the redistribution of these resources. When this happens, fertility will decline as the natural result of social and economic development.

Still other nations viewed the concern over population as nothing more than a continuing effort by the nations of the capitalist, developed world to exploit Third World nations. Developing nations are very suspicious that the industrial world does not wish to have additional countries industrialized. There are racial overtones in these fears in addition to economic considerations. Since much of the Third World lies in black Africa and oriental Asia, some see population control as an attempt by the white European or North American world to keep the black or oriental populations "in check."

In spite of differing nationalistic, political, and regional views relating to the issue of population growth and control, the accumulated data clearly indicate an increase of people. As we review this data, it is important to question just how many people the Earth can accommodate. Resources are not infinite and are being depleted at a rapid rate.

The present world population is about 5.5 billion people. Growth continues at about ninety-five million individuals each year. Ninety-five percent of this growth is occurring in the developing Third World nations. By the turn of the century, world population is expected to increase to over six billion. The present doubling rate, or the amount of time that will elapse at the present growth rate before the number of people doubles, is about thirty-five years.

The most dramatic increase of the population growth rate has occurred in this century. There were only a quarter of a billion people in the world from the beginning of humankind until the end of the fifteenth century, when the Americas were discovered. Population doubling to a half billion did not occur until more than 150 years had elapsed (about 1650). It took nearly two centuries, until about 1850, for the world's population to double again, reaching the one billion mark. The doubling period for the next billion was only eighty years; the two billion figure was reached about 1930. The world's population reached four billion in the mid-1970s, and five billion in 1987 (figure 4.1).

Many concerns must be considered in analyzing the problems of population growth. The regions of the world with the greatest population growth rates are also the poorest and most economically underdeveloped. In some African and Asian nations, the growth rate surpasses 3 percent per year. In some instances there is a doubling rate of under twenty years. In most of these nations, this population growth is compounded by illness, poverty, and a lack of resources vital to healthful and productive living.

Another problem is that in much of the Third World the population is very young. Nearly half the population in Latin America, Africa, and Asia is under twenty-one years of age. This means that a large sector of the

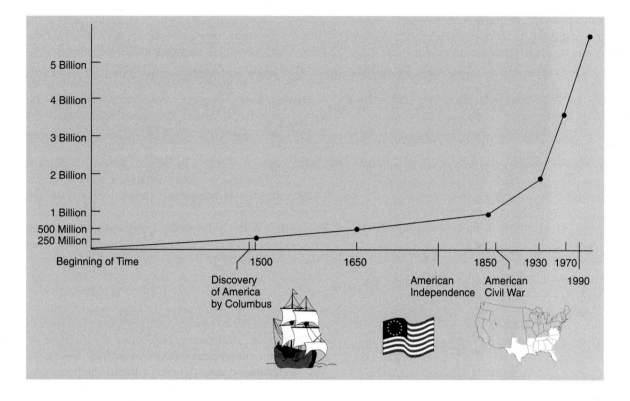

Figure 4.1 The population of the world has skyrocketed in the past century. There is little evidence that this growth will subside in the near future.

population is of childbearing age. Even with major efforts at population control in these nations, an overall population leveling will not occur until well into the twenty-first century. Unless the average number of children per family is dramatically reduced, the worldwide population explosion will not abate in the near future.

It has been estimated by the United Nations Fund for Population Activities that in spite of the decline in the world population rate, zero population growth cannot be reached worldwide until the year 2110.[15] There are several reasons for this. Longevity has increased in many parts of the world, especially in the developed nations. With increased longevity and lower death rates, population rises.

Less than a century ago the infant mortality rate in the United States surpassed one hundred per one thousand live births. Today this statistic is less than eleven per one thousand. Improved communicable disease control

measures, better infant and child health care services, and better nutrition have all contributed to reducing the levels of infant mortality in the United States. As a result, population growth has accelerated. This pattern has occurred in all the nations of the industrial, developed world.

Until the mid-1800s death rates were high, the result of many different diseases. But with the identification of specific disease-causing microorganisms and the development of the germ theory of disease, death rates have been greatly reduced. Today smallpox, diphtheria, and many other communicable diseases are either eradicated or significantly diminished because of immunization programs for young children.

It is no easy task to develop population control programs because of the barriers to their success. In many areas of the world, children are a kind of "social security" as old age approaches. People wish to have a number of children so that they will have help in farming the land and thus increased economic security.

Another reason that family planning is relatively ineffective is that in many Third World nations the infant mortality rate is still very high. Many parents see as many as one-half of their children die from disease, hunger, or other conditions before reaching the age of five. If they are to have the size of family believed to be necessary and desirable, it means having many more children. These additional children are "insurance" that there will be enough hands to do the work. Therefore, it is nearly impossible to achieve family planning among these people.

Religious teachings and practices are yet another barrier to population control, especially in countries where the Roman Catholic and the Islamic religions are practiced. The Roman Catholic faith prohibits the use of artificial birth control measures. This presents serious problems in many already overcrowded areas of the world where the Catholic faith is strong, as it is in the Latin American countries. The teachings of the Islamic religion also oppose birth control measures. This could lead to the population doubling in many Middle Eastern nations within twenty years.[16]

In many countries governmental policy supports population growth. These countries see population expansion as an overall part of the economic growth of the nation. Additional numbers of people are actually desired. In a study conducted by the Population Commission of the United Nations Economic and Social Council, most nations in the world felt that a higher rate of population growth was desirable or that the current rate was satisfactory. Only one-third of the nations considered a lower population growth rate desirable.

Another very important obstacle to population control programs is illiteracy. Teaching illiterate people to practice effective birth control measures is very complex since the reproductive process must be explained. Getting poor, illiterate people to understand and practice birth control measures, even relatively easy-to-learn procedures, requires effective communication and learning strategies.

Pure Water Supply

In thousands of rural villages scattered throughout the world, the source of water is a watering hole shared by both people and animals; it is a slow-moving stream polluted by sediment and human and animal excrement; or it is located several miles from the place where people live. The water supply may be contaminated by human excrement resulting from improper, or a complete lack of, sanitation. It is not unusual for public water supplies to not be available to people living in slum communities. If public water is available, often the costs are greater than what the regular city dwellers must pay. As a result, a great number of people have no access to an adequate, pure water supply.

The World Health Organization, through extensive studies, has estimated that in many of the world's poorest nations over 80 percent of the population lacks a fresh water supply.[17] In some Third World nations the percentage is less, but in most instances it still means that more than half of the population lacks pure water.

Millions of people throughout the world suffer from disease caused by impure water. The problem is so widespread that the World Health Organization has estimated that impure water supplies cause nearly 80 percent of all diseases in the world.[18] Many are the result of ingestion of microorganisms found in the water. For example, gastroenteritis, typhoid, and cholera are commonly found in areas where water is contaminated. Usually this contamination is linked to poor hygiene—the failure of people to use sanitary latrines.

Parasitic diseases are often endemic to areas having poor water supplies. Many parasites live in water and, without proper water purification, are ingested by the local inhabitants. Parasites are also able to burrow through the skin and enter the bloodstream of individuals who walk barefoot in the water. Examples of two such parasitic diseases are schistosomiasis and dracunculiasis. Schistosomiasis is carried by snails that reside in slow-moving or stagnant water; dracunculiasis is carried by the guinea worm.[19]

Communicable diseases are also transmitted by impure water. An example is trachoma, which causes blindness in thousands of individuals who wash in the dirty water.

Another contributing factor associated with impure water is that mosquitoes, which are carriers of malaria, breed in stagnant water such as ponds, open sewage systems, and water in outdoor cooking pots. At one time (the 1950s) it was felt that malaria would be eradicated with the use of the pesticide DDT. But today malaria

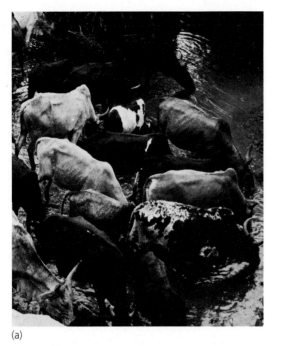
(a)

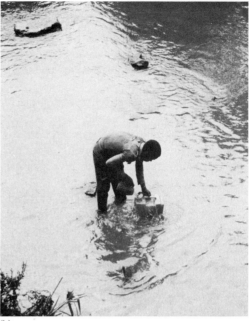
(b)

A common cause of many health problems is the contamination of water. (a) Cattle are found in a river. (b) The same watering hole is later used by a man as a water source for himself and his family.

is at epidemic proportions in many areas of the world. Mosquitoes have built up a resistance to DDT, and their breeding grounds—stagnant waters—are still common.

Any effort to improve water supply in a community must include measures to stop the pollution of the water source. Sanitary latrines must be introduced as an alternative to the streams and rivers. However, in communities where latrines have been introduced, the people frequently do not use them. They fail to understand the relationship between improper sanitation, impure water supply, and disease. These people must be taught the appropriate behaviors necessary for good health and well-being.

Another reason water supplies are polluted is that they are used as garbage "dumps." Many times the garbage from the local village is emptied directly into the river or stream. Unfortunately, people living downstream draw their drinking water from this same source. This demonstrates that an improved water supply is not the task of a single isolated community. The efforts of all

who use the same water supply must be coordinated from village to village, city to city, and country to country.

The problem of a pure water supply has no easy solution. National and international conferences have been held to develop resolution strategies. These conferences have been less than effective overall, but improvements have occurred in some countries. Positive action has taken place where the people of the area have been educated about and convinced of the need for pure water as a means to prevent disease, sickness, and debilitation. The government, too, has seen the need for action and has been committed to pure water programs.

The 1980s were designated as the International Water Supply and Sanitation Decade by the United Nations Water Conference in 1977. The goal of this effort was to make available fresh water for all people in the world by 1990. Many nations demonstrated a commitment to the idea of improved water supply for the people of their communities by establishing goals for 1990. However, their intentions were seldom matched by the funding necessary to carry out the plans.[20] Even though some successes were reported during this decade, in 1991 the World Health Organization reported that 1.2 billion people in the world still lacked the availability of a safe water supply and 1.8 billion individuals were without appropriate sanitation.[21]

How successful such an effort will be in the future remains to be seen. It requires the cooperation of many multinational organizations and agencies. Governments must set water supply as a high priority, both programmatically and economically. Also, creative measures need to be designed for educating people.

Programs to improve the quality of the water supply will not be effective unless similar efforts are made to improve sanitation. Sources of drinking water must be free from contamination both by humans and by animals.

Lack of fresh water is closely related to the problem of malnutrition and hunger. Physiologically, the human body needs water just as it requires food. Hunger and malnutrition reduce the body's resistance to disease and infection. Thus, a malnourished body is more susceptible to the illnesses caused by impure water. Diarrhea often accompanies many of these diseases and leads to a loss of body fluids, compounding the problem of malnutrition.

If the goal of providing safe drinking water (safe both chemically and bacteriologically) was achieved, the immediate result would be healthier, more productive people. There would be less mortality and morbidity. A safe water supply would virtually eliminate all pathogenic conditions that are the result of impure water. Improved health status and productivity would no doubt play an important role in the social and economic stability of the nation.

AIDS: A Worldwide Concern

The spread of HIV/AIDS has become a global problem. The World Health Organization estimates that there are more than two million cases of AIDS worldwide.[22] As many as ten million people worldwide are infected with the HIV virus.[23] Projections are that the number of cases will increase by the year 2000.

AIDS cases have been reported in 162 different countries. The majority of these cases have been in Africa and the Americas, with the sub-Saharan region of Africa being hardest hit. However, AIDS is reported to be expanding throughout Asia and in Latin America. In all likelihood thousands of HIV positive cases go unreported in many Third World countries with poor national disease-reporting systems.

The World Health Organization has projected that by 2000 more cases of AIDS will be found in Asia than in Africa. The HIV virus has been spreading rapidly in South Asia and Southeast Asia since 1990. When it is realized that more than half of the world's population is located in countries in these areas, the potential for an epidemic of frightening proportions is awesome.

It is suspected that the majority of this spread of disease will be by heterosexual contact. Such development will result in more women being affected than has been the case in other parts of the world. This has serious implications not only for the health of women, but also for the health of infants and children.

Worldwide as many as one million children have been born with HIV infection. Early in 1990 the world medical community became aware of a widespread pediatric AIDS epidemic in Romania. Several hundred infants with AIDS were identified. These cases were related to the practice of reusing needles when injecting blood into infants with low birthweights. This governmental policy was designed to reduce costs. Owing to food shortages during the 1980s, many infants were born to malnourished mothers and were of low birthweight. Thus, many babies were infected by HIV positive blood donors.

The social fiber and economic dynamics of many nations will become seriously strained in the next decade as the result of AIDS. Already overburdened and inadequate health care systems in Third World nations will be impacted. Many Third World nations have not openly addressed the increasing problem of AIDS because of fear of the impact upon their economy. This is particularly the case where significant income results from foreign tourism.

AIDS has resulted in tragic upheaval of family structures in many localities throughout Africa. The death of thousands of young and middle-aged adults in such countries as Uganda has left millions of orphaned children and dependent elderly without any kind of personal and economic support system.

In 1985 the World Health Organization drafted a global strategy for AIDS prevention and control. The following very broad objectives for this initiative were identified:

Prevent the spread of HIV infection—focus on education strategies.

Reduce the impact of AIDS on individuals and society—emphasize support for AIDS victims and their families.

Coordinate worldwide strategies—bring together the medical and social resources of the nations.

Educational initiatives have been developed and are being carried out in many nations. As in the United States, many different mass communication and educational strategies are being used to inform the public about AIDS. This is not always easy. For example, in Africa the majority of people live in rural areas. Many are illiterate and have minimal access to the mass media. The most effective strategies for bringing about behavioral change among these population groups still need to be determined.

Since 1988 the World Health Organization has sponsored World AIDS Day. Initiatives have been carried out in many of the world's nations. Ten concepts regarding AIDS have been highlighted for dissemination on this day.

Deforestation, Drought, and Desertification

There are numerous environmental factors that impact community health programming. On a global scale hundreds of millions of people have been affected by problems related to the destruction of the tropical rain forests, drought, and the extension of the world's deserts. These three global environmental matters are closely intertwined in many ways.

Deforestation

Since the beginning of recorded history vast regions of the tropics have been covered by forests. In many instances these tropical rain forests have been uninhabitable. Where humans did reside in these forests and jungles they were usually isolated from the developed civilization.

However, in recent years thousands of square miles of forests have been destroyed in the name of economic development and advancement of civilization. Though the destruction of the world's tropical rain forests has taken place in several countries, the most destruction has occurred in Brazil and Colombia in South America, in Mexico, and in Indonesia. It has been suggested that should destruction of the forests continue at the same pace as has occurred throughout the 1980s and into the 1990s, all rain forests will be destroyed within the first or second decade of the twenty-first century.

Economic development has been a principal reason for the destruction of the forests. The sale of wood worldwide has been a major reason that loggers have cut millions of acres of forests. Timber brings foreign currency to economically hard-pressed governments. For example, Nicaragua sold one-eighth, nearly one million acres, of its forests to Taiwan. Taiwan paid $30 million to help Nicaragua eliminate its national deficit.

Increasing population pressures have contributed to the destruction of the forests. Because of the need for more land as the numbers of individuals in a nation increase, land is being cleared for settlement. The land has also been cleared so that it can be used for subsistence farming and for cattle ranching. Some Latin American countries have offered economic incentives to those who will establish cattle ranches. This is in part due to the increased demand for meat products by people in both the developed and developing nations. Unfortunately, the increasing numbers of cattle, sheep, and other grazing animals can rapidly destroy marginal grasslands.

In some of the poorer nations people depend on firewood as a major source of energy. For example, at one time Haiti was a nation covered by forests. Today many of the hills and mountains are completely denuded as people have cut down trees and shrubs to use as firewood for cooking and for heat in their houses. This has occurred in many regions of Africa as well.

Thousands of square miles of forests have been destroyed by cutting and burning. This has been the principle strategy used in the Amazon rain forests. Loggers tend not to cut selectively, but practice clear-cutting in which everything is removed for miles. Burning of the forests adds millions of tons of carbon dioxide into the atmosphere. In the presence of vegetation, trees and bushes use carbon dioxide during the process of photosynthesis. With the destruction of forests, more carbon is being released and less removed from the atmosphere. Many believe this is one significant contribution being made to the problem of global warming.

Drought

Drought has seriously affected a number of localities throughout the world in recent years. This has been particularly the case in Africa. In southern Africa several countries that have historically been grain producing regions have experienced drought since early 1991. As a result there has been a loss of as much as 90 percent of maize and other grain in some countries.[24]

As areas are faced with water shortages, not only is food production affected, but so are other factors affecting the life of the inhabitants. For example, diarrhea, cholera, skin and eye infections, and meningitis are some of the human infirmities impacted by drought in such localities. With the shortage, or absence, of normal water levels thousands of cattle die. This results in further depletion of possible sources of protein for people already suffering from nutritional diseases and thirst.

Cattle, sheep, goats, and other animals, like humans, need water to survive. Often in arid regions the only water available is a watering hole. The animals come to these spots to drink and soon eat all the surrounding vegetation. The land is left denuded, erosion results, the watering hole becomes polluted, and since the vegetation renewal cycle is very slow in arid regions, the area is destroyed for future productivity. Therefore, the cattle are moved to another productive watering hole and the unfortunate cycle repeats itself.

An unfortunate related human factor in several parts of the world where drought has been most severe has been the combined presence of war between tribal and political factions within the regions. War causes displacement of people and loss of crops, livestock, and water. Warfare also destroys much of the infrastructure by which relief food is able to be brought to hungry and starving populations affected by the civil war. Lack of security to be able to grow crops in fields surrounding villages and towns make the planting of grain and other possible foodstuffs an impossibility. As a result civil war has contributed to epidemics, hunger, starvation, and the displacement of tens of thousands of people throughout the world, particularly in Africa.

Desertification

As vegetation coverage is destroyed in the rain forests, soil is then used for farming and ranching. In time, with overuse and misuse, there is a resulting loss of nutrients and fertility of the land. When tree roots that once helped to hold soil in place are removed, the land becomes eroded. As eroded, once fertile soil is exposed to rain, heat, and wind, it disappears. Each year millions of acres of land are turned to desert or reduced to zero economic productivity. This process of desert encroachment and

Hunger, overpopulation, disease, infant mortality, poverty—the world health problems are overwhelming. It seems as though there is little room for optimism. One college student, after study of the many issues relating to world health, concluded that it seemed as though the world was "going to hell." In the face of such a gloomy forecast, an individual might be tempted to accept the theoretical concepts of lifeboat ethics.

Lifeboat ethics suggests that the poor, underdeveloped nations should not be helped by the industrial, developed world. In short, lifeboat ethics proponents suggest that each developed country is a lifeboat. These countries have limited resources and will only be able to survive if these resources are kept and used for those in "the lifeboat." Only those "in the boat" will survive and live; all others will be lost to starvation, hunger, and death. The United States and other industrialized nations should not try to feed the entire world nor provide health care to the poor of the Third World nor spend time and money to help the needy.

Lifeboat ethics theorists point out that improvement of certain problems will only compound other problems in the future. For example, any efforts to control communicable diseases, to reduce infant mortality, or to reduce death rates will result in greater numbers of people. This, in turn, will cause more food shortages, greater incidences of hunger, and more poverty. This theory raises many questions. If you have ever visited, lived in, or worked in a Third World nation, you may find it hard to accept the idea that the people you have come to help and befriend might be those doomed to "sink" in the sea of life.

Can you look on the world scene from your lifeboat of luxury and resources and permit little children, your friends and acquaintances, or just simple well-meaning people to drown? Does the concept of "lifeboat" ethics have any meritorious features in your judgment? What would be the ultimate outcome in the world if the concepts of lifeboat ethics were applied? Would world conditions improve or get worse?

---

land deterioration is known as *desertification.* Desertification causes land to become so denuded that it cannot sustain agriculture or human habitation.

Desertification occurs on all the world's continents. In North America, sheep farming on the Navajo Indian Reservation combined with poor range management has destroyed much of the marginally productive land. In South America, the Atacama Desert in Chile has expanded, and today cacti are found where more tropical vegetation used to be. This, too, has been caused by overgrazing of cattle and sheep.

Possibly the most widespread encroachment of desert lands has taken place in the Sahara Desert of North Africa. All along the southern boundaries of the Sahara, the desert has expanded. Aerial photography has shown that these boundaries have shifted southward an average of ninety to one hundred kilometers (fifty to sixty miles) since the late 1950s.[25] This desert movement has affected all the countries immediately south of the Sahara known as the Sahel: Gambia, Niger, Sudan, Chad, and Burkina Faso.

Desertification compounds the problems of food and hunger. In many arid areas of the world the inhabitants are nomads. With the loss of productive land for growing crops, the people either must go without adequate food or are forced to leave their nomadic life-styles and move to urban areas. In the cities, they live in already overcrowded conditions, and few have the skills to make a decent living.

The continuing loss of productive land has broader implications. This situation often means that a nation becomes dependent upon other nations to feed its population. This creates an inflationary food cost spiral so that many people cannot afford even basic nutrients. The outcome, of course, is malnutrition and hunger.

Whether the process of desertification can be slowed, halted, or reversed is uncertain. Most experts suggest that the root cause is human-made.[26] If this is true, then people must seek ways to solve the problem. Many ideas, theories, and suggestions for solutions have been discussed. However, many of the possible solutions only create other environmental problems which, in turn, contribute to the original problem.

Summary

A review of health conditions in the world reveals some seemingly insurmountable problems. Disease, lack of adequate and appropriate health care, hunger, malnutrition, overpopulation, lack of pure water supplies, and environmental pollution are but some of the serious problems faced by humanity. Throughout history, numerous conferences have been held and many organizations and programs designed to improve the health of people have been established. These efforts have met with varying degrees of success.

In 1948, the World Health Organization was founded as an agency of the United Nations. Through WHO's programming, with its six regional offices, some positive measures have been taken. For example, a major worldwide program, organized and conducted by the World Health Organization, has eradicated smallpox; established international standards for foods, drugs, and vaccines; and educated many health professionals, particulary from Third World nations. Although the World Health Organization's priorities and program efforts change as new situations and problems arise, not all their programs are successful. Malaria is still a worldwide problem in spite of efforts to eradicate it.

In most Third World nations, health care providers and facilities are not made available to the poor. Attempts to correct or improve this condition have not been particularly successful.

Changing concepts have led the World Health Organization to place greater emphasis on primary health care. This emphasis resulted in an international conference at Alma-Ata, USSR, in 1978. This conference produced a document that now serves as an important guide to the World Health Organization and to other international agencies and organizations in setting program goals, priorities, and efforts throughout the world.

An important reason for health problems in many nations of the world is the inadequate health care facilities and work force. This is particularly true in rural areas and among the poor in urban localities. Governmental efforts to combat the problem have included mandatory service in underserved regions by physicians, nurses, and other health providers. The integration of traditional medical healers with modern medicine has also received increasing support. Another approach at meeting the health needs of the world population has been the integration of health care strategies with community development efforts, where the village health worker is a primary health care provider.

Though there are many world health problems, three are especially critical: world hunger, population growth, and the lack of pure water sources. Each of these three negatively affects the health, well-being, and lifestyle of millions of people throughout the world. None can be totally isolated from the other, although international efforts, conferences, and programs have been designed to focus upon improvement of each.

HIV/AIDS has become a worldwide health concern, with reported cases in 162 nations. Initiatives being carried out by individual nations as well as the World Health Organization have focused on education, care, and research. Prevention is possibly the most important measure in curbing the spread of this disease.

The world's resources are not infinite, and nowhere is this more obvious and relevant to world health problems than in the availability of land for agricultural purposes. In many countries of the world destruction of the tropical rain forests and drought have resulted in some of the most serious environmental problems in human history. As thousands of square miles of forests are burned and destroyed and as lack of adequate rainfall for agricultural production falls in many parts of the world, useable land for raising crops is diminished. Each year the deserts continue to encroach upon marginal farmland, leading to an uprooting of millions of people and adding to problems of hunger, malnutrition, and starvation.

Discussion Questions

1. What relationships exist between the United Nations and the World Health Organization?

2. What are some of the program initiatives being carried out by the World Health Organization?

3. In what ways does the World Health Organization join with other international agencies in conducting activities?

4. Discuss the areas of emphasis of the *Facts for Life* program.

5. What has been the value of the declaration of the conference on international health at Alma-Ata?

6. Give an illustration of the meaning of primary health care.

7. Explain the significance of the 1982 statement of UNICEF on the state of the world's children.

8. What have been the results of using oral rehydration therapy?

9. What can be learned from using cardboard growth charts?

10. Do you feel it is possible to integrate the practices and concepts of traditional medicine with those of modern medical practice? Explain your position.

11. What are some of the things that a village health worker can do that contribute to improved health in his/her community?

12. Explain some of the causes of the present world food crisis.

13. Identify some of the problems associated with getting food aid to the people who are most in need of it. How can these problems be solved?

14. What examples of programs of the World Food Programme can you identify?

15. What was the basic position expressed nearly two hundred years ago by Malthus regarding food, hunger, and population?

16. In your view, is there a world population crisis? Explain the reasons behind the position you have taken.

17. Why do some nations desire not to encourage population reduction?

18. What are some of the problems that are related to impure water supplies?

19. Discuss the relationships between water supply and sanitation of the local environment.

20. Explain the current pattern of the spread of AIDS worldwide.

21. Discuss various reasons for the serious economic impact of AIDS upon nations.

22. What kinds of activities have been designed to cope with AIDS on an international basis?

23. Discuss the World Health Organization strategy for AIDS prevention and control.

24. For what reasons is destruction of the tropical rain forests considered to be an environmental health problem?

25. What effect does drought have on health of humans?

26. Identify some of the factors associated with warfare and hunger, starvation, and malnutrition.

27. What are some of the factors that have contributed to the problem of desertification?

28. What is your position on lifeboat ethics?

Suggested Readings

Numerous articles on issues related to international health can be found in the following World Health Organization publications: *World Health,* and *World Health Forum.*

Anderson, Alastair. "Oncho: A Concerted Effort." *World Health* (March 1986): 14–15.

Diarrhoeal Diseases Control Programme. "Diarrhoeal Dehydration: Easy to Treat But Best Prevented." *World Health Forum* 10, no. 1 (1989): 110–15.

Ellis, William S. "Africa's Sahel: The Stricken Land." *National Geographic* 172, no. 2 (August 1987): 140–79.

Forman, Martin J. *Nutritional Aspects of Project Food Aid.* Rome: Food Policy and Nutrition Division, FAO, 1986.

Fox, Robert W. "The Population Explosion: Threatening the Third World's Future." *Futurist* 26, no. 1 (1992): 60.

"Global AIDS Update." *World Health Forum* 13, no. 1 (1992): 92–93.

Halpern, Judy Stoner. "Oral Rehydration Therapy: The Best Response to Diarrheal Dehydration." *Journal of Emergency Nursing* 17, no. 2 (April 1991): 99–101.

Hudson, Hugh. "Money Trees in Pakistan." *Refugees* 89 (May 1992): 16–17.

International Conference on Primary Health Care, Alma-Ata, USSR. *Primary Health Care*. Geneva: World Health Organization, 1978.

Kates, Robert W., and Viola Haarmann. "Where the Poor Live: Are the Assumptions Correct?" *Environment* 34, no. 4 (May 1992): 4–11, 25–28.

Lewis, Gwyneth, Joel Finlay, and Roy Widdus. "AIDS Programmes in Transition." *World Health Forum* 12, no. 3 (1991): 297–301.

Mann, Jonathan. "Global AIDS into the 1990s." *World Health* (October 1989): 6–7.

McNamara, Robert S. "The Population Explosion." *Futurist* 26, no. 6 (1992): 9–13.

Mpofu, B., and others. "Combating Drought: Food for All." *World Health Forum* 9, no. 1 (1988): 92–96.

Narayan-Parker, Deepa. "Low-Cost Water and Sanitation: Tasks for All the People." *World Health Forum* 9, no. 3 (1988): 356–60.

Okware, Samuel I. "Giving AIDS a New Face." *World Health* (October 1989): 18–20.

"Polio Eradication: Part and Parcel of EPI." *World Health* (December 1989): 6–9.

Sayagues, Mercedes. "The Parched Earth: Drought in Southern Africa. *Refugees* (July 1992): 4–7.

Skeet, Muriel. "Community Health Workers: Promoters or Inhibitors of Primary Health Care?" *World Health Forum* 5 (1984): 291–95.

Sze, Szeming. "WHO: From Small Beginnings." *World Health Forum* 8, no. 1 (1988): 29–34.

United Nations Children's Fund. *The State of the World's Children 1993*. Oxfordshire, UK: Oxford University Press, 1993, 90 pp.

"WHO and the Global AIDS Strategy." *World Health* (October 1989): 4–5.

Endnotes

1. "Sessions of the WHO Regional Committees." *WHO Chronicle* 39, no. 6 (1985): 223.

2. Henderson, Donald A. "Smallpox—Epitaph for a Killer." *National Geographic Society Magazine* 154, no. 6 (December 1978): 800.

3. *Ibid.*, 797.

4. Anderson, Alastair. "Oncho: A Concerted Effort." *World Health* (March 1986): 14–15.

5. World Bank. *Health: Sector Policy Paper*. Washington, D.C.: World Bank, 1980, pp. 10–46.

6. Report on the International Conference on Primary Health Care. Alma-Ata, USSR. *Primary Health Care*. Geneva: World Health Organization, 1978, pp. 24–25.

7. UNICEF. *State of the World's Children Report*. New York: UNICEF, 1982.

8. UNICEF. *The State of the World's Children, 1993*. Oxfordshire, UK: Oxford University Press (1993).

9. *Ibid.*, 4.

10. *Ibid.*, 22.

11. The subject of breast-feeding and infant formula is discussed in chapter 19.

12. Newell, Kenneth W., ed. *Health by the People*. Geneva: World Health Organization, 1975.

13. Sayagues, Mercedes. "The Parched Earth: Drought in Southern Africa." *Refugees* (July 1992): 4.

14. "A Report on Bucharest," *Studies in Family Planning* 5, no. 12 (December 1974): 362–64.

15. United Nations Fund for Population Activities. *World Health* (November 1981): 31.

16. Raymond, M., and Susan Ueber. *Health and Policymaking in the Arab Middle East*. Washington, D.C.: Georgetown University, 1978, p. 47.

17. Guest, Iain. "The Water Decade 1981–1990." *World Health* (January 1979): 3.

18. *Ibid.*

19. Parasitic diseases are discussed in more detail in chapter 10.

20. World Health Organization. *The Work of WHO 1984–1985*. Geneva: World Health Organization, 1986, p. 145.

21. Reported in the 44th World Health Assembly Report in 1991.

22. "Global AIDS Update." *World Health Forum* 13, no. 1 (1992): 92–93.

23. *Ibid.*

24. Sayagues, "The Parched Earth," 4–7.

25. Eckholm, Erik, and Lester R. Brown. "The Spreading Desert." *War on Hunger* 12, no. 8 (1975): 4.

26. Tolba, Mostafa Kamal. "Desertification: A Man-Made Process." *World Health* (July 1977): 2–3.

CHAPTER FIVE

The Private Sector

Of Increasing Importance in Community Health

Programs funded and operated by the government are in the public domain; that is, governmental activity is open to review by the general public. Nongovernmental activity is in the private domain, or private sector. Any organization or agency that is not tax supported is considered "private."

Despite governmental programs designed to improve the health status of a nation, many activities sponsored, funded, and conducted by the private sector play important roles in community health. Nowhere in the world is this more true than in the United States. Some of the most important medical advances in history have been funded by private organizations. These organizations also provide a number of health services to various segments of society. They are responsible for health promotion efforts targeted at every conceivable audience.

Private sector programs were overshadowed in the 1960s and 1970s by increased governmental programming in the health fields. Legislation, particularly at the federal level, as well as combined federal and state projects, received more attention in most American community health circles than did the private organizations.

During the 1980s a major reversal of this trend occurred. With reductions in governmental funding for health-related programs and the elimination of many federal health and social service projects and activities, the role of the private sector assumed increased importance in meeting the health needs of the nation. The result has been that many health needs that were the focus of governmental programming in the 1960s and 1970s are now being met by private sector programs.

Three community health groupings constitute the private sector: (1) voluntary health organizations, (2) private foundations, and (3) religious organizations.

Each of these groups can be subdivided into a number of organizations and agencies. Each has a definite focus with specific goals and objectives. Some programming efforts do overlap, but others are quite specific or unique. Though not coordinated by any central agency, they all play an important role in achieving a healthy United States.

Voluntary Health Organizations

Voluntary health organizations are unique American institutions. Although such agencies can be found in other countries, only in the United States do they play a vital role in society's health programs. These agencies are non-governmental, non-tax-supported organizations that rely heavily upon volunteer services to accomplish their program goals.

The voluntary health movement began with the founding in 1892 of the Anti-Tuberculosis Society in Philadelphia. This organization has since been renamed the National Tuberculosis Association, then the National Tuberculosis and Respiratory Disease Association (NTBRD), and later, in 1973, the American Lung Association.

These name changes exemplify the evolutionary process that often occurs within voluntary health organizations. Such organizations usually come into being because of a specific health problem. The resources of the organization, both finances and personnel, are mobilized for the purpose of eliminating or neutralizing that specific problem. When the particular disease is "conquered," the focus of the health organization often changes. Rarely does a voluntary health organization disband when its primary objective has been reached. Instead, it develops new goals.

This is what occurred in the case of the original Anti-Tuberculosis Society. At the end of the nineteenth and the beginning of the twentieth century, tuberculosis was a grave concern in the United States. But when it ceased to pose a serious threat to the health of the general public, the program and objectives of the organization shifted to a broader spectrum. Today the American Lung Association is concerned not only with tuberculosis but with all lung diseases, including emphysema, pneumonia, silicosis, pneumoconiosis, asbestosis, asthma, as well as lung cancer. Because of the relationship between smoking and lung disease, particularly lung cancer and emphysema, one major program centers on antismoking initiatives.

Another example of the evolution in voluntary health organizations is seen in the National Foundation for Poliomyelitis. This organization, founded in 1938 by President Franklin D. Roosevelt, had as its original goal the prevention of polio. In the 1940s and the early 1950s, when polio was a great concern, the National Foundation for Poliomyelitis was at the forefront of the "battle against polio." Many researchers, including Dr. Jonas Salk, were recipients of grants from this organization. After Salk's discovery of the polio vaccine and the elimination of polio as a major health problem in the United States, the National Foundation for Poliomyelitis became known as the National Foundation/March of Dimes. Today the activities of this organization are directed toward the prevention of congenital malformations, commonly called birth defects.

The American Heart Association is an example of a voluntary health organization that has maintained its original emphasis since its formation in 1916 as the Association for the Prevention and Relief of Heart Disease. This agency, which later became known as the New York Heart Association, originally admitted only physicians and scientists as members. By 1924 interest and program had expanded to the point that a national heart association was established, known as the American Heart Association. However, not until 1948 was membership opened to nonmedical persons. Through the years and through these minor changes in membership, the American Heart Association has maintained its original and primary objective, the prevention of cardiovascular disease.

The National Society for the Prevention of Blindness has also had the same emphasis—to reduce needless cases of blindness—since its founding in 1908. Members of this organization believe that half of all blindness in the United States can be prevented. For this reason the activities of the National Society for the Prevention of Blindness are not directed toward blind people, but toward the general public.

Voluntary health agencies range from national or international in scope with large budgets and programs to small, local agencies interested in just one isolated problem. The voluntary health organizations can be classified according to the specific focus or concern of each agency:

1. A specific disease entity—American Cancer Society, Arthritis Foundation, American Diabetes Association, National Leukemia Association, Cystic Fibrosis Foundation, Multiple Sclerosis Society

2. Health problems affecting specific organs and structures of the body—American Heart Association, American Lung Association, National Society for the Prevention of Blindness

3. Problems of special groups or matters related to a large sector of the population—National Safety Council, Planned Parenthood Association, National Association for Mental Health

Structure

Most voluntary health organizations that operate at the national level have state and local affiliate agencies. Efforts to provide direct local services are more effective when there are these affiliates at the "grass roots" level.

The American Heart Association has fifty-seven affiliated heart associations, one in each state. There are also heart association affiliates in the District of Columbia, Puerto Rico, and in the cities of New York, Chicago, Los Angeles, Philadelphia, and Cleveland. Each acts independently, which permits programming tailored to the particular needs of the given geographic location. There are also many Heart Association chapters located in various communities throughout the country, each with specific programs focusing upon the prime objective of this voluntary health organization—the reduction of cardiovascular disease. Each American Heart Association chapter reports to the state or regional affiliate in the area in which it is located.

Not all organizations so thoroughly cover the nation. Whereas the American Heart Association has affiliates in every state, the National Society for the Prevention of Blindness has only twenty-two state affiliates.

Organization differs from one agency to another. The typical pattern includes a board of directors with a paid executive director, paid professional staff, and numerous volunteer workers. These volunteer workers from all walks of life donate time and talent to the program.

The members of the board of directors usually serve in a voluntary capacity. These people have most likely already served as volunteers for many hours, and often contributed many dollars, to the agency. Their responsibility is to establish policy and provide direction for the organization. The board is also primarily responsible for determining how the agency activities will be financed. The executive director, employed by the board and usually a board member, directs the activities of the agency as determined by the board.

Professional personnel are employed by most voluntary health organizations. These individuals carry on the day-to-day work of the agency. Some staff members have responsibility for program planning and implementation. Since many voluntary health organizations have educational programs and a need to evaluate them, the professional staff usually includes an individual with research skills. This person develops evaluation designs, conducts statistical analyses, and recommends changes based on the findings.

Volunteer workers help an agency to function efficiently and effectively. They provide professional and supportive services, conduct fund-raising campaigns, and perform a variety of other activities essential to the workings of the agency.

Organizational Activities

There are several kinds of activities in which the voluntary health organization participates: health services provision, research support, sponsorship of educational programs, and service as a lobbying agent in the legislative process.

Services

Various types of health services are rendered by voluntary health organizations. For instance, Planned Parenthood services include Pap tests and breast examinations for women, blood testing, physical examinations, and male sterilization.

A number of services for cancer patients and their families are provided by the American Cancer Society volunteers. Many who have themselves been treated for cancer assist other patients. For example, volunteers are active in the International Association of Laryngectomees, which provides speech training to those cancer patients who have lost their vocal cords. Another volunteer service program is Reach to Recovery, which teaches exercises to mastectomy patients. This program is conducted by women volunteers who have had mastectomies. Ostomy patients receive rehabilitative services.

Personal management of diabetes is very important. Therefore, the American Diabetes Association helps the diabetic to accept, understand, and cope with problems associated with the disease.

The American Lung Association provides respiratory rehabilitation services to individuals suffering from pulmonary diseases such as emphysema, chronic bronchitis, and asthma.

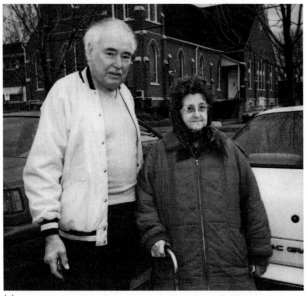
(a)

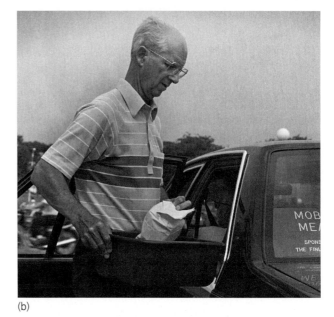
(b)

A broad range of services is provided by the voluntary health organizations. (a) Volunteer transportation has enormous value in the American Cancer Society service program. It plays no small part in saving lives. The men and women who donate their automobiles and their time to driving cancer patients to treatments provide a vital link in the cancer program.
(b) Meals are provided to people, elderly and disabled, by mobile meals on wheels programs.

A wide range of services is provided by the American Red Cross. Two of the better-known functions are (1) providing services to the families of military personnel and (2) disaster service. When it is necessary for one's family to contact a member of the military on active duty, the American Red Cross has the facilities to carry out this function.

In times of natural disasters the American Red Cross undertakes relief activities to alleviate suffering caused by the disaster. When a disaster occurs, the personnel of the American Red Cross are available on a twenty-four-hour-a-day basis providing food, clothing, emergency medical care, and shelter. All Red Cross help to disaster victims is provided at no cost to the recipient. Even though the American Red Cross provides relief assistance when there is a major flood, hurricane, tornado, or other widespread disaster, most relief actions involve helping victims of fires and accidents in local communities.

The National Easter Seal Society provides various types of direct services for people with orthopedic, neurological, and neuromuscular disabilities and their families. This organization makes available speech, hearing, and audiological services along with physical and occupational therapy. Children with learning and developmental problems are an important target population of this organization. Needed equipment is supplied on loan, and respite care and transportation to social and medical services are provided.

Help for children with asthma and their parents is given by the Asthma and Allergy Foundation of America. How to recognize the warning symptoms of an asthma attack, how to cope with it, and other needed information, along with services, are available.

Research

Extensive research efforts are supported by voluntary health organization funds. Several billion dollars have been given to medical and scientific researchers to further their efforts in understanding and curing illnesses.[1]

The American Cancer Society has spent more than $1.4 billion on cancer research since the first funding in 1945. In a recent year, $94 million was distributed to medical schools, hospitals, universities, and other institutions for research programs. These programs include

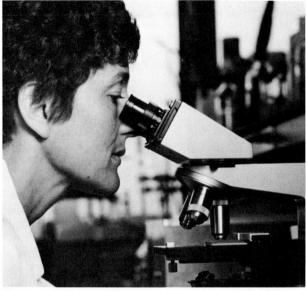
(a)

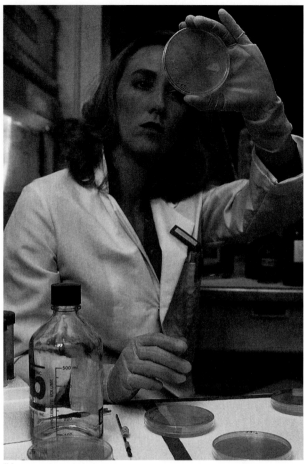
(b)

Support from the voluntary health organizations plays a major role in medical research. (a) The American Cancer Society funds basic research into all kinds of malignancies. (b) Studying cell cultures helps the researcher determine risk assessment.

molecular biomedical research into cancer and epidemiological studies of large population groups.

The American Heart Association also actively supports research. It has provided almost $1 billion for research since 1949. An American Heart Association policy is that 60 percent of its national budget must be allocated to research efforts. Some of these efforts have led to the development of artificial heart valves and pacemakers, as well as the surgical repair of congenital and acquired heart defects. Investigations into the control of high blood pressure and the relationship of exercise to the prevention of heart diseases have also been conducted. Also, the first studies as to how people could be saved by using CPR were supported by AHA research monies.

Research funded by the American Diabetes Association has added to the store of knowledge on the nature and causes of diabetes. Identifying effective methods of treating this disease, in addition to research aimed at the prevention and cure of the disease itself, has been important.

The National Foundation/March of Dimes funds have helped identify the causes of congenital diseases and the effective prevention and treatment of birth defects.

March of Dimes financial support has also led to the establishment of the Salk Institute in San Diego, California. Here researchers study the growth of both normal and abnormal cells, reproductive biology, virology, and genetics. Grants are made available to young medical students to encourage them to enter careers as medical specialists in birth defects.

Educational Programs

The most noticeable voluntary health organization activities are educational. Programs designed to promote well-being and to help patients with specific health problems are directed at a variety of audiences. These programs are widely conducted and use many educational strategies— including films, literature, community classes, educational exhibits, and speakers. Radio and television

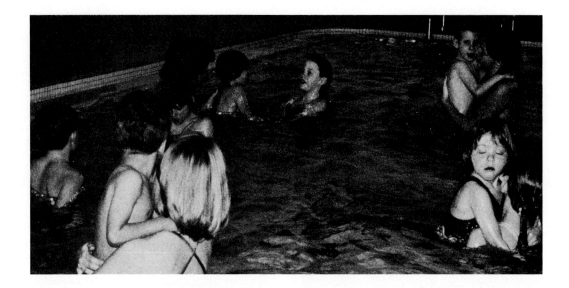

Educational programs sponsored by the voluntary health organizations teach skills that will help the individual having a particular health problem to better function in everyday activities. The American Lung Association sponsors swimming instruction for children with asthma.

announcements, news releases, and documentaries are also used to inform the public about the concerns of a voluntary health organization.

The American Heart Association conducts educational programs to inform the general population about cardiovascular diseases. Its *Schoolsite Program* is a school program focusing upon the behavioral patterns that contribute to good cardiovascular health. This program has components for preschool children, as well as for elementary and junior and senior high school students. Programs on proper nutrition, exercise, and the detrimental effects of smoking are also part of the educational activities of the Heart Association.

Another important Heart Association activity has been its cardiopulmonary resuscitation (CPR) training program. This program instructs people to recognize cardiac arrest and to apply CPR skills.

The *Open Airways for Schools* program is a six-lesson curriculum for children ages eight to eleven prepared by the American Lung Association. This curriculum makes use of group discussion, stories, games, role playing, and other procedures to teach children about asthma. It teaches children how to cope with asthma and presents

measures to help asthmatics overcome anxieties related to their problem. The curriculum includes material for parents, also.

A number of important community educational programs are conducted by the American Red Cross. The American Red Cross is probably best known for its instructional programs in first aid and CPR, and a broad range of water safety programs, including swimming skills, lifesaving, and water safety instruction. In recent years the Red Cross has developed instructional modules relating to nutrition and weight control as well as substance abuse. Other classes include instruction about family health and home nursing, stress management, and parenting. All these educational endeavors are taught by individuals specifically prepared as instructors by the Red Cross.

The American Red Cross has been involved in major educational initiatives centered on AIDS. Because of the historic role of the Red Cross in blood banks and transfusions, this organization has been particularly concerned about AIDS education.

Some voluntary health organizations offer educational programs for people with a specific health problem. The program objective is to help the individual cope with

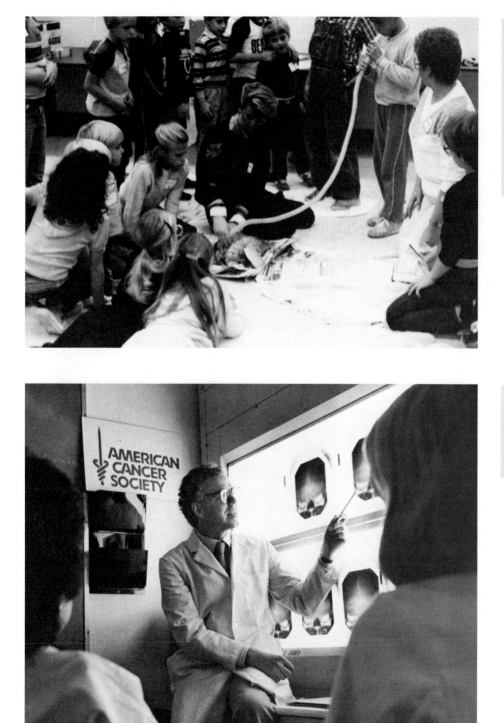

Asthma is the most common chronic childhood lung disease. The American Lung Association conducts a week-long summer camp, Camp Superkids, for children with asthma. The children participate in a number of activities and also receive instruction about their condition. A pig's lungs are used as part of this instruction because they most closely resemble the human lungs in structure and function.

Educational programs supported by the American Cancer Society are aimed at many different audiences. Physicians share cancer information with other health professionals.

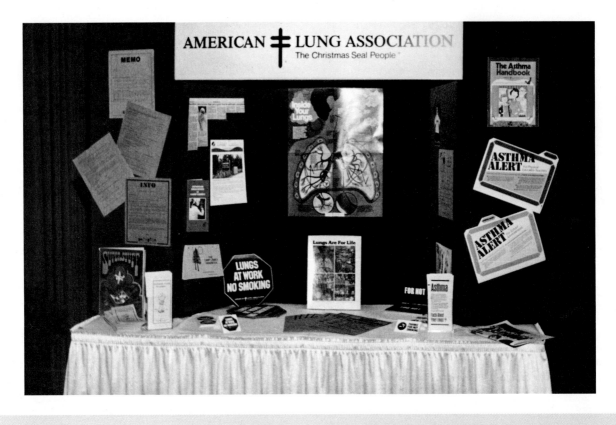

Information about lung diseases is provided to the public by the American Lung Association.

the illness, to reverse the problem if possible, and to teach the family how to assist the individual in coping with or reversing the disease. These programs are conducted in homes, factories, churches, schools, community clubs, or other appropriate settings; and they employ a number of educational strategies.

Several voluntary health organizations have developed a variety of educational programs for presentation in the corporate and industrial setting. The March of Dimes has a program for industries called *Babies and You*. This program is designed to educate employees and their spouses about the factors that affect pregnancy. Smoking cessation clinics are available from the American Lung Association.

An American Heart Association program that has been used with employee worksite health promotion activities is the *Heart at Work Program*. This program can be a useful part of health promotion programs at the workplace.

It is composed of five modules to enhance health behaviors relating to smoking, exercise, the warning signals of heart problems, nutrition and weight reduction, and basic emergency care. There are several different modules that focus on behavioral modification.

The American Lung Association conducts very effective emphysema and asthma clinics for patients and their relatives. The patient learns about the nature of the illness and how to live with this respiratory health problem.

Besides those services mentioned earlier, Planned Parenthood also conducts many sessions for sexually active or pregnant teenagers. These sessions instruct the participants in the use of effective birth control or, in the case of the pregnant teenager, in the basics of good prenatal care.

The *Glaucoma Alert Program* (GAP) of the National Society for the Prevention of Blindness promotes its cause through several activities. For example, one film has been shown on over a hundred television stations. Radio spots, printed literature, and the glaucoma information kit have also been widely used.

Since 1977 one day in November has been set aside for the American Cancer Society sponsored program, the *Great American Smokeout.* This program is designed to encourage cigarette smokers and individuals who use smokeless tobacco to refrain from tobacco use for a period of twenty-four hours. Communitywide activities are carried out. Media coverage is widespread, there is distribution of education materials to businesses and industries, various programs are conducted in schools, and other creative activities are organized for this day. Smokers are encouraged to quit "cold turkey" for one day. It is felt that if they can quit for one day, they can refrain from use of tobacco for longer periods of time.

Many voluntary health organizations provide research data to medical professionals to keep these health providers informed of recent developments. Educational workshops, seminars, periodicals, and audiovisual materials are included in professional education efforts of such organizations as the American Lung Association, the American Cancer Society, the American Heart Association, and the National Foundation/March of Dimes. The American Diabetes Association, in addition to conducting seminars and conferences, publishes a monthly professional journal on diabetes. Some national voluntary health organizations have annual conferences where health professionals are informed of the most recent knowledge concerning the specific disease or health problem. The American Cancer Society provides fellowships in chemical oncology for physicians and scholarships in cancer nursing.

Some agencies tailor their educational programs to a special population group not directly associated with the disease. For example, the American Diabetes Association has educational programs for teachers, police, and fire fighting personnel. Teachers must know how to cope with the special problems of the diabetic in the classroom. Emergency personnel often deal with diabetics. Failure to recognize diabetic symptoms may result in the false diagnosis of alcohol intoxication. Such an error could be damaging or fatal to the victim.

The American Heart Association also trains teachers, as do the National Dairy Council and numerous other voluntary health organizations. The American Lung Association has been instrumental in developing and disseminating a health education program for students in grades kindergarten through three in a number of school districts.

Political Lobbying

The voluntary health organization is often active and frequently effective as a political lobby agent. In this capacity, its purpose is to influence legislation that is of specific concern to that agency. One reason that voluntary agencies have been effective at lobbying is that a large number of volunteers with definite interests and concerns can be mobilized successfully. These volunteers write letters and contact appropriate legislators at both the federal and state levels.

The American Lung Association has been active in lobbying for antismoking legislation. Nationally this organization was active in supporting the passage of the National Clean Air Act and has been very instrumental in lobbying for reauthorization of this legislation. This interest in clean air relates to the American Lung Association's concern for efficient pulmonary functioning.

The National Society for the Prevention of Blindness has worked for laws that would protect eyes in hazardous environments. The society has also been active in obtaining the governmental prohibition of a number of potentially dangerous consumer products such as fireworks, toy guns, and other weapons, in addition to many toys with sharp edges or projections. The society has also lobbied for the mandatory use of protective eyewear in industrial settings. This concern has now expanded to include the wearing of eyeglasses during sports activities, especially racket sports such as tennis, racquetball, handball, and squash. These increasingly popular sports are a leading cause of sports-related eye injuries.

Financing

The voluntary health agency is financially supported by means other than governmental tax funds. However, some local voluntary agencies may receive government grants for specific programs. Some agencies provide certain services for which a fee is charged, though support is usually obtained through private contributions and donations.

These contributions come from a variety of sources. Monies are made available to voluntary health organizations from foundation grants, gifts from corporations or estates, memorial gifts, and large and small individual donations. Much of an agency's operating funds are generated by special fund-raising events, including golf and tennis tournaments and exhibitions, bowling contests, running and cycling marathons, and other athletic events. Musical concerts are held, and the funds that are raised support various voluntary health agency programs.

Communitywide fund-raising campaigns are conducted in most localities. The campaign may be either a joint community effort with many agencies participating or the individual effort of a single agency. There are advantages and disadvantages to both approaches.

The joint venture combines the efforts of the agencies within a community. A specific budgetary goal for each agency is determined. When all the goals are combined, an overall objective for the entire community fund-raising project is identified, and the community is mobilized to reach the established financial objective. This joint project, often called the United Way, United Appeal, or Community Chest, eliminates numerous calls on individual citizens during the year. Overhead and administrative expense for the fund-raising effort are shared and thus reduced.

Some voluntary health organizations do not participate in community fund-raising campaigns. They feel that their specific identity is lost in a joint appeal. These organizations argue that one of the objectives of the fund-raising campaign, in addition to obtaining funds, is to educate the public about the services rendered by the particular agency and about the health problem with which they are concerned.

Many local voluntary health organizations submit a large portion of their received funds to their state and national affiliate offices. The local community United Way is opposed to this practice and will not include such agencies in community fund-raising programs.

Nationwide television appeals have been used quite effectively to raise funds. One of the best-known is the "Jerry Lewis Telethon for Muscular Dystrophy" held every Labor Day weekend.

Many unique and creative fund-raising initiatives are carried out by different voluntary health organizations. For example, the American Cancer Society had a program where several community leaders were stopped as they drove to work. They were "arrested by the Cancer Society" and taken to a "jail" at a local mall, where a bank of telephones was installed. The "arrested" individuals had to call friends, relatives, and professional contacts to raise pledges, "bond," for the American Cancer Society. Bond was set by the Cancer Society, and the individual was released upon raising the given amount.

Problems

The voluntary health organizations provide vital services to the comprehensive community health program. However, they do encounter special problems. Often there is a tendency to duplicate services and programming when a community is served by several agencies. One example is the antismoking campaign. At least three national voluntary health organizations found in most communities—the American Cancer Society, the American Heart Association, and the American Lung Association—are involved in programs to combat smoking. The increasing formation of community coalitions designed to work together on a similar problem has helped to reduce program duplication.

Another problem facing the voluntary health agency movement is economic. In times of economic pressure, it is very difficult to raise funds. Therefore agency programming is often at the whim of the financial status of the community. This often leads to fluctuations in program emphases based on economic constraints, rather than on the health needs of the people in the community.

Unfortunately, the staff must often spend much time in fund-raising in some voluntary health organizations instead of on direct services, research, and educational initiatives. The employees often find their emphasis must be on raising money. On occasion, program activities completely stop for several weeks while the funding campaign is in progress.

In spite of the problems facing voluntary health organizations today, they have and will continue to have a vital role in the community health programs of our nation. Possibly you, as a citizen, may become involved in one of these organizations. Volunteers are always needed, and financial support is never refused.

Philanthropic Foundations

There are more than three thousand philanthropic foundations in the United States. These are nonprofit funding foundations in the private sector that support a broad range of educational, humanitarian, and health and social services. Hundreds of millions of dollars are distributed annually by these organizations for the support of projects and activities.

There are five different categories of philanthropic foundations:[2] national foundations, special interest foundations, corporate foundations, family foundations, and community foundations. Foundations in each of these categories vary as to their program goals and emphases. The largest in terms of assets and grants provided are the national foundations. The program support interests of these foundations usually are not limited by geographic boundary. They also receive the greatest number of requests for funding each year. The special interest foundations have a specific issue or problem of concern as their sole reason for existing. The Robert Wood Johnson Foundation is an example of a special interest foundation. The sole support of this foundation is focused upon health programs.

More than four hundred foundations have been established by corporations. These foundations vary widely as to their areas of funding support. An individual or agency seeking funding from these foundations must review very closely their program goals before submitting a request for support to assure that the request is related to the goals of the foundation.

The largest number of foundations are family foundations. These foundations have been established by individuals and/or families from their personal financial resources. Generally these foundations provide less individual amounts than do the other foundations. The W. K. Kellogg Foundation is an example of a family foundation having health as a primary program support.

There are more than three hundred community foundations. These foundations are established to provide support within a specific geographic region. They will not fund projects and programs outside of an identified community area.

Health has been the subject of specific interest of a number of foundations. This interest usually results in the provision of health care to people in medically underserved areas, and in health program planning, development, and research. It would be impossible to review all foundations with health care and health promotion as a goal. Several will be presented as examples; each of these has provided major, if not exclusive, support for health agencies, organizations, and programs.

Rockefeller Foundation

One of America's largest foundations is the Rockefeller Foundation. Since its establishment in 1913, this foundation has appropriated $1.5 billion in support of projects throughout the world.[3] The principal program objective of this foundation is the reduction of human suffering and need.

As a means of achieving this goal, public health measures have long been an important focus of this foundation. The development of public health programs and support of disease eradication programs for such ailments as hookworm, yaws, schistosomiasis, malaria, and yellow fever were some early foundation activities. Today the foundation's scope of interest, plus funding, has broadened to include the arts, humanities, and international relations. But activities designed to alleviate and solve the problem of worldwide hunger are still vital Rockefeller Foundation programs.

The "conquest of hunger" program involves a number of Latin American and Asian projects designed to increase food production and distribution. In addition, agricultural research focusing on plant breeding and control of animal diseases is an important part of the hunger program.

The Rockefeller Foundation has long had an interest in the problem of population growth. The program established to study this problem has three components:[4]

1. Research in reproductive biology
2. Research on new contraceptive technology
3. Policy studies to understand the determinants and consequences of fertility and the socioeconomic factors affecting population

During its nearly eighty years of existence, the foundation has supported a number of programs designed to control diseases. Though communicable diseases are no longer the serious problem they once were in the United States, they still afflict millions of people worldwide, particularly in the Third World. Malaria, trypanosomiasis, and infant diarrhea are examples of diseases that this foundation is studying. Specifically, biomedical research to develop a malaria vaccine and to study infant diarrhea in Haiti has been supported by the Rockefeller Foundation.

Particularly in the Third World nations, the foundation has supported educational training programs for such primary health workers as epidemiologists, laboratory technicians, and nurse practitioners. In addition to basic biomedical research and training programs, the Rockefeller Foundation has funded field studies in many parts of the world. These studies have involved pharmacology, biochemistry, and clinical field work.

Henry J. Kaiser Family Foundation

This foundation has supported many programs in health and medicine since it was established in 1948. In fact, the annual fund distribution exceeds $23 million.[5] This foundation was established by industrialist Henry J. Kaiser and his wife out of concern for the unmet health care needs of many in our society. This foundation has set five specific program outcomes for support: (1) research, (2) development of new health care approaches, (3) application of innovative methods of health care, (4) project evaluation, and (5) dissemination of information to improve health care.[6]

Present initiatives of this foundation are to provide support for programs that are designed to improve primary health care. Monies from this foundation are used to encourage the expansion of health maintenance organizations. Support has been provided for nutrition programs for Hispanics. Also, in recognition of the need to prevent teen pregnancy, this foundation has supported several teen pregnancy prevention programs.

Scholarships for minority students in medicine and dentistry are made available. In addition, planning, delivery, and improvement of health care receive financial support. Another area of increased support has been encouraging creative efforts focused on health needs of the elderly, particularly the frail elderly. The Henry J. Kaiser Foundation usually does not finance institutional construction or laboratory or clinical research.

The Robert Wood Johnson Foundation

Supporting projects designed to improve access to health care, this foundation was established in 1972 from the estate of General Robert Wood Johnson. More than $128 million a year are made available by this foundation to a broad range of medical institutions, schools, and health care facilities. Funding priorities include improving the availability and quality of health care for population groups at risk for inadequate care.[7] Foundation support is directed chiefly toward (1) specific diseases and threats to the health and well-being of Americans, (2) identified vulnerable populations, and (3) national health issues.

The Robert Wood Johnson Foundation initiated a major nationwide effort in the latter part of the 1980s to support programs in AIDS prevention and services for AIDS patients. One such initiative is the production of an hour-long documentary on AIDS designed to provide accurate information for medical practitioners, public policymakers, and the general public. Other AIDS-related programs included direct services to AIDS patients and assistance for their families, and informational packages for public policymakers, schools, and other organizations.

Three other specific concerns were the focus of this foundation funding in recent years. These concerns included a variety of psychiatric diseases among children, the nation's substance abuse problem, and the need for daycare centers for elderly suffering from such disorders as Alzheimer's disease.

The Robert Wood Johnson Foundation has also directed its support toward several specific vulnerable population groups: the elderly, mothers and infants, children and youth, Native Americans, and the medically indigent. Support has been provided for programs in rural communities as well as in urban settings. Initiatives designed to remove barriers to needed health care for these population groups have been of particular interest.

Funding has also been provided to medical schools in order to help increase the number of general medical practitioners: pediatricians, doctors in family practice, and medical generalists. The funded medical schools have introduced a number of initiatives in the curriculum, established residency training to emphasize general practice, and made specific efforts to attempt to recruit students into general medical practice.

A nationwide study has been supported by the Robert Wood Johnson Foundation to study trauma. Of particular concern has been an attempt to learn why some physicians are reluctant to treat trauma patients. Measures that can help health care providers to better cope with emergency medicine are hoped-for outcomes of this project.

The foundation has been interested in several broad problems of national significance. The increasing shortage of nursing personnel in hospital and clinical settings has been one. More than $26 million was made available for programs to redesign the hospital as an effective workplace for nurses. The foundation has also encouraged people from minority groups to train for the medical and health professions, including physicians, dentists, and nurses.

The foundation has supported research, project development, and demonstration projects as means of attaining these goals. Grants have been made available to a number of hospitals for the purpose of developing primary care group practices. Many people, particularly the disadvantaged, depend on a local hospital as the primary source of health care. The objective of primary care group practices in hospital settings is to offer preventive health care to these individuals.

Research interests have centered on the health and medical status of African Americans. This foundation has also supported research directed at identifying factors associated with teenage pregnancy.

Another important health need funded by the Robert Wood Johnson Foundation is a program that expands and strengthens the inner-city health service programs developed and operated by municipal governments. Access to health care in rural areas has also received support. Efforts to develop nonprofit group medical practices in these medically underserved localities have been financed.

Institutions that train professionals in primary health care have been supported by this foundation. The foundation has supported primary care training programs for nurses—especially faculty education—and for emergency care nurses. It has also encouraged the preparation of rural nurse practitioners, the preparation of physicians for careers in family practice, and training programs for physicians' assistants. Funds have also been generated to establish a graduate program at a midwestern university to prepare speech and language pathologists to pursue careers in treatment of infants at risk for communication disorders.

Foundation concerns also include the health needs of infants, children, and adolescents. This interest has led to the development of a school health service system, and a preventive dentistry demonstration program for school age children. The foundation has been actively supportive of school-based health clinics. Over $16 million was awarded for the establishment of about twenty clinics designed to provide students with a comprehensive range of medical services. The specific focus of this initiative has been the health needs of children in lower socioeconomic communities.

Another program interest of the foundation has been assisting the physically disabled. In 1990 a program designed to help such individuals live independently was announced.

W. K. Kellogg Foundation

This foundation also supports health programs. W. K. Kellogg, upon creating this foundation in 1930, said that its objective was to "help people to help themselves." The foundation continues to pursue this objective today. Its support is limited to activities in agriculture, education, and health. In addition to supporting programs in the United States and Canada, the Kellogg Foundation funds

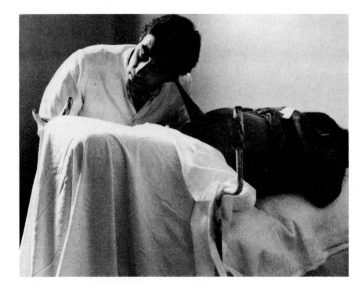

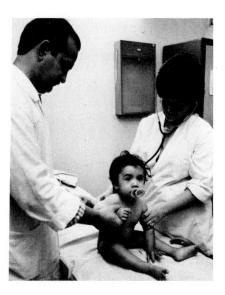

In Latin America, community health projects funded by the W. K. Kellogg Foundation are helping to bring medical care to urban and rural communities alike. Efforts are concentrating on infectious diseases, unsanitary living conditions, dental caries, outdated medical curricula and practices, and basic inaccessibility of health services.

"help people help themselves" in Latin America, the Caribbean, and southern Africa. The foundation does not fund research efforts; rather, it supports projects that apply existing knowledge to specific needs.

Foundation support for health includes programs that fall into four categories:

1. Programs that enhance the comprehensiveness and continuity of health care
2. Activities and projects that are aimed at cost containment and increased productivity of health care
3. Activities related to health promotion, disease prevention, and public health efforts
4. Efforts to ensure quality health care and health professional education[8]

The programs designed to enhance the comprehensive nature of health care include the establishment of several holistic health centers. Those programs designed to cut costs offer grants to hospitals to combine the skills of several health care providers into a single service.

Though the Kellogg Foundation supports a diversity of initiatives, recent interest has focused on community primary care programs. Infants and children and the elderly are two population groups who experience the special concern of this foundation. The needs of the urban poor, rural families, and minorities have been a recent emphasis.

The foundation's interest in health promotion, disease prevention, and public health has resulted in programs for several different populations. One such project was the development of a secondary school health education curriculum in a New England community. Other projects have involved nursing education and medical school family practice programs. Yet another project supported by the Kellogg Foundation involved the diffusion of health promotion activities to the inhabitants of one mid-western state.

Funds have been provided by this foundation to improve the health of Native Americans. Two particular programs receiving recent support are initiatives to help Native Americans who are at high risk for pregnancy and the establishment of a comprehensive vision care program.

With increased numbers of people being homeless in the United States in recent years, the need for health education and health care services for this population has increased. The Kellogg Foundation has supported programs designed to help this population in most of America's urban localities.

A current program priority of the foundation is nutritious food production. This has been important for improving the life of rural citizens. Encouraging research, teaching and extension work in human nutrition has also been a focus, including educational initiatives concerning nutrition and food production. One such program of support was the development of a model nutrition and health education program for urban African-American women and children.

The Kellogg Foundation has expanded its interest in programs designed to help the frail elderly population. Because of increased mobility in the United States, many senior citizens live apart from family support. When in need of health care related to serious illness or surgery, these people often are without adequate assistance. The foundation has supported demonstration projects designed to meet this growing need.

One can see that this foundation actively supports a number of programs. Some funds help in the establishment of programs. Other monies provide for the enlargement of already existing projects. Demonstration projects, continuing education activities, and curriculum development and improvement are of special interest. These programs are costly, too. Since its founding, the Kellogg Foundation has distributed nearly $2 billion. In one recent year, expenditures exceeded $151 million, with over 50 percent supporting health-related projects.[9]

Ford Foundation

A major program focus of the Ford Foundation has been the problems of urban and rural poverty. It supports programs throughout the United States as well as in the developing Third World nations. This foundation's budget exceeded $644 million in a recent year.

An emphasis of this foundation has been the problem of teenage pregnancy among the poor and the support of activities to reduce infant mortality and childhood sickness in this population group. Funds have been provided to develop prevention projects to help children in middle school avoid pregnancy, especially educational programs that help students make responsible choices about sexual behavior. Funds have also been made available for treatment of sexually transmitted diseases and gynecological infections.

The Ford Foundation is currently interested in improving health, nutrition, and intellectual development of poor children in the United States. Community outreach workers contact women early in their pregnancies and help them obtain appropriate health care and nutritional information. For example, in rural Appalachia paraprofessional home visitors advise expectant mothers regarding prenatal care, breast-feeding, and infant development.

The problem of population growth has been another interest of the Ford Foundation. Various programs designed to improve family-planning and fertility control methods, research to develop new methods of contraception, and information dissemination programs have been supported.

The increasing need for good child care in the United States has been another program focus of this foundation. It has supported programs for evaluating child care models in which community schools provide education, health, and social services for young children.

Since 1987 the Ford Foundation has set aside specific funding for programs relating to AIDS, including programs of education, community care, and public policy. Educational initiatives have focused on preventive measures as well as strategies for AIDS patients and caregivers. In foreign countries, several measures designed to identify patterns of the spread of AIDS have received support.

In addition, the Ford Foundation has supported field projects in several Third World nations to provide a safe, effective water supply.

Religious Organizations

Playing important roles in health programming in many areas are religious organizations. Interest is usually focused on health care in a given locality for a special population group, such as those located in a rural mountain community where there are inadequate resources to meet certain health or other personal needs. Religious organizations have also been active in meeting the social needs of the poor living in inner-city locations. To help inner-city teenagers cope with problems of substance abuse, some churches have established drug counseling and rehabilitation programs. In Washington, D.C., with the support of Ford Foundation funds, one church has operated a community service center. This center was established to help young African-American males enhance their health, education, and self-esteem.

In the African-American community, churches have been used effectively for health intervention programs.[10] Such initiatives have been successful because the church and the clergy often play a leadership role within the African-American community.

In some instances health promotion activities are conducted within the religious facility. The health departments and religious institutions act as partners. Some churches have health outreach programs as part of their ongoing activities. For example, hypertension is a particularly serious problem among African-American children, and the church has been shown to be a useful location where information regarding this problem can be given and blood pressure measured.[11] Other services such as cancer screenings may also be carried out. Health fairs have been held in some churches.

The Ford Foundation has provided grants to church organizations to prepare materials on teen pregnancy, sex education, and family values. Youth conferences focusing on these matters have also been conducted.

Many relief efforts are designed, administered, and carried out by religious organizations. In situations where a natural catastrophe has occurred, the personnel and services of these organizations move into the area and provide needed medical assistance.

Throughout the United States many hospitals, nursing homes, and other health care institutions are operated by religious groups. The largest number are operated by the Roman Catholic Church. In addition, numerous protestant denominations and Jewish religious centers have developed and operate health care facilities.

The increased numbers of homeless individuals in the United States have led to a need for more shelter and food sources. Many religious organizations have "soup kitchens" to feed the homeless. These facilities are often the only places where the homeless can come for food and for protection from inclement weather.

Several religious agencies have also been involved in helping refugees relocate to the United States. Usually sponsors—individuals or interested church groups—are found to assist the family upon their arrival in this country.

Many more religion-sponsored programs in the health sector are carried out in countries other than the United States. Health care provision has been a major goal of missionary agencies. The health clinic, nurse, and

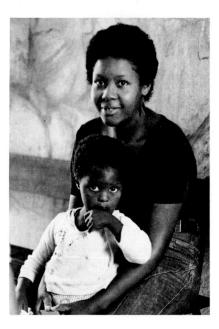

In communities throughout North Carolina, a project to improve the health of southern African-Americans is being headed by the General Baptist State Convention of North Carolina, Inc. (GBSC), with support from the W. K. Kellogg Foundation. With the help of the medical profession, the GBSC is training pastors and lay leaders in churches throughout the state to convey vital health information to their congregations.

medical missionary provide health care to many people, particularly in the Third World. In recent years such agencies have become involved in coordinating rural community development projects, including health care, preventive health, and agriculture.

With the increased interest in health promotion in the United States, churches, mosques, synagogues, and other religious facilities provide strong potential as sites for health promotion activities.[12] Several reasons can be given for the effectiveness of churches in promoting health:

1. Religious organizations are found in nearly every community.

2. Religious organizations are able to draw on volunteers to carry out their program activities.

3. Religious organizations can have an influence on whole families.

4. Religious organizations usually own facilities that have space for use in health programming.[13]

Summary

The private sector plays an important role in community health. Three private sector groups are involved in the health field: (1) voluntary health organizations, (2) private philanthropic foundations, and (3) religious organizations.

Though voluntary health organizations differ in emphasis, size, and organizational structure, there are some similarities between them. All are funded by nongovernmental sources. They are administered by a board of directors with a professional staff that conducts the day-to-day activities of the agency. In addition, volunteer workers carry out professional services, supportive services, and fund-raising activities.

The activities of most voluntary health organizations include provision of health services, support for research, both general public and professional educational programs, and service as a lobby agent in the legislative process. Fund-raising efforts include media coverage, athletic events, charity performances, and community fund-raising campaigns.

A number of philanthropic foundations provide funding for the planning and development of health care projects. Support is usually allocated for services to people residing in medically underserved localities. Biomedical research and both medical professional and general community health education programs also receive support.

Though not nearly as extensive nor as well known, various religious organizations play an important role in community health programming. Activities include operating health care facilities such as hospitals and nursing homes, assisting in relief and disaster efforts, and organizing refugee placement in the United States.

Discussion Questions

1. Discuss the role that the private sector plays in community health programming in the United States.

2. In what ways do voluntary health organizations differ from official governmental health organizations?

3. Identify the ways in which the program priorities of voluntary health organizations have changed through the years.

4. What types of health services are provided by the various voluntary health organizations?

5. Identify the advances in medicine and health care made by private sector-funded research through the years.

6. Discuss the differences and similarities in programming between three voluntary health organizations.

7. What is the Great American Smokeout?

8. What are some educational initiatives that are carried out by voluntary health organizations?

9. In what ways do voluntary agencies work with the legislature in health-related legislation?

10. How are funds raised to support voluntary health organizations?

11. Explain the characteristics of the five different types of philanthropic foundations.

12. Identify three different foundations with specific interest in health programming.

13. What are some of the differences between a voluntary health organization and a philanthropic foundation?

14. Discuss the different ways in which the philanthropic foundations interested in health have become involved in primary health care.

15. What roles in community health programming do religious agencies play in your community?

16. Why are religious organizations often effective in providing primary health care?

17. How do religious organizations and the philanthropic foundations work together to improve the health of certain population groups in our communities?

Suggested Readings

The annual reports of voluntary health organizations are useful in providing information on the specific organization. These annual reports can be obtained by writing the voluntary health organization.

The annual reports of philanthropic organizations provide current information about the program initiatives of each foundation. These annual reports can be obtained by writing the specific foundation.

One of the best sources of information about how to locate foundations with program interest in community health related concerns is: R. R. Rowker, *Annual Register of Grant Support: A Directory of Funding Sources,* 26th ed. (1993), Reed Publishing Company.

Other readings:

Bardack, Michelle A., and Susan H. Thompson. "Model Prenatal Program of Rush Medical College at St. Basil's Free People's Clinic, Chicago." *Public Health Reports* 108, no. 2 (March/April 1993): 161–65.

Department of Health and Human Services. *Churches as an Avenue to High Blood Pressure Control.* NIH Publication No. 92–2725 (May 1992): 97 pp.

Hatch, John, and Steve Derthick. "Empowering Black Churches for Health Promotion." *Health Values* 16, no. 5 (September/October 1992): 3–9.

Hatch, John. "Viewpoints: Promoting Black Health." *Health Aims* 4, no. 1 (Spring 1988): 5.

Jackson, Anita Louise. "Operation Sunday School—Educating Caring Hearts to be Healthy Hearts." *Public Health Reports* 105, no. 1 (January/February 1990): 85–88.

Lasater, Thomas M., and others. "The Role of Churches in Disease Prevention Research Studies." *Public Health Reports* 101, no. 2 (March/April 1986): 125–31.

Shapes, Cecil G. "Review of the National Preventive Dentistry Demonstration Program." *American Journal of Public Health* 76, no. 4 (April 1986): 434–45.

Tobin, Sheldon S., and others. "Enhancing CMHC and Church Collaboration for the Elderly." *Community Mental Health Journal* 21, no. 1 (Spring 1985): 58–61.

Endnotes

1. Data in this section on research was provided by each specific agency's annual report.
2. R. R. Rowker. *Annual Register of Grant Support: A Directory of Funding Sources,* 26th ed. (1993): 2–5.
3. R. W. Lyman. "The President's Review" in *The President's Review and Annual Report, 1980.* New York: The Rockefeller Foundation, p. 24.
4. *Ibid.,* 71.
5. Information provided in correspondence with the Henry J. Kaiser Family Foundation, 525 Middleford Road, Menlo Park, California 94025.
6. Annual Report, Henry J. Kaiser Family Foundation, 1985.
7. *Robert Wood Johnson Foundation Annual Report, 1988.* Princeton, N.J., 1989.
8. W. K. Kellogg Foundation. *1990 Program Information and Guidelines.* Battle Creek, Mich., 1990.
9. Rowker, *Annual Register of Grant Support,* 84.
10. John Hatch. "Viewpoints: Promoting Black Health." *Health Aims* 4, no. 1 (Spring 1988): 5.
11. Jackson, Anita Louise. "Operation Sunday School—Educating Caring Hearts to be Healthy Hearts." *Public Health Reports* 105, no. 1 (January/February 1990): 85–88.
12. Lasater, Thomas M., and others. "The Role of Churches in Disease Prevention Research Studies." *Public Health Reports* 101, no. 2 (March/April 1986): 125–31.
13. *Ibid.,* 126.

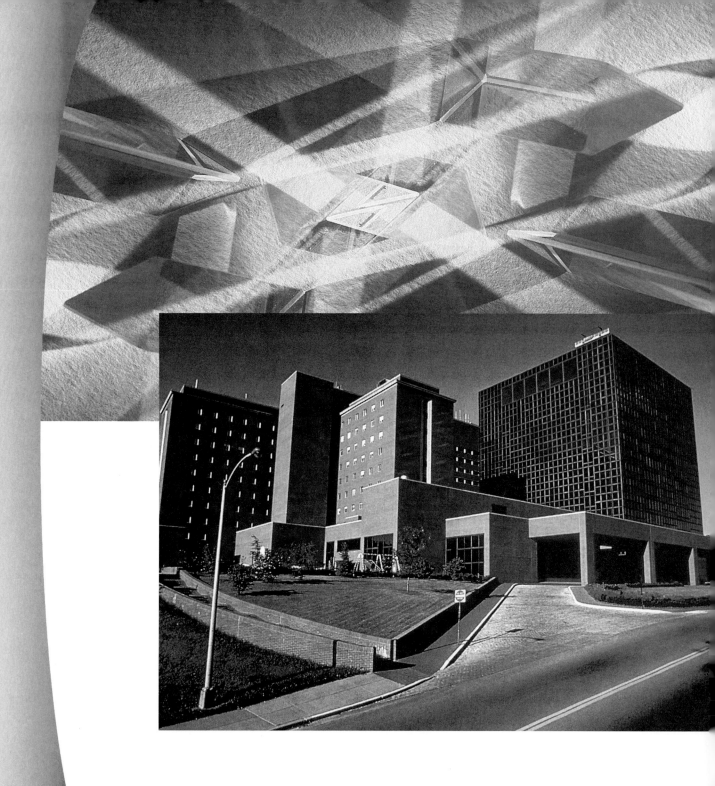

TWO

Health Care and Community Health

CHAPTER **SIX**

Health Care:
Socioeconomic Factors and Cost Containment

"Medical care, once seen as outside the realm of public health . . . is increasingly seen . . . as part of our fabric, integral to public health."[1]

Cost of Health Care

Skyrocketing costs, expensive medical technology, companies providing less health insurance for their employees, more and more people without the financial resources to pay for their health care! Health care costs in the United States are rising dramatically, and most individuals are affected in some way by this continuing problem. A visit to a physician's office with a minor problem such as a fever or rash may cost as much as fifty to seventy-five dollars. The cost of a hospital room in many communities approaches a thousand dollars a day, and the average hospital stay ranges from five to seven days. The bill for minor inpatient surgery followed by a couple of days of treatment and care may be over five thousand dollars.

Health care costs have continued to rise at twice the overall economic inflation rate during the early 1990s. Medical expenditures have soared in all areas of health care: hospital expenses, physicians' costs, and the cost of pharmaceuticals, rehabilitation services, and both inpatient and outpatient services. This steady, often dramatic, rise in health care costs is illustrated on the accompanying graph. National expenditures for health care in the United

National Health Expenditures

Date	Total (in billions)	Per Capita	Percent GNP
1970	74.4	346	7.3
1975	132.9	592	8.3
1980	250.1	1063	9.2
1985	422.6	1710	10.5
1990	666.2	2566	12.2
1995 (est)	800		

Source: U.S. Bureau of the Census. *Statistical Abstracts of the United States, 1992.* 112th ed. Washington, D.C.: 1992, p. 97.

108

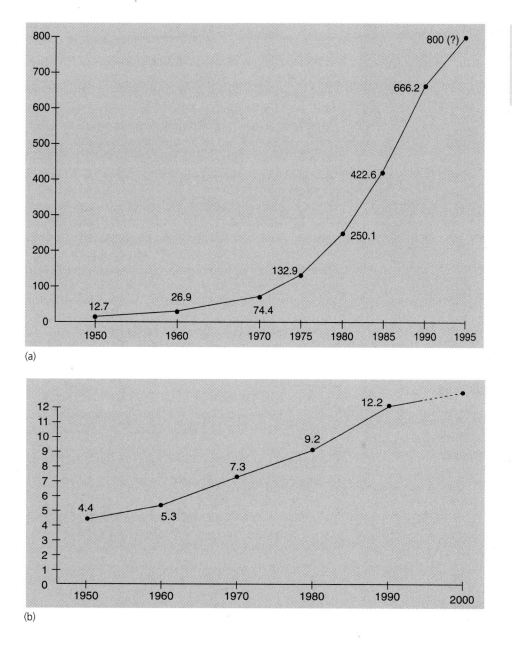

Figure 6.1 (a) National Health Expenditures, United States, in billions of dollars. (b) Health expenditures, United States, percent of GNP.

(a)

(b)

States have increased from a total of $12.7 billion in 1950 to over $800 billion by the mid-1990s. That amounts to nearly two billion dollars a day (see fig. 6.1).

Expressed in more personal terms, this sum equals a per capita outlay for health care of more than $2,500 per year. The percentage of the gross national product (GNP) spent on health care in the early 1990s was more than 12 percent, up from 4.4 percent in 1950.[2] Hospital costs account for 42 percent of the health care costs, the largest single expenditure. Another 29 percent pays for professional physician and dental services.[3] Projections suggest that by the year 2000 the cost of health care

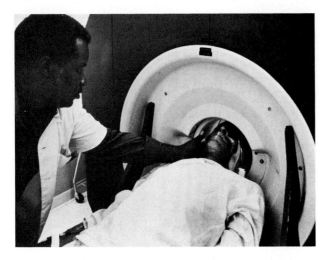

New technology has contributed to the increased cost of health care. For example, this computerized tomography (CT) scanning machine is an instrument that allows physicians to take a detailed visual slice, or tomograph, of the brain.

Legal problems in the medical field are another contributing factor. Very large settlements have been awarded in malpractice suits against health care providers. Thus, medical malpractice insurance premiums have greatly increased throughout recent years. Concern over the possibility of malpractice litigation has led most physicians to practice defensive medicine. This means authorizing more tests for patients than was the case in the past. Physicians want to be sure that the likelihood of charges of malpractice being leveled at their care is minimized.

The use of hospital emergency rooms for primary care by many economically disadvantaged individuals is another factor contributing to the increasing expenditures for health care. In some of these cases Medicaid has traditionally picked up the bill. In other instances the uninsured are provided care. Most people who go to emergency rooms for primary care do not receive primary preventive care services. This results in increased illness and disease, and thus health care costs are raised.

Another factor that has impacted the expenditures on health care in the 1990s has been the AIDS epidemic. Patient care is extremely expensive, and with increasing numbers of AIDS cases the expenditures have escalated.

These, and probably many more, factors have all played a part in the increasing health care costs in recent years. Until some workable solutions can be agreed upon, curtailing this very serious economic problem in American society is not going to be easy.

Cost Containment

Most individuals will agree that the rising costs of health care experienced in the United States since the end of World War II must be brought under control in some way. Unfortunately there is no simple solution to this problem.

There has been little reason in the past to control hospital costs, shorten hospital stays, or limit the use of technology. As long as people who are covered with adequate health insurance have had their costs paid for, and when much of the premiums have been paid for by employers, there has been little concern by most people. However, cost containment and shifts in public sentiment have become focuses of public policy. Increasingly the hospitals, physicians, and pharmaceutical companies

in the United States will exceed $1.5 trillion. This will mean an average per capita expenditure of $5,551, or 15 percent of the GNP.

Many reasons have been given for the continuing escalation of health care costs. Greater demand for high-tech medical equipment has been one contributing factor. No hospital wants to be without the most up-to-date, and expensive, equipment. Therefore, although it may not be economically efficient to buy these items, they are purchased in any case. Obviously these costs are passed along to patients using the facilities of the health care institution.

The U.S. population is becoming an older population. People are living longer and thus are using more health services. As one becomes older, there are more chronic health problems which usually demand longer and more expensive services.

Basic salary structures and resource costs have contributed to the overall rise in health care costs. For example, hospitals must employ many other workers besides those directly involved with patient care, including maintenance personnel and food service workers. Salary expectations of all these people continue to rise. The costs of energy, such as oil, gas, coal, and electricity, also have an impact on charges for health care recipients.

are finding themselves confronted with challenges to their payment systems by government, business, and industry, as well as the individual person.

How cost containment of health care can be achieved is a subject open to much political debate and discussion.[4] Anyone's answer depends a great deal on his or her political, economic, and social views, as mentioned in the first chapter of this text.[5] There will be no simple solution found that will have the support of every American. Yet many considerations have received attention. Two major ideas that have been tried in the past have been the implementation of nationwide comprehensive health planning and the encouragement of development of managed care delivery systems.

Health Planning

The need for comprehensive health planning has been advocated by many who have examined health care issues in the United States. The development of high-tech medical facilities for treating health problems has been an important contributor to the increase in health care costs. Besides being very costly, this technology is often underused and poorly distributed geographically within a locality. In many instances expensive health care facilities, equipment, and services are duplicated. On the other hand, health care services for the economically disadvantaged, the handicapped, those living in rural areas, and minorities are often inadequate. The basic purpose of health planning is to provide coordination at the local and state levels to correct these and other problems related to the distribution and provision of health care.

The original concept of health planning had its beginning in the 1920s.[6] At that time the New York Academy of Medicine issued a report stating that there was an adequate number of beds in New York hospitals. Other studies looked at other localities to determine the adequacy of hospitals to meet community needs.

The Hospital Survey and Construction Act, better known as the Hill-Burton Act, was passed by Congress in 1946. This legislation, while providing federal funds for local hospitals, also mandated the implementation of planning measures. Each state was required to survey its hospital facilities and to develop a state hospital plan. Before a state could receive federal funds for hospital construction, a survey of existing institutions and a construction plan had to be submitted to the appropriate federal agency.

Between 1946 and the 1960s, all states developed plans and determined hospital facility construction and renovation priorities. In 1954, the Hill-Burton program was expanded to include nursing homes, outpatient facilities, public health centers, rehabilitation services, and chronic disease facilities. Owing to this expansion, over twelve thousand health facility construction and modernization projects were funded by the Hill-Burton program. However, though some planning occurred, little effort was made to adhere to the Hill-Burton requirements. The activities of hospital facilities and other regional health care facilities were not being coordinated. Thus, the proliferation of health programs during this period only compounded problems.

Throughout the 1960s and the early 1970s several federal legislative attempts were made that were designed to require planning components before federal funds could be used for specific programming. For instance, the Regional Medical Program was established to create regional care centers for heart disease, cancer, and stroke patients. The Comprehensive Health Planning and Public Health Services Act provided federal funds for comprehensive health planning at the state and regional levels.

Despite these programs health planning was not considered successful by the early 1970s. In 1974 Congress passed the National Health Planning and Resource Development Act (P.L. 93-641). This legislation required that each state governor designate "health service areas." A planning system involving both regional and state health agencies was established. The local Health Systems Agency had to develop a regional plan. Also, the state health planning agency was required to develop a state plan that integrated the various health plans of the Health Systems Agencies within the state. The state plan then had to be submitted to the governor for approval.

These Health Systems Agencies had the responsibility to collect and analyze data concerning health care resources and programs in their regions. The data were reviewed and a health systems plan having long-range goals as well as specific annual implementation suggestions was written. The plan was to be approved at the state planning level. Through the process of review and comment, the Health Systems Agencies recommended the approval or denial of requests for federal funding applications.

By 1980 most Health Systems Agencies had developed plans that addressed the problems of cost containment, health promotion and prevention, and maternal and child health. However, political thinking changed during this time and, in the movement to reduce the control of federal government regulations, comprehensive health planning was greatly reduced by the mid-1980s. Whatever health planning that was to occur would have to be done by the individual states.

State regulatory programs of review and approval by health planning agencies of capital expenditures by hospitals and other health care facilities are known as *certificate of need* (CON) programs. Under certificate of need programming a health care facility cannot build a capital expenditure project without review and approval by the state planning agency. Individual states now determine to what degree they wish to be involved in health planning. They must determine what will be the functions of certificate of need programs, how they should be structured, and how and to what degree they will be funded.

Since the early 1980s eleven states have repealed CON laws. However, with increased concern about health care cost containment by the early 1990s, several of these states have taken measures to revive CON planning.[7] A majority of states still have certificate of need programs. This has led to a great diversity in programs. For example, in one state reviews are not required where capital expenditures will not substantially affect patient costs.[8] In some states review approval for purchase and operation of expensive medical equipment is not necessary unless the annual costs exceed a given sum of money. A few states have maintained effective state certificate of need review programs.

Managed Care Delivery Systems

A health care system that brings together the health care providers, health care facilities, and the insurers into an integrated system involving both the delivery and the financing mechanisms has been defined as managed care delivery.[9] Arrangements with providers within this system are to provide comprehensive health care to members. Management of the system is directed toward cost effectiveness. There are a variety of models of managed care delivery systems. The oldest type of managed care is the health maintenance organization (HMO).

There are two basic types of health maintenance organizations: (1) the individual practice association (IPA), and (2) the prepaid group practice. Another managed care delivery system is the preferred provider organization (PPO).

Health Maintenance Organizations (HMOs)

The basic concept of health maintenance organizations is that payment is made in advance on a fixed contract-fee base by a certain population. This payment is used to cover the costs of a comprehensive range of medical services including hospital visits, clinic care, and professional and technical personnel care. Usually there is a small out-of-pocket charge for each visit.

Health maintenance organizations are founded on several principles. An HMO is an organized system of health care. As such, a set of comprehensive services is available to a specifically identified population group. These individuals provide payment on a prepaid contractual basis. Enrollment in the HMO is voluntary. There are specified enrollment periods when a person can join, either as an individual, as a family, or as part of a group. If the HMO has group enrollment, the membership must also have alternative health care options. The employee is then free to select which plan she or he wishes to join. Some HMOs operate on a nonprofit basis, but most are investor-owned for-profit corporations.

The individual practice association (IPA) model is the result of an agreement among a number of independent physicians to treat patients who are enrolled in an HMO. The health maintenance organization then reimburses the physicians on a fee-for-service basis. Though the consumer prepays, the health care is provided by individual physicians in their private offices as in the traditional fee-for-service system. The HMO management organization markets the plan, collects premiums, and pays the bills.[10] Physicians that are part of an IPA work more independently than those in the group prepaid HMO model, and they continue to serve non-HMO patients as well.

In contrast, the physicians and other health care providers in the prepaid group practice HMOs are salaried. Their services are provided in facilities owned or leased by the health maintenance organization, not in their own individual offices. The providers not only provide the normal types of curative health care, but they are also encouraged through program incentives to keep the enrollees healthy.

Benefits of Enrollment

Why would a person select membership in an HMO? The individual enrolled in a health maintenance organization has a broad range of comprehensive health services available. With the comprehensive services provided, the consumer knows exactly where the particular care can be obtained. All records and control of the patient's care are housed in one organization.

Another benefit of belonging to an HMO is that health care is always available. Regardless of the time of day or the day of the week, a subscriber is guaranteed access to a health care system. This type of security is most valuable for those living in medically underserved locations.

The emphasis on prevention is another benefit of HMOs. In an effort to help control the costs of long-term chronic illnesses, various preventive measures are encouraged, and paid for, by HMOs. These include regular physical examinations of adults and the provision of prenatal and postnatal medical care and immunizations of infants and children.

Those who perceive a cost benefit will join HMOs. HMO costs are lower than those of more traditional health insurance programs. Health maintenance organizations have been shown to provide good care at 28 percent less than fee-for-service systems.[11] However, there does not seem to be evidence that the rise in health costs for HMO enrollees is any less than that found in overall medical care provision.[12]

Problems with HMOs

With the number of benefits that HMOs provide and the federal legislation that encourages their development, it is important to analyze why they have not become as widespread as had been forecast a decade or more ago. For many people the HMO seems impersonal. There often is no guarantee than an individual will be able to see the same physician with each visit. This is particularly the case in the group prepaid plan HMO. Hence there is less

Health Maintenance Organizations			
Date	Total	Group (GPP)	IPAs
1976	175	134	41
1980	236	139	97
1985	393	212	181
1991	556	208	348

Source: U.S. Bureau of the Census. *Statistical Abstracts of the United States: 1992.* 112th ed. Washington, D.C.: U.S. Government Printing Office, 1992, p. 106.

likelihood that a close physician-patient relationship can develop, though this is somewhat compensated for in the HMO-IPA model.

Health maintenance organizations tend to be very limited geographically. Whenever one is residing or traveling in areas other than their home locality and they do not have access to the health care providers within their HMO, problems can occur. Emergencies usually can be covered as long as the primary care provider is contacted and recommends emergency treatment. However, college students have had difficulties receiving care when away from their home community attending school. For example, a young man was in need of follow-up care for a fractured bone that occurred at college. The emergency care costs were covered by his family's HMO. When the physician in the community where the student was attending college recommended follow-up treatment, the HMO refused to cover those expenses unless he returned home and was treated by physicians enrolled in the HMO. This can present very difficult problems for individuals that are unable to return to their home areas when in need of health care.

The health maintenance organization concept has not been accepted by some of the medical profession. Some physicians will not work within this framework. They do not like being salaried nor practicing in the more structured format. It is their belief that their independence is reduced in the group prepaid HMO setting. These negative viewpoints are often overcome with the HMO-IPA model. Growth of the IPAs has led increasing numbers of physicians to participate in HMOs.

Another problem in HMO development has been the high start-up costs. This usually results in large financial deficits during the first few years of operation. These costs are rarely offset by the federal monies made available for HMO establishment. It has not been unusual for a new HMO to begin and a couple of years later to go out of business because of economic problems. This, obviously, does little to develop confidence in HMOs among consumers.

HMOs: Good or Bad?

What conclusions can be drawn about health maintenance organizations? Conceptually, they appear to be a positive alternative to the traditional fee-for-service provision of medical care. Politically, there has been governmental support for their development. But there has not been popular support.

A Louis Harris survey showed that most HMO members—91 percent—are satisfied with the health care received through a health maintenance organization.[13] This finding serves to indicate a positive view toward health maintenance organizations by those who have joined.

A major concern expressed about HMOs relates to the quality of care provided by health maintenance organization providers. Some people view the care received as being inferior to the fee-for-service approach. However, some studies have concluded that the quality of care received in HMOs is equal to that received through the conventional plans.[14]

The health maintenance organization approach to receiving health care is a different concept for millions of Americans. As with many things in our society, that which is new, different, and untried often is not readily received by the public. Whether there will be a continuing increase in this form of health care provision in the future remains to be seen.

Preferred Provider Organizations (PPOs)

The basic concept of the preferred provider organization (PPO) is rather simple. A self-insured employer, an independent insurance company, or a public organization negotiates a low fee-for-service with selected hospitals and health care providers in a specific area.

Group insurance costs are reduced in exchange for a guaranteed pool of patients. The fee schedule negotiated between providers and consumers is an attempt to create a uniform price for services delivered. Employers looking for an overall cost savings can channel a significant number of employees to cost-effective hospitals and physicians. The competitive price for services is possible because the provider charges are discounted by as much as 20 percent.[15]

When employees (consumers) use the PPO facilities and providers, they have 100 percent coverage with no deductibles or coinsurance to be paid. Should the individual select a hospital or physician that is not on the PPO list, they pay all or part of these costs.

The only way participating consumers and providers are bound together is through the negotiated fee. The consumers are not required to go to a PPO participant, and each service is handled separately. The consumer retains the right to return to regular insurance coverage at any time.

The first PPOs established in the early 1970s were designed for hospital employees. Since then they have expanded and developed in various ways throughout the country. There are several common characteristics of PPOs. There is a limited grouping of hospitals and physicians who agree to provide services for specified negotiated discounted fees. For the consumer, there are no co-payments or deductible costs if they receive health care services through the listed providers. A major attraction for hospitals and physicians is the rapid payment of PPO claims. The efficient claims processing of a PPO has made for low administrative costs.

All PPOs have some type of utilization review system. The mechanisms vary, with some having physician peer review and others having instituted preadmission certification and concurrent ongoing review. Utilization review provides assurance that care has been rendered in an effective and cost-efficient manner. Proper use of hospital services can result in long-term cost savings.

Into the early 1990s PPOs have continued to increase in growth. There are nearly eight hundred reported PPOs with about 48 million people enrolled.[16] Whether PPOs will increase in development in the years ahead will depend on several variables. Possibly the most important will be whether they will be an effective competitor in the reduction of health care costs. PPOs can be a major factor in health care planning of the future if the government includes some aspect in a national health program, if the corporate world becomes convinced of their cost-efficiency, and if the employees come to accept the concept of receiving services from PPO providers.

Poverty and Health Care

Within the American society the provision of health care has been geared to middle- and upper-class needs, values, and standards. However, there are many individuals with values, education, and health habits quite different from the "mainstream." This population group encompasses people of all ages, races, cultural groups, and both sexes. These are the economically disadvantaged, the poor. The nature of poverty and its effects on our nation's health must be understood. Only as such understanding takes place will effective programming for these groups result.

Much has been said and written about the relationship between poverty and the status of health and well-being in the United States. The poverty level, as established by the United States government, varies depending on such factors as family size, sex and age of family head, number of children under the age of eighteen, and location of residence. It was developed by the Social Security Administration in 1964 and revised in 1969. By the mid-1990s, for example, the poverty level for a family of four was $13,359.[17] It is estimated that more than 14 percent of the American population are living in poverty.

It is well known that the poor in this country usually do not experience the same level of health as do those individuals who have the financial means to receive proper health care. The problem is more than an inability to afford the cost of health care. The poor person tends to feel less at ease in medical care settings than does the more affluent individual. The poor, as a group, usually have less understanding of how the medical system operates and are less likely to seek treatment or preventive care.

As a result of this discomfort, the poor tend to make less use of health facilities. They seek the services of a physician less often than do those in the middle and upper classes. These individuals are much less likely to have available the services of a general, family practitioner to whom they can turn for minor health concerns.

In many areas where the economically disadvantaged reside, particularly in metropolitan areas, the primary source of health care is the emergency outpatient department of the city hospital or the public health department clinic. Not having a physician who can be contacted when there are health needs, the economically disadvantaged have no other place to turn. They often are thrust into the health care system at a time of urgent need, with little or no familiarity with the health care provider.

Vital statistics demonstrate the disparity in well-being between the economically disadvantaged and the middle and upper class in American society. Mortality rates for the poor are more than a third greater than those for the nonpoor. Birth rates are greater among the poor. Among the economically disadvantaged, infant mortality is twice that of the middle- and upper-class population. Maternal mortality is three times greater.[18]

Poor people are not usually oriented to the concepts of preventive health. Instead, these individuals tend to be crisis oriented. Too often the poor are reluctant to seek health care because of a feeling of not needing or being able to afford it. The person may deny that he or she is susceptible to a specific condition or may not even perceive the seriousness of the situation. When poor people become ill and need proper medical care, they are likely to try some home remedy, or to ask the advice of friends and relatives, rather than go to a doctor or a health clinic.

Health usually does not rank as a high-priority item among the poor. Instead, finding acceptable living conditions and employment have top priority. Only when health limits activities through debilitation or pain does health become a priority.

The child born in poverty is often handicapped from birth because the mother suffered from malnutrition or did not have proper prenatal care. A mother who has inadequate prenatal care is much more likely to give birth to a premature baby or a child with below average birthweight. Premature births are those in which the child at birth weighs less than 2,500 grams or five and one-half pounds.[19] These infants are more likely to experience serious health problems needing extensive medical care and treatment.

Children born in poverty are less likely to receive such preventive care as immunizations for the basic childhood diseases. They are also less likely to receive the recommended number of postnatal well child visits. The American Academy of Pediatrics recommends eight visits during the first two years and annual checkups afterward. This is not accomplished in a majority of cases of economically disadvantaged children.

Malnutrition is all too common among the poor. Two population groups are particularly affected by malnutrition: children and the aged. Studies have shown that the normal growth of children from low socioeconomic environments is often impaired by as much as six months to a year because of poor nutrition. This is of particular concern during the early years when normal brain development is affected. It is now believed that retardation may occur because of malnutrition during early childhood.

Closely related to problems of malnutrition is dental health. Tooth decay and periodontal disease are very common problems among children living in poverty. As many as two out of every three children living in poverty in the United States never see a dentist for preventive purposes.

The Medically Uninsured or Underinsured

A growing number of Americans do not have any kind of health insurance. It is estimated that as many as thirty-seven million people are uninsured. This accounts for approximately 17 percent, or one in six, of the U.S. population.[20] Many people, because of escalating health care costs and a lack of insurance, have little or no access to health care.

One may ask, who are these uninsured? Though the majority tend to be of lower socioeconomic status, most are not unemployed but work in low-salary, service-oriented jobs with no fringe benefits. A large proportion of minorities, particularly African-Americans and Hispanics, are included in this population.

As many as one-third of the uninsured are young adults in the nineteen-to-twenty-four-year age group.[21] These individuals are no longer covered by the health insurance of their parents. They tend to have entry-level, low-paying jobs where health insurance coverage is not provided by the employer. Many in this population group are not employed full-time. They may be working part-time while going to school.

Increasingly, businesses and industries are hiring personnel for the lower-paying jobs only on a part-time basis. These persons are not being provided with the fringe benefits of full-time employees. Many companies employ individuals on this basis in order to save money.

Small businesses, companies employing fewer than ten people, are less likely to provide health insurance for their workers. As many as one-third of the uninsured population are employed by small companies and industries. These companies often are not unionized, and employees have not organized to demand certain fringe benefits. People in the repair, entertainment, and personal service fields tend to be in this category.[22]

Individuals employed as seasonal agricultural workers usually do not have insurance coverage. Many are Hispanic and are continually moving with the agricultural season. Thus, they usually do not live in a specific location long enough to qualify for federal Medicaid insurance.

Many self-employed individuals do not have health insurance. Purchasing an individual insurance policy is more costly than a group plan. People who have started their own businesses often feel they cannot afford the high cost of personal health insurance coverage at a time when they are faced with many expenses involved in operating their businesses.

Where do the uninsured people go when in need of health care? They are most likely to receive health care in institutional settings. The hospital emergency room or outpatient clinic receives many of these individuals. Originally the hospital emergency room was conceived of as a place to treat trauma and acute health conditions. In recent years it has become more of an outpatient care facility and clinic for the economically disadvantaged and the uninsured.

This development has placed undue pressures on hospital emergency room facilities. It has meant that these facilities are often used for nonemergency treatment when they should be available for the emergency patients. In addition, hospitals have been faced with decisions about providing care to individuals who have no insurance. Though some hospitals have been willing to take "charity" cases, far too many deny care to the uninsured.

Homelessness

Causes of Homelessness

There have always been people who live on the streets, in parks, and in slum buildings of America's cities. The "tramp," the "wino," or the "bum" has been a part of the landscape of many urban communities since the founding of the nation. However, in recent years there has been an increasing number of homeless people. The homeless population has become younger, many having a history of psychiatric hospitalization. Whereas the homeless have traditionally been males, there is an increasing number of women and children and families found on the streets of our cities.

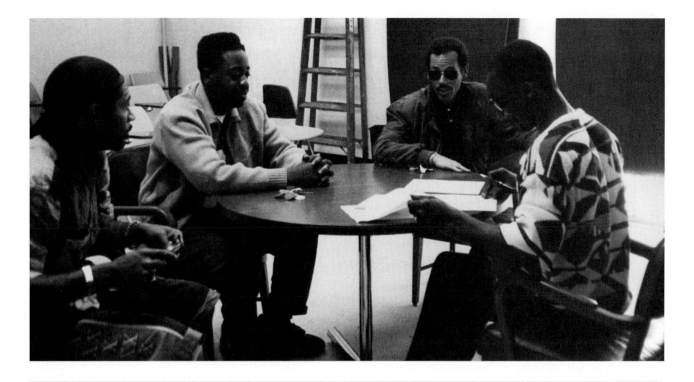

Many homeless centers provide various types of programming to help their clients overcome their problems. Some programs provide alcohol and drug rehabilitation, others are educational in nature, and some include occupational rehabilitation opportunities.

The number of such people has risen quite dramatically in recent years. It is difficult to define or to obtain an accurate count of the homeless in America today. The Department of Housing and Urban Development estimates the number to be between 250,000 and 350,000. Other estimates range as high as two to three million.[23]

The homeless tend to fall into one of three categories. (1) Some are individuals who have had recent economic setbacks. (2) Others are persons who have had severe personal crises. (3) A large number of the homeless are the chronically mentally ill.

In the early 1990s many people found themselves unemployed, often as a result of economic recession, plant closings, bankruptcies, and expanded high technology in the industrial world. Inability to find work or being released from employment after years of seniority with a company often causes extreme frustration. Anxiety and depression, manifested by various physical symptoms, are often seen among these individuals.[24] Those who are homeless because of economic problems increasingly are families, the fastest-growing segment of the homeless population.

Most families seeking shelter are headed by single women with young children. They have been evicted from their homes for failure to pay the increasing costs of rental and ownership. Their homelessness is often due to marital breakup, being without a job, and lack of public assistance. Low-cost housing in many cities has been demolished to make way for new business and residential developments; thus, hundreds of people have lost their homes. Migration to other locations in attempts to find employment has been another factor contributing to homelessness.

Deinstitutionalization has resulted in neglect of the chronically mentally ill. Many of the social welfare, housing, and other support system needs of these individuals have not been provided.

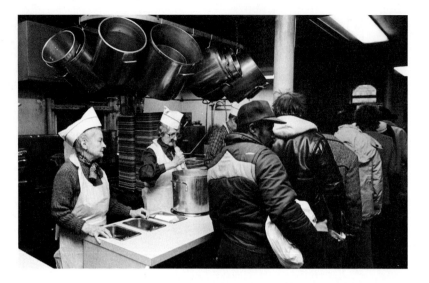

Numerous community agencies provide meals for the homeless. For most homeless individuals, this is the major source of nutrition they obtain each day.

The original concept of deinstitutionalization was that services would be made available outside of the mental health hospital and back in one's community. This concept in theory was good in that people would be cared for in community mental health centers. In reality this is not what has happened. During the early 1980s, funding cutbacks reduced community mental health services. Many communities are now without community mental health facilities and personnel. Needed ambulatory care and adequate case management are not available in many localities.

As a result, thousands of the mentally ill have become homeless or are living in substandard conditions owing to the absence of follow-up, rehabilitative services and help from the community. They have shifted from one place to another with little help being available.

Runaway children compose another category of homeless individuals. There is a serious increase of adolescents now living on the streets of America's cities. These young people have numerous physical as well as emotional health problems. Many children run away from their homes because of physical and sexual abuse. Running away is their only alternative to an otherwise unbearable living condition. Substance abuse by parents and other adults in the home often causes circumstances which lead to the young person leaving. Sickness and school problems are other factors that result in children running away. In some circumstances young people are thrown out of the home and told not to return.

Health Problems

Numerous health problems are found among the homeless. Much untreated illness and disease is noted. Respiratory infections are much more common than among the nontransient population. Numerous skin problems and nerve disorders have been observed among the homeless.

Trauma is an all too prevalent occurrence among street people. Muggings, fights, and rape often occur, resulting in lacerations, skin injuries, fractures, and additional emotional distress.

A variety of different nutritional disorders are found among these individuals. Lack of money usually prohibits the purchasing of adequate nutritious meals. An increase in the risk of malnutrition is often noted. Many homeless people depend on shelters, fast-food restaurants, and garbage cans for their food. The nutritional quality is often low. Even though the food quality is adequate in many kitchens serving the homeless, there is a shortage of these facilities in many communities.

Hypothermia is another health problem found among the homeless. During cold winters in many large, urban communities the street people will often have no place to get out of the extremely cold temperatures and weather elements. Once they lie down to rest or sleep, they experience a reduction of body temperature which can lead to frostbite or freezing to death.

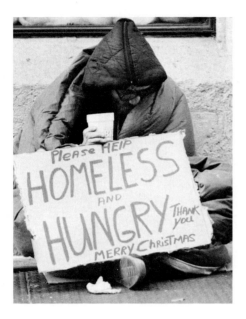

Alcohol use is common among the homeless. Whether alcohol is a cause of the problems that lead to one's homelessness or a result of the homelessness is a subject of debate and discussion. In all probability, it is a combination of both. Alcohol abuse affects most of the health problems of street people. It is a major cause of malnutrition. Drunkenness results in violent behavior and related trauma injuries. Alcohol abusers are prone to hyperthermia and hypothermia because perception of temperature changes becomes less acute, particularly among older individuals.

Substance abuse has been another important factor contributing to homelessness. Of particular importance has been the increased use of cocaine and amphetamines. The use of crack cocaine is seen as a major factor resulting in homelessness in many localities.

The homeless usually experience a lack of access to needed health care. Most have no health insurance. Without a permanent address it is difficult to obtain Medicaid coverage. People will usually go to a public hospital or a free clinic, or will not seek medical attention when needed. All too often they fail to seek care until the specific health problem is serious, painful, or debilitating. Medically speaking, the problem of establishing continuity of care is always a concern, owing to the transient nature of the homeless.

Many homeless rely on overcrowded emergency rooms of general community hospitals for whatever medical care they might seek. Some communities have established mobile medical units located throughout the area to help provide some care for these individuals.

As there are increasing numbers of children who are homeless, attention needs to be focused on their health conditions. Because they lack health care and good nutrition, these children experience poor weight gain and physical development, often accompanied by stomach disorders.[25] Many experience such chronic problems as asthma, ear infections, anemia, and lead poisoning. In addition, these children often have not been immunized and tend to develop communicable diseases.

Most homeless people experience severe stress, which results in emotional and psychological problems. When basic needs such as food, shelter, and health care are not available, depression, anxiety, and hopelessness often follow. Living in welfare hotels and various strange settings often traumatize the individual, resulting in stress. All too often the homeless do not have any social support to help them in meeting their needs. Loneliness and lack of close ties with family and friends lead to isolation.

Unfortunately, many runaway, homeless adolescents turn to prostitution. This often leads to a variety of sexually transmitted diseases. HIV/AIDS has been reported among this population group.

Services for the Homeless

Government, both local and federal, has not been particularly effective in assisting the homeless. Providing shelters has been the major focus of government efforts. In many communities private agencies, nonprofit and religious organizations, have been the principal source of shelter and food for the homeless. Many feel that the problem of homelessness will not be resolved until measures are taken to provide affordable housing for the poor and lower-middle class. In the meantime, the health care needs of the homeless must be met in an orderly and effective way.

The National Institute of Mental Health has established several areas of research to cope with the problems of homelessness.[26] Epidemiological studies are being conducted to reach agreement on a definition for homelessness, including the nature and extent of the homeless and how chronic mental illness results in homelessness. The National Institute of Mental Health is working with health professionals so they can effectively help the chronically mentally ill homeless person.

In 1987 the federal government passed legislation that provided funds to the states for community mental health services for the homeless.[27] These funds were to be administered through the Mental Health Services for the Homeless block-grant program. In order to be able to receive funding under this block-grant program, states must provide: (1) outreach services to the homeless, (2) referral for hospital and substance abuse services, (3) diagnosis, crisis intervention, and rehabilitation services, (4) training for outreach workers, and (5) supportive services in residential settings. Several community mental health services demonstration programs have been funded under provisions of this legislation. These programs provide comprehensive mental health services to homeless mentally ill adults and to severely emotionally disturbed children and adolescents.

Community Health Centers

A major public health program to improve access to medical care for the poor has been the establishment of community health centers. Primary health care for low-income families in both rural and urban settings is provided at these facilities. Two-thirds of the people served by community health centers are minorities.

In many urban communities, the major health care facility for low-income residents has been the local hospital. The hospital, however, is an inappropriate source of primary health care. The services available at the hospital clinic are treatment oriented and not preventive in nature. The development of community health centers has helped to reduce this reliance on hospital care.

The community health center delivers accessible, comprehensive, integrated, and family-oriented health care. The kinds of services available vary from one locality to another, but medical, pediatric, surgical, nutritional, and dental services are usually available.

The central location of community health centers helps overcome an important barrier to obtaining health care—travel. The proximity of the needed facilities encourages these residents to procure health care when needed.

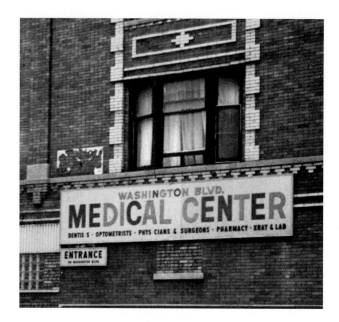

Many economically disadvantaged urban residents obtain their health care at neighborhood health centers.

It is important that community residents understand what services are available and the procedures for obtaining them, so that minor hospitalizations can be avoided. Many citizens often are not aware of the services available, so they continue to use the more expensive outpatient department of the local hospital. They do not know that quality care can be provided at another location. It has been difficult to encourage people to turn from the traditional health care facility—the hospital—to a different type of health care facility, even though it can be shown that effective service is provided at the community health center.

There are 347 community health centers providing care at about 1,400 sites throughout the nation. More than half of these centers are located in nonmetropolitan areas. In 1990 about six million people received care in these facilities. Funding for the centers relies on federal money and patient fees. Federal support of community health centers is provided through the block-grant program. As a result, states are increasingly having to operate and provide matching funds for these centers. Increasing financial pressures on state governments leave the future operation level of community health centers in question.

Summary

The cost of health care in the United States has risen consistently throughout the 1980s and 1990s. More than 12 percent of the GNP is spent on health care. It is estimated that unless major changes occur these costs will continue to escalate in the years ahead.

Much has been said about taking measures to contain the costs of health care. Various procedures, programs, and activities have been developed with cost containment in mind. One program with this goal in mind has been comprehensive regional health planning. At present the responsibility for health planning rests with specific state governments.

Expansion of managed health care systems has been another attempt to reduce the costs of health care. Expansion and development of health maintenance organizations (HMOs) and preferred provider organizations (PPOs) have occurred with cost containment in mind. Two types of HMOs, the group prepaid model and the individual practice association (IPA), have expanded in recent years. The HMO is an organized system with an identified population of enrollees receiving comprehensive health care from salaried health providers. The PPO is another organized approach to health care involving the provision of health services at a prearranged reduced cost.

The high cost of health care is a particular burden to the economically disadvantaged. This population usually does not experience as high a level of well-being as does the general population. This lower level of health is evidenced by malnutrition, increased respiratory disease, and an overall lack of physical and emotional wellness. Because their limited financial resources are not spent on health unless it is absolutely necessary, health promotion and disease prevention measures are not particularly important to the poor, so illness and other medical problems are usually in the advanced stages by the time treatment is sought.

The poor often do not have access to needed health care facilities and services. For many, the emergency outpatient department of the hospital or the health clinic of the public health department is the entry point to the health care system.

A number of factors have contributed to an increase in homelessness in the United States. Unemployment, economic setbacks, personal crises, and deinstitutionalization of the mentally ill have been major contributing factors. All population groups are included in the homeless category. Many are single parent families and their young children. Often shelter, food, health care, and other social services to assist the homeless are lacking in many communities.

Discussion Questions

1. Discuss some of the factors that have contributed to the continuing rise in the cost of health care.

2. What are some of the factors that have contributed to the fact that a large segment of the U.S. population is without health care insurance coverage?

3. Explain what is meant by managed health care.

4. Identify the similarities and differences between the two different basic kinds of health maintenance organizations.

5. Explain some of the problems associated with belonging to a health maintenance organization.

6. Would you join an HMO for your primary source of health care? Discuss the reasons for your answer.

7. Explain how preferred provider organizations (PPOs) might make a contribution to containing health care costs.

8. Discuss some of the relationships observed between poverty and the status of health and well-being of a population group.

9. Why do the poor tend to make less use of health care facilities than do the middle and upper class?

10. Explain why health is not a high priority among the poor.

11. Identify some of the factors that have contributed to the increase in the numbers of homeless individuals.

12. In what ways has deinstitutionalization had an impact on the problems of homelessness?

13. What are some of the health problems associated with the homeless?

14. Present several ideas that you would recommend for resolving the problem of homelessness in the United States.

15. What were principal features of the 1987 federal legislation designed to help states with the problems of homelessness?

16. How do community health centers meet the health needs of low-income families?

Suggested Readings

Axelson, L., and others. "The Changing Character of Homelessness in the U.S." *Family Relations* 37, no. 4 (October 1988): 124–28.

Bowdler, J. Ensign. "Health Problems of the Homeless in America." *The Nurse Practitioner* 14, no. 7 (July 1989): 44–51.

Drake, Mary Anne. "The Nutritional Status and Dietary Adequacy of Single Homeless Women and Their Children in Shelters." *Public Health Reports* 107, no. 3 (May/June 1992): 312–19.

Harris, Louis, and Associates, Inc. *A Report Card on Health Maintenance Organizations: 1980–1984.* Conducted for the Henry J. Kaiser Family Foundation, study no. 844003, 1984.

Hutchins, Vince, and Charlotte Walch. "Meeting Minority Health Needs through Special MCH Projects." *Public Health Reports* 104, no. 6 (November/December 1989): 621–26.

Kinchen, Kraig, and James D. Wright. "Hypertension Management in Health Care for the Homeless Clinics: Results from a Survey." *American Journal of Public Health* 81, no. 9 (September 1991): 1163–65.

Leshner, Alan I. "A National Agenda for Helping Homeless Mentally Ill People." *Public Health Reports* 107, no. 3 (May/June 1992): 352–55.

Morganthau, Tom, and Andrew Murr. "Inside the World of an HMO." *Newsweek* (April 5, 1993): 34–40.

Sherman, Deborah J. "The Neglected Health Care Needs of Street Youth." *Public Health Reports* 102, no. 4 (1992): 433–40.

Stroetzel, Donald, and Diana Stroetzel. "HMOs: What You Need to Know." *American Health* 12, no. 5 (June 1993): 77–81.

Winkleby, Marilyn A, and others. "The Medical Origins of Homelessness." *American Journal of Public Health* 82, no. 10 (October 1992): 1394–98.

Endnotes

1. Sidel, Victor W. 1985 Presidential address of the American Public Health Association, November 18, 1985, Washington, D.C. Reported in the *American Journal of Public Health* 76, no. 4 (April 1986): 373.

2. United States Department of Commerce, Bureau of the Census. *Statistical Abstracts of the United States, 1992,* 112th ed. Washington, D.C.: U.S. Government Printing Office (1992): 97.

3. *Ibid.,* 98.

4. This topic is discussed in chapter 7.

5. See chapter 1 for a discussion of procompetitive debate regarding health care.

6. Braverman, Jordan. *Crisis in Health Care.* Washington, D.C.: Acropolis Books, 1980, p. 123.

7. "Certificate of Need: An Idea Whose Time Has Come—Again?" *State Health News,* November 30, 1992.

8. Simpson, James B. "State Certificate-of-Need Programs: The Current Status." *American Journal of Public Health* 75, no. 10 (October 1985): 1126.

9. Health Insurance Association of America. *Source Book of Health Insurance Data, 1991,* p. 18.

10. Harris, Louis, and Associates, Inc. *A Report Card on Health Maintenance Organizations: 1980–1984.* Conducted for the Henry J. Kaiser Foundation, study no. 844003 (1984): 6.

11. Manning, W. G., and others. "A Controlled Trial of a Prepaid Group Practice on Use of Services." *New England Journal of Medicine* 310 (1984): 1505–11.

12. Luft, Harold S. "Assessing the Evidence on HMO Performance." *Milbank Memorial Fund Quarterly, Health and Society* 58, no. 4 (1980): 508.

13. Harris, Louis, and Associates, Inc., *Report Card on HMOs.* 142.

14. Wolinsky, Fredric D. "The Performance of Health Maintenance Organizations: An Analytic Review." *Milbank Memorial Fund Quarterly, Health and Society* 58, no. 4 (1980): 544.

15. Ellwein, Linda, and David D. Gregg. "Interstudy Researchers Trace Progress of PPOs." *FAH Review* (July/August 1982): 20.

16. United States Department of Commerce, Bureau of the Census. *Statistical Abstracts of the United States, 1992,* 112th ed. Washington, D.C.: U.S. Government Printing Office.

17. *Ibid.,* 456–57.

18. Rudov, M. H., and N. Santangelo. *Health Status of Minorities and Low-Income Groups.* Washington, D.C.: U.S. Government Printing Office, 1979, p. 6.

19. These topics are discussed in chapter 18.

20. Short, Pamela Farley, Alan Monheit, and Karen Beauregard. *Uninsured Americans: A 1987 Profile.* Rockville, Md.: National Center for Health Services Research and Health Care Technology Assessment (1988).

21. *Ibid.*

22. *Ibid.*

23. Frazier, Shervert H. "Responding to the Needs of the Homeless Mentally Ill." *Public Health Reports* 100, no. 5 (September/October 1985): 462–69.

24. Linn, Margaret W., and others. "Effects of Unemployment on Mental and Physical Health." *American Journal of Public Health* 75, no. 5 (May 1985): 502–6.

25. Axelson, L., and others. "The Changing Character of Homelessness in the United States." *Family Relations* 37, no. 4 (October 1988): 124–28.

26. National Institute of Mental Health. *National Leadership Workshop on the Homeless Mentally Ill: Proceedings of the Workshop.* Rockville, Md.: National Institute of Mental Health, 1985.

27. P.L. 100-77, Homeless Assistance Act, 1987.

CHAPTER **SEVEN**

Health Care
What Kind of Payment Program? And Who Pays?

Fee-For-Service Concept

In purchasing almost any commodity an individual will pay for the item upon making the choice of which item he or she wishes to purchase. This is a very basic concept regardless of what economic principles are central to a society. Everyone expects to have to pay something when buying a product or when receiving services provided by another person.

This concept when applied to the provision of health care services is known as fee-for-service. The concept is very simple: When in need of the services of a health care provider, whether it be a physician, dentist, pharmacist, hospital, clinic, or other, an individual receives the care needed. In return the person is billed for the services received. In theory, the amount charged is based to a great degree on the economic principle of supply and demand.

Fee-for-service has historically been the principle way that people have been charged and in turn have paid for their health care. Problems with fee-for-service arise when one begins to consider whether the provision of health care is the same as purchasing commodities, such as automobiles, clothes, groceries, and other domestic items.

It is the belief of many that health care should not be considered the same as buying things (commodities). Health care is considered to be something necessary when one is sick or debilitated. Economic inability to pay should not be a limiting factor to an individual being able to obtain that which is necessary. In other words, do all people have a right to adequate health care regardless of the ability to pay? This question has been central to many discussions and differences of opinion as to whether fee-for-service is appropriate as it relates to the economics of obtaining health care services.

Unfortunately, for many people it becomes difficult, if not impossible, to pay out-of-pocket for health care costs. This is particularly true when the required care becomes long-term, necessitating expensive medical procedures or for those people who are economically disadvantaged.

Third-Party Payment

If an individual were forced to pay out-of-pocket for all health care costs, some would become bankrupt and many would find it impossible to seek and obtain needed care. Most Americans do not have the cash on hand to cover the cost of necessary health care. Because of this, the role of a third party, or health insurance carrier, takes on major significance in the lives of most Americans.

Of all Americans, 83 percent have some type of hospital or medical health insurance coverage.[1] Despite this figure, less than three-quarters of all health care costs are covered by third-party payment. This is because many people do not carry major medical insurance which covers long-term, chronic illnesses. Also, most insurance policies have deductibles, copayments, and upper limits. In all these situations, people who think their medical expenses are covered discover they must pay from their own financial resources for these noncovered provisions.

More than eight hundred private insurance companies in the United States have health insurance programs, with the largest being the Blue Cross/Blue Shield Plan. They offer many different options to the individual. Some companies are involved only in health insurance, whereas others offer comprehensive coverage—life, auto, and house insurance, in addition to health coverage. Many people obtain health insurance coverage as part of a group plan. These are usually a part of the wage and benefit packages provided by employers. Premiums for the health insurance coverage are paid by both the employer and the employee. Other people must purchase health insurance on an individual basis. This is often necessary when one is self-employed or when a group program is not available. There are also health insurance programs that combine group coverage with individual coverage.

The first *accident* insurance plans in the United States were established in the 1850s and 1860s. The first *group health* insurance policy was offered by the Montgomery Ward Company in 1910.[2] Other types of individual, prepaid, hospital benefit plans were established in the 1920s. In 1929 a hospital prepayment plan was started to help public school teachers pay for their health bills at Baylor University Medical Center. The cost for each enrollee was fifty cents per month. This provided payment of six dollars per day for twenty-one days of hospital care. This program was established at the beginning of the Great Depression, a time of high unemployment and the financial collapse of many economic institutions, and was the beginning of the present Blue Cross program.

Today there are hundreds of health insurance schemes available to the consumer. To make a knowledgeable decision about appropriate insurance coverage, the individual must understand something about health insurance programs and their specific provisions. Regardless of whether the health insurance is an individual or a group program, there are several kinds of coverage: hospital, room and board, surgical, physician, major medical, income disability, and dental.

Insurance covering the cost of hospital expenses, primarily room and board, is a necessity for most Americans. The type of hospital insurance coverage varies, depending on the services and other supplies the patient receives.

Hospitalization insurance is usually sold in combination with surgical insurance. Surgical insurance covers the cost of surgical procedures (including anesthesia) related to sickness or accident. Usually a schedule of surgical costs will indicate the maximum benefit for each specific type of operation.

Payment for physician services is covered by physician's expense insurance. This covers nonsurgical care that is provided in the hospital or the physician's office. Nonsurgical benefits also include such items as outpatient care and home care. Usually the policy indicates which benefits are covered and the maximum amount of payment provided.

Serious health problems needing expensive long-term care and resulting in large medical expenses can ruin the economic status of most Americans. Major medical insurance is designed to provide protection against such expenses. Maximum benefits are indicated, usually ranging from ten thousand dollars to unlimited coverage. Major medical insurance plans have some deductible provisions as well as coinsurance requirements. *Coinsurance* refers to a cost-sharing procedure whereby the individual pays a certain percentage of the total cost and the insurance carrier covers the remaining cost. For example, the patient may pay 20 percent of the costs, with the insurance company paying the remaining 80 percent. The coinsurance percentages vary from one policy and type of coverage to another.

S hould health insurance provide coverage for preventive measures such as mammogram screening?

All too often health insurance programs only cover curative medical expenses. This is true of most private insurance programs as well as Medicare and Medicaid. Payment is available only for treatment of sickness and injury and for hospitalization.

In the case of mammogram screening, it is known that regular screening of women after age forty-five could reduce death rates by more than 20 percent. Yet Medicare will only pay for a mammogram if it is ordered for specific medical reasons. In other words, the physician must find a lump in the breast and suspect cancer before Medicare will provide payment. It seems logical that health insurance programs, both private and public, should be encouraged to cover preventive screening for breast cancer as well as many other conditions.

Do you have coverage for preventive screenings under your health insurance program? If your answer is no, why haven't you made an issue of this matter?

Doesn't it seem logical, and cost efficient, for health insurance programs to focus more on preventive screening? Do you think that this will become the norm in the 1990s?

Serious illness often means that an individual is unable to work, creating grave economic consequences. Disability insurance, available on either a short-term or long-term basis, provides partial replacement of income lost as a result of accident or illness. Short-term coverage is available for a period of up to two years; long-term insurance extends beyond two years to a specified time.

Dental insurance provides coverage for most dental services, including oral examinations, extractions, oral surgery, root canal therapy, and orthodontics. Most dental insurance is provided as part of a group health insurance program.

Millions of individuals have inadequate health insurance. To reduce their rising costs of health insurance coverage, many companies have cut the amount and kinds of coverage available to their workers. In particular large corporations are now requiring their employees to pay a portion of their health care insurance. For example the automotive industry estimates that $900 to $1,000 of the cost of a motor vehicle results from the industry's annual expenditures for health care coverage. More than half of America's largest companies now require employees to pay some part of their premiums. Many people who previously had complete health insurance are now only partially covered for health costs.

Whereas in the past the family of the employee was usually covered by the company-provided health care plan, today limitations are being placed on this coverage.

For example, some now do not cover one's spouse if that person is employed full-time. The company feels that the spouse's employer should be responsible for paying for that individual's health care insurance.

One strategy many companies are using to shift health insurance costs onto the worker is requiring the employee to pay a greater share of the premiums. Other employers are providing less of the copayment share of the benefit.

Another tactic is to provide a selection of coverages to each employee. Workers can choose to reduce coverages for care that they might not need or wish to have provided. Because the copayment of the benefit premiums is rising, employees are faced with decisions about the extent of coverage that is appropriate. Unfortunately, the decision often rests on the amount of money employees feel they can afford to pay, not on a need that may occur some time in the future.

Federal Government Involvement

Historical Dimensions

In the United States, health insurance coverage has principally been a private enterprise activity. The federal government has not become involved in any type of comprehensive national health insurance for the general public. The first federally funded medical care for persons other than those in the military began in 1798 when the Marine

Hospital Service provided a compulsory national sickness insurance program for sick or disabled merchant seamen. The Marine Hospital Service later became the Public Health Service.

An early attempt to develop a government-funded health insurance system for a broader segment of the population was made by the American Association for Labor Legislation (AALL) in the first part of the twentieth century. It was then that workers' compensation laws were passed by the states, providing protection for work-related accidents and injuries. Subsequently, the AALL proposed the establishment of state insurance programs to cover the costs of non-work-related medical services. Opposition from the American Medical Association defeated such a proposal, and so little further action was taken at that time.

Not until the mid-1930s were other attempts made to introduce the concept of national health insurance. Opposition from the private insurance industry and from the organized medical and hospital professions again negated any effective governmental initiative. It was the feeling of private industry, particularly the insurance and hospital industries, that such action interfered with private enterprise. The medical profession considered any type of national health insurance to be "socialized medicine"—unacceptable in a free, democratic society.

Following World War II, President Harry S. Truman proposed the establishment of a national health insurance program to Congress. However, continued opposition by various groups through the 1950s and into the 1960s defeated several such federal legislative proposals.

It was not until the mid-1960s that the federal government instituted two medical health insurance programs, Medicare and Medicaid. These programs resulted from increased concern at that time for the social conditions of the economically disadvantaged and the elderly.

Medicare

After years of debate, in 1965 the United States Congress passed legislation establishing a federal health insurance program for the elderly (people aged sixty-five and over). The establishment of Medicare inaugurated the first government payments for health services to a segment of citizens other than federal government employees. The basic purpose of Medicare is to make quality health care available to the elderly. Senior citizens who are entitled to

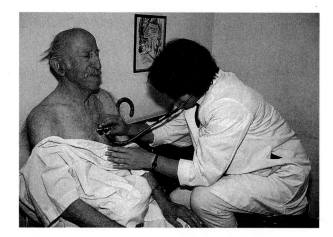

Skyrocketing health care costs are a concern for all Americans, but particularly for the elderly existing on fixed incomes. Often the elderly incur charges that require out-of-pocket expenditures since Medicare will not cover them.

Social Security or railroad retirement benefits are entitled to receive health insurance coverage under this program.

There are two parts to the Medicare program: *Part A* provides coverage of hospital expenses, and *Part B* provides medical insurance.

Medicare hospital insurance (Part A) covers four types of medically necessary care: inpatient hospital care, inpatient care in a skilled nursing facility following a hospital stay, home health care, and hospice care. The patient must pay a deductible, but Medicare covers all other costs for the first sixty days. This deductible is currently $652.[3] For the next thirty days of hospitalization (days 61–90) Medicare pays for all covered services except for a deductible of $163 per day.[4]

Medicare will pay for up to twenty-one consecutive days of full-time home care. These services must be ordered and reviewed by a physician. Two hundred and ten days of hospice care are provided for under Medicare.

The medical insurance (Part B) helps pay for the services provided by physicians, outpatient hospital services, outpatient physical therapy and speech pathology, home health care, and other health services and supplies. The medical insurance part of Medicare is voluntary. An individual chooses to have this coverage, and a monthly premium is deducted from the individual's Social Security check. After receiving any covered services, the beneficiary pays a deductible and 20 percent

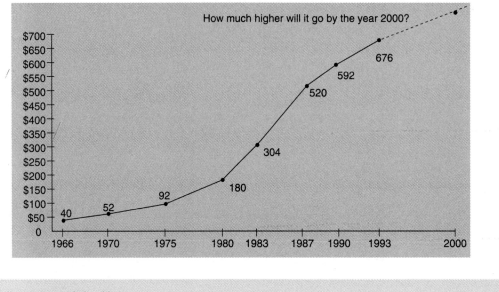

Figure 7.1 Medicare—Part A deductible.

of the remainder. Medicare pays the remaining 80 percent of the medical and surgical charges. Medicare also pays for prescription drugs that are administered while the patient is hospitalized.

Several health services are not covered by Part B of Medicare: routine physical examinations, eye examinations, eyeglasses, mammography screenings, and dental care.

Opinions concerning the effectiveness of the Medicare program differ. Without question, it has provided for the health care of many of America's elderly population. However, many problems have been noted by the opponents of Medicare. Since its inception in 1965, Medicare has contributed significantly to the inflationary rise in health care costs. In 1967, $4.5 billion in benefits was paid out. This amount continued to rise significantly so that by the mid-1990s more than $130 billion in benefits had been paid by Medicare.[5] It is estimated that this sum will double by the turn of the century.

The individual cost to the senior citizen for Medicare coverage has risen dramatically since 1965. The developers of Medicare established a deductible and co-payment provision for Part A and required a premium payment for Part B. When the program started, the monthly payment for Part B was $3 per month. By the early 1990s the premium cost had risen to $36.60 per month. The deductible portion of Part A has increased more than fifteenfold from $40 in the late 1960s when the program started to $676 in 1993 (see fig. 7.1).

These increases in deductibles and premium costs have meant that individuals must continue to pay more out of their savings or from other resources each year. On fixed retirement incomes, this presents serious problems for many.

In order to provide some protection for the elderly, a type of insurance referred to as Medigap policies, has been created by private insurance carriers. These policies are designed to supplement Medicare. They cover the expenses for deductibles and the first day of hospital stay. More than 35.5 million senior citizens are covered by such policies. In order to provide protection against fraudulent sales of Medigap policies, the Health Care Financing Administration oversees state regulation of these policies. By regulatory law any company selling a Medigap insurance policy must include a basic policy offering a "core package" of benefits. Also, the elderly cannot be denied Medigap insurance or charged higher premiums because of health problems.

Problems Associated with Medicare

There has been a lot of reported waste, fraud, and abuse of the Medicare system. Some health providers have abused the Medicare system by charging for services not rendered as well as for unnecessary surgical procedures. Another reported abuse is "gang" visits to nursing homes, where a number of patients not seen by the physician are billed for a visit. Also, some health care providers have referred their patients to long-term nursing care facilities in which they (the specific physician) have financial investment. This procedure was banned by government regulation in the early 1990s.

To combat some of the abuses, Congress passed the Medicare-Medicaid Anti-Fraud and Abuse Amendments in 1977. This legislation was designed to reduce health provider abuses. Legal penalties for defrauding the government in either the Medicare or Medicaid programs were imposed. Such abuse was considered a felony, with conviction subject to a maximum sentence of five years imprisonment, a twenty-five thousand dollar fine, or both.

Another problem with Medicare is that in some localities, physicians will not participate in the program. They refuse to accept Medicare patients. Thus, many senior citizens are unable to obtain needed health care.

Prospective Payment System

In 1983 an amendment to the Social Security Act changed the way Medicare reimbursed hospitals for their services. The basic purpose of this legislative action was to control the increasing costs of health care supported by the federal government through Medicare. The legislation requires hospitals to charge patients at a predetermined rate, which is based on the average cost of treating a particular diagnosis. Prior to this, payment was on a retrospective basis, determined by the bill at discharge. There was no economic incentive to contain costs. The health providers—hospitals and physicians—were reimbursed on a "reasonable" charge basis. They set the fees and Medicare paid the bill.

This prospective payment system provided for the establishment of *Diagnosis Related Groups*. A rather complicated formula is used to determine the reasonable costs for services offered at health care facilities. The DRG system was derived by taking all possible diagnoses and classifying them into twenty-three major diagnostic categories based on organ systems. These are further divided into 474 different illness categories that are referred to as diagnostic related groups, or DRGs. The DRGs are differentiated by age, principal diagnosis, types of procedures performed, secondary diagnosis, and discharge disposition.

Upon providing service to the patient, the hospital is paid a certain amount depending on the specific DRG, regardless of how long the individual must stay in the hospital. DRG cost allowances are predetermined based on the average cost for treating a given illness. If the patient is treated for less cost than the DRG allowance, the hospital will make money. On the other hand, if the expenses exceed the DRG cost allowance the hospital will lose money.

When a patient is admitted to the hospital the physician must give an admitting diagnosis. This diagnosis is a preliminary one. As diagnostic and therapeutic results are received, the physician revises the admitting diagnosis and makes a secondary diagnosis. A record of surgical procedures is entered, and when the patient is discharged the physician completes a discharge summary. At this point the physician indicates the principal and secondary diagnoses and all surgical procedures performed. Then by way of a coding system the number of the DRG and the preestablished rate are identified.

The Health Care Financing Administration establishes the payment rates for each DRG classification. A variety of factors goes into determining these rates. A specific DRG weight is multiplied by a standard payment amount. This sum is adjusted for the specific hospital wages in the locality, the percentage of low-income patients, and other factors.

This prospective payment system has raised many questions about its effect on the quality of care being rendered. Physicians are under pressure to maintain an average length of stay and to use an average number of ancillary services. If they exceed these amounts, they will need to modify their patterns of practice. Many believe that this system leads to the reduction of diagnostic testing and therapeutic strategies provided in an attempt to keep costs down.

Medicare requires external review organizations to monitor the financial incentives that could cause abuse and negatively affect the quality of care delivered. Federal legislation passed in 1982 created Professional Review

Organizations (PROs) for this purpose. The PROs review admission patterns to check for inappropriate admissions, look at records for unnecessary days and/or services provided, and verify DRG assignment for accuracy, use, and completeness of information. Penalties may be imposed if clinical information is found to be inaccurate or if other evidences of abuse are noted. The Health Care Financing Administration requires professional review organizations to deny payment to hospitals for medically unnecessary admissions and unnecessary procedures.

Medicaid

Title XIX (Title Nineteen) of the Social Security Act, known as Medicaid, became law in 1965. Medicaid provides health insurance for certain economically disadvantaged people in the United States. In order to be eligible for Medicaid benefits, an individual must be on welfare, have dependent children, or receive supplemental security income for the aged, blind, or disabled.

Medicaid does not provide medical assistance to all economically disadvantaged people. This program is administered by each state and is funded jointly with state and federal monies. The federal government establishes guidelines and regulations that must be met before funds are made available. The state determines the eligibility requirements for welfare program participation and, therefore, eligibility for Medicaid. States can set more restrictive standards than those recommended by the federal government. In 1988 Congress passed a law requiring states to cover pregnant women and children with incomes up to 100 percent of the poverty level under the Medicaid program. Some states vary their standard to as much as 185 percent.

The share that the federal government contributes to Medicaid ranges from 50 to 75 percent, based on a formula that considers the state's per capita income. If a state's per capita income is low, the federal contribution is greater than if it is high. State participation in the Medicaid program is optional.

A number of services must be provided before a state Medicaid program qualifies to receive federal money. An approved state plan must include inpatient and outpatient hospital services, laboratory and x-ray services, nursing services, home health care services, family planning, and physicians' services, as well as early and periodic screening, diagnosis, and treatment of children under twenty-one. Each state determines the scope of services covered by its Medicaid program. In some states there are no limitations on inpatient hospital coverage, whereas in others there are limitations such as length of hospital stay and days of coverage per year.

Payment for physician's services also varies. Some states limit physician visits to ten per month; another sets a limit of two per month; others set only certain conditions under which reimbursement can be made.

In addition to those that are federally mandated in a state Medicaid program, some states provide additional services. For example, podiatric services, chiropractic services, optometric services, physical therapy, and emergency hospital services are covered in some states but not in others.

Payment for services is made directly to the health provider under Medicaid. The provider must process all forms, submit them for reimbursement, and accept the reimbursement figure determined by Medicaid as payment in full.

The cost of the Medicaid program has risen significantly since its inception. In 1969, the cost was slightly over $4 billion. By the early 1990s more than $65 billion was being spent annually on Medicaid payments. The number of Medicaid recipients has slightly more than doubled in this same period of time, from about twelve million in 1969 to nearly twenty-five million at the present time.[6]

How effective has Medicaid been? There are a number of responses to this question. Many feel that Medicaid, though effective in providing health insurance to a segment of the American population not previously covered, has been too costly. This program, along with Medicare, has played a major role in the escalation of federal government spending for health in the past two decades. Some go so far as to suggest that Medicaid should be eliminated. These individuals consider it poorly managed and too costly. They contend that the federal government should get out of the health insurance business altogether.

Still others feel that Medicaid needs only to be reorganized to make it more efficient. As with Medicare, there have been many instances of fraud and abuse in the Medicaid program. Some health providers have filed for services that were never performed or have done multiple filing.

Federal Financial Outlays for Health in Billions of Dollars		
Date	Medicare	Medicaid
1967	$ 4.5	$ 3.4 (1968)
1970	$ 7.0	$ 4.8
1975	$ 15.5	$12.2
1980	$ 35.7	$23.3
1985	$ 70.5	$37.5
1990	$108.7	$64.8

Source: U.S. Department of Commerce, Bureau of the Census. *Statistical Abstracts of the United States, 1992*. 112th ed. Washington, D.C.: U.S. Government Printing Office, 1992, pp. 101 and 103.

Another major problem with Medicaid is the diversity in the programs and coverage from state to state. The states with the greatest percentage of the economically disadvantaged population have the least Medicaid coverage. The more industrial and wealthier states tend to have better Medicaid coverage, resulting in a disparity in state Medicaid programs. Much recent discussion has centered on the recommendation that national standards, rather than state, should be established.

Another negative aspect of Medicaid is that not all poor people are covered. Only about half of the people with incomes under the poverty line are included. Only those dependent upon public assistance are eligible, and since that decision is made by the state, many are not covered by Medicaid. All too often these are the same people that have no private health insurance. Measures should be taken to include all individuals with incomes below the poverty line.

The future of Medicaid continues to remain in question. An acceptable replacement system that would eliminate all the negative features of the present program is unknown at this time. A number of different ideas and proposals have been discussed.

Health Care Reform

Rising health care costs and the increasing numbers of people lacking some type of health insurance have led to a widespread examination of the health care system in the United States. Calls for change and reform have been issued from many throughout the nation. Organized labor in 1989 announced a campaign to work for development of a national health program. Business and industry have also expressed interest in some type of health care reform. Large corporations are concerned about the lack of controls on health care costs. The costs of health care benefits that corporations pay for employees have increased between 13 and 17 percent per year during the latter part of the 1980s and the early part of the 1990s. Health care benefits cost businesses an average of $3,105 per year per employee. Such costs are eating into wage increases and are having a serious impact upon company profits.

State governments have become very concerned about the rising costs of health care. Medicaid is the greatest health cost expense confronting the individual states. As a result, many states have passed legislation designed to improve access to health care for residents in their states and to implement measures to control costs, especially of Medicaid. Measures have also been examined to improve access to health care in rural areas, to fill in gaps in insurance coverage for citizens of the state, to provide universal health coverage for children, and to provide a basic benefit package for everyone in the state.

Concern over health care reform has increased at the federal government level. The national election in 1992 saw the election of a president committed in his campaign statements and in the party platform to creation of a national health reform program.

State Health Care Plans

Throughout the 1980s and into the 1990s state governments have been confronted with increasing financial demands for programs for their citizens. By the early 1990s many states were facing serious economic problems. Some states had incurred very high budget deficits. Others, unable by law to become involved in deficit spending, were forced to cut major programs. State, city, and local governments had to increase every type of tax to pay for the demands of an ever more costly society. Though health care was not the only factor causing these problems, it became a major concern. Of particular importance to state legislatures was the escalating cost of the Medicaid program.

As a result, several states passed comprehensive health care reform legislation in 1992. These programs were designed to improve access to health care for residents of the states. They also were legislated for the purpose of controlling costs, especially in Medicaid. More

Corporate Health Premiums

Some corporations are beginning to individualize the amount of health premiums they are willing to pay for each employee. Determination of the monthly premium the company is willing to pay is based on the personal life-style of the individual. For example, the company will pay more of the premium if an individual practices positive health behaviors, such as exercising regularly, controlling weight, and not smoking. The individual who smokes, is overweight, or does not exercise regularly is required to pay a greater portion of the monthly health premium.

This practice of basing the payment of premiums upon healthy life-style practices has been challenged by some on the grounds of fairness and invasion of privacy. Should employees be required to report their smoking, drinking, eating, and other personal habits to their employer? It has also been argued that workers with unhealthy habits are penalized in ways that do not relate to their ability to perform on the job.

Some companies have implemented reward-penalty systems. For example, one company reported that those employees with good fitness and healthy life-style patterns could save as much as $100 per month on their health insurance premiums. Do you believe this is discriminatory?

On the other hand, it must be asked if those who do practice healthy life-styles should be expected to help subsidize long-term illnesses such as cancer, chronic pulmonary respiratory diseases, and cardiovascular diseases. Many of these diseases result from negative health behaviors. Much of the 15 percent or more increase in health care costs results from care for such conditions.

than half of the states have entertained some type of health care reform legislation.

As various states implement individual state initiatives, a broad divergence of approaches and programs is seen from one state to another. For example, one state has instituted a program to establish pediatrics clinics throughout the state. These will be placed in public access areas. All children will be able to receive care. However, this will not be the case in other states. On the other hand, many states are not taking any action at this time. They are waiting to see what type of program will come from the federal government.

During 1992 the state legislatures of Minnesota, Florida, and Vermont passed health care reform laws. Each of these has a unique focus; however, all were implemented with the goal of doing a better job of getting health care to the people of the state. In each case the law provides for universal access to health care for all state residents.

The basic feature of the Minnesota program was to reform insurance practices within the state and finance a plan that would give health care access to everyone in the state at an affordable cost. This was considered to be particularly helpful to people with modest incomes who were not eligible for coverage under Medicaid. Subsidies for the uninsured would be provided for low-income families with children. Premiums are to be deducted from state income tax.

The state of Florida passed legislation designed to provide access for all Floridians to basic health care services by 1995. It required that health insurers must offer a basic health plan to employers who employ from three to twenty-five employees. Because of its large senior citizen population the legislation called for the establishment of standards for long-term care insurance and Medigap insurance coverage.

In Vermont legislation expanded Medicaid coverage for children within that state. A financial restructuring for health care was to be implemented with strict certificate of need and hospital budget reviews being mandated. It is hoped that these measures will result in more cost-effective health services to residents of the state.

A controversial proposal in Oregon would ration health care to certain economically disadvantaged people with long-term problems, so that health coverage could be provided to uninsured residents. The federal government, after initially rejecting this proposal, reversed itself in 1993 and permitted implementation of the proposal.

Massachusetts Health Security Act   In 1988 the state of Massachusetts passed the Health Security Act. This legislation was to have been implemented by 1992. It would have provided mandatory, employer-subsidized insurance for everyone. However, due to economic recession during this time, political conflict within the state, and lack of support by small businesses, the program has not been implemented.

Hawaii Health Care Plan   The state of Hawaii has had a statewide health care plan in place since 1974 which has drawn the attention and interest of many people concerned about national health care reform. In 1974 legislation was passed which requires most employers to provide health insurance for all employees who work at least twenty hours a week. Exempted from this requirement are seasonal farm workers and certain self-employed salespeople who work on a commission basis.

In 1989 a state insurance plan was implemented for the working poor and for individuals who are employed part-time. The state pays for participants in this program. About 20 percent of the population is covered by this program. All members of this plan are placed in the same insurance risk pool. No one is charged higher premiums because of age or illness.

Evidence suggests that this plan has been successful in providing health care coverage for most of the population. Also it is reported that emergency room visits are less frequent than in the nation as a whole. Also there are one-third fewer surgeries in the state than in the nation as a whole.

National Health Program

As early as 1912 Theodore Roosevelt ran on a platform calling for a system of social health insurance adapted to American use. Roosevelt lost, and the issue did not surface again for several decades. In 1945, following World War II, President Harry Truman presented a plan for universal health care coverage. This plan was blocked by many opponents who spoke of such governmental health initiatives as being socialistic, un-American, and communistic. The label "socialized medicine" used by the plan's opponents was enough to scare away many people.

Through the years various approaches for a national health program have been discussed. Generally speaking most of the suggestions that have been proposed for Congressional action follow one of three different models: the private market model, the employer-based model, and the government-based model.

Three Models

Under provisions of the *private market model* people would purchase health insurance either through their employer or by themselves. Upon receiving health care, the provider bills the individual, or the third-party insurance carrier. Those who are self-employed must purchase their own individual health insurance plan. These individuals would be able to receive tax deductions for the costs they incur for purchase of health insurance.

This model builds on the current health care system. Medicare and Medicaid would remain as they have operated for the past several years. Price controls would be assured through competition among the various insurance companies. Individuals would be expected to shop around for the insurance coverage offering the best rates and medical care coverage. Under this model there would be no long-term care coverage.

The *employer-based model* has been referred to as the "play or pay" model. Under this model everyone would be covered by health insurance which would be provided from either one's employer or a government insurance program. Each employer must provide health insurance for all workers or pay a tax to finance a government insurance pool. All businesses and industries would be required to provide a basic health insurance plan for each employee. Current private health insurance programs would be permitted to continue. This is the "play" component of this model. Small companies would be given tax breaks to help them afford to provide insurance for employees.

Government would create a public plan that would cover the unemployed and those individuals who are not provided with health insurance by their employers. A tax would be placed on employers who do not provide coverage for their employees that would provide coverage through the public plan. This is the "pay" component of this model. Taxation would provide funds to cover those individuals who are unemployed.

Generally preventive care is included by those who support this model, as is long-term care. No preexisting conditions would be prerequisite for inclusion in this program. Medicare would remain, but Medicaid would not be necessary and would be eliminated under provisions of this model.

The *government-based model* would guarantee access to health care for everyone through the provision of a national health insurance program. Under this model, government is the sole payer of all health services. Private health insurance plans would be eliminated, resulting in a lack of competition.

Under this system, preventive care and long-term care are provided for. Regardless of where one lives in the country or one's status of employment, she or he is covered. Individuals would have the option of choosing the health care provider they desire. A medical card would be presented upon entering the health care facility.

Funding for this program would come through government taxation. The government would control costs by setting strict payment rates for services rendered. Some proposals for national health insurance would require that individuals pay some level of premiums and that deductibles and copayment provisions be a part of the program.

Federal Government Legislative Proposals

Through the years more than thirty legislative proposals have been submitted in Congress for the establishment of a national health program. Each proposal has been a spin-off to some degree of one or more of the models just described. No proposal has received enough support to be seriously considered for passage as of the early 1990s. It would be impossible to present the features, supporters, detractors, and issues involved in each proposal submitted since World War II; however, several will be mentioned to show the range of positions that have been presented.

One proposal that would have resulted in major change in the health financing system was sponsored by Senator Edward Kennedy. Benefit coverage under this proposal would have been compulsory for all citizens and would have covered all health care services. Financing of this program, which would have carried no maximum limits, no deductibles, nor any coinsurance provisions, would have been by payroll taxes and general revenue monies. The program would have been administered by an agency of the federal government created by federal legislation. This proposal would have eliminated the need for private health insurance carriers.

Without question, this plan would have led to a major change in health care funding in the United States.

Also, the role of the federal government in the field of health care would have been greatly enlarged, leading to expanded governmental regulation and control. The cost of this program to the taxpayers would have been extensive. On the other hand, all citizens would have been able to obtain health care when needed. Cost would no longer be a limiting consideration. However, this proposal was opposed by the American Medical Association, the insurance industry, the business community, and most conservative economists and politicians.

Another proposal, which would have had a less radical effect on the health care system in the United States, was one sponsored by the American Medical Association. This plan would have used a system of tax credits to encourage the purchase of health insurance from current health insurance carriers. Medicare and Medicaid would have been reformed, tax credits would have been made available for small businesses that provide insurance to employees, risk pools would have been established for the uninsured, and catastrophic care coverage would have been included. The private health insurance system would have remained as it had been. The delivery of health care would not have changed.

Between these extremes there have been a number of other proposals. One proposal would have encouraged the establishment of health care corporations. The employer would be required to purchase a comprehensive health insurance plan for all employees and to pay at least 75 percent of the premium. If the employee joined a health care corporation, a federal subsidy of a specified percent would apply to the insurance premium. This proposal would have failed to meet the insurance needs of the economically disadvantaged and the unemployed.

Another proposal would have made use of tax incentives to encourage employers to buy health insurance for their employees. This did not—nor did any other proposal—receive widespread public, political, and economic acceptance.

Many people interested in changing the health care system of the United States have looked to the system that Canada has had in place for two decades. In 1989 a Louis Harris poll reported that a majority of Americans wanted a health plan similar to Canada's in which the government pays insurance costs out of taxes and sets all physician and hospital fees.[7] This desire for change extended across various segments of the population.

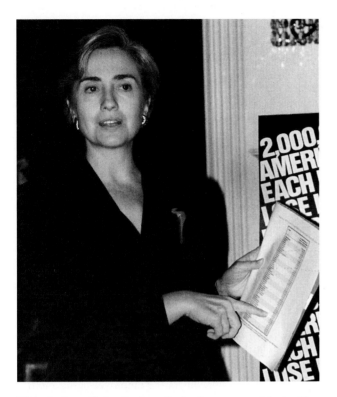

Hillary Rodham Clinton has been the leading proponent for health care reform. Her activities have taken her to numerous health care facilities and seen her involvement in many different committee settings in the attempt to "sell" a program of national health care reform.

The Canadian health insurance system provides coverage for all people, and it pays for all medically necessary services. Each province has its own insurance program, which must meet requirements and standards set by the federal government. The federal government negotiates fee schedules; extra charges on behalf of the health care facility or physician are prohibited.

The Clinton Plan

Upon being elected president of the United States in 1992 William J. Clinton announced that within the first several months of his new administration a national health care program proposal would be submitted to Congress and the nation. In a national speech to both houses of Congress the president outlined his Health Security Plan.[8] There were six basic principles that the president outlined in his proposal. First, everyone would be entitled to a standard package of benefits. In other words, there would be universal access for health care coverage for all Americans. No one would be excluded due to preexisting conditions. This comprehensive coverage would include prescription drugs. Second, measures would be taken to control health care costs. In order to accomplish this, limits on the amount that an insurance premium can be raised would be established. Also, competition in the health care field would be encouraged to keep prices from rising. Third, the president called for simplifying the paperwork involved in health care as a cost reducing function. To do this it was suggested that everyone will have a health security card and one single claim form would be developed. Fourth, employers would be required to provide coverage for all employees. Where necessary the federal government would subsidize small businesses. Fifth, the proposal called for an emphasis upon preventive care. In addition, incentives would be introduced to encourage health care providers to locate in medically underserved areas. There were proposals to permit all citizens a choice of the health care provider they wished to go to and a choice of health plan to join. Last, a health care reform program would be based on the concept of managed competition. The president concluded that health care was the responsibility of everyone, not just the government.

Managed competition has different meanings for different people. As used and supported by President Clinton it referred to "a purchasing strategy to obtain maximum value for money for employers and consumers."[9] Competition among health providers would be encouraged. In theory this would control costs. Under such a system government would regulate prices in various regions of the country.

Health networks would be established that would contract with hospitals, physicians, nursing homes, laboratories, and other providers of health care to provide services at fixed annual rates. These groups would be called Health Insurance Purchasing Cooperatives (HIPCs). Consumers would have a wide range of choices as to what doctors, hospitals, and other professionals they wish to have provide their health care. Cost-effective arrangements could be negotiated. Employers and individuals would negotiate with a range of health plans to obtain the best coverage possible considering one's health needs and economic status.

Among the many concerns about a national health care program is the question of its cost and how it is to be financed. The president said that the system could be funded by savings on Medicare and Medicaid, savings from federal employee health care costs, the introduction of certain taxes, and initiatives designed to reduce the rate of growth of the health industry.[10]

Months of study, discussion, and debate have revealed that there is little consensus as to what form the American health care system should take. Many different vested-interest groups have contributed to the problem of finding consensus. The answer awaits compromise, willingness to change, and a recognition that business as usual in health care is not possible.

Summary

Fee-for-service has been the basic way that health care services have been paid for upon receiving care from health care providers in the United States. Payment for health care costs by a third party (health insurance carrier) has increased since the early years of this century. Today many health expenses, including hospital, surgical, physician, major medical, income disability, and dental expenses are paid by some type of health insurance. The amount of coverage under each category, deductibles, and extent of copayment vary from one health insurance carrier to another.

Payment for health care in the United States has been a private enterprise activity, seldom involving governmental resources. However, since 1965 the U.S. government has funded two health insurance programs, Medicare and Medicaid. Medicare provides hospital insurance and medical coverage for the elderly, while Medicaid covers the cost of health care for certain economically disadvantaged people.

Increasing concern about the cost of health care and the inability of many Americans to obtain adequate health care has led to calls for health care reform. Many segments of the American population during the past decade have spoken out for change and governmental involvement in the health care system. Business and industry as well as labor have become concerned. Also state, local, and federal governmental initiatives have been designed to solve the nation's health care problems.

There have been attempts to introduce legislation that would create a national health insurance program for all citizens of the nation. Several models have been the basis of more than thirty proposals submitted to Congress during the past two decades. Some proposals support the private market model, others the employer-based model, and still others the government-based model. There has been much interest in a national health insurance system similar to that which has been in Canada since the 1970s.

The presidential election in 1992 focused much attention on the need for immediate action in health care reform. Whatever program becomes law will need to have cost containment strategies, allow universal access for all Americans, and be built to some degree on the concept of managed competition.

Discussion Questions

1. What is the meaning of fee-for-service when referring to health care costs?

2. Explain what is meant by third-party payment.

3. What are some of the differences between hospital insurance and major medical insurance?

4. What is Medicare?

5. What kinds of coverage are provided under Part A of Medicare? Part B?

6. Explain the purposes behind the development of Medigap insurance policies.

7. What is the significance of the prospective payment system?

8. What groups of people are covered by Medicaid?

9. Discuss some of the problems associated with Medicaid.

10. What are several reasons for concern about health care reform in the United States?

11. Explain some of the health care reform legislation passed in recent years by individual state governments.

12. Discuss some of the basic features of the Hawaii Health Care Plan.

13. Explain the differences between the three different models for a national health program.

14. What is meant by "play or pay" as it relates to development of a national health program?

15. What have been some of the differing positions regarding the development of a national health insurance program in the United States?

16. Upon what principles has the Canadian health insurance system been built?

17. Explain what is meant by managed competition.

18. What are the specific provisions included in the Clinton administration health proposal?

Suggested Readings

Angell, Marcia. "How Much Will Health Care Reform Cost?" *New England Journal of Medicine* 328, no. 24 (June 17, 1993): 1778–79.

Aswad, Charles N., and Mario V. Menghini. "Medical Society of the State of New York Universal Health Plan: A Proposal for Improving the United States Health Care System." *New York State Journal of Medicine* 92, no. 2 (February 1992): 45–48.

Brown, Barry. "How Canada's Health System Works." *Business and Health* 7, no. 7 (July 1989): 28–30.

Brown, E. Richard. "Access to Health Insurance in the United States." *Medical Care Review* 46, no. 4 (Winter 1989): 349–85.

Brown, E. Richard. "Principles for a National Health Program: A Framework for Analysis and Development." *The Milbank Quarterly* 66, no. 4 (1988): 573–617.

Clinton, Bill. "The Clinton Health Care Plan." *New England Journal of Medicine* 327, no. 11 (September 10, 1992): 804–7.

Coughlin, Kenneth M. "While Congress Debates, the States Legislate." *Business and Health* 10, no. 11 (1992): 24–30.

Dougherty, Charles J. "Ethical Perspectives on Prospective Payment." *Hastings Center Report* 19, no. 1 (January/February 1989): 5–11.

Enthoven, Alain C. "Commentary: Measuring the Candidates on Health Care." *New England Journal of Medicine* 327, no. 11 (September 10, 1992): 807–9.

Enthoven, Alain C. "The History and Principles of Managed Competition." *Health Affairs* 12, Supplement (1993): 24–48.

Guterman, Stuart, and others. "The First Three Years of Medicare Prospective Payment: An Overview." *Health Care Financing Review* 9, no. 3 (Spring 1988): 67–77.

Hagen, Ron. "Medigap Insurance: Pitfalls and Progress." *Business and Health* 3, no. 5 (April 1986): 25–30.

Johnsson, Julie. "Managed Health Care in the 1990s: Providers' New Role for Innovative Health Delivery." *Hospitals* (March 20, 1992): 26–30.

Johnsson, Julie. "State Health Reform." *Hospitals* (October 5, 1992): 26–28.

Jordahl, Gregory. "Oregon Continues to Push Its Health Care Reform Plan." *Business and Health* 10, no. 11 (1992): 31–35.

Levey, Samuel, and James Hill. "National Health Insurance—The Triumph of Equivocation." *The New England Journal of Medicine* 321, no. 25 (December 21, 1989): 1750–54.

Lewis, John C. "Hawaii—A Blueprint for Health Care Reform." *Business and Health* 10, no. 11 (1992): 55–56.

Linton, Adam L. "The Canadian Health Care System." *The New England Journal of Medicine* 322, no. 3 (January 18, 1990): 197–99.

McCarthy, Carol M. "DRGs—Five Years Later." *New England Journal of Medicine* 318, no. 25 (June 23, 1988): 1683–86.

Mitchell, Mark R. "Universal Health Insurance in Canada: Are There Lessons for the United States?" *Health Matrix: The Quarterly Journal of Health Services* 7, no. 1 (Spring 1989): 74–79.

Price, Kurt F. "Pricing Medicare's Diagnosis-Related Groups: Charges versus Estimated Costs." *Health Care Financing Review* 11, no. 1 (Fall 1989): 79–90.

Resnick, Rosalind. "Florida Grapples with Universal Health Care." *Business and Health* 10, no. 8 (1992): 56.

Short, Pamela Farley, Alan Monheit, and Karen Beauregard. *Uninsured Americans: A 1987 Profile*. Rockville, Md.: National Center for Health Services Research and Health Care Technology Assessment, 1988.

Simmons, Henry E., and others. "Comprehensive Health Care Reform and Managed Competition." *The New England Journal of Medicine* 327, no. 21 (November 19, 1992): 1525–27.

Simpson, James B. "State Certificate-of-Need Programs: The Current Status." *American Journal of Public Health* 75, no. 10 (October 1985): 1225–29.

Sloan, Frank A., and others. "Effects of the Medicare Prospective Payment System on Hospital Cost Containment: An Early Appraisal." *The Milbank Quarterly* 66, no. 2 (1988): 191–220.

Wellstone, Paul D., and Ellen R. Shaffer. "The American Health Security Act." *New England Journal of Medicine* 328, no. 20 (May 20, 1993): 1489–93.

"What You Should Know About Medigap Policies." *Consumers' Research* 76, no. 1 (January 1993): 27–30.

Zedlewski, Sheila R., and others. "Play-or-Pay Employer Mandates: Potential Effects." *Health Affairs* 11, no. 1 (Spring 1992): 62–83.

Endnotes

1. Short, Pamela Farley, Alan Monheit, and Karen Beauregard. *Uninsured Americans: A 1987 Profile.* Rockville, Md.: National Center for Health Services Research and Health Care Technology Assessment, 1988.
2. Health Insurance Association of America. *Source Book of Health Insurance Data, 1986.* Washington, D.C.: HIAA, 1986, p. 91.
3. Information provided by personal correspondence from Health Care Financing Administration, Department of Health and Human Services, 1993.
4. *Ibid.*
5. Data from Health Care Financing Administration, Department of Health and Human Services, 1992.
6. Department of Health and Human Services. *Health, United States, 1991.* Washington, D.C.: U.S. Government Printing Office, 1992, p. 297.
7. Reported in the American Public Health Association (A.P.H.A.) monthly news publication *Nation's Health,* March 1989.
8. Department of Commerce. *The President's Health Security Plan—Preliminary Summary.* Springfield, Va.: U.S. Department of Commerce, September 22, 1993, 30 pp.
9. Enthoven, Alain C. "The History and Principles of Managed Competition." *Health Affairs* 12, Supplement (1993): 29.
10. Department of Commerce, *The President's Health Security Plan.*

CHAPTER **EIGHT**

Health Personnel and Facilities

The Resources of Health Care

The health care industry is no small enterprise. In terms of personnel, the health care field is the third largest industry in the United States. Some 5 percent of the total nation's labor force are involved in health care in some way.[1] The growth in the health care industry has been exceptional in the past two decades. Many new jobs created during the past decade have been related to health care.

Despite this growth in the number of individuals involved in the health professions and related health activities, problems do exist in the health work force. One area that has received widespread discussion, debate, and evaluation in the past decade concerns the adequacy, in terms of number, of health personnel. Are there enough physicians, dentists, nurses, and related health professionals to meet the health demands of the U.S. population? How can health care providers be more equitably distributed on a geographical basis? Can a greater number of minorities and women be brought into the health care industry as health care providers?

When the matter of health personnel is discussed, the number of physicians is often the first focus of interest, yet other health professionals must also be considered. In recent years a group of nonphysician health care providers has developed: physician's assistants and nurse practitioners. In addition to these individuals, numerous other health workers are found in the various health-related professions.

Medical Education Programs

During the 1960s and 1970s increased federal financial support resulted in greater numbers of health professional school graduates and in the expansion of existing professional programs. Numerous new medical, dental, nursing, and allied or related health schools and training programs plus schools of public health were developed. However, throughout the 1980s there was a slight, but steady, decline in the number of applicants to health professions schools.[2]

What Is Podiatry?

Podiatry is a branch of medicine that is concerned with the diagnosis, treatment, and prevention of abnormal conditions of the feet. The podiatrist conducts surgical procedures, prescribes drugs, and prepares the use of corrective devices as needed for problems of the feet. Also the podiatrist treats skin and nail conditions of the feet and toes. Injuries to the bones, tendons, muscles, and joints relating to the feet are cared for by this individual. Corns and callouses as well as deformities such as clubfoot are commonly cared for by the podiatrist.

The education and training of the podiatrist usually involves four years of study in podiatric medicine after completion of four years of college. Most podiatrists tend to be found practicing in urban areas in solo practice. As with medical doctors, very few podiatrists are females or minorities.

Physicians

By the latter 1980s there were approximately 571,000 physicians in the United States.[3] Present consensus seems to be that the existing medical schools will prepare an adequate number of physicians for the future. It has been projected that physician supply will continue to increase into the 1990s.

There is general agreement that an adequate number of physicians is available in the United States. But what continues to be a problem is an inadequate distribution, both geographically and by medical specialty, of existing medical personnel. If you have ever been in need of a physician and have been unable to find one, you have some idea of the problems of health care access.

There is a significant shortage of primary care physicians in the United States. Approximately 30 percent of the nation's physicians are in primary care or general practice.[4] Primary care includes family or general practice, osteopathic general practice, and general internal medicine. Sometimes pediatrics and obstetrics are classified as primary care. The majority of all physicians (nearly 70 percent) practice specialized medicine and are not available for routine medical care and treatment. The number of these medical specialists has continued to increase in recent years as new specialities have been established.

The reduction in available primary-care physicians has resulted in shortages in certain localities. Shortages are particularly acute in rural communities and in the inner-city areas. This lack of primary health-care providers and related facilities becomes a serious burden for the nation's economically disadvantaged living in these localities. It is a seemingly never-ending circle: the medical provider chooses not to live in these localities for several reasons, one being that the poor are less likely to be able to pay for health care. As the poor individual is not as likely to have resources to pay for preventive health care, the chance becomes greater that the services of a physician will not be sought. The services provided by local health departments often are the principal source of medical care for many of these individuals.

Several measures have been taken for the purpose of attempting to encourage greater numbers of physicians to go into primary health care. Some states have assumed medical school loans of physicians who enter primary care. The Robert Wood Johnson Foundation has provided financial support programs to institutions that have developed strategies to increase the numbers of medical generalists. These include provisions of medical school scholarships and debt forgiveness for individuals who enter primary health care practice.

In 1990 a long-term study of medical work force needs was announced. This study will update projections into the year 2010 for such medical specialties as family practice, pediatrics, obstetrics/gynecology, internal medicine, general surgery, and psychiatry.

Other Health Professions

The supply of other health care providers, such as dentists, optometrists, podiatrists, and pharmacists, appears to be adequate. The problem of geographic distribution of these health providers is similar to that of physicians. Urban areas tend to have the greatest concentration of providers.

Today there are 58 dental schools throughout the United States. There are over 158,000 dentists in the United States. Nearly two-thirds of the total dental care work force are auxiliary personnel, dental hygienists and dental assistants, who provide many dental services.[5]

I
is known that the health status of economically disadvantaged minorities is not as good as the general U.S. population and that the poor are not as likely to practice preventive health measures.

Although minority health care personnel are more likely to serve in communities and localities where minority health needs are the greatest, professionally trained minorities are seriously lacking in the various health care fields.

The lack of minorities in the health care professions is shown by the following information:

| | Percentage of | | | |
	Total Population	MD/DOs	Dentists	Nurses
African-Americans	12%	3%	5%	7%
Hispanics	7%	4%	2%	2%

What can be done to get more medically trained minorities into the health care industry? Where does the responsibility lie for recruiting, preparing, and educating minorities to become health care providers?

There are thirteen schools of optometry, five schools of podiatry, and seventy-two colleges of pharmacy. Owing to the increasing number of professional schools and the increased enrollments in already existing schools during the past decade, there seems to be no need to establish additional health professional schools in the immediate future.

Imbalance of Race and Gender

In spite of the assumed adequate supply and projected future oversupply of health care personnel, there is an imbalance of both race and gender in all health professions. Over 90 percent of dentists, optometrists, podiatrists, and pharmacists are white males.

Though still proportionally underrepresented, there has been an increasing percentage of women in the medical professions. Today nearly half of all medical school students are female. It is projected that by the year 2000 approximately one-fourth of all physicians will be female.[6] Though still in the extreme minority, the percentage of female dentists has nearly doubled in the past decade.

Admission to the medical professions has been limited for many minority groups, such as African-Americans, Native Americans, and the Spanish-speaking population. Minorities have been poorly recruited, have historically experienced a general denial of access into

Dentists

Date	Number	Dental Schools
1960	105,000	47
1965	112,000	49
1970	116,000	53
1975	127,000	59
1980	141,000	61
1985	156,000	60
1990	186,000	58

Source: U.S. Bureau of the Census. *Statistical Abstracts of the United States.* 1993. 113th ed. Washington, D.C.: U.S. Government Printing Office, 1993, p. 118.

medical and dental schools, and have had, in general, inadequate academic backgrounds. These factors combined with the existence of few minority role models have often created a lack of awareness among minority adolescents of the opportunities in medicine.

Other Medical Practitioners

The medical doctor (MD) is educated in what is known as the allopathic medical model. Thousands of people receive treatment every day in the United States by medical practitioners other than these. Best known are the osteopathic physician (DO) and the doctor of chiropractic medicine.

Osteopathic Medicine

The underlying philosophy of *osteopathic medicine* originated in the late 1800s with the concepts of Andrew Still. According to this philosophy of medicine, impairment of nerve function—pinching of the nerves as they leave the spinal column—results in musculoskeletal disturbance, which places stress on the body. Manipulative therapy is used to restore "structural integrity" of the skeletal system.

Osteopathic medicine is based on the concept that all body systems are interdependent. A disturbance in one body system causes altered functions in other body systems. This emphasis on the relationship between body structure and organic functioning leads to holistic medical care and treatment.

Osteopathic medicine has gradually modified many of its original concepts. Today the doctor of osteopathic medicine (DOs) uses the same methods of treating disease and injury as the allopathic physician. This includes the use of drugs, surgery, radiation, and other physical modalities plus manipulation of the musculoskeletal system.

Over half of the DOs in the United States are involved in primary care medicine. There are specialists in such fields as anesthesiology, surgery, psychiatry, and internal medicine. About two-thirds of all DOs practice in rural and small-town communities. They are often the sole source of health care in these settings.

Today there are fifteen schools of osteopathic medicine. Each has an affiliation with a teaching hospital of osteopathic medicine.

Osteopaths are licensed to practice in all fifty states after passing the same examination as is given to the medical doctor. Most DOs practice in osteopathic hospitals. However, increasing numbers now have medical staff appointments in general community hospitals.

Chiropractic Medicine

Another healing modality that attracts many patients every year is *chiropractic medicine,* which is based on a theory originally put forth in 1895 by Daniel Palmer. This theory is that health is determined by the "structural integrity" of the bones of the vertebrae. Disease results from improper alignment or derangement of the vertebrae, known as spinal subluxation. These derangements cause a disturbance of the nervous system that "is often a primary or contributing causative, provocative and extending factor in the pathological process of many common and at times seemingly intractable human ailments."[7]

The chiropractor detects spinal subluxations by using x-rays, palpation, and thermeter readings. Palpation is the careful feeling of the spine and associated muscles and joints with the fingers to detect abnormalities. A thermeter measures temperature differences on either side of the spine. These measurements can give evidence of subluxation.

The doctor of chiropractic medicine uses manipulation or adjustment to return the vertebrae to proper alignment. These procedures restore nerve transmission and normal functioning of body parts. The chiropractor employs clinical nutrition, physical therapy, basic hygienic practices, and other measures directed toward the prevention and treatment of disease.

Historically, chiropractic medicine has been opposed by allopathic medicine. However, in 1980 the American Medical Association approved the referring of patients to chiropractors. This measure was taken in part because of the threat of lawsuits claiming monopolistic practices by medical doctors in the health care field. In a 1987 court decision the American Medical Association was found guilty of conspiracy to destroy chiropractic medicine as a health care profession. The court indicated that chiropractors should be allowed to practice in hospitals and that chiropractors and medical doctors should cooperate, with mutual referrals being encouraged.

Several trends in chiropractic medicine occurred in the latter part of the 1980s. The chiropractor has become a "limited practitioner" of medicine with the same status as dentists and podiatrists. Their practice is restricted to certain back and musculoskeletal problems caused by mechanical, not organic, disorders. All states now license and recognize chiropractic medicine as a health care profession. Thus both Medicare and Medicaid will pay for chiropractic care. In addition, most health insurance companies reimburse for chiropractic services. Coverage is also available through all state workers' compensation programs.

Alternative Medicine

As many as one-third of all Americans use alternative medicine.[8] It is estimated that as many as sixty million Americans use at least one such therapy. Though it is rather difficult to find agreement as to what constitutes this type of health care, usually it tends to include the use of what are considered to be unorthodox healing modalities and therapies by the health care industry. The treatment modalities most often used include relaxation techniques, therapeutic massage, special diets, and megavitamins.[9] Research has shown that alternative medicine is used for many different types of health problems. Back pain, headache, arthritis, insomnia, anxiety, and depression are the most common ailments for which individuals seek such procedures.[10] For many years people tended to seek these types of therapies principally when experiencing life-threatening conditions, as in the case of terminal cancer. However, there is increasing evidence that the effectiveness of alternative medicine is not limited to life-threatening circumstances and that more people seek this type of care for primary, preventive care.

Not every population group seeks the use of alternative medicine equally. Generally, white Americans from the middle economic class tend to use these treatment modalities more than do members of the lower socioeconomic population. Also, these persons' personal medical doctors are normally not aware of the visits to unconventional therapy.

It has been estimated that over ten billion dollars a year is spent for alternative medical therapies and treatments. More than half of the payment for such care is not covered by third-party payment. People pay for service out-of-pocket, rather than rely on insurance payment. Insurance policies do cover some alternative therapies, such as biofeedback, use of herbal therapists, and purchase of megavitamins.

There are several nontraditional alternative medical practitioners. The *naturopath* uses a system of healing that includes therapies of sunlight, manipulation, exercise, water, air, organic foods, nutrition supplements, and naturally occurring drugs in the promotion or restoration of normal body processes. The *homeopath* treats diseases by giving drugs in small doses. The *naparapath* subscribes to a system of therapeutics based on the theory that diseases are caused by connective tissue and ligament disorders. The *Christian Science practitioner* makes use of religious concepts and beliefs in healing modalities.

The ancient Chinese art of *acupuncture* has received increasing interest in the United States. Acupuncture is the procedure of treating diseases by the insertion of fine needles into the human body at specific points. Research is ongoing to learn how acupuncture works to relieve pain and treat disease.

Nursing

Nursing has a rich heritage in the United States. It is estimated that there are over 1.6 million actively employed registered nurses in this country. The Public Health Service estimates that there are more than two million registered nurses throughout the nation.[11]

Working in a variety of settings, nurses are found in any inpatient health care facilities and in most outpatient clinical settings. They care for patients in hospitals, nursing homes, and other health care institutions. Many nurses provide home health care services. They also are found working as public health nurses and in industrial settings. Nurses also provide very important services to children in the schools. Others work in private doctors' offices.

Whether there are an adequate number of registered nurses is open to question. It is more important to consider whether an adequate number of nurses with specific skills work in certain clinical settings. Despite the fact that two-thirds of all nurses work in hospitals, there is little question that a shortage of nurses willing to work in the hospital setting exists. This is obvious from the job advertisements in the newspapers, where many openings for nursing employment are listed. This shortage has been noted by the American Hospital Association and the National League of Nursing. The American Hospital Association reported in 1992 that as the result of increased recruitment and retention initiatives, nurse shortages in hospitals had been reduced. However, continued growing demand still necessitates the need for recruitment of

Registered Nurses

Date	Number	Nursing Programs
1960	517,000	1,128
1965	621,000	1,182
1970	750,000	1,340
1975	961,000	1,362
1980	1,273,000	1,385
1990	1,715,000	1,470

Source: U.S. Bureau of the Census. *Statistical Abstracts of the United States,* 1993. 113th ed. Washington, D.C.: U.S. Government Printing Office, 1993, p. 118.

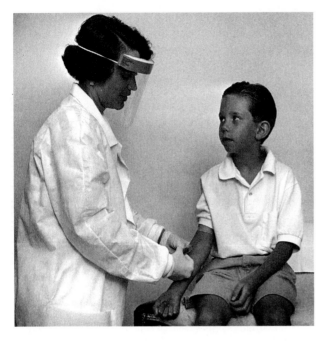

The nurse can provide a broad range of tasks in the clinical setting.

stressed the importance of nurses being assigned fewer non-nursing tasks. They also feel that more long-term professional opportunities are needed.

Several changes have been noted that would alleviate the nursing shortage. Better financial reimbursement for services rendered would encourage greater interest in this profession. Also, more respect on behalf of the medical community and the opportunity to experience more meaningful responsibilities are necessary. The education required for a nurse in this day of advanced technology must be upgraded.

Two other significant pressures on nursing are the increasing demand for long-term care necessary for AIDS patients and for the elderly. AIDS has placed a growing demand on all health care personnel, but particularly on nurses who must provide the majority of AIDS patients' daily care. Nursing is the largest group of health care providers caring for HIV infected people. They serve as care givers, case managers, educators, and counselors. A great need exists for additional in-service training and education of nurses in the care of HIV/AIDS patients. As the number of cases of AIDS increases in the years ahead, so will the demand for more nurses.

Nurses provide much care to the elderly in long-term care nursing facilities. As the elderly population in the United States increases, the need for nurses working with long-term care conditions will expand.

Nursing education has gone through a variety of changes in recent years. The number of nursing graduates and nursing schools has greatly expanded in the past two decades. This increase is due in part to the several different training programs for nurses. The hospital-based programs as well as the associate-degree programs prepare the nurse primarily for institutional nursing service. Most hospital-based programs are two or three years in duration and expose the student to a variety of clinical experiences in the hospital setting. These programs are being phased out throughout the country because of cost on the part of the hospital and the present feeling in the nursing profession that all nurses should hold either the associate degree or the bachelor of science in nursing (BSN) degree.

The associate degree program is a two-year program usually offered by a junior or community college. The curriculum emphasis tends to be more academic than clinical. Though there are clinical learning experiences, they are limited compared with the hospital-based programs.

more nurses. The base for nurse recruitment needs to be broadened in order to make nursing a more attractive career. This particularly suggests the need to encourage more males to enter nursing. In 1993 only 11 percent of first-time nursing students were male. Also, the numbers of minorities in nursing, as in the other health care professions, is extremely low.

The turnover of nurses in hospitals is very high and so contributes to a lack of continuity in work relationships. Although the number of men entering the nursing profession has increased, it has basically been women who are nurses, and many do not stay in the work force for extended periods of time. It is still common for nurses to leave the active practice of nursing when their children are young, or to work only part-time during the years that their children are at home. Increasingly, nurses are finding work opportunities in settings other than hospitals.

A perceived lack of status and input about hospital working conditions causes many nurses to find work in other settings, such as in public health, in industry, or in schools. Members of the nursing profession have been striving for a greater shared responsibility with physicians in the practice of health care in the hospital and in other inpatient facilities. The nursing profession has

A third type of nursing education program is the baccalaureate degree program which usually combines a strong hospital-based clinical experience with the educational requirements of a four-year degree institution. Graduates of these programs receive the BSN (Bachelor of Science in Nursing).

The general trend in nursing education today is toward the four-year degree program. This is in part owing to the increased need for an in-depth education and also the prestige that a degreed individual has in U.S. society. Also, the degreed nurse is usually able to command a greater salary than the nondegreed individual.

Nurses with advanced degrees, such as the MSN or the PhD, remain in short supply. These individuals are needed to fill teaching positions in nursing education programs and for administrative work both in the academic world and in the institutional setting, as well as to conduct research in the field of nursing.

Nonphysician Health Care Providers

Many of the health problems of people who seek primary care can be managed by nonphysician health-care providers. These individuals are trained to perform services traditionally offered only by physicians. They perform medical services under the supervision of a physician. Two types of nonphysician health-care providers have developed since the mid-1960s: (1) the physician's assistant (PA) and (2) the nurse practitioner (NP). A third type of nonphysician health-care provider is the nurse-midwife.

Physicians' Assistants and Nurse Practitioners

These nonphysician health care providers are trained to perform selected tasks that were, in the past, usually performed by physicians. These tasks are actually an extension of the nursing role. But in addition to regular nursing duties, various primary care medical services are performed.

The physician's assistant and nurse practitioner provide primary care in a variety of settings. They have been useful in meeting the need for health care personnel in the inner cities and in other medically underserved localities. The physician's assistant program has been somewhat successful in servicing small communities. Three-fourths of all physicians' assistants are working in

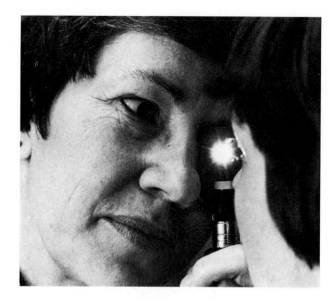

The nurse practitioner is important to many occupational health programs. Here a nurse practitioner conducts an eye examination as part of the health evaluation for each Kimberly-Clark employee in the company's Health Management Program.

primary care, and half of these are in rural communities. Nurse practitioners are not as likely to settle in rural areas, preferring larger cities.

Both the physician's assistant and nurse practitioner programs originated in 1965. The first physician's assistant program was introduced at Duke University. The nurse practitioner program began at the University of Colorado when a nurses' training program expanded the scope of practice to develop the pediatric nurse practitioner. The physician's assistant programs often enroll older students with previous health care experience in some related field. Former military corpsmen along with various related health profession technicians have become PAs.

The training programs for these occupations differ in both curriculum and program completion time from one institution to another. Both physician's assistant programs and nurse practitioner training programs range anywhere from one to two years.

Duties

As stated earlier, the nonphysician health care provider performs a number of services that were formerly physician responsibilities. These include taking a health history, performing routine medical examinations, and providing emergency medical care.

In addition to traditional advanced nursing duties, both the physician's assistant and the nurse practitioner are able to perform some diagnostic procedures, assess health status indicators, perform health maintenance tasks, and, generally, better assist sick patients. Because these individuals are active in health care, ambulatory care services can be extended to more people. Some of these providers are even trained to perform minor surgery such as suturing. They also provide various types of rehabilitative medical services.

Patient education and health counseling are other important roles played by the nonphysician health care provider. If the patient is informed of his or her problem and shown how to cope with it, a better sense of wellness and adaptation results.

Since the primary duties of the nonphysician health care provider involve caring for the well and treating minor illnesses, the physician should be able to spend more time with, and so better care for, the chronically and more seriously ill.

Specialties

Both the physician's assistant and the nurse practitioner may be trained in a number of specialized roles. The family nurse practitioner serves mothers and children. This practitioner is able to deal with infant diseases, as well as injuries and most emergency situations involving infants and children.

Other nurse practitioner specialists include the gerontological nurse practitioner, who works with the elderly in both private and public settings, usually as part of a team. Many geriatric nurse practitioners are found in nursing homes. A number of school districts throughout the country employ a school nurse practitioner. The pediatric nurse practitioner cares for expectant mothers and children, and advises parents in telephone conversations about home management of minor pediatric problems. He or she also provides care and assistance for newborn infants and their parents. Most of the problems dealt with by the pediatric nurse practitioner are not serious enough for the child to be seen by the physician, yet still require the input of a medical person. Physician's assistant specialists can be found in a broad range of medical practice.

Issues

A number of issues and concerns have developed over the physician's assistant and the nurse practitioner programs. One important concern is whether the consumer will accept this health care provider in place of the physician. Would you go to a physician's assistant or receive the services of the nurse practitioner rather than see a physician? For the most part, people in the United States are so philosophically oriented to the physician as the predominant and sole health care provider that acceptance of the nonphysician provider has been limited. In spite of the reluctance to accept this new type of medical care personnel, the nurse practitioner has proved to be an effective provider of primary care.[12] As patients have had more exposure to these individuals as a source of medical care, they have become more receptive to them.[13]

For the nurse practitioner and the physician's assistant to be even more widely and effectively employed, it is important that they receive greater physician acceptance. Only 20 percent of nurse practitioners are employed in private physicians' offices. Slightly more than one-fourth are employed in health departments and with governmental agencies. Others are found working in HMOs, in business and industry, at college and university health centers, and in general hospital care settings. Many physicians do not understand the role or responsibilities of this type of health provider. Some physicians even view the nonphysician health care provider as a threat to their practice, both economically and professionally. Perhaps, though, exposure to these new health professionals during medical training will encourage physicians to accept them.[14] The future physician needs to learn the value of the nurse practitioner and the physician's assistant and develop an appreciation of the interactive roles they can play in health care. Physicians who employ nurse practitioners have come to value them.[15]

A number of legal questions have been raised concerning this type of health care provider. The appearance of the nonphysician health care provider has forced many states to reexamine and change statutes regarding medical practice and procedures. Medical supervision of both groups, especially the physician's assistant, is necessary. However, the definition of acceptable supervision has been controversial. Must the physician's assistant work in direct proximity to the physician? All states require some type of direct supervision. The question of whether the nurse practitioner is practicing medicine without a license has gone to court in one state.[16] That court ruled that they were. Obviously, many difficult and unanswered legal questions still exist in various localities.

Whether the nonphysician health care provider has been successful at improving the availability of health care to the poor, the elderly, and those in medically underserved localities is open to question. For example, less than one-third of nurse practitioners are employed in medically underserved areas. This is partly owing to reimbursement patterns and legal factors. Because many states do not allow nurse practitioners to provide services unless under the direct supervision of a physician, they cannot work in rural or economically depressed areas unless a physician is present.

Reimbursement

Pay for services provided by the nonphysician health care provider also presents problems. For example, the nurse practitioner should receive greater reimbursement than the traditional RN or BSN nurse. The training is more extensive and the individual is capable of performing a much greater range of services to the patient. However, many medical clinics and physicians do not employ nurse practitioners for that reason, choosing instead to pay the lower salaries of traditional registered nurses.

The services of the nonphysician health care provider should reduce costs to the patients. In theory, certain health care should be provided by a nonphysician in the outpatient, clinical, or office setting at a reduced price. However, in practice, when the nonphysician health care provider is employed by a physician or group practice, it is not uncommon for the costs to be greater. This is because the physician's assistant or nurse practitioner is considered a member of the health care team and, as such, the cost of his or her employment must be passed on to the consumer. There is no evidence that the nonphysician health care provider has helped to reduce health care costs.

Third party insurance programs have not always reimbursed for services provided by the nonphysician health care provider. Federal legislation passed in 1990 allows Medicaid to pay pediatric and family nurse practitioners directly for family health services. However, there are many other services that are not presently reimbursable.

Nurse-Midwives

A registered nurse who has completed additional education and training beyond the basic nursing program may be a certified nurse-midwife. This additional education prepares the nurse to provide health care for women and their babies during pregnancy, labor, delivery, and the postnatal or postpartum period. They also provide gynecologic care for nonpregnant women.

The nurse-midwife provides such prenatal care as the early diagnosis and initial physical examination of pregnancy. The nurse-midwife is also involved in all aspects of managing a normal delivery, including staying with the patient until the delivery is over. Other important services offered by the nurse-midwife include postpartum care, care to the newborn, family-planning advice, and health counseling.

The nurse-midwife works in association with physicians, usually with an obstetrician/gynecologist or general practice physician. The physician must permit the nurse-midwife to perform those tasks he or she is prepared to handle, that is, most cases of pregnancy and childbirth; but a patient with high-risk complications is referred to the physician.

Nurse-midwifery was first introduced into the United States in 1925.[17] The first educational program to train the nurse-midwife was established in 1931 in New York City.[18] Currently there are twenty-five nurse-midwife educational programs in the United States. There are more than three thousand certified midwives in the United States, with the greatest numbers residing in California, New York, and Florida.[19] Though some nurse-midwives work in private practice, most are affiliated with hospitals or with public health facilities. In addition to their educational requirements, they must pass a certification examination prepared by the American College of Nurse-Midwives.

Midwives have traditionally been found in localities where there is a lack of physicians to serve the economically disadvantaged. In recent years their services have been sought by middle- and upper-class couples desiring more personal involvement in the pregnancy and birthing process.

The nurse-midwife is not as common in the United States as in other countries throughout the world. In fact, in some European countries, most deliveries are managed by the nurse-midwife.

There are still a number of unanswered questions about the future role of nonphysician health care providers. Since an important reason for their existence has been to make health services available in medically underserved areas, it will be important to observe whether they remain in these geographical localities. Will they continue to work and live in the rural communities or the inner cities, or will they seek employment in medically overexposed areas as doctors have? It seems that the appearance of these new health care providers is timely, since their services will increase the availability of health care for the needy in this country.

Allied Health Personnel

Allied health personnel constitute the majority of all persons working in the health care professions. They work in all types of health care—primary, acute, tertiary, and chronic—and in a multiplicity of settings, such as physicians' and dentists' offices, HMOs, freestanding health care facilities, and hospitals, as well as in providing home health care. In some instances they are in independent practice. The allied health worker has specific skills to contribute to the care, treatment, and rehabilitation of the health consumer.

Some allied health personnel perform tasks that in the past were the responsibility of physicians, dentists, or nurses. For example, dental hygienists today clean teeth, perform initial examinations, and take x-rays. They play an important role in preventive dental health. Radiologists today must administer CAT scans, conduct MRI imaging, and be skilled in the use of ultrasound. Laboratory technicians are expected to carry out increasingly more sophisticated laboratory procedures.

Included in the allied health professions are various health technologists and technicians, therapists, laboratory workers, administrators, dieticians, and nutritionists. Technical advances in the health care field have led to the establishment of many new health occupations. The increasingly sophisticated technology of health care has created a demand for better-trained and more knowledgeable workers. Technologists, such as inhalation and respiratory therapists, are trained to operate diagnostic and monitoring equipment and to perform rehabilitative services. A greater need for rehabilitation services has resulted in a growing demand for occupational and physical therapists.

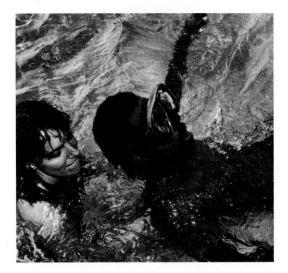

The physical therapist helps the injured, handicapped, and disabled person to regain physical movement if possible and to adapt to the handicapped conditions. Here a VA hospital physical therapist assists a disabled veteran in preparing for the National Veterans Wheelchair Games, one of the recreational services sponsored by the Veterans Administration and other veterans service organizations.

More than three million health workers, or approximately 60 percent of all health personnel, are considered allied health personnel. There are over one hundred occupational titles in the health field, but nearly 90 percent of the total personnel employed in the allied occupations are among the following:[20]

Dental assistants

Dental hygienists

Dental laboratory technicians

Dietitians and dietetic technicians

Health and medical record technicians, assistants, and aides

Medical laboratory technologists, technicians, and assistants

Occupational and physical therapists

Radiology technologists, technicians, and assistants

Respiratory therapists

Speech pathologists and audiologists

The demand for increasing numbers of individuals in the allied health professions depends on a number of variables. The past decade has witnessed significant need in most of the professions. Projections indicate that this need will continue to be greater in the 1990s than was the case in the 1980s. Shortages in these professions have been expressed by various state health agencies, by professional health associations, as well as by the many hospital vacancies being reported. As the American population becomes older there will be increasing need for the services of many of the allied health professions.

With increased outpatient care the role of various allied health therapists and technologists will grow during the 1990s. The greatest shortages in the allied health professions are in physical therapy, occupational therapy, medical lab technology, respiratory therapy, dental hygiene, and speech pathology.[21]

Physical therapists plan and administer treatment to individuals in need of pain relief, to persons with limited disabilities, to those who need improved mobility, and to cardiac patients. Their services are provided in both inpatient and outpatient settings and in the patients' homes. The need for physical therapists has been enhanced since workers' compensation now covers payment for their services. Occupational therapists help individuals to develop skills necessary to perform daily tasks. Their services are provided on an outpatient basis and in patients' homes as well as in the medical care institutions.

Medical lab technologists carry out a variety of laboratory tests. There has been an increasing specialization of medical lab personnel. For example, today lab techs are trained in microbiology, cytotechnology, and histology. The respiratory therapist works under medical supervision to assist the patient having respiratory problems. This individual plays a major role in the treatment of post-surgical patients. Also care is rendered to individuals suffering from asthma and emphysema.

As is true with medical care providers, more minorities must be recruited into the allied health professions. Young people from minority populations need to be informed about the opportunities available. Many have little knowledge and understanding of the broad range of positions available and the education and training required for entry into these professions.

The allied health professional must be seen as part of the overall health team. These individuals must understand how their contributions fit into the health care system. More research relating to the factors associated with the various allied health professions must be conducted, and financial reimbursement must be increased in many of these positions. Retention in some of the allied health professions has been low for many of the same reasons as in nursing: low pay, poor professional image, and lack of opportunity for long-term professional growth.

Education and Training

The professional education and training of allied health personnel takes place in many different settings, including hospitals, vocational schools, and colleges. Clinical teaching and experience are the major thrusts of most allied health education programs. In these clinical settings students learn, while under close direct supervision, to evaluate the condition of the patient and to carry out the treatment modalities they are being taught.

Originally, allied health professions were developed as outgrowths and expansions of the provision of medical care. As the role and responsibilities of various allied health personnel have become more complex, the education required has become more academic. This greater emphasis on academics in addition to clinical training has led to more programs being in colleges and universities. The number of college and university allied health programs has grown from 2,000 to 6,900 since the mid-1960s.[22]

Many allied health training programs are offered by two-year colleges. The student receives clinical experiences in the hospital or other health care facilities, but the basic academic education takes place in the college or university setting. Some programs are hospital-based throughout the entire training period. The allied health programs most frequently found in hospitals include clinical laboratory, radiologic technology, administration, mental health, and dietetic and nutritional services.[23]

Some allied health training programs are offered by vocational training institutions. Usually, the programs found in these settings train students in medical office assistance, dental assistance, nursing aid, dental and medical laboratory technology, and radiologic technology.[24]

Many medical schools have departments of allied health. Here allied health personnel receive education and degrees beyond those offered by the two-year college program. In some instances, graduate degrees can be earned at these institutions.

Licensure and Certification

Some allied health personnel must obtain either state or national credentials, or both, before they are able to practice. Usually these credentials are in the form of either a license or a certificate. These indicate that the individuals have fulfilled certain educational and skill requirements and are endorsed to work in a given locality. Some allied health fields require formal registration as well as certification.

Licensing for some allied health professions is performed under the mandates of state law. Dental hygienists, physical therapists, physicians' assistants, and occupational therapists are examples of this pattern of licensing. Medical record administrators and technicians, dietitians, respiratory therapists, and cardiopulmonary resuscitation technologists are certified by their respective professional societies.

Another method by which the student obtains state or federal permission to practice is through the accreditation of the educational institution or training program. An institution or a training program must meet specific standards established for the academic curriculum, faculty, institutional resources, and facilities. An institution seeking certification for its program must conduct an in-depth self-study, including an examination of program goals, objectives, resources, and curriculum. This self-study is submitted to the accrediting agency prior to the visit of the evaluation team, which then either approves the program or makes recommendations for change. The approval is granted for a specific period of time, after which recertification is required. All students graduating from the program will have the necessary credentials to practice. The process of obtaining credentials, whether on an individual or institutional basis, results in a degree of standardization from one locality to another throughout the nation.

Professional Associations

The various health professions are represented by a number of professional health associations. These associations are usually national in scope, often having state and local affiliates, and play several different roles. In-service education and updating of knowledge and skills are major concerns of the meetings conducted for the association membership. These professional meetings provide opportunities for presenting research of interest to the profession and for the membership to debate and approve policy statements and professional resolutions.

A number of the professional associations have established standards of training and certification and/or licensing for those entering the specific health profession. For example, such standards have been established for physicians (American Medical Association, 535 No. Dearborn St., Chicago, Ill. 60610), nurses (National League of Nursing, 10 Columbus Circle, New York, N.Y. 10019), and dentists (American Dental Association, 211 E. Chicago Ave., Chicago, Ill. 60611), to name just a few.

The scope and interest of a professional organization may be quite broad. The principal professional health association for those involved in community health is the American Public Health Association (APHA, 1015 15th St. NW, Washington, D.C. 20005). Membership in this association includes representatives from all fields working in community health—physicians, nurses, environmentalists, sanitarians, health planners, and dietitians, plus a host of others. The annual meeting of the American Public Health Association provides hundreds of sections from which the membership can choose to attend. The major publication of the American Public Health Association is the *American Journal of Public Health,* published monthly. In an attempt to keep the membership updated about current happenings in community health, a monthly newspaper, *The Nation's Health,* is made available to all members.

Many of the professional health associations provide a much narrower span of professional interest. For example, the American Academy of Pediatrics (P.O. Box 927, 141 North West Point Road, Oak Grove Village, Ill. 60007) has basically one objective: to improve the health of children. The American Physical Therapy Association (1156 15th St. NW, Washington, D.C. 20005) is the professional association for those certified in physical therapy. The American Association of Respiratory Care includes support, certification, and identification for individuals trained as respiratory therapists. The American School Health Association is composed of health educators and nurses interested in school health programs.

Selected Professional Health Associations

American Society of Allied Health Professions 1101 Connecticut Ave. NW Suite 700 Washington, D.C. 20036	American Optometric Association 7000 Chippewa St. St. Louis, Missouri 63119	National Association of Sanitarians 1550 Lincoln St. Denver, Colorado 80203
American Dietetic Association 840 No. Lake Shore Drive Chicago, Illinois 60611	American Osteopathic Association 142 E. Ontario St. Chicago, Illinois 60611	National Dental Association 5506 Connecticut Ave. NW Washington, D.C. 20015
American Hospital Association 840 No. Lake Shore Drive Chicago, Illinois 60611	American Psychological Association 1200 17th St. NW Washington, D.C. 20036	National Medical Association 1012 Tenth St. NW Washington D.C. 20001

Many of these associations have played important roles in effecting change in community health. The American Dental Association, for instance, has been a leading proponent of community programs for fluoridation of public drinking water.

Health Care Facilities

Health care diagnosis and treatment are generally performed in the office of a health care provider (physician, dentist, podiatrist, optometrist, etc.), in a clinic that is funded and operated by public monies (local health department, community health center, etc.), in hospitals, or in an increasing variety of outpatient health care facilities. The private office may be a single operation where the physician, dentist, or other provider works on an independent basis. But an arrangement where the health care provider merges with other providers to form a group clinic is increasingly common. The provision of health care is still on an individual practice basis. However, administrative overhead costs, facility costs, and other expenditures are pooled for economic benefit.

Most local and state health departments provide health care in public clinics that are funded by tax monies. The type and extent of services provided in these clinics vary from one locality to another. A number of community health centers and other public health service facilities have been established to provide health care, particularly in medically underserved areas.

Hospitals

In the United States, hospitalization most often takes place in community hospitals—any nonfederal hospital that provides both short- and long-term general and specialized care. When patients are hospitalized for care and treatment, it is known as inpatient care.

Most short-term hospitalization in the United States takes place in community hospitals. There are three classifications of these hospitals, determined by ownership and management: (1) private, nonprofit; (2) public owned, government-operated; and (3) proprietary, for-profit.

The private, nonprofit hospitals provide health care for the general public. These hospitals are usually governed by a board of trustees and are operated by religious organizations, community nonprofit corporations, or philanthropic agencies. Private, nonprofit hospitals provide nearly 70 percent of all hospital beds, even though just over half of all community hospitals are so operated.

The nonprofit hospitals qualify for exemption from federal taxation. This tax exempt status permits the hospitals to solicit and accept contributions that are deductible by donors. The nonprofit hospitals are faced with financial pressures to raise operating capital. They cannot raise money for capital expenditures as can the proprietary hospitals, but must rely on philanthropy, governmental grants, or other measures in the private sector.

The prospective pay system is causing increasing budgetary pressure and competition for all hospitals, particularly the nonprofit facilities. With the rise of economic competition in health care, these hospitals have had to undergo substantial changes.

Government-owned hospitals are tax supported and operated by local or state health agencies and offer a range of services. Often they are found in large cities and provide the only health care for large segments of the poor population. Owing to financial restrictions, these hospitals are often understaffed. They have 17 percent of all hospital beds in the United States, yet provide more than 40 percent of uncompensated health care.[25]

The proprietary, for-profit hospital is privately owned and established as a profit-making organization. It is managed by a board of directors, and policy is determined by the owners, often stockholders who have invested in the corporation.

Prior to the 1980s, for-profit health care facilities were usually rather small and localized, often owned by a group of physicians. However, during the 1980s a significant change occurred. Health care became a growth industry with investment potential. Increasingly for-profit health care facilities have been taken over by large multihospital, investor-owned corporations. These management companies own nursing homes, HMOs, freestanding surgical centers, emergency clinics, and pharmaceutical and health care supply companies, in addition to hospitals. Approximately one-fourth of all hospitals in America today are owned and operated by for-profit corporations.

The largest investor-owned hospital corporation is the Hospital Corporation of America—its hospitals have more than fifty thousand beds.[26] Other well-known health care corporations are Humana Health Corporation, National Medical Enterprises, and the American Medical International Corporation. Investor-owned corporations have moved beyond the provision of direct health care services into areas of research and new product development. For example, the Humana Health Corporation has done much work on artificial heart surgery.

Obviously, monetary profit is a principal goal of such corporations. Some estimates are that by the latter 1990s close to half of all health care in the United States will be performed in investor-owned corporation facilities. Thus profit will be an increasing factor in the future shape of the United States health care delivery system. These large corporations will continue to purchase smaller hospitals and other health care facilities as they grow larger.

Those who support the expansion and growth of the for-profit health care delivery system suggest that investor-owned health management companies provide a more efficient delivery system. They are able to attract capital for expansion, development, and growth. It is felt that better quality health care can be provided and that industrial management principles will assure better health care.

On the other hand, opponents of this development question the basic motives of the for-profit movement. Should the motive for provision of health care be monetary return on investment? It is felt by many that everyone's health needs cannot be met adequately by corporations with a profit motive. Those individuals who cannot afford the costs of the investor-owned facilities will be forced to go to public and voluntary hospitals for their health care. This will add serious pressures to this segment of the health care delivery system. Public hospitals could become health care facilities basically for the economically disadvantaged population. How will funds be raised to meet the demands of such a development? Will the quality of health care for the economically disadvantaged be similar to that found in the for-profit facility, or is this leading to a "two-track" health care system in the United States?

Rural Hospitals

Nearly one-half of all hospitals in the United States are small or rural facilities with fewer than one hundred beds.[27] A majority of these smaller hospitals are located in rural settings and have often been the primary source of health care for many people living in a large geographical region.

In recent years, owing to financial pressures, a number of these rural community hospitals have been forced to close, form alliances with larger urban hospital centers, or sell out to for-profit health care corporations. Seven out of ten rural hospitals lost money in recent years. A number of factors have contributed to these problems.

One major reason has been that the elderly constitute a large part of those needing hospital care in these locations. Rural hospitals are paid less under the DRG system than are their urban counterparts. Because of this underfunding by Medicare and Medicaid, these hospitals lose money when they treat patients covered by these programs. In addition, the elderly suffer from many chronic conditions that must be provided for.

The closing of a hospital in a rural community has a number of negative effects. The most obvious is the reduced access to care for local residents. Rural

America is not always a healthy place to live. Occupations such as agriculture, forestry, and mining are among the most dangerous in America. Employees in these jobs, usually found in rural locations, are at risk for accidents and injury.

The rural hospital plays other roles in the community besides being a provider of health care. The hospital is often one of the community's largest employers and as such is important in the local economy. Closing the hospital can have a serious detrimental effect on the economic status of many of the local citizens. The depressed economy of rural America during the latter 1980s and the early 1990s was a related factor to the problems faced by rural medical care facilities.

Rural medical care facilities have attempted to diversify their services to make better use of their resources. Often this has resulted in providing long-term care facilities. However, with a smaller population than in urban centers, there tend to be fewer ways to develop and expand. Hospitals that are members of multihospital systems are more likely to stay open. The independent for-profit hospital in a rural location is more likely to close.

In order to help primary health care physicians deliver a broader range of services in rural hospitals, new technologies have been designed to link the rural facility with large urban medical complexes. For example, telecommunication satellite and fiber-optic links with specialists at the urban facilities now give direct information to the physician at the rural hospital. Consultation can take place with the needed medical specialist and care be given to the patient without having to transport the individual from the rural setting.

Linkage between facilities hundreds of miles apart has been accomplished in some instances. Medical facilities in Seattle have been linked with rural clinics in the remote sections of Alaska. Such procedures have potential for providing health care to many Native Americans living in isolated villages throughout the north.

Teleconsulting in internal medicine is an example of recent types of developments. By means of such telecommunications an ophthalmologist can see the inside of a patient's eye at the same time that the on-site primary care provider does. The specialist can provide instruction as to what appropriate measures should be taken with the patient.

Outpatient Health Care Facilities

When the patient receives medical care in a health care facility but does not stay overnight, it is referred to as outpatient care. An increasing amount of health care is being provided in outpatient health care facilities. They constitute the nation's fastest-growing groups of health care providers. The future will involve more health care away from the hospital—in the community.

Outpatient care facilities include emergency centers (urgent care centers) where emergency and other primary care services are provided. Freestanding ambulatory surgical facilities (surgicenters) provide surgery for conditions for which it is not necessary that the patient be kept overnight. These facilities include hospital outpatient clinics, community mental health clinics, as well as home care programs.

There are many reasons for the increased development of these facilities. Cost reduction has been a major motivation for obtaining health care in these settings. Some have been established by large hospital corporations for the purpose of providing care to geographical localities often lacking in health care services. Rural setting and inner city localities are common locations for these facilities.

Cost Containment Strategies and Hospitals

With the increase in health care costs during the past two decades, hospitals have been experiencing increasing pressures to hold down costs. This has resulted in a number of major changes in medical care as it relates to all health care facilities, particularly hospitals.

One important change has been the decrease in use of hospital inpatient services and the corresponding increase in outpatient, ambulatory health care. Procedures which in the past would have meant inpatient hospitalization for a couple of days are now often performed on an outpatient basis, the result being less cost to the consumer than if one were to be treated on an inpatient basis. The increased interest in outpatient services has been encouraged by cost containment patterns of governmental insurance programs, by hospital insurance coverages provided by business and industry, and by insurance companies.

Advances in medical technology have also been a factor in the growth and expansion of ambulatory surgical health care. For example, cataract removal used to

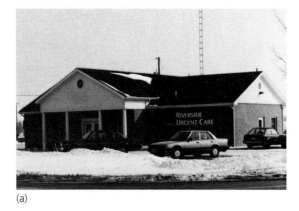

(a)

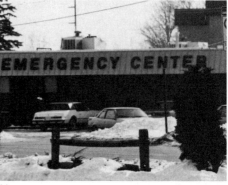

(b)

Many people today go to outpatient ambulatory care centers for medical care. Hospitals now provide outpatient services in a variety of different settings. (a) This facility is housed in a renovated gasoline station. (b) Free-standing emergency trauma centers, separate from any hospital, are rapidly developing facilities in many cities.

require several days of immobilization. This surgical procedure now takes less than a half hour because of new technologies that eliminate most of the radical cutting and suturing.

Health maintenance organizations and preferred provider organizations are contracting with freestanding outpatient surgery centers. As these centers expand, they will be able to purchase better equipment and perform more complete forms of surgery on an outpatient basis.

This switch from inpatient care has resulted in a lower hospital occupancy rate. Hospitals have been forced to reduce bed facilities and staff. Staffing reductions have involved both part- and full-time personnel. Despite this change in hospital inpatient care, overall hospital costs have continued to rise. Individuals having minor problems receive outpatient care; those patients being cared for in hospitals tend to have more serious problems necessitating long-term care and need more expensive, technologically sophisticated procedures. Increased malpractice insurance premium costs have also added to the financial stresses on hospitals.

To be competitive and to be able to survive economically, hospitals are making numerous changes in their operations. Departments must be cost-effective; if they are not, they may be eliminated.

Increased marketing of services is now seen. Hospitals are developing new or expanded services, many of which are designed to make use of facilities no longer occupied at full capacity. Programs are being developed that will result in economic profit, such as health promotion programs, alcoholism treatment, and substance abuse rehabilitation programs. Today, one sees advertisements in the mass media and on community billboards for various hospital programs. This was unheard of several years ago.

Diversification is occurring in many hospitals, particularly the smaller ones. Facilities previously used for acute care have been converted to provide such services as long-term care, ambulatory care, and retirement housing. Another idea is to place nursing homes near hospitals so that hospital patients who require long-term care can be transferred to the nursing home. If an acute episode arises, the patient can quickly be returned to the hospital.

Charity Needs

Who should pay the health care bills of individuals with no health insurance? The cost of charity hospital care has more than doubled in recent years. The hospitals most affected by the pressures of providing such care are government-owned county or municipal facilities. These facilities are most commonly located in rural communities or in the inner city.

The medically indigent are persons who have no private health insurance. They often are employed, but by small businesses or in part-time positions where no health insurance coverage is provided by the employer. These marginally employed individuals are no longer covered by Medicaid.

Hospitals serving the medically indigent must find ways to cover the losses they suffer from providing care to this population group. Some turn to private philanthropy for assistance. Hospitals also become involved in "cost shifting," the process of charging greater prices for reimbursable services to cover the areas of economic loss.

One might ask why hospitals accept the medically indigent. Part of the answer to this is that hospitals that accepted Hill-Burton monies for construction are required to provide a certain amount of free care each year to indigent patients. This is mandated for a certain number of years. However, the number of hospitals obligated to provide this care has declined in recent years. Thus, "patient dumping" is all too common. This is the process of transferring patients to public hospitals or other institutions willing to provide free health care.

Resolutions for the problems associated with charity hospital care will be complex. As long as millions of Americans are without any type of health insurance and the for-profit medical care industry continues to grow and does not accept these individuals, the pressures on government-operated facilities will continue.

Summary

The health care industry is the third largest industry in the United States. Seven-and-a-half million people are employed in some profession or occupation related to the provision of health care. Physicians and other health care providers account for about one-third of these employees, while nearly two-thirds are allied, or related, health personnel.

In spite of growth in the health care industry, some still question the adequacy of the number now employed in the field. Are there enough physicians, dentists, nurses, and other health care personnel? What is an adequate number? Most studies of health personnel report that the supply of health providers has greatly increased in the past two decades. It has been shown that there is a surplus of most medical specialists. On the other hand, there continues to be a need for general practice physicians. Also, a serious lack of women and minorities in the various medical care professions continues to exist.

The majority of persons in the health care industry are allied health personnel. There are over one hundred occupational titles with over three million employed persons that fall into this category. These persons are trained to contribute to the care, treatment, and rehabilitation of the patient. The education and training of allied health personnel have become more academic, and a number of allied health fields now have state and national standards for obtaining credentials. Most of the health professions have some type of professional association for membership of those certified in the given field.

Health care personnel work in medical offices, clinics, and outpatient facilities, as well as in hospitals and other long-term inpatient settings. Most hospitalization in the United States occurs in community hospitals. The trend in hospital development in recent years has been toward larger, more comprehensive facilities, with many being owned by for-profit health care corporations.

Growing economic stresses have had an impact on the operation of most hospitals in America in the past decade, with smaller, rural hospitals experiencing much of the impact. Many of these facilities have had to close, leaving large segments of the rural U.S. population without a hospital.

Discussion Questions

1. What are some of the issues relating to the physician work force?

2. Discuss some of the reasons for the shortage of primary care physicians in the United States.

3. What medical specialities are usually classified as general, primary care?

4. What are reasons for the lack of female and minority health care providers?

5. Identify some of the specific characteristics of osteopathic and chiropractic medicine.

6. What have the courts stated concerning the status of chiropractic medicine?

7. Identify the basic characteristic of naturopathy, homeopathy, and naparapathy.

8. What are some reasons for the shortage of nurses interested in working in the hospital setting?

9. Discuss reasons why the AIDS epidemic has contributed to the need for increased numbers of nurses and allied health personnel.

10. Identify and discuss the trends in nursing education.

11. What are some of the issues that surround the employment of the nonphysician health care provider?

12. Discuss the legal status of the nonphysician health care provider.

13. What are the actions that the nurse-midwife is licensed to perform?

14. Discuss the role that allied health personnel play in the American health care system.

15. Explain the differences between physical therapy and occupational therapy.

16. What are several specialities of medical lab technology?

17. What are some of the trends in the education and certification of allied health personnel?

18. Identify some of the activities and roles played by professional health associations.

19. Identify some of the factors that have contributed to the growth of for-profit hospitals.

20. What are some of the questions raised by the increase in operation of hospitals by large, for-profit, health care corporations?

21. Discuss some of the issues concerning rural hospitals.

22. How did the interest in containing health costs affect hospitals in the 1980s?

23. What is diversification as it relates to hospitals?

24. Discuss services provided in outpatient health care facilities.

25. In your opinion, how can the needs of the economically disadvantaged be met when hospitalization is required?

Suggested Readings

Adams, Constance J. "Nurse-Midwifery Practice in the United States, 1982 and 1987." *American Journal of Public Health* 79, no. 8 (August 1989): 1038–39.

Batey, Marjorie V., and Jeanne M. Holland. "Prescribing Practices among Nurse Practitioners in Adult and Family Health." *American Journal of Public Health* 75, no. 3 (March 1985): 258–62.

Bowman, Marjorie A. "Family Physicians: Supply and Demand." *Public Health Reports* 104, no. 3 (May/June 1989): 286–90.

Campion, Edward W. "Why Unconventional Medicine?" *New England Journal of Medicine* 328, no. 4 (January 28, 1993): 282–83.

Eisenberg, David M., and others. "Unconventional Medicine in the United States: Prevalence, Costs, and Patterns of Use." *New England Journal of Medicine* 328, no. 4 (January 28, 1993): 246–52.

Elwood, Thomas. "Overview of Allied Health Personnel Shortages." *Journal of Allied Health* 20, no. 1 (1991): 47–62.

Executive Summary. "Healthy America: Practitioners for 2005." *Journal of Allied Health* 21, no. 4 (Fall 1992): 3–66.

Henry, Marie O. "How Many Nurse Practitioners Are Enough?" *American Journal of Public Health* 76, no. 5 (May 1986): 493.

Higgins, Linda C. "Rural Docs." *Medical World News* (December 11, 1989): 32–38.

"How Each State Stands on Legislative Issues Affecting Advanced Nursing Practice." *The Nurse Practitioner* 15, no. 1 (January 1990): 11–18.

Institute of Medicine, National Academy of Sciences. "Allied Health Services: Avoiding Crisis." *Journal of Allied Health* 18, no. 4 (Summer 1989): 335–47.

Pattison, Robert V., and Halliem Katz. "Investor-Owned and Not-For-Profit Hospitals." *New England Journal of Medicine* 309, no. 6 (August 11, 1983): 347–53.

Public Health Service. *Minorities and Women in the Health Fields.* Washington, D.C.: U.S. Government Printing Office (1990).

Public Health Service. *Seventh Report to the President and Congress on the Status of Health Personnel in the United States.* Washington, D.C.: U.S. Government Printing Office, 1990. DHHS Pub. #HRS-P-09-90-1.

Rogers, Bonnie, Sue Sweeting, and Barbara Davis. "Employment and Salary Characteristics of Nurse Practitioners." *The Nurse Practitioner* 14, no. 9 (September 1989): 56–63.

Schlesinger, Mark. "The Rise of Proprietary Health Care." *Business and Health* 2, no. 3 (January/February 1985): 7–12.

Schroeder, Steven A. "Physician Supply and the U.S. Medical Marketplace." *Health Affairs* 11, no. 1 (Spring 1992): 235–43.

Shanks-Meile, Stephanie L., and others. "Changes in the Advertised Demand for Nurse Practitioners in the United States, 1975–1986." *The Nurse Practitioner* 14, no. 9 (September 1989): 41–49.

Simpson, Clay E., and Remy Aronoff. "Factors Affecting the Supply of Minority Physicians in 2000." *Public Health Reports* 103, no. 3 (March/April 1988): 178–84.

Stoll, G. Alan. "Accreditation in the Allied Health Professions." *Journal of Allied Health* 18, no. 5 (Fall 1989): 425–35.

Thibodeau, Janice A., and Joellen W. Hawkins. "Nurse Practitioners: Factors Affecting Role Performance." *The Nurse Practitioner* 14, no. 12 (December 1989): 47–52.

Tootelian, Dennis H., and Ralph M. Gaedeke. "The Changing Role of Pharmacies in the 1990s." *Journal of Health Care Marketing* 6, no. 1 (March 1986): 57–63.

Endnotes

1. U.S. Bureau of the Census. *Statistical Abstracts of the United States,* 1992, 12th Ed., Washington, D.C.: U.S. Government Printing Office, 1992.

2. Public Health Service. *Seventh Report to the President and Congress on the Status of Health Personnel in the United States.* Washington, D.C.: U.S. Government Printing Office, 1990, p. II-1.

3. *Ibid.,* p. II-1.

4. Public Health Service. *Eighth Report to the President and Congress on the Status of Health Personnel in the United States.* Washington, D.C.: U.S. Government Printing Office, 1991.

5. National Health Insurance Association. *Source Book of Health Insurance Data,* n.d., p. 77.

6. Public Health Service, *Seventh Report to the President and Congress.*

7. National College of Chiropractic. *Fact Sheet on Chiropractic.* Lombard, Ill.: The College (n.d.).

8. Campion, Edward W. "Why Unconventional Medicine?" *New England Journal of Medicine* 328, no. 4 (January 28, 1993): 282–83.

9. *Ibid.*

10. *Ibid.*

11. Public Health Service, *Eighth Report to the President and Congress,* IV-C-2.

12. Mauksch, Ingeborg G. "The Nurse Practitioner Movement—Where Does It Go from Here?" *American Journal of Public Health* 68, no. 11 (November 1978): 1074.

13. Henry, Marie O. "How Many Nurse Practitioners Are Enough?" *American Journal of Public Health* 76, no. 5 (May 1986): 493.

14. Weinberger, Morris, and others. "Changing Nurse Staff Attitudes toward Nurse Practitioners during Their Residency Training." *American Journal of Public Health* 70, no. 11 (November 1980): 1206.

15. Henry, "How Many Nurse Practitioners?" 493.

16. Hayes, Eileen. "The Nurse Practitioner: History, Current Conflicts, and Future Survival." *Journal of College Health* 34, no. 3 (December 1985): 145.

17. Rooks, Judith Bourne, and Susan H. Fischman. "American Nurse-Midwifery Practice in 1976–1977: Reflections of 50 Years of Growth and Development." *American Journal of Public Health* 70, no 9 (September 1980): 990.

18. *Ibid.,* 990.

19. Information provided by American College of Nurse-Midwives.

20. Department of Health, Education, and Welfare. *A Report on Allied Health Personnel,* DHEW Pub. No. (HRA) 80-28, PHS, Health Resources Administration, Bureau of Health Manpower, 1980: 1–2.

21. Elwood, Thomas. "Overview of Allied Health Personnel Shortages." *Journal of Allied Health* 20, no. 1 (1991): 49.

22. Department of Health, Education, and Welfare. *A Report on Allied Health Personnel,* III-1.

23. *Ibid.,* III–5.

24. *Ibid.,* III–6.

25. U.S. Bureau of the Census, *Statistical Abstracts,* 112.

26. Friedmam, Emily. "The For-Profits." *Medical World News* (February 27, 1989): 36.

27. Higgins, Linda C. "Rural Docs." *Medical World News* (December 11, 1989): 32–8.

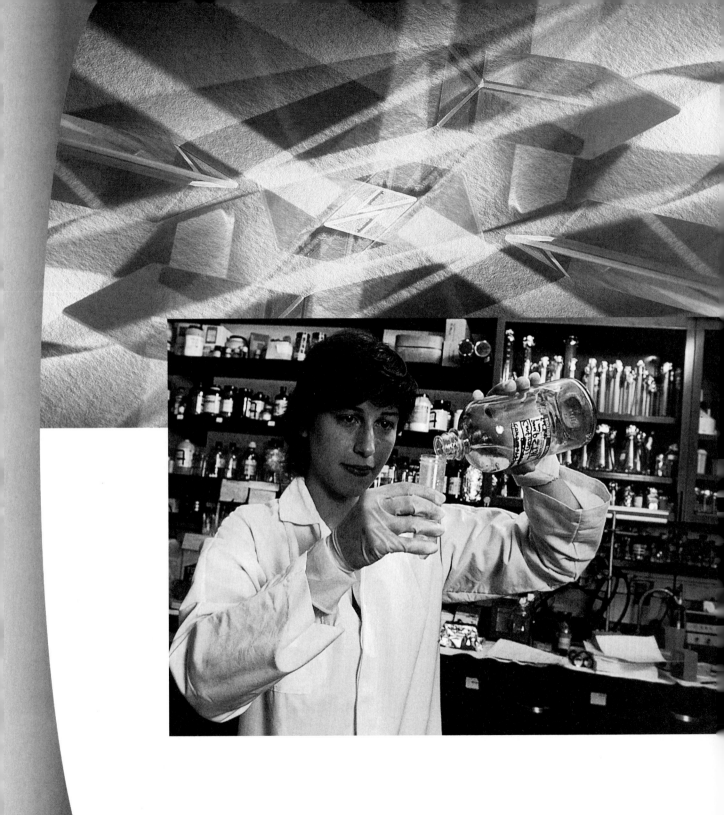

Programming for Community Health

CHAPTER   **NINE**

Epidemiology

Counting and Analyzing for Planning and Programming

What Is Epidemiology?

Historically, the study of the occurrence of diseases in human populations has been known as epidemiology. The term *epidemiology* is derived from the two Greek words *epi* and *demos, epi* meaning "among" and *demos* meaning "people." Hence, the work of epidemiology looks at such factors as the distribution of disease and injury and the determinants of these conditions among people. Epidemiological study is focused upon groups of persons, not separate individuals.

Investigation of disease occurrence is not new. It is likely that humankind first began to study disease causation and distribution by asking simple questions. What is causing sickness in our family? Why is there an increase in illness among our people? Is there a reason why adults do not get certain illnesses they had when they were children?

The more formal development of epidemiology came about as a result of studying the great communicable disease epidemics of the past, such as smallpox, yellow fever, cholera, the plague, and numerous other infectious diseases. The primary emphasis has been on identifying the *etiology* or cause of specific diseases.

The findings of epidemiological study can be used for many purposes. One use is to determine the magnitude of diseases or other conditions and their impact on certain populations. Information gathered from the epidemiological process can be used in setting community health program priorities, in evaluating the effectiveness of current programs, and in determining what type of treatment facilities may be needed in the future.

Through the years the procedures of epidemiology have been applied to a broad range of problems other than infectious diseases. For example, early studies in this century looked at problems of malnutrition. Lack of certain nutrients among population groups resulted in such conditions as scurvy and pellagra. More recently the procedures and techniques of epidemiology have focused on chronic illnesses, such as malignant diseases, cardiovascular diseases, diabetes, the various types of arthritic conditions, and a host of other chronic ailments. The

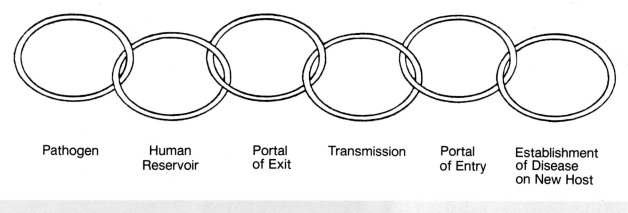

Figure 9.1 The chain of infection.

process of epidemiological study has been applied to injury causation and prevention. It has been used widely in occupational safety and health studies, in studies of health services needs, in the measurement of health risks, and in health planning. Epidemiological methods are also applied to family planning, congenital defects, mental illness, and drug addiction.

Epidemiology asks what characteristics that seem to contribute to a given disease can be identified within a population group. It also looks at the role that environmental factors play in certain people getting a specific disease or injury. Epidemiology looks at frequencies of diseases in groups of people and identifies factors that influence these frequencies. It also provides a procedure for identifying specific concerns when trying to resolve a particular problem.

The Epidemiological Model

The epidemiological model involves the interaction of three different factors influencing disease: (1) the *causative agent,* (2) the *host,* and (3) the *environmental factors.* Epidemiological research is directed toward one, two, or all three of these factors with the hope of breaking the "chain of infection." A change in any of the three components can affect the factor under study.

The Chain of Infection

In the case of infectious diseases, a host may be an individual, an animal, or a plant. Our concern is primarily with diseases where humans are the host. Pathogenic microorganisms, or pathogens, leave the host reservoir through a route of discharge, known as a *portal of exit.* Examples of portals of exit are discharges from the mouth and the nose by coughing, sneezing, breathing, and speaking. Other portals of exit are fecal wastes, saliva, blood, mucous membranes, semen, open wounds, sores, and insect bites.

Once the pathogen comes into contact with a new host, it enters by what is known as a *portal of entry.* Usually the portal of entry and portal of exit are part of the same body system. For example, microorganisms that leave a host reservoir by way of the nose and mouth, such as by a cough or sneeze, enter another host who breathes the air droplets containing the pathogen. Pathogens that leave a host by way of human feces work their way back into the food or water chain and so into the digestive system when food or water are ingested. This communicable disease chain of infection is pictured in figure 9.1. Communicable disease control measures are effective if they break any one of the links in this chain of infection.

Pathogenic microorganisms are transmitted between the host reservoir and a new host in several different ways: by direct contact, by indirect contact, by airborne transfer, and through the action of a vector (figure 9.2).

Direct contact transmits disease when a new host comes into contact with the infected skin or mucous membrane. This is the case in sexually transmitted diseases; the microorganisms of syphilis, gonorrhea, and AIDS are transferred through the direct contact of sexual partners.

Figure 9.2 Pathogen transmission from host to host.

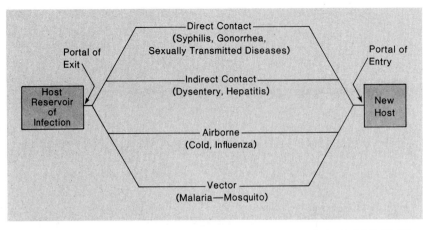

Indirect transmission involves an intermediate object as the mode of transmission between hosts. Diseases that are spread by the ingestion of contaminated food, milk, and water are considered to be the result of indirect transmission. This is also the case when the pathogenic microorganism is present on towels, bedding, hypodermic needles, and other objects—all known as *fomites*—that are used by a diseased person. The disease is transmitted to another individual who uses the same objects. Serum hepatitis is an example of an indirectly transmitted disease. The microorganisms remain on hypodermic needles so that when drug addicts share unsterile utensils, the disease is transmitted from one host to another. This occurs in AIDS transmission also.

Another means of communicable disease transmission between hosts is through *airborne transfer*. Disease organisms are spread on either air droplets or dust from one locality to a host. The common cold and influenza are spread in this way.

Vectors are arthropods that transmit pathogenic microorganisms from one host to another. Many insects spread disease by biting the host and transferring the pathogen. Others carry the pathogenic organisms on their body and contaminate food ingested by hosts. The fly is a common vector of disease.

The most widespread communicable disease in the world is malaria. This disease is caused by a parasite, a one-celled protozoan, and transmitted by the *Anopheles* mosquito. This parasite spends part of its life cycle in human red blood cells and the other part in the female *Anopheles* mosquito.

Malaria

The Most Widespread of the World's Diseases

Several factors come into play in developing control programs for malaria. Malaria can be controlled by destroying the mosquitoes and their breeding places. This is not an easy task and is unlikely to succeed. Swamps must be drained, breeding places sprayed with pesticides such as DDT to destroy the larvae, and all sources of standing water eliminated.

Malaria transmission occurs primarily between dusk and dawn. This is because of the nocturnal feeding habits of *Anopheles* mosquitoes. Therefore, individuals need to stay in well screened areas, use mosquito nets, and wear clothes that cover the entire body.

Chloroquine has been the primary drug in treating malaria attacks. It is used both to cure and to provide protection against malaria. But the microorganism that causes malaria has become increasingly resistant to chloroquine in much of the world. This has led to an increase in the number of cases in the United States, as well as worldwide.

Since 1982 the Centers for Disease Control and Prevention has recommended the combined use of chloroquine and Fansidar for those traveling in chloroquine-resistant areas, but Fansidar may have adverse side effects. Individuals who have histories of reaction to sulfa drugs should not use this medication.

Research has attempted to find alternative drugs for providing protection from malaria. Most have been of limited value or cause adverse reactions. A new drug, mefloquine, is now being used with some success.

Communicable Disease Control

The control of communicable disease requires action to break the chain of infection. This action may involve the human host, as when an individual is immunized before being exposed to a disease, or it may mean taking drugs for protection against the pathogens, as when individuals take chloroquine as protection against malaria.

Control measures may be taken to reduce the possibility of pathogen transmission between hosts. For instance, a condom can be used during sexual intercourse to protect against the spread of sexually transmitted diseases. In addition, any disease control program administered by a community health agency is usually designed to reduce or eliminate disease vectors.

In determining the needed communicable disease control measure or measures, it must first be decided where the focus would be most effective: on the host, the reservoir of infection, the microorganism, or the means of transmission. Economy, effectiveness, education, and available resources are all factors in this decision.

Acquired Immunodeficiency Syndrome (AIDS) and the Chain of Infection

To bring about control of or to eradicate a disease, the chain of infection must be broken. This is true for the most minor of the communicable diseases as well as those occurring at epidemic proportions throughout the world. During the 1930s and 1940s poliomyelitis caused extensive debilitation and death throughout the United States. It wasn't until the mid-1950s when a vaccine was developed that this feared disease was brought under control. This control effort has been directed at protecting the *host*. Similarly, worldwide initiatives to eradicate smallpox began in the latter part of the 1960s and extended through the 1970s. This disease had disfigured millions and killed additional millions, and smallpox epidemics had even affected the course of history. Eradication has occurred because various initiatives have eliminated the *reservoirs of infection* for this disease.

During the 1980s another disease, acquired immunodeficiency syndrome (AIDS), became a worldwide epidemic. At present, there is no known measure that effectively breaks the chain of infection, and the number of cases and deaths continues to escalate.

Innumerable initiatives are being undertaken in order to resolve this issue. Scientific, medical, epidemiological, and social research is being conducted throughout the United States and other countries of the world. Applying the epidemiological model of disease control indicates the measures most likely to succeed in eventually eliminating AIDS.

The disease is spread from a reservoir of infection (a person who has the HIV virus) to another individual (a host) in several ways. The two most commonly identified modes of microorganism transmission are through direct person-to-person sexual contact and through common use of blood-infected drug needles. What procedures might be considered for controlling or eradicating AIDS by focusing on the reservoir of infection?

It is known that the causative agent of AIDS is the *human immunodeficiency virus (HIV)*. Knowledge about viruses indicates that it is impossible to find a cure for this disease by the development of effective vaccines as might be possible if the causative agent were a bacterium.

Disease control initiatives directed toward the reservoir of infection have shown to be of little value. Unfortunately, once an individual has AIDS there is no cure. No medication can bring about a cure or remission. Scientists have experimented with some pharmaceuticals, with azidothymidine (AZT) being the most successful. However these drugs have only slowed the progress of the disease or alleviated the symptoms. As a cure, none has been effective.

Are there other measures that could be directed at the reservoir of infection? On occasion some individuals have made rather outlandish suggestions, such as placing all AIDS patients in confinement. Certainly quarantine has been used in the past for control of some diseases; however, it is considered most unsatisfactory as a control measure for AIDS because of infringement of individual rights.

Because the chain of infection is unlikely to be broken at the reservoir of infection, the next step is to consider the prospective host. This is the uninfected person who is likely to get the disease when exposed. The basic measures of transmission of the disease are by sexual contact and use of infected IV drug needles, so the chain of infection could be broken by refraining from activities that allow infection. For some this is readily accomplished by abstaining from illicit sexual activity and the use of illegal drugs. In the value system of many Americans, this is a logical solution to the problem. From a public health perspective, abstinence alone will not resolve the problem since many people choose different behavior.

The development of a vaccine that will protect the host, as has occurred with numerous other diseases such as polio, is also receiving much attention and research. It is likely that, in time, this will happen.

However, the scientific community currently believes this is at least a decade away. In the meantime, the number of AIDS cases continues to mount.

At present, preventive measures are the only truly effective means for breaking the chain of infection of AIDS at the host. Such practices as using a condom during sexual intercourse, having sex with only one partner, and not using infected IV needles are appropriate actions.

However, these measures do not resolve the problem—the control and/or eradication of AIDS. The answers to the questions concerning where on the chain of infection major initiatives and resources should be directed have become a leading political issue and are not easy to determine. Nevertheless, such decisions are most important if we are going to break the chain of infection for the most serious disease of the 1990s—AIDS.

Noncommunicable Disease Applications

The application of the epidemiological model has broadened to a number of areas other than infectious diseases. Currently, it is widely used within the community health, health care, and injury prevention fields, as well as in studies of chronic disease risk factors, disabilities, and personal and group health practices.

The epidemiological model has been used in the study and prevention of unintentional injuries. This model was first suggested as an approach to accident prevention in 1948.[1] When the focus is directed toward the person (the host), various actions can be taken to reduce the risk of an accident. For example, the development of driving skills or bicycle riding skills helps reduce the possibility of injury. The agent of causation of an industrial or home injury may be one of a number of different possibilities. It may be a piece of metal that flies into the eye of an individual running a lathe in a factory, or it may be a knife resting in a drawer that cuts a finger when one reaches in. The agent of injury may be the flame from a grill or a fire. Measures need to be taken to reduce the possibility of the causative agent coming into contact with the individual. This may mean purchasing a car with a padded dashboard or a shatterproof windshield. It means putting sharp tools in storage racks or wearing eye protection devices.

Environmental health studies make extensive use of the epidemiological model. For example, Three Mile Island, Chernobyl, the Love Canal, and hundreds more other environmental accidents have been investigated using this model to determine their effects on human health. Studies of environmental toxic exposures often warrant long-term, continuing surveillance.

Possibly the most widespread use of epidemiology today is the study of risk factors associated with chronic diseases. Cancer, cardiovascular diseases, diabetes, and many other chronic conditions are focuses for every type of epidemiological study. Various factors that might be linked to the specific cause of the disease and individual health behaviors of the population under study are explored. The etiology of chronic diseases often involves multiple risk factors. Also, the time period between exposure and actual presentation of the signs and symptoms of the chronic disease is usually lengthy. Because of these two factors the application of the epidemiologic model to chronic disease control is very complex, often necessitating long-term data collection and analysis before interventions can be identified to cope with the chronic disease. Any review of the medical, epidemiological, and community health literature will reveal innumerable studies involving the epidemiological model.

For example, in studying the relationship between the use of smokeless tobacco and oral cancers, the epidemiologists might direct attention toward the individual using tobacco (the host), the tobacco itself (the agent), or the means of obtaining the product (the environment). It is first beneficial to ascertain the most efficient focus. For instance, programs designed to educate the host about the dangers associated with chewing-tobacco products have been developed. It is doubtful that measures directed toward the elimination of the agent, the tobacco, are effective. Some ordinances and regulations have been established to discourage its purchase. However, most disease control professionals have concluded, by using the epidemiological model, that the best way to reduce this "cycle of disease" is to focus on the host.

Types of Epidemiological Studies

Analysis and study of data leads to the establishment of a hypothesis or several hypotheses about the causative agent. Once the hypothesis is established, it is necessary to test it. Epidemiologists conduct such tests either by observational or experimental study.

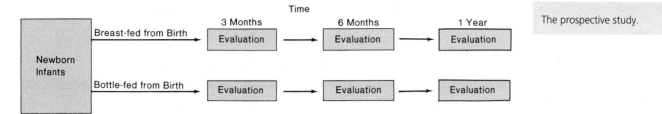

Cohort—Newborn Infants
Factor under Study—Breast-feeding Compared with Bottle-feeding and the Effect on Growth and Development
Time Factor—Selected Time Intervals
Evaluation—Weight Gain at 3 and 6 Months and One Year
   Physiological Development at 3 and 6 Months and One Year
   Motor Development at 3 and 6 Months and One Year

Observational Studies

Not involving the manipulation of a population, these kinds of epidemiological investigations focus on events in a field setting, such as a community, hospital, clinic, school, worksite, or other environmental setting. Grouping of a specific population for analysis is on the basis of certain identified characteristics such as age, race, gender, occupation, or other demographic variables.

There are three different kinds of observational studies: (1) prospective, (2) retrospective, and (3) cross-sectional. A *prospective study* begins with a group of people who are free of the disease or problem under investigation and share common experiences. This grouping is referred to as a *cohort*. The individuals vary in the degree of exposure to a given factor being studied. The different groups are followed over a period of time to ascertain the effect of exposure to the given factor.

For example, in a study to ascertain the effect of breast-feeding compared with bottle-feeding on child development, a specific number of pregnant women are selected. Certain information is gathered concerning the women's attitudes and knowledge relating to breast-feeding. Data might be collected about risk factors during the pregnancy. After the birth of the infants, both groups, those bottle-fed and those breast-fed, are identified and data is collected. Selected time factors will be established (i.e., 3 months, 6 months, 1 year). A variety of data might be evaluated, such as weight gain, physiological development, and basic motor skills development. Comparisons

are made and conclusions drawn about the role of breast-feeding or bottle-feeding in child development.

A prospective study involves group identification before the disease or factor under consideration develops. Though one particular factor is usually designed into the study, observations of a variety of outcomes can often be obtained from this type of study. For example, if a group of young adults was being studied for several years to ascertain the effectiveness of regular exercise in reducing hypertension, it is most likely that a number of other measurements could also be made relating to such factors as cholesterol levels, triglycerides, and overall weight control.

The prospective study usually is long-term, expensive, and time-consuming. It is often very difficult to maintain controls because the cohort group must have a large number, resulting in rather large-scale projects.

One of the best-known prospective studies in the United States has been the Framingham, Massachusetts, cardiovascular disease study, which was started in 1948 and conducted by the United States Public Health Service. The primary goal was to ascertain the relationship of a number of different factors to the development of heart disease. More than six thousand individuals between the ages of thirty and sixty-two were initially selected to be studied over a period of twenty years. During this time all participants were given a physical examination every other year in order to obtain information about factors related to heart disease, such as serum cholesterol, blood

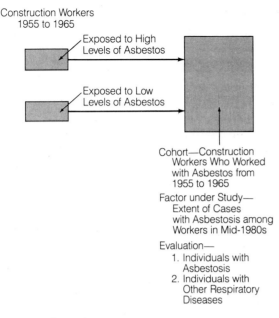

Construction Workers
1955 to 1965

Exposed to High
Levels of Asbestos

Exposed to Low
Levels of Asbestos

Cohort—Construction
Workers Who Worked
with Asbestos from
1955 to 1965

Factor under Study—
Extent of Cases
with Asbestosis among
Workers in Mid-1980s

Evaluation—
1. Individuals with
   Asbestosis
2. Individuals with
   Other Respiratory
   Diseases

The retrospective study.

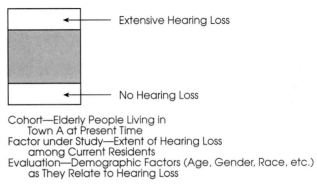

Extensive Hearing Loss

No Hearing Loss

Cohort—Elderly People Living in
Town A at Present Time
Factor under Study—Extent of Hearing Loss
among Current Residents
Evaluation—Demographic Factors (Age, Gender, Race, etc.)
as They Relate to Hearing Loss

The cross-sectional study.

pressure, weight, and cigarette smoking. Great amounts of information about risk factors and heart disease were acquired.[2] The Framingham Study has been used as a prototype for similar long-term studies in other localities.

A second type of observational study is the *retrospective study*. This type of study looks at population groups that include individuals with or without the disease. The past history of these people is analyzed in order to ascertain what factors, either personal life-style, environmental, or other, might have led to the cause of the health problem under consideration and why others in the study were not affected. In this type of study the individuals who have the disease or problem under examination are referred to as "cases," while those that do not have the problem are "controls."

One might wish to study those factors that contributed to the development of asbestosis among a certain population group. A selected sample of employees who worked with asbestos in the construction industry over a given period (maybe from 1955 to 1965) are chosen for the study. These individuals are similar with respect to other factors except for the specific exposure under study. Comparisons are made with regard to the presence of asbestosis at the present time, and conclusions are formulated about what factors might have caused this

disease. Retrospective studies are less expensive to conduct and are less time-consuming. It is also possible to look at more than one risk factor in this type of study.

Another type of study often used in epidemiological study is the *cross-sectional study*. In this procedure exposure of two groups being compared is limited to their current situations. The cross-sectional study does not establish a sequence of events leading to findings. It is simply a survey of present status, which is the simplest form of observational study. Survey studies are undertaken to describe the distribution of disease or other factors of concern. They are easy to accomplish, and can be done in a rather short period.

For example, a study might be conducted to ascertain the extent of hearing loss among elderly people living in a given community. Certain criteria are established as to what will be considered acceptable hearing levels and what will be considered serious hearing loss. Procedures for measuring hearing levels are identified, and those involved in the study are tested. A variety of demographic factors may be of interest as they relate to hearing loss, including age, gender, race, location of residence, and occupation.

Experimental Studies

Unlike observational studies, where the epidemiologist only observes and records, experimental epidemiology involves a manipulation or intervention of human populations. The conditions of the study can be controlled. This type of study seeks to identify cause-and-effect relationships.

In experimental research some action is taken within a population group. It may be the withholding of a treatment, a drug, or other factor from an identified group to ascertain certain relationships and causes. On the other hand, it may be exposing the experimental group to medication, a vaccine, or something that has an uncertain effect. Experimental epidemiology can be divided into (1) clinical studies and (2) community studies.

There are three types of *clinical studies:* (1) therapeutic trials, (2) intervention, and (3) preventive. The *therapeutic study* attempts to determine whether a therapeutic procedure is effective in relieving symptoms of a disease or whether its use will improve the specific conditions relating to the disease. Probably the most common type of therapeutic study involves the study of the effects of a new healing modality or a new drug.

Intervention studies involve the application of some intervention modality in an attempt to improve the chances that disease risk can be reduced. For example, many studies have been conducted to ascertain the effect of exercising in reducing risk for cardiovascular disease, hypertension, and stroke.

The *preventive study* involves the application of some measure designed to prevent disease. Probably the most common preventive epidemiological studies are vaccination programs. Vaccines are applied to a population group to prevent diseases such as tuberculosis, malaria, and the childhood diseases.

In medicine and public health, experimental studies are not always feasible. For example, if a study looking at the relationships of chewing tobacco and oral cancer were being conducted, it would be necessary to randomly assign individuals to two groups. One group would be required to chew tobacco for a given period of time, the other would not be permitted to use any tobacco products. Obviously, using human subjects to intentionally cause illness, disease, or debilitation is unacceptable. Random selection to the chewing-tobacco group would be considered unethical. One can see that many human experimental studies are not possible. Therefore, much experimental research must be performed in the laboratory with animals.

Animal research is also the setting in which many early effects of drugs are first studied. Only where there is a strong possibility of success can human research take place.

The experimental epidemiological research study must be controlled if it is to provide useful information. This type of study involves identifying at least two equally assigned groups. In the development of an experimental study individuals are assigned to specific groups for study. It is important that the groups to be studied are comparable. Two groups are usually identified: (1) the *control group,* which will not be given the particular factor, and (2) the *experimental group,* which will be given the specific treatment under study. The researcher should randomly assign subjects to specific study groups. It is also possible to conduct experimental studies using several groups. In these situations several different types or amounts of the treatment may be tested.

A second type of experimental study is the *community study.* Rather than the subjects being individually selected and assigned to a study group, a population group is selected for involvement in the study. Individuals residing in the community of selection are studied. One of the classic public health community experimental studies was begun in 1945 in New York state to ascertain the effectiveness of preventing tooth decay by placing fluoride in the public drinking water. In that study two communities located about thirty-five miles apart, Newburgh and Kingston, New York, were selected. The communities were about equal in population. Sodium fluoride was added to the drinking water of Newburgh, while the drinking water of Kingston was left unchanged. For ten years children of various ages were examined for tooth decay in the two communities. It was concluded after ten years of study that the fluoridation of public drinking water is an effective and safe measure for reducing the incidence of tooth decay. Data supporting fluoridation as a safe and effective dental caries preventive strategy continues to be collected.[3]

Measurement Used in Epidemiology

Quantitative data is used to identify the incidence of a disease or specific factor being studied in a selected population. Biostatistics, or counts of individuals, are the basic data used in epidemiology.

Presentation of Data

Data that are collected in epidemiological studies must be presented in a useful manner. Initially one has simply a frequency count. For example, one may have fifteen persons in a factory who were injured last month, or twelve college students who sought assistance of the university health center physicians for food poisoning in the past two weeks. How serious are these numbers? Do we have a problem of epidemic proportion in either case? To make decisions about the extent of the problem it is necessary to have additional information and to break the raw numbers down into useful data.

Frequency counts are the simplest, most often used statistical procedure in epidemiology, but they are of little value in and of themselves. In order to be useful, data must be presented as proportions or rates, which put data into some perspective in relationship to the population under consideration. Rates (R) are usually expressed as the number of people with a given problem in relation to the number of persons in the population at risk, and are obtained by dividing the number of cases of the problem under study by the population in the study.

$$R = \frac{\text{Number of Cases}}{\text{Population under Study}}$$

In order to be able to use data for analysis and decision making it is important that the ratios being used have been gathered with regard to similar time periods. Two types of data rates are used: prevalence rate and incidence rate. It is important in vital statistical analysis to know whether the data being used consist of prevalence or incidence rates. These statistics are not comparable. It is like the "apples and oranges" analogy. They are not similar, and any comparison between them has no place in community health work.[4]

Prevalence rate. Data can be presented as the number of persons with a given problem *at a particular point in time*. This is known as the *prevalence rate*. The prevalence rate indicates the number of people out of the considered population who have the disease at a specific time. The prevalence rate is determined by dividing the number of existing cases by the total population involved in the study. This result should be multiplied by 1,000, 10,000, or 100,000 depending on what ratio for comparison one wishes to use. When considering prevalence rates, the ratio is usually expressed per 1,000 population.

Formula for Prevalence Rate

$$\frac{\text{Number of Existing Cases}}{\text{Total Population}} \times 1,000$$
(At a specific point in time)

For example, in a school district with 7,540 students, there were 69 absent on February 16 with colds. The prevalence rate on February 16 was 9.15 (per 1,000).

$$\frac{69 \ (\text{existing cases})}{7,540 \ (\text{total school population})} = 0.00915 \times 1,000 = 9.15$$

Incidence rate. Another type of statistic used by epidemiologists is the *incidence rate*. This measures the number of cases that developed *over a specific period of time*. It reflects the number of new occurrences that developed in ratio to the total population at risk. The formula for determining incidence rate involves dividing the number of new cases by the number of individuals in the population at risk over a given period of time. This decimal is multiplied by whatever ratio for comparison is going to be used (i.e., 1,000, 10,000, or 100,000).

Formula for Incidence Rate

$$\frac{\text{Number of New Cases}}{\text{Population at Risk}} \times 1,000$$
(Over a given period of time)

For example, in a given community of senior citizens during the months of November and December, 36 people developed influenza to the extent that it necessitated a visit to the physician. The population at risk for this study, senior citizens, numbers 6,121. The incidence rate for the common cold during these two months was 5.88.

$$\frac{36 \ (\text{new cases of the common cold})}{6,121 \ (\text{senior citizens at risk})} = 0.00588 \times 1,000 = 5.88$$

Sources of Data

Data that are used in epidemiological work come from a variety of different sources. Much information is available from data collected every ten years in the national census. The recording of vital data by the local and state health departments provides a vast array of information for use in epidemiology. Also, morbidity information can be obtained from many other sources in the community such as hospitals, clinics, physicians, schools, and the courts.

Census Data

In the United States a census, that is, a gathering of information on the entire national population, has been conducted by the Federal Bureau of the Census every ten years since 1790. Census data that are useful to epidemiological studies include age, gender, race, marital status, and other factors such as geographical distribution. Use is made in epidemiology of census data to determine the vital health events as rates.

Vital Statistics

The major source of information about the health of a population lies in the collection of vital statistics. The individual state and local health departments are required to collect and register vital data on citizens within their jurisdictions. These vital statistics include births, deaths, marriages, divorces, and morbidity from various diseases.

Data are collected by the local health department and are then relayed to the state health department for compilation and statistical analysis. Legal responsibility for registration of vital data lies with the state governments. The vital statistics section of the state health department handles the recording of the data. The official record is filed permanently in that office. When an individual needs to obtain a copy of a birth certificate or other personal document, a copy may be obtained from the state health department.

Statistical information collected by state health departments is transmitted to the National Center for Health Statistics in Washington, D.C., where nationwide vital statistics are compiled and disseminated. This center was established in 1960 to provide data—to any agency, organization, or persons needing such data—regarding births, deaths, illnesses, disability, health services, marriages, and divorces. In addition to these data, it now has an extensive body of information regarding health status, utilization of health resources, and health care expenditures in the nation. It became part of the Centers for Disease Control in 1987. Each year the National Center for Health Statistics publishes an annual report entitled *Vital Statistics of the United States.*

Vital statistics are helpful in community health program planning. From the study of such data, it is possible for health officials to determine where specific problems exist and to tailor corrective action accordingly.

Live Births By law all live births must be recorded and a certificate of live birth registered. A standard certificate of live birth has been developed by the National Center for Health Statistics. This certificate contains two parts. The first part identifies the name of the child and the parents, and the second part is designed for "medical and health use only." Information in this section—about maternal age, race, birthweight, marital status and education of parents, plus the pregnancy history of the mother—is useful for epidemiological investigations.

In 1989 the National Center for Health Statistics made several changes in the birth certificate. A standard certificate was designed that is to become the basis for state certificates. This newly developed certificate is expanded from previous ones to include additional information relating to health promotion and disease.

The new birth certificate now incorporates information on sixteen risk factors that can affect pregnancy outcome including tobacco and alcohol use and weight gain during pregnancy. These can be noted and checked on the certificate. Information about obstetric procedures, the method of delivery, and abnormal conditions of the newborn can also be checked and noted.

The standard statistical datum used for stating birth rates is the *crude birth rate*. This statistic is arrived at by dividing the number of live births during the year by the average population at midyear. In formula it looks like this:

$$\text{Crude Birth Rate} = \frac{\text{Number of Live Births during the Year}}{\text{Average Population at Midyear}}$$

The usual factor for expressing birth rate is per one thousand population.

A live birth has been defined as:

. . . the complete expulsion or extraction from its mother of a product of human conception, irrespective of the duration of pregnancy, which, after such expulsion or extraction, breathes, or shows any other evidence of life such as beating of the heart, pulsation of the umbilical cord, or definite movement of voluntary muscles, whether or not the umbilical cord has been cut or the placenta is attached.[5]

This definition, which is based upon the 1950 World Health Organization definition, is used in most states of

Ohio Department of Health
VITAL STATISTICS
CERTIFICATE OF LIVE BIRTH

Reg. Dist. No. _____
Primary Reg. Dist. No. _____

Registrar's No. _____

Birth No. 134 —

TYPE OR PRINT IN PERMANENT BLACK INK.

CHILD

1. CHILD - NAME First Middle Last | 2. SEX | 3a. DATE OF BIRTH (Month, Day, Year) | 3b. TIME OF BIRTH M

4a. FACILITY NAME (If not institution, give street and number) | 4b. CITY, VILLAGE OR LOCATION OF BIRTH | 4c. COUNTY OF BIRTH

5. PLACE OF BIRTH
☐ Hospital ☐ Freestanding Birthing Center ☐ Clinic/Doctor's Office ☐ Residence ☐ Other (Specify)

6. REGISTRAR'S SIGNATURE | 7. DATE FILED BY REGISTRAR (Month, Day, Year)

ATTENDANT

8a. I certify that the above named child was born alive at the place and time and on the date stated above. | 8b. DATE SIGNED | 8c. ATTENDANT – ☐ M.D. ☐ D.O. ☐ C.N.M.
SIGNATURE ▶ | | ☐ Other Midwife ☐ Other (Specify)
8d. ATTENDANT - NAME (Type or Print) | 8e. MAILING ADDRESS (Street or R.F.D. No., City or Village, State, Zip)

MOTHER

9a. MOTHER'S NAME (First, Middle, Last) | 9b. MAIDEN SURNAME | 10a. DATE OF BIRTH (Month, Day, Year) | 10b. AGE

11. BIRTHPLACE (State or Foreign Country) | 12a. RESIDENCE - STATE | 12b. COUNTY | 12c. CITY, TOWN, OR LOCATION

12d. STREET AND NUMBER | 12e. INSIDE CITY LIMITS? (Yes or No) | 13. MOTHER'S MAILING ADDRESS (If same as residence, enter zip code only)

FATHER

14. FATHER'S NAME (First, Middle, Last) | 15a. DATE OF BIRTH (Month, Day, Year) | 15b. AGE | 16. BIRTHPLACE (State or Foreign Country)

INFORMANT

17. I certify that the personal information provided on this certificate is correct to the best of my knowledge and belief.
Name or Signature of Parent or Other Informant ▶

INFORMATION FOR MEDICAL AND HEALTH USE ONLY

18. OF HISPANIC ORIGIN? (Specify No or Yes - If yes, specify Cuban, Mexican, Puerto Rican, etc.) | 19. RACE — American Indian, Black, White, etc. (Specify below) | 20. EDUCATION (Specify only highest grade completed) | 21. OCCUPATION AND BUSINESS/INDUSTRY (Worked during last year)

Elementary/Secondary (0-12) | College (1-4 or 5+) | Occupation | Business/Industry

MOTHER
18a. ☐ No ☐ Yes Specify: | 19a. | 20a. | 21a. | 21b.

FATHER
18b. ☐ No ☐ Yes Specify: | 19b. | 20b. | 21c. | 21d.

22. PREGNANCY HISTORY (Complete each section) | 23. MOTHER MARRIED? (At birth, conception, or any time between) (Yes or no) | 24. DATE LAST NORMAL MENSES BEGAN (Month, Day, Year)

LIVE BIRTHS (Do not include this child) | OTHER TERMINATIONS (Spontaneous and induced at any time after conception) | 25. MONTH OF PREGNANCY PRENATAL CARE BEGAN - First, Second, Third, etc. (Specify) | 26a. TOTAL PRENATAL VISITS (If none, so state)

26b. CITY | 26c. COUNTY

22a. NOW LIVING | 22b. NOW DEAD | 22d.
Number ___ | Number ___ | Number ___
☐ None | ☐ None | ☐ None

27. BIRTH WEIGHT IN GRAMS | 28. CLINICAL ESTIMATE OF GESTATION (Weeks)

22c. DATE OF LAST LIVE BIRTH (Month, Year) | 22e. DATE OF LAST OTHER TERMINATION (Month, Year) | 29a. PLURALITY - Single, Twin, Triplet, etc. (Specify) | 29b. IF NOT SINGLE BIRTH - Born First, Second, Third, etc. (Specify)

30. APGAR SCORE | 31a. MOTHER TRANSFERRED PRIOR TO DELIVERY? ☐ No ☐ Yes If yes, enter name of facility and city transferred from.
30a. 1 Minute | 30b. 5 Minutes | 31b. FACILITY NAME | 31c. CITY

31d. INFANT TRANSFERRED? ☐ No ☐ Yes If yes, enter name of facility and city transferred to.
31e. FACILITY NAME | 31f. CITY

32a. MEDICAL RISK FACTORS FOR THIS PREGNANCY (Check all that apply)
Anemia (Hct. <30/Hgb. <10) .... 01 ☐
Cardiac disease .... 02 ☐
Acute or chronic lung disease .... 03 ☐
Diabetes .... 04 ☐
Genital herpes .... 05 ☐
Hydramnios/Oligohydramnios .... 06 ☐
Hemoglobinopathy .... 07 ☐
Hypertension, chronic .... 08 ☐
Hypertension, pregnancy-associated .... 09 ☐
Eclampsia .... 10 ☐
Incompetent cervix .... 11 ☐
Previous infant 4000+ grams .... 12 ☐
Previous preterm or small-for-gestational-age infant .... 13 ☐
Renal disease .... 14 ☐
Rh sensitization .... 15 ☐
Uterine bleeding .... 16 ☐
None .... 00 ☐
Other .... 17 ☐
(Specify)

32b. OTHER RISK FACTORS FOR THIS PREGNANCY (Complete all items)
Tobacco use during pregnancy .... Yes ☐ No ☐
Average number cigarettes per day ____
Alcohol use during pregnancy .... Yes ☐ No ☐
Average number drinks per week ____
Weight gained during pregnancy ____ lbs.
Pre-Pregnancy weight ____ lbs.

33. OBSTETRIC PROCEDURES (Check all that apply)
Amniocentesis .... 01 ☐
Electronic fetal monitoring .... 02 ☐
Induction of labor .... 03 ☐
Stimulation of labor .... 04 ☐
Tocolysis .... 05 ☐
Ultrasound .... 06 ☐
None .... 00 ☐
Other .... 07 ☐
(Specify)

34. COMPLICATIONS OF LABOR AND/OR DELIVERY (Check all that apply)
Febrile (>100°F. or 38°C.) .... 01 ☐
Meconium, moderate/heavy .... 02 ☐
Premature rupture of membrane (>12 hours) .... 03 ☐
Abruptio placenta .... 04 ☐
Placenta previa .... 05 ☐
Other excessive bleeding .... 06 ☐
Seizures during labor .... 07 ☐
Precipitous labor (<3 hours) .... 08 ☐
Prolonged labor (>20 hours) .... 09 ☐
Dysfunctional labor .... 10 ☐
Breech/Malpresentation .... 11 ☐
Cephalopelvic disproportion .... 12 ☐
Cord prolapse .... 13 ☐
Anesthetic complications .... 14 ☐
Fetal distress .... 15 ☐
None .... 00 ☐
Other .... 16 ☐
(Specify)

35. METHOD OF DELIVERY (Check all that apply)
Vaginal .... 01 ☐
Vaginal birth after previous C-section .... 02 ☐
Primary C-section .... 03 ☐
Repeat C-section .... 04 ☐
Forceps .... 05 ☐
Vacuum .... 06 ☐

36. ABNORMAL CONDITIONS OF THE NEWBORN (Check all that apply)
Anemia (Hct. <39/Hgb. <13) .... 01 ☐
Birth injury .... 02 ☐
Fetal alcohol syndrome .... 03 ☐
Hyaline membrane disease/RDS .... 04 ☐
Meconium aspiration syndrome .... 05 ☐
Assisted ventilation <30 min .... 06 ☐
Assisted ventilation ≥30 min .... 07 ☐
Seizures .... 08 ☐
None .... 00 ☐
Other .... 09 ☐
(Specify)

37. CONGENITAL ANOMALIES OF CHILD (Check all that apply)
Anencephalus .... 01 ☐
Spina bifida/Meningocele .... 02 ☐
Hydrocephalus .... 03 ☐
Microcephalus .... 04 ☐
Other central nervous system anomalies (Specify) .... 05 ☐
Heart malformations .... 06 ☐
Other circulatory/respiratory anomalies (Specify) .... 07 ☐
Rectal atresia/stenosis .... 08 ☐
Tracheo-esophageal fistula/Esophageal atresia .... 09 ☐
Omphalocele/Gastroschisis .... 10 ☐
Other gastrointestinal anomalies (Specify) .... 11 ☐
Malformed genitalia .... 12 ☐
Renal agenesis .... 13 ☐
Other urogenital anomalies (Specify) .... 14 ☐
Cleft lip/palate .... 15 ☐
Polydactyly/Syndactyly/Adactyly .... 16 ☐
Club foot .... 17 ☐
Diaphragmatic hernia .... 18 ☐
Other musculoskeletal/integumental anomalies (Specify) .... 19 ☐
Down's syndrome .... 20 ☐
Other chromosomal anomalies (Specify) .... 21 ☐
None .... 00 ☐
Other .... 22 ☐
(Specify)

37a. ☐ PARENT(S) REQUEST ISSUANCE OF A SOCIAL SECURITY NUMBER FOR THIS CHILD.

38. NAME OF PROPHYLACTIC USED IN EYES OF CHILD | 39. DATE OF APPROVED TEST FOR SYPHILIS, IF NONE STATE REASON | 40. DATE OF APPROVED TEST FOR GONORRHEA, IF NONE STATE REASON

Certificate of live birth.

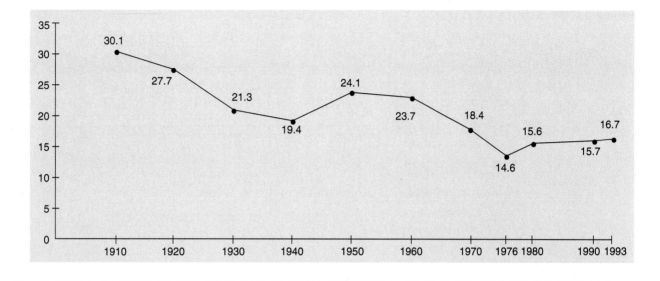

Birth rates, United States: number of live births per 1,000 population.

the United States in determining the start of life. A few states use a shortened definition.

Birth records give some indication of population growth. Birth rates are influenced by a number of variables, the most important of which is the number of women of childbearing age. The birth rate in the United States dropped to an all-time low of 14.6 in 1976, but since then has risen to the present rate of 16.7. The United States Bureau of the Census projects that the number of women of childbearing age will continue to increase into the 1990s. As this happens, there is a strong possibility that a similar rise in birth rates will occur.

Mortality   A statistic that can tell much about the health conditions of a given population is the mortality rate, or number of deaths per one thousand population. This is particularly true if there is a decrease in the mortality rate, since a decrease is indicative of overall improvement of the health of a population. The presence of a large number of elderly individuals in the population produces a rise in the mortality rate. This is one reason that these rates are more valuable when they are age adjusted or when specific age groups are presented separately.

In the United States death registration is based on individual state law. Death certificates are filed and maintained in the offices of state vital statistics. They are the primary source of information about mortality. Generally, the Standard Certificate of Death is revised about every ten years. In 1989 the National Center for Health Statistics made several changes in this certificate. It now seeks information to better clarify the medical cause of the death. The occupation of the deceased and whether the deceased is Hispanic are also now recorded.

In most cases, information certifying the cause of death is provided by the attending physician or coroner. The funeral director provides demographic information such as age, race, and sex. It is usually the funeral director's responsibility to file the death certificate with the state.

Mortality rates are often expressed in relation to the specific cause of death. Death rates are published in terms of age, gender, race, cause of death, and geographical location. This kind of data is useful in keeping abreast of causes of death. Nearly 90 percent of all deaths are currently attributable to the ten causes listed in table 9.1.

Ohio Department of Health
VITAL STATISTICS
CERTIFICATE OF DEATH

Reg. Dist. No. _____

Primary Reg. Dist. No. _____

State File No. _____

Registrar's No. _____

DO NOT WRITE IN MARGIN RESERVED FOR ODH DATA CODING

a. _____
b. _____
c. _____
d. _____
e. _____

DECEDENT

1. DECEDENT'S NAME (First, Middle, LAST)	2. SEX	3. DATE OF DEATH (Month, Day, Year)

4. SOCIAL SECURITY NUMBER	5a. AGE - Last Birthday (Years)	5b. UNDER 1 YEAR		5c. UNDER 1 DAY		6. DATE OF BIRTH (Month, Day, Year)	7. BIRTHPLACE (City and State or Foreign Country)
		Months	Days	Hours	Minutes		

8. WAS DECEDENT EVER IN U.S. ARMED FORCES? ☐ Yes ☐ No	9a. PLACE OF DEATH (Check only one) HOSPITAL: ☐ Inpatient ☐ ER/Outpatient ☐ DOA OTHER: ☐ Nursing Home ☐ Residence ☐ Other (Specify)

IF DEATH OCCURRED IN INSTITUTION, GIVE RESIDENCE BEFORE ADMISSION →

9b. FACILITY NAME (If not institution, give street and number)	9c. CITY, VILLAGE, TWP., OR LOCATION OF DEATH	9d. COUNTY OF DEATH

10. MARITAL STATUS - Married, Never Married, Widowed, Divorced (Specify)	11. SURVIVING SPOUSE (If wife, give maiden name)	12a. DECEDENT'S USUAL OCCUPATION (Give kind of work done during most of working life. Do not use retired.)	12b. KIND OF BUSINESS/INDUSTRY

13a. RESIDENCE - STATE	13b. COUNTY	13c. CITY, TOWN, TWP., OR LOCATION	13d. STREET AND NUMBER

13e. INSIDE CITY LIMITS? (Yes or No)	13f. ZIP CODE	14. WAS DECEDENT OF HISPANIC ORIGIN? (Specify No or Yes - If yes, specify Cuban, Mexican, Puerto Rican, etc.) ☐ No ☐ Yes Specify:	15. RACE - American Indian, Black, White, etc. (Specify)	16. DECEDENT'S EDUCATION (Specify only highest grade completed.)
				Elementary/Secondary (0-12)	College (1-4 or 5+)

PARENTS

17. FATHER'S NAME (First, Middle, Last)	18. MOTHER'S NAME (First, Middle, Maiden Surname)

INFORMANT

19a. INFORMANT'S NAME (Type/Print)	19b. MAILING ADDRESS (Street and Number or Rural Route Number, City or Town, State, Zip Code)

DISPOSITION

20a. METHOD OF DISPOSITION ☐ Burial ☐ Cremation ☐ Removal from State ☐ Donation ☐ Other (Specify)	20b. PLACE OF DISPOSITION (Name of cemetery, crematory, or other place)	20c. LOCATION - City or Town, State

20d. DATE OF DISPOSITION	21a. NAME OF EMBALMER	21b. LICENSE NUMBER

22a. SIGNATURE OF FUNERAL DIRECTOR OR OTHER PERSON ►	22b. LICENSE NUMBER (of Licensee)	23. NAME AND ADDRESS OF FACILITY

REGISTRAR

24. REGISTRAR'S SIGNATURE ►	25. DATE FILED (Month, Day, Year)

f. _____
g. _____
h. _____
i. _____

26a. SIGNATURE OF PERSON ISSUING PERMIT ►	26b. DIST. No.	27. DATE PERMIT ISSUED

CERTIFIER

28a. CERTIFIER (Check only one)	☐ CERTIFYING PHYSICIAN To the best of my knowledge, death occurred at the time, date, and place, and due to the cause(s) and manner as stated.
	☐ CORONER On the basis of examination and/or investigation, in my opinion, death occurred at the time, date, and place, and due to the cause(s) and manner as stated

28b. TIME OF DEATH M	28c. DATE PRONOUNCED DEAD (Month, Day, Year)	28d. WAS CASE REFERRED TO CORONER? ☐ Yes ☐ No

j. _____
k. _____

28e. SIGNATURE AND TITLE OF CERTIFIER ►	28f. LICENSE NUMBER	28g. DATE SIGNED (Month, Day, Year)

l. _____
m. _____
n. _____
o. _____
p. _____
q. _____
r. _____
s. _____
t. _____
u. _____

29. NAME AND ADDRESS OF PERSON WHO COMPLETED CAUSE OF DEATH (Type/Print)

CAUSE OF DEATH

30. PART I. Enter the diseases, injuries, or complications that caused the death. Do not enter the mode of dying, such as cardiac or respiratory arrest, shock, or heart failure. List only one cause on each line. TYPE OR PRINT IN PERMANENT INK	Approximate Interval Between Onset and Death
IMMEDIATE CAUSE (Final disease or condition resulting in death) → a. ____ DUE TO (OR AS A CONSEQUENCE OF):	
Sequentially list conditions, if any, leading to immediate cause. Enter UNDERLYING CAUSE (Disease or injury that initiated events resulting in death) LAST b. ____ DUE TO (OR AS A CONSEQUENCE OF):	
c. ____ DUE TO (OR AS A CONSEQUENCE OF):	
d.	

SEE INSTRUCTIONS ON OTHER SIDE

PART II. Other significant conditions contributing to death but not resulting in the underlying cause given in Part I.	31a. WAS AN AUTOPSY PERFORMED? ☐ Yes ☐ No	31b. WERE AUTOPSY FINDINGS AVAILABLE PRIOR TO COMPLETION OF CAUSE OF DEATH? ☐ Yes ☐ No

32. MANNER OF DEATH ☐ Natural ☐ Pending Investigation ☐ Accident ☐ Suicide ☐ Could not be Determined ☐ Homicide	33a. DATE OF INJURY (Month, Day, Year)	33b. TIME OF INJURY M	33c. INJURY AT WORK? ☐ Yes ☐ No	33d. DESCRIBE HOW INJURY OCCURRED
	33e. PLACE OF INJURY - At home, farm, street, factory, office building, etc. (Specify)			33f. LOCATION (Street and Number or Rural Route Number, City or Town, State)

HEA 2717 5152.06 (Rev. 2/89)

TYPE OR PRINT IN PERMANENT INK

Certificate of death.

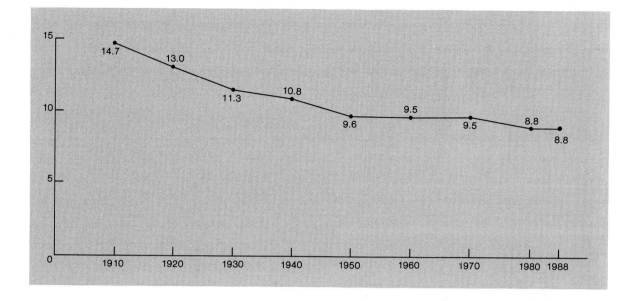

Death rates, United States: number of deaths per 1,000 population.

Table 9.1 Ten Leading Causes of Death, United States

Rank	Cause
1	Heart disease
2	Cancer
3	Cerebrovascular diseases
4	Bronchitis/Emphysema
5	Injury
6	Pneumonia/influenza
7	Diabetes
8	AIDS
9	Suicide
10	Homicide

Source: National Center for Health Statistics, CDC, (Fall 1993).

$$\text{Crude Death Rate} = \frac{\text{Number of Deaths during the Year}}{\text{Average Population at Midyear}}$$

The basic indication of mortality is the *crude death rate,* determined by dividing the number of deaths during the year by the average population at midyear. The crude death rate is expressed in ratio per one thousand population. This rate has continued to decline since the early years of this century to a rate of 8.6 per 1,000. The crude death rate has been very consistent, ranging between 8.5 and 8.8 since the mid-1970s.

Several specific kinds of mortality data are collected and used in analyzing the health conditions of a population. Most of this data concerns mother and child health.

Infant Mortality The number of deaths that occur in infants under one year of age, excluding fetal deaths, is the infant mortality rate. This statistic is one of the most widely accepted measures of estimating the health of a population. The survival of an infant during the first year of life also reflects the health of the mother and the health condition of the newborn's environment.

Infant mortality rates are expressed in terms of the number of incidences per one thousand live births. Currently this rate in the United States is 9.2 (see table 9.2).[6] The Department of Health and Human Services has set as an objective for the nation by the year 2000 an infant mortality rate of seven.[7]

Table 9.2 Infant Mortality Rates, United States.

Year	All	Whites	All Other
1940	47.0	43.2	73.8
1950	29.2	26.8	44.5
1960	26.0	22.9	43.2
1965	24.7	21.5	40.3
1970	20.0	17.8	30.9
1975	16.1	14.2	24.2
1980	12.6	11.0	21.4
1985	10.6	9.3	15.8
1990	9.2	7.7	14.4

Source: U.S. Bureau of the Census. *Statistical Abstracts of the United States.* Washington, D.C.: U.S. Government Printing Office, 1993, p. 89.

$$\text{Infant Mortality Rate} = \frac{\text{Number of Deaths in Calendar Year among Infants Less than One Year of Age}}{\text{Number of Live Births during Calendar Year}} \times 1,000$$

Table 9.3 Fetal Death Rates, United States.

Year	Rate
1950	19.2
1960	16.1
1970	14.2
1980	9.2
1990	7.5

Source: U.S. Bureau of the Census. *Statistical Abstracts of the United States.* Washington, D.C.: U.S. Government Printing Office, 1993, p. 89.

Table 9.4 Neonatal Death Rates, United States.

Year	Rate
1940	28.8
1950	20.5
1960	18.7
1970	15.1
1980	8.5
1990	5.8

Source: U.S. Bureau of the Census. *Statistical Abstracts of the United States.* Washington, D.C.: U.S. Government Printing Office, 1993, p. 89.

Table 9.5 Maternal Mortality Rate,* United States.

Year	All	Whites	All Other
1940	376.0	319.8	773.5
1950	83.3	61.1	221.6
1960	37.1	26.0	97.9
1965	31.6	21.0	83.7
1970	21.5	14.4	55.9
1975	12.8	9.1	29.0
1980	9.2	6.7	19.8
1985	7.8	5.2	18.1
1990	8.2	5.4	19.1

Source: U.S. Bureau of the Census, *Statistical Abstracts of the United States.* Washington, D.C.: U.S. Government Printing Office, 1993, p. 89. *(Per 100,000 live births)

Fetal Death Commonly referred to as *stillbirth*, fetal death is defined formally as follows:

. . . death prior to the complete expulsion or extraction from its mother of a product of human conception, irrespective of the duration of pregnancy; the death is indicated by the fact that after such expulsion or extraction the fetus does not breathe or show any other evidence of life such as beating of the heart, pulsation of the umbilical cord, or definite movement of voluntary muscles.[8]

This definition, like that of live birth, is based on the World Health Organization determination set forth in 1950. Most states use this definition; however, some differences do exist on the length of gestation. To be classified as a fetal death, a stated or presumed gestation period of twenty weeks or more is necessary. United States fetal death rates are shown in table 9.3.

Neonatal Death When an infant death occurs within the first twenty-eight days after birth, it is recorded as a neonatal death. Data of neonatal deaths do not include fetal deaths (see table 9.4).

Maternal Mortality The death of a woman due to childbirth, the complications of pregnancy, and puerperium (the woman's condition after birth) is referred to as maternal mortality. The National Center for Health Statistics defines maternal death as "death from any maternal condition in which the date of onset of the condition was within one year prior to the date of death."[9] On the other hand, the National Vital Statistics System defines maternal death as "the death of any woman while pregnant or within 42 days of termination of pregnancy. . . ." It is for this reason that one often finds differences in maternal mortality rates upon analyzing federal governmental data (see table 9.5).

This statistic, unlike other indices of mortality, is expressed as a ratio per 100,000 live births. Maternal mortality was quite common in the early part of this century, but in the 1930s its incidence began to drop. For example, the maternal mortality rate in the 1920s was about 700 per 100,000, but today, the ratio has dropped to about 8 per 100,000. This decline has not been equal among the white and nonwhite population. Maternal mortality in the early 1990s for the white population was about 5, while for the nonwhite population it was about 19.

$$\text{Maternal Mortality Rate} = \frac{\text{Number of Deaths in Calendar Year Due to Childbirth}}{\text{Number of Live Births during Calendar Year}} \times 100,000$$

The federal government has established the goal of decreasing maternal mortality by the year 2000 to no more than 3.3.[10] In order for this objective to be achieved, major initiatives must be instituted toward improving the health of women during pregnancy among the African-American population.

The incidences of material mortality fall into four major categories: (1) deaths related to pregnancies with abortive outcomes, (2) deaths related to complications of the puerperium, (3) deaths related to complications of the delivery, and (4) deaths related to complications of pregnancy.[11] Deaths from abortive outcome pregnancies tend to be either a result of induced abortions or ectopic pregnancies. Deaths due to illegally induced abortions have been virtually eliminated with the legalization of abortion in the United States. Ectopic pregnancies occur in situations where women have damaged fallopian tubes due to bacterial infections and the use of contraceptive agents, particularly IUDs. Deaths in the puerperal period are mainly due to embolisms. The chief cause of fatality among the complications of delivery is hemorrhage, which can be caused by premature separation of the placenta, retained placenta, uterine rupture, or postpartum hemorrhage. Deaths due to complications of the puerperium are mostly attributed to hypertensive diseases such as toxemia.

Abortion States are now required to report induced and spontaneous abortions. For consistency between states, induced termination of pregnancy has been defined as ". . . the purposeful interruption of pregnancy with the intention other than to produce a liveborn infant or to remove a dead fetus and which does not result in a live birth."[12]

A spontaneous fetal death is ". . . the expulsion or extraction of a product of human conception resulting in other than a live birth and which is not an induced termination of pregnancy."[13]

The increase in numbers of abortions since 1972, when the Supreme Court legalized abortion in the United States, can be seen by analyzing vital data. In 1972 the rate of abortions per 1,000 women in the United States was 13.2; by the early 1990s it was slightly above 27.[14]

Marriages and Divorces The record of the number of marriages and divorces is not a direct indicator of the health status of a population. These statistics are more likely to have socioeconomic value. Both are expressed in ratio per one thousand population. Often the number of marriages reflects the age group composition of a locality. A higher marriage rate is often found in a community with a university or college, whereas a retirement community in Florida or Arizona is likely to have a lower marriage rate. The national marriage rate in the latter 1980s was 9.7.[15]

The divorce rate has risen dramatically in the past two decades. The National Center for Health Statistics reported that the divorce rate was 5.0 per one thousand population in the 1980s, a rate nearly two and a half times that of the early 1960s. The divorce rate peaked in 1981 and has dropped slightly since, to 4.7/1,000 population.[16]

Reportable Diseases

In 1878 Congress passed legislation that required the Public Health Service to collect morbidity reports on certain diseases.[17] At that time the diseases of concern were cholera, smallpox, plague, and yellow fever. In order to be able to develop these reports, it was necessary for the individual states to submit data to the federal government. However, it was not until 1925 that all states were reporting information about certain diseases on a regular basis.

Today these data are submitted to the Centers for Disease Control and Prevention. This information is compiled and published weekly, and a summary of reportable diseases is published annually.

The responsibility for initiating the reporting of these diseases belongs to the individual health care provider and medical facility. The physician and the hospital or clinic staff are required to report to the local health department all instances of these diseases. This information is reported to the state health department, which then reports to the Centers for Disease Control and Prevention. The Epidemiology Program Office of

Issue—Case Study
Epidemiological Study of Influenza

The state health department has been collecting data on the number of cases of influenza reported during February. In one northern county of the state, 295 cases were identified and reported. Another region of the state reported 202 cases, and in the southeastern section of the state 168 cases were reported.

While analyzing the population densities of the regions, the state recognized that the northern county has two major cities with a combined population of 258,000. The southeastern section includes two-and-a-half counties.

All villages in this area are small, with an estimated total population of 62,000. The other region under consideration is the eastern half of one county, which has a population of 159,000.

As you analyze these reports, what conclusions can you draw? Your department director indicates that there are resources for working in only one of the areas at this time. Which localities within the state would you recommend for immediate aid or programming?

Notifiable Diseases in the United States

Acquired Immunodeficiency Syndrome (AIDS)	Measles
	Meningococcal infections
Amebiasis	Mumps
Anthrax	Murine typhus fever
Aseptic Meningitis	Pertussis
Botulism	Plague
Brucellosis	Poliomyelitis
Chancroid	Psittacosis
Cholera	Rabies (animal and human)
Diphtheria	Rheumatic fever
Encephalitis	Rocky Mountain spotted fever
Gonorrhea	Rubella
Granuloma inguinale	Salmonellosis
Haemophilus influenzae	Shigellosis
Hansen's disease	Syphilis
Hepatitis (A and B)	Tetanus
Legionellosis	Toxic shock syndrome
Leptospirosis	Trichinosis
Lyme disease	Tuberculosis
Lymphogranulome venereum	Tularemia
Malaria	Typhoid fever
	Varicella (chicken pox)

Source: Centers for Disease Control. "Summary of Notifiable Diseases, United States, 1992." *Morbidity and Mortality Weekly Report* 41, no. 55 (September 1993).

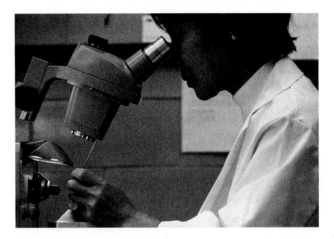

The microbiologist plays an important role in epidemiologic studies where the etiologic agent is unknown.

CDC has the responsibility of bringing together all the data and publishing the information for the public.

It must be understood that data on the more severe conditions (such as AIDS and rabies) are usually very accurate, whereas milder diseases (such as salmonellosis or mumps) are less likely to be reported. The accuracy of the data also is dependent upon the priorities established by state and local health departments. Only as these departments submit information and data do national data reports reflect the true extent of each notifiable disease.

Data are also collected on a number of nonreportable diseases. These diseases may be no less serious, but for various reasons they have not been added to the required reportable list. Diseases in this nonreportable category include infectious mononucleosis, Reye's syndrome, histoplasmosis, pelvic inflammatory disease (PID), and a broad range of occupational diseases.

An Interdisciplinary Team

The work of epidemiology necessitates the expertise and input of a number of different fields of study. The skills and contributions of basic biological scientists, anatomists, physiologists, and microbiologists are necessary to disease-related work. Pathology and immunology

176   Unit 3 Programming for Community Health

are also necessary since much epidemiological study of disease causation centers around immunization. Also, clinical medicine and preventive medicine are important as groups of individuals are studied. Studies have little meaning without analysis of statistical data. The skills of biostatistics and research methodology must be a part of any epidemiology work.

Summary

The study of occurrence of diseases in human populations is epidemiology. Epidemiological study attempts to identify the cause of diseases. The procedures of epidemiology historically were directed toward solving the epidemics of infectious diseases. In more recent years the procedures of epidemiology have been applied to a broad range of problems in community health other than infectious diseases.

Epidemiological study involves use of the epidemiological model. This model looks at the interaction of three factors influencing health and well-being: (1) the causative agent, (2) the host, and (3) the environmental factors.

Two basic methods are used in epidemiology: observational study and experimental study. Observational studies may be prospective or retrospective. Prospective studies start with a group of individuals who are followed for a period of time to ascertain the effect of a factor being studied. The retrospective study examines the historical records of a population group to ascertain what factors might have led to the cause of a given health problem under study.

Experimental studies are different in that the epidemiologist manipulates the study population. The study population is placed into two equal study groups: the control group and the experimental group. Experimental studies may be clinical or community-involved examinations.

Analysis of data collected in epidemiological studies must be presented so as to be useful. The basic data is placed into ratios which then can be used for comparisons and projections. Data that are important in community health are obtained from many different sources. Census data, vital statistics, and data of reportable diseases are all widely used in epidemiological work.

Epidemiology makes use of a number of different professional fields. All must work together so that the epidemiological investigations are useful and of value.

Discussion Questions

1. What is meant by the concept of "epidemiology"?
2. Explain the ways in which epidemiology is useful in community health.
3. Discuss the relationships of the host, the causative agent, and the environmental factors as they relate to a given disease problem.
4. What is meant by the chain of infection?
5. At what point in the chain of infection do you feel success will eventually come in the treatment and cure of AIDS? Explain your position.
6. If you were responsible for developing a malaria eradication program, to which component of the epidemiological model would you direct the major resources? Explain your answer.
7. In what ways is the epidemiological model useful in environmental health programming?
8. Can epidemiology be as effective in studies of chronic diseases as in communicable diseases? Demonstrate your answer with examples.
9. Explain the basic differences between the prospective study and the retrospective study.
10. What is the cross-sectional epidemiological study?
11. Describe how the experimental study differs from the observational study.
12. Explain some of the ethical issues concerning experimental studies.
13. How does the incidence rate differ from the prevalence rate?

14. Why can prevalence data not be compared with incidence data?

15. In an industry with 2,341 employees, 16 were absent from work on March 3 owing to respiratory illnesses. What is the prevalence rate in this company for this disease? State the rate in relation to 1,000 population.

16. What use is made of census data in epidemiological studies?

17. Describe the various uses of vital statistics.

18. What kind of information is found on a birth certificate? a death certificate?

19. Trace the flow of data from the local health department to the National Center for Health Statistics.

20. What can one learn from reviewing the statistical data on marriages and divorces?

21. Explain the differences between infant mortality, fetal death, neonatal death, and maternal mortality.

22. Explain what is meant by notifiable diseases.

Suggested Readings

American Academy of Pediatrics and the American College of Obstetricians and Gynecologists. "Standard Terminology for Reporting of Reproductive Health Statistics in the United States," *Public Health Reports* 103, no. 5 (September/October 1988): 464–71.

Ahlbom, Anders, and Staffan, Norell. *Introduction to Modern Epidemiology.* Chestnut Hill, Mass.: Epidemiology Resources, Inc., 1984, 97 pp.

Berkelman, Ruth L., and James W. Curran. "Epidemiology of HIV Infection and AIDS." *Epidemiologic Reviews* 11 (1989): 222–28.

Flanders, W. Dana, and Thomas R. O'Brien. "Inappropriate Comparisons of Incidence and Prevalence in Epidemiologic Research." *American Journal of Public Health* 79, no. 9 (September 1989): 1301–3.

Fox, L. P. "A Return to Maternal Mortality Studies: A Necessary Effort." *American Journal of Obstetrics and Gynecology* 152, no. 4 (June 1985): 379–86.

Friedman, Gary D. *Primer of Epidemiology.* New York: McGraw-Hill Book Company, 1980, 288 pp.

Kaunitz, A. M., J. M. Hughes, and others. "Causes of Maternal Mortality in the United States." *Obstetrics and Gynecology* 65, no. 5 (May 1985): 605–12.

Koonin, Lisa M., and others. "Maternal Mortality Surveillance, United States, 1980–1985." *Morbidity and Mortality Weekly Report* 37, no. SS-5 (December 1988): 19–29.

Mausner, Judith S., and Shira Kramer. *Epidemiology—An Introductory Text.* Philadelphia: W. B. Saunders Company, 1985, 361 pp.

Novick, L. F., C. Greene, and R. L. Vogt. "Teaching Medical Students Epidemiology: Utilizing a State Health Department." *Public Health Reports* 100, no. 4 (July/August 1985): 401–5.

Orenstein, Walter A., and others. "Assessing Vaccine Efficacy in the Field." *Epidemiologic Reviews* 10 (1988): 212–41.

Rieder, Hans L., and others. "Epidemiology of Tuberculosis in the United States." *Epidemiologic Reviews* 11 (1988): 79–98.

Smith, J., and others. "An Assessment of the Incidence of Maternal Mortality in the United States." *American Journal of Public Health* 74, no. 8 (August 1984): 780–83.

Thacker, Stephen B., and Ruth L. Berkelman. "Public Health Surveillance in the United States." *Epidemiologic Reviews* 10 (1988): 164–90.

Thomas, Patricia. "New Framingham Algorithm Tells CAD or Stroke Risk." *Medical World News* (August 14, 1989): 21–22.

Thompson, W. Douglas. "Statistical Criteria in the Interpretation of Epidemiologic Data." *American Journal of Public Health* 77, no. 2 (February 1987): 191–99.

Waters, W. E. "Ethics and Epidemiological Research." *International Journal of Epidemiology* 14, no. 1 (1985): 48–51.

Endnotes

1. Gordon, J. E. "The Epidemiology of Accidents." *American Journal of Public Health* 39, no. 4 (1948): 504–15.

2. Dawber, T. R., G. F. Meadors, and F. G. Moore, Jr. "The Epidemiological Approach to Heart Disease: The Framingham Study." *American Journal of Public Health* 41 (1951): 279–86.

   Gordon, T., and W. B. Kannel. "The Framingham, Massachusetts Study, Twenty Years Later." In *The Community as an Epidemiologic Laboratory: A Casebook of Community Studies,* edited by I. I. Kessler and M. L. Levin. Baltimore, Md.: The Johns Hopkins Press, 1970, 123–46.

   McGee, D., and T. Gordon. *The Framingham Study: The Results of the Framingham Study Applied to Four Other U.S. Based Epidemiologic Studies of Cardiovascular Disease.* Washington, D.C.: U.S. Government Printing Office, 1976.

3. V. Kumar, Jayanth, and others. "Trends in Dental Fluorosis and Dental Caries Prevalences in Newburgh and Kingston, New York." *Public Health Reports* 79, no. 5 (May 1989): 565–69.

4. Flanders, W. Dana, and Thomas R. O'Brien. "Inappropriate Comparisons of Incidence and Prevalence in Epidemiologic Research." *American Journal of Public Health* 79, no. 9 (September 1989): 1301–3.

5. Department of Health, Education, and Welfare. *Model State Vital Statistics Act and Model State Vital Statistics Regulations,* 1977, Revision, Publication no. (PHS) 78–1115.

6. An in-depth discussion of infant mortality is presented in chapter 19.

7. Department of Health and Human Services. *Healthy People 2000: National Health Promotion and Disease Prevention Objectives.* Washington, D.C.: U.S. Government Printing Office, 1991, p. 368.

8. Department of Health, Education, and Welfare. *Model State Vital Statistics.*

9. Smith, Jack C., and others. "An Assessment of the Incidence of Maternal Mortality in the United States." *American Journal of Public Health* 74, no. 8 (August 1984): 780–83.

10. Department of Health and Human Services, *Healthy People 2000,* 373.

11. Rochat, R. W. "Maternal Mortality in the United States of America," *World Health Statistics Quarterly* 34, no. 1 (1981): 267.

12. Department of Health, Education, and Welfare. *Model State Vital Statistics.*

13. *Ibid.*

14. United States Bureau of the Census. *Statistical Abstracts of the United States,* 1992, 112th Ed. Washington, D.C.: U.S. Government Printing Office, p. 74.

15. United States Bureau of the Census, *Statistical Abstracts,* 1992, 90.

16. *Ibid.,* 90.

17. "History of Morbidity Reporting and Surveillance in the United States." *Morbidity and Mortality Weekly Report, Annual Summary, 1984* 33, no. 54 (March 1986): 9

CHAPTER **TEN**

Disease Control

Concern for Communicable Diseases

A significant change in disease patterns in the United States has occurred during the 1900s. At the turn of the century, communicable diseases were the principal health problems, causing serious illness and death. Today many of these once common communicable diseases are no longer a threat. In fact, chronic diseases, not communicable diseases, are now the major health problem faced by millions of people.

An analysis of the leading causes of death indicates that chronic diseases now pose a more serious health threat to most Americans than communicable diseases. Today the four leading causes of death are (1) heart disease, (2) cancer, (3) injuries, and (4) stroke. By comparison, the three most life-threatening diseases in 1900 were (1) influenza and pneumonia, (2) tuberculosis, and (3) diarrhea and related diseases.[1] The latter diseases, though still health problems among certain populations, are not a serious concern for most Americans today. Safe drinking water, public water purification systems, and public sanitation systems have effected this change.

Of the three leading causes of death in 1900, only influenza and pneumonia still rank high—sixth—as a cause of

Leading Causes of Death, United States

1900	1990s
1. Influenza and pneumonia	1. Heart disease
2. Tuberculosis	2. Cancer
3. Diarrhea and related diseases	3. Stroke
4. Heart disease	4. Chronic lung disease
5. Stroke	5. Injury

Source: Department of Health and Human Services. National Center for Health Statistics (Fall, 1993).

death today. For the general population, influenza and pneumonia do not pose a serious threat because medication and good personal health care normally counter them. For the elderly whose general health has declined, influenza and pneumonia pose serious threats.

Ten Leading Causes of Death and Related Risk Factors, 1990s

Cause of Death	Risk Factors
1. Heart disease	Smoking, diet, lack of exercise, hypertension, stress
2. Cancer	Smoking, diet, environmental carcinogens
3. Stroke	Smoking, diet, hypertension, stress
4. Chronic lung disease	Smoking, air pollution
5. Injuries	Alcohol, smoking, (fires), drug use
6. Pneumonia/influenza	Smoking, vaccination status
7. Diabetes	Obesity
8. AIDS	Unprotected sex, drug abuse
9. Suicide	Stress, alcohol, drug abuse
10. Homicide	Drug use, alcohol, social problems

Source: Department of Health and Human Services. National Center for Health Statistics (1993).

Disease Organisms

Communicable diseases are caused by small living organisms, plant or animal, that are invisible except when viewed through a microscope. These organisms, referred to as microorganisms or microbes, are found in the body and throughout the environment. Many microorganisms play important roles in the maintenance of good health and in the stability of ecosystems. For example, microbes in the digestive tract aid digestion, and microorganisms in the soil increase fertility by causing decay.

Some microorganisms, known as pathogens, invade the human body and cause disease. This invasion can occur in several different ways. The pathogen may enter the host through a wound or a break in the skin; the microorganism can be transmitted from an infected animal to a human host; or infection can be spread from one person to another.

The major pathogenic microorganisms are bacteria, viruses, fungi, protozoa, rickettsiae, and metazoa. *Bacteria* are small, single-celled microorganisms that are visible only under a microscope and appear in three dif-

ferent shapes: (1) spiral, (2) spherical, and (3) rod. They constitute the most common cause of human disease. Diseases caused by bacteria include cholera, diphtheria, gonorrhea, syphilis, tetanus, typhoid fever, trench mouth, tuberculosis, and yaws.

The *virus* is the smallest pathogen. It can only be seen with an electron microscope and relies upon other living cells to complete its life cycle. Viruses are found in various sizes and shapes. They are known to cause the common cold, influenza, measles, rabies, smallpox, chicken pox, polio, yellow fever, herpes, and acquired immunodeficiency syndrome (AIDS).

Fungi are plantlike organisms that vary in size from a single cell to large multicellular structures such as mushrooms and toadstools. They include yeasts and molds, and because they contain no chlorophyll, they do not carry on photosynthesis. Thus, the fungus lives on or in another organism. This type of relationship is termed *parasitism.*

Fungal infection results in two types of diseases: (1) superficial skin diseases that affect the skin and hair, such as athlete's foot and ringworm of the scalp, limbs, or trunk, and (2) systemic infections of the respiratory and intestinal tract. Systemic infections can be very serious and occasionally fatal. Histoplasmosis and blastomycosis are systemic fungal infections. Another mycosis, candidiasis, affects the skin and mucous membranes of various parts of the body. Lesions caused by this fungus appear in the mouth, vagina, urinary tract, and other parts of the body where moisture, which favors growth of the fungus, is present.

Protozoan are single-celled microscopic animal forms. Though microscopic, the protozoa are larger than bacteria, and some forms even feed on bacteria. Pathogenic protozoa in humans cause several diseases, the most common of which is malaria. Dysentery and African sleeping sickness are other communicable diseases caused by protozoa.

Rickettsiae, small microorganisms that resemble bacteria and viruses, are usually transmitted to animals and humans by fleas, lice, or ticks. These microorganisms are smaller than bacteria and grow within the cells of the host. Rocky Mountain spotted fever and Q fever are diseases caused by this pathogen.

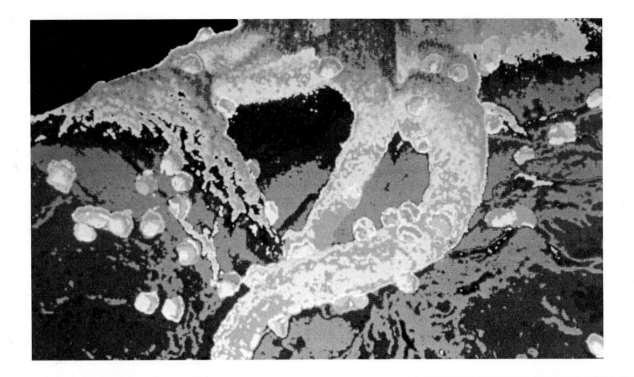

The AIDS virus on a lymphocyte.

Typhus is another disease caused by a rickettsia (*Rickettsia prowazekii*). This disease is spread by the body louse. Lice become infected when they feed on the blood of a person with typhus fever and then transmit the microorganism to another person through their feces. The lice usually defecate at the time of feeding. The individual becomes infected by rubbing the feces and crushed lice into the body through the wounds made by the bites.[2] Treatment requires medical care with administration of appropriate drug therapy. Measures to prevent an outbreak of typhus include improved sanitation, insecticide use to reduce lice, and frequent bathing and washing of clothes. Immunization for typhus is available and recommended for individuals living and traveling in high-risk areas.

Multicellular animals (*metazoa*) that infect humans are parasitic in nature. One example is *helminths*. These pathogens, not considered microorganisms, usually enter the body when the human consumes food and fluids containing them. Tapeworms in beef and pork are examples of this pathogen.

Natural Disease Defense

The human body has several natural defenses against disease-causing organisms. The skin and mucous membrane linings of the body serve as barriers to microorganisms. Thus, a cut or wound that interferes with this barrier can result in an invasion of the body by pathogens. The cilia of the respiratory system help keep disease-causing organisms from entering the lungs. In the digestive system, the acidity of the stomach is resistant to pathogenic microorganisms. In the bloodstream the leukocytes destroy foreign organisms; and lysozyme, a chemical found in human tears and saliva, dissolves the cell walls of certain bacteria.

When illness and infection are present, the body temperature often rises. This elevated body temperature is also an important protection against pathogens. High body temperature, or fever, tends to have a negative effect on the pathogen's ability to carry on normal metabolism. Hence, body temperatures above one hundred degrees Fahrenheit counter the disease-causing ability of pathogens.

Recommended Schedule for Immunization of Infants and Children

Age	Vaccine
2 mo.	DPT (#1), OPV (#1)
4 mo.	DPT (#2), OPV (#2)
6 mo.	DPT (#3)
15 mo.	DPT (#4), OPV (#3), MMR
18 mo.	Influenza
4–6 yrs.	DPT (#5), OPV (#4)
14–16 yrs.	Diphtheria and tetanus

Adapted from: Centers for Disease Control. "General Recommendations on Immunization." *Morbidity and Mortality Weekly Report* (April 7, 1989): 205–28.

A newborn infant is able to resist disease as ably as its mother. This immunity is obtained directly from the mother as maternal antibodies (protein substances) cross through the placental membranes and enter the baby's blood. This protection is potent for only a short period of time. Therefore, it is important for infants to begin receiving immunization at about two to three months of age.

Immunity

Resistance to the pathogenic microorganism of a disease is known as immunity. In the presence of specific disease-causing microorganisms, the body produces antibodies. These antibodies neutralize and destroy the pathogens and, as a result, the individual overcomes the illness. This ability to produce antibodies is referred to as natural acquired immunity, and is often obtained when a person has a given disease. The body produces the antibodies to counter the infection, and when the pathogens for the disease invade the body, the antibodies immediately function and the individual does not develop the signs and symptoms of the disease.

Immunity without contracting the disease is acquired by *immunization*. Immunization involves administering a vaccine containing preparations of a killed or weakened strain of the pathogenic microorganism. With the introduction of this vaccine, the body produces antibodies without the observable signs and symptoms of the disease. Toxoids are also used to provide immunity against disease. Toxoids are preparations of altered bacterial poisons or toxins that do not cause the disease.

Immunization is a widely accepted disease control procedure in the United States. Vaccines have been developed for diphtheria, pertussis (whooping cough), polio, mumps, rubella (German measles), rubeola (measles), tetanus, typhus, yellow fever, cholera, plague, and rabies. Some vaccines have also been developed for influenza and pneumococcal pneumonia.

For certain diseases, often referred to as the "childhood diseases," all fifty states require immunization before the child is permitted to enter school. The immunizations most commonly required for school admittance include those for diphtheria, pertussis, tetanus, mumps, polio, measles, and German measles. In the past, smallpox vaccination has been included in this listing but is no longer a requirement. The worldwide eradication of smallpox led to the recommendation by the World Health Organization and the medical profession that this vaccination was no longer needed.

In 1921 there were more than two hundred thousand cases of diphtheria in the United States, with about 5 percent being fatal. In 1988 there were only two cases reported, thus demonstrating the effectiveness of immunization for this disease. During the latter part of the 1980s there were about fifty cases of tetanus a year. Two out of every three were among individuals over fifty years of age.[3] By 1988 there were only three reported cases. This fact highlights the importance of tetanus immunizations when one realizes that the protective levels of this vaccine last for about ten years. In 1952 there were over fifty-seven thousand reported cases of polio in the United States. By 1991, because of immunization programs, only six cases were reported.[4]

Despite immunization programs, populations at risk must be under constant surveillance. During the 1980s an increase in the number of measles cases began to occur. By the early 1990s there were more than 27,000 reported cases.[5] These outbreaks tended to be among unvaccinated preschool-aged children living in the inner city and adolescents, mostly between twelve and nineteen, who had been vaccinated prior to one year of age.

Many of these children improperly vaccinated for measles receive their immunizations by the public sector. Many public clinics require physician referral in well baby clinics before the children are eligible for immunization. Also many clinics lack adequate staff to carry out measles immunization programs. These factors support the importance of tying immunization programs with other child care settings, such as WIC or Head Start.

Comparison of Number of Cases of Childhood Diseases

	Peak Year	1988	Goal for Year
	1950s/1960s	*1988*	*2000*
Diphtheria	5,796 (1950)	2	0
Mumps	152,209 (1968)	4,866	No more than 500
Pertussis	120,718 (1950)	3,450	Less than 1,000
Polio	57,879 (1952)	0	0
Rubella	49,371 (1968)	225	0
Rubeola	763,098 (1958)	3,058	0
Tetanus	524 (1954)	3	0

Source: Department of Health and Human Services. *Healthy People 2000: National Health Promotion and Disease Prevention Objectives* (1991): 513.

The dramatic impact of immunization is demonstrated by the data in the accompanying chart. The number of cases of childhood diseases has dropped significantly since the 1950s and 1960s, before effective vaccines were available, and the ultimate goals established for the year 2000 are certainly within reach.

It is important that children begin to receive the immunizations as infants. Most medical doctors recommend that babies be given the first DPT (diphtheria, pertussis, and tetanus) immunization and the first oral polio feeding as early as two to three months of age. Unfortunately, many parents fail to have their children immunized as recommended. This is particularly true among the economically disadvantaged. Because of the cost of injections, many simply do not have it done. In some poor inner-city areas, the government estimates that the immunization rate is less than half.

Many children, particularly the poor, are immunized at the local health department or community health center. Funding for these programs has been made available through various federal programs. As funding has been reduced for these programs, many are concerned that the national level of immunization of children may become a serious health problem.

The Centers for Disease Control and Prevention has established a program designed to improve access to immunization by the second year of life.[6] Activities are coordinated with state and local health departments to develop programming, particularly among urban populations. These initiatives include making use of mobile immunization clinics which move into areas where there are large numbers of unimmunized children. They also include establishing walk-in immunization clinics and on-site immunization centers in public housing developments. A computerized system of tracing Medicaid eligible children has been established to facilitate and locate children needing immunization.

It is important that mothers of newborn infants receive instruction about immunization schedules. Education of the public should help to increase the percentage of children who are immunized. Also, school immunization regulations must be enforced. In many communities, children are permitted to enroll and attend school when they have not had the full complement of injections.

Adult Immunization

In 1985 the immunization committee of the American College of Physicians reported the importance of giving attention to the immunization of adults.[7] The National Coalition for Adult Immunization, consisting of professional, public, and voluntary organizations, was established in 1988 to develop program initiatives to encourage immunization of adults.

Most individuals fail to consider the necessity of checking their personal immunization records as they reach adulthood. The Centers for Disease Control and Prevention reports that many American adults are not protected against communicable diseases for which there are appropriate, effective immunizations. Not only does this include the traditional childhood diseases such as diphtheria, tetanus, measles, mumps, and polio but also hepatitis, influenza, and pneumonia.

Adults should receive ten-year boosters for diphtheria and tetanus. Many adults have not been vaccinated for rubella and rubeola nor have they had the disease. This is particularly important for young adults, as recent

Vaccines Available in the United States

BCG (Bacillus of Calmette and Guerin)
Cholera
DPT
  D—Diphtheria
  P—Pertussis
  T—Tetanus
Hepatitis B
Haemophilus influenza B
Influenza
IPV (inactivated poliovirus vaccine)
Measles
Meningococcal
MMR
  M—Measles
  M—Mumps
  R—Rubella
Mumps
OPV (oral poliovirus vaccine)
Plague
Pneumococcal
Rabies
Rubella
Tetanus
TD
  T—Tetanus
  D—Diphtheria
Typhoid
Yellow fever

Adapted from: Centers for Disease Control. "General Recommendations on Immunization." *Morbidity and Mortality Weekly Report* (April 7, 1989): 205–28.

outbreaks of measles have occurred on a number of high school and college campuses throughout the nation.

Adult cases account for 86 percent of all instances of hepatitis B, yet a vaccine is available to provide protection. This vaccine should be given to health care workers who are at risk for hepatitis. A series of three doses is assumed to be satisfactory for giving lifetime protection. A major barrier to the use of this vaccine is that it is rather expensive. If an individual is planning to travel abroad to areas where polio is endemic, it is necessary to be completely protected for this communicable disease.

Immunizations among the elderly for influenza and pneumonia should also be of concern. Standard procedure is that anyone over sixty-five years of age should be given yearly influenza shots, as should other people with such chronic health conditions as heart disease, lung disorders, and diabetes. These vaccines are usually made available through local health departments, medical care facilities, and individual physicians.

A number of measures need to be encouraged to increase the level of immunization among adults. All adults, young and old, should analyze their immunization records to ascertain the diseases for which they lack protection. Institutions of higher education should require all entering students to meet certain immunization standards. In addition, many adults, particularly elderly individuals, would be more likely to obtain necessary immunizations if payment was provided by health insurance carriers. Physicians serving adults need to be more involved in seeing that their patients have current, updated immunizations.

Respiratory Diseases

Respiratory illnesses, especially if acute, are frequently the cause of short-term debilitation and sickness. It is estimated that as many as 250 million people fall victim to acute respiratory diseases each year in the United States.[8] These illnesses account for a minimum of 400 million days in bed, 125 million days lost from work, and 125 million days of absence from school.[9]

Respiratory infections follow a similar pattern. Each begins when the pathogenic microorganism, the virus or bacteria, invades the host. The period from this time of invasion until the first appearance of symptoms is known as the *incubation period*. The incubation period varies in length from one disease to another. It may last only a day or two, as in the case of the common cold and influenza, or, as with rubella and rubeola, it may be much longer. Because there are no disease symptoms during the incubation period, the individual is unaware of infection. As a result, the person will continue to work or attend school, so spreading infectious organisms to others.

The symptoms of respiratory infections vary. However, the initial symptoms are usually fever, chills, headache, sweating, and general aches and pains. These symptoms occur for only a short period, known as the *prodromal period*. This period ends when the specific disease symptoms appear. During the prodromal period, the respiratory infection is very contagious. For effective disease control, individuals experiencing symptoms of a slight cold should be kept away from school, work, and other locations where the disease could spread to others.

As the specific disease signs and symptoms develop to their fullest intensity, the *acme stage* of the disease is reached.[10] The disease is communicable during this stage, although the patient is usually not well enough to move in settings where the disease can be easily spread. The individual is either home in bed or hospitalized, and under the care of a physician.

The defense mechanism of the body, the development of antibodies, and various drug therapies reduce the effect of the pathogens. In many instances the sick person also receives treatment for specific symptoms— fever, sore throat, or chills.

The last stage of a respiratory disease is the *convalescence stage*. During this time the disease subsides and the host's body returns to normal. There are times after recovery, however, when the host may still be a reservoir of infection. Even though there is no outward indication of the disease, the host may be a *carrier* of the pathogenic microorganisms and is capable of transmitting the disease to another human host. During this stage the overall body resistance is also weakened. If the person is not particularly careful, a relapse can occur. For this reason, the patient should not return to work or school until certain that the infection is no longer present.

There are numerous respiratory diseases that affect people of all ages, races, and localities. The common cold, influenza, and pneumonia are examples of infectious respiratory diseases that cause a great deal of illness and debilitation.

Common Cold

Possibly the most prevalent respiratory disease is the common cold, which is caused by a number of different viruses classified as rhinoviruses. The common cold is a highly contagious disease of the upper respiratory tract, affecting particularly the nose and throat. The pathogens involved can be easily transmitted to another individual by coughing, sneezing, talking, and even breathing.

The incubation period of the common cold is from one to three days, and the greatest period of communicability is at the onset of the disease. However, the length of illness varies, often lasting up to two or more weeks.

The principal care and treatment of a person with the common cold involves symptom relief. Bed rest and liquids are usually recommended. Aspirin may be helpful in relief of fever and pain, although there is no drug therapy that will cure the common cold. Antibiotics, such as penicillin, are not effective against the viruses.

Though some measures can be taken to prevent the common cold from developing, there is no guarantee of protection. Vaccination is ineffective because of the number of viruses (possibly one hundred or more) that cause colds; protection against one virus does not protect against all others.

Influenza

Another infectious respiratory illness is influenza, which is more severe than the common cold. Four different types of viruses cause influenza. These viruses are spread by direct contact (as by kissing) and by the common use of objects, such as cups, glasses, and towels. The influenza viruses are most likely transmitted by droplets on these objects that have been expelled by coughing, sneezing, and breathing.

The influenza incubation period is from one to two days. The early symptoms include high fever (101 to 104 degrees Fahrenheit), chills, headache, sore throat, aches and pains, and exhaustion. In addition, a dry cough may appear.

Influenza often occurs in epidemic patterns in a specific geographical area. Historically, pandemics (worldwide incidences) of influenza have caused the death of millions of people. It is estimated that the influenza pandemic in 1918 caused the death of more than twenty-one million people. But such widespread epidemics have been reduced with the development of vaccines that are effective in the prevention and control of influenza. Public health policy today is to vaccinate those populations at greatest risk: individuals over 65 years of age, those with chronic medical conditions, and children and adults with other respiratory problems.[11]

The normal treatment of influenza includes bed rest, plentiful liquids, regular doses of aspirin, and warmth. As with the common cold, the use of drugs is not effective in combating the influenza viruses.

Pneumonia

The sixth leading cause of death is pneumonia combined with influenza. Approximately 2.4 million cases of pneumonia occur each year, causing an estimated 40,000 deaths.[12]

Pneumonia is an acute inflammation of the lungs caused by bacteria, viruses, or mycoplasmas. It can be an original infection or it can be the result of a complication of some other illness. For example, pneumonia often develops after a person has had the common cold or influenza. Because of lowered body resistance, the pathogenic microorganisms gain control, multiply, and spread; pneumonia develops.

The signs and symptoms of pneumonia include high fever, chills, sweating, and chest pain. In many instances breathing may be difficult and the victim may cough up colored sputum.

Treatment of bacterial and mycoplasma-caused pneumonia includes the use of antibiotics, though antibiotics are not effective against the viral infection. As with other respiratory diseases, treatment is symptomatic. Measures are taken to lower the high body temperature caused by fever, since sustained high body temperature can cause convulsions and severe brain damage. If the person is having difficulty breathing, oxygen intake must be assisted. Relief from coughing is also important, as is rest.

There are vaccines available for some types of pneumonia. New vaccines are under research and development. In spite of the availability of vaccines it is estimated that only about 20 percent of adults take advantage of these vaccines.[13] For this reason the federal government has called for an increase in vaccination for pneumonia, particularly among high-risk populations, by the year 2000.[14]

Prevention is extremely important in limiting the spread of the common cold, influenza, and pneumonia. Good health habits are more helpful than the use of vaccines in preventing these respiratory diseases. Proper diet, adequate rest, and good hygiene provide resistance to respiratory diseases. Prompt remedial action is also important whenever the initial signs of a respiratory disease appear.

Tuberculosis

One of the most feared of all respiratory diseases has been tuberculosis. At the beginning of the twentieth century tuberculosis was as dreaded as AIDS is today. This disease has caused millions of deaths since the beginning of human history. Despite the fact that tuberculosis is no longer a problem of epidemic proportion in the United States, over twenty thousand cases are reported annually, and of these, nearly two thousand victims die.[15] Currently the tuberculosis incidence rate is 9.3 per 100,000 population.[16] The United States government has set 3.5 per 100,000 as the objective for the nation by the year 2000.[17] Worldwide the incidence of tuberculosis is much higher, about three million people die from tuberculosis each year.[18]

By the early 1980s the tuberculosis rate in the United States had reached the lowest in modern history. This was the result of improvements in nutrition, hygiene, and hospital care through the years. However, in 1985 the incidence of tuberculosis started to rise and has continued to increase each year since. Most of the new cases are occurring among the poor minority populations living in large urban cities. These cases are found principally among individuals with AIDS, drug abusers, homeless persons living in shelters, diabetics, prison inmates, and immigrants coming to the United States from countries having high tuberculosis incidence. For most of these people, poor nutrition, crowded living conditions, high levels of stress, and lack of adequate medical care are particular risk factors.

There has been an increased incidence of tuberculosis among individuals with AIDS. Tuberculosis is not caused by AIDS. However, the individual who is HIV positive has a weakened immune system and as a result has a greater chance of developing tuberculosis.

Antitubercular drugs will almost always cure tuberculosis. As symptoms begin to disappear, many infected individuals stop taking the medication and do not finish treatment. When treated in a tuberculosis treatment facility or general hospital there has usually been assurance that the person would stay on the medication. However, with the increasing use of outpatient care, control is reduced and many of the economically disadvantaged do not continue with their medication.

In 1989 the Centers for Disease Control and Prevention (CDC) adopted a plan for the elimination of tuberculosis in the United States by the year 2010. The CDC suggested that such a goal could be reached by implementing three action steps:[19]

1. More effective use of existing preventive and control measures among high-risk populations.

2. Development of better technologies for tuberculosis treatment, diagnosis, and prevention.

3. Use of newly developed technologies in clinical and public health practice.

In setting this goal, the CDC called for improved surveillance and reporting of cases to health departments. More effective preventive screening was identified as a means of reaching the objective. Education of the public about tuberculosis was also noted as being important.

The primary cause of tuberculosis is the tubercle bacillus *Mycobacterium tuberculosis*. Though this disease primarily affects the lungs, it can spread to other parts of the body, such as the bones, joints, kidneys, and skin. Most people's immune system keeps the tuberculosis bacterium, when present, from becoming active. When the immune system breaks down the bacteria start to multiply and spread throughout the body.

There are a number of secondary causes of tuberculosis. Throughout history it has been closely associated with poverty. Tuberculosis is frequently found in overcrowded environments, in locations having poor hygiene and sanitation, and in settings where there is poor ventilation. It is associated with malnutrition, inadequate sleep, and emotional stress. In the United States, tuberculosis is concentrated among the economically disadvantaged in urban ghettos, in Appalachia, among Native Americans, and in the Southwest among Hispanics.

The majority of tuberculosis in the United States today is found among the elderly. Most of these individuals were infected years ago and are experiencing a recurrence of old infections. Most cases of tuberculosis among children occur in minority populations.

There are two commonly used measures for detecting tuberculosis in humans: (1) the tuberculin skin test and (2) the chest x-ray. The tuberculin skin test indicates the presence of the tuberculosis bacillus in the body. If the reaction is positive, it indicates that the individual has the bacillus. However, this does not indicate whether the case is active or dormant.

The chest x-ray indicates the infection's degree of activity. It is the most accurate procedure for detecting pulmonary tuberculosis as well as the extent of the development and spread of the infection.

Treatment of active tuberculosis often involves hospital inpatient care as well as extended outpatient medical supervision. The need for extended hospital care has been reduced in recent years largely because of drug treatment. The use of drugs to combat and cure tuberculosis has been very successful. Such drugs as isoniazid (INH), rifampin, streptomycin, and ethambutol do not kill the tubercle bacillus, but keep it from multiplying so that the body can more effectively counter the disease organism. Many of the cases that have been diagnosed recently are being caused by microorganisms that seem to have developed a resistance to the traditional drugs of choice for treating tuberculosis. This is causing much concern by physicians and public health authorities.

A vaccine, called the BCG (Bacillus Calmette-Guerin) vaccine, has been developed for tuberculosis. This vaccine provides a degree of active immunity. It also makes the person "TB-positive" and thereby destroys the usefulness of the tuberculin skin test as a diagnostic screening device. As a result, the vaccine is only used in the United States among populations at risk for tuberculosis, such as the elderly, the poor, and certain medical care providers. The BCG vaccine has been used extensively in some nations with high incidences of tuberculosis and where a large number of people have already tested positive for the disease.

Tuberculosis is a disease that is best combated by providing better living conditions for the population at risk. Improved housing and living conditions for the poor, better nutrition, and the development of positive health habits can be very effective in reducing tuberculosis incidence. It is felt that the current need is to develop better diagnostic, treatment, and preventive procedures.[20] A need exists for biotechnological development of methods that involve simple, rapid, and low-cost tests to diagnose the disease.

Gastrointestinal Diseases

Many communicable diseases are spread through the gastrointestinal tract. The pathogenic microorganisms enter the individual through the digestive system—they are present in the food or water that is ingested—and usually leave the body through the feces or urine.

Worldwide, the principal cause of such diseases is impure, unsanitary water supplies. Millions of people do not have access to a pure water supply. Their basic source of drinking and cooking water is a stream used by cattle, by other members of the community for bathing and washing of clothing, and by other polluters. A number of different diseases affect people as a result of these poor sanitary conditions.

Dysentery affects millions of people. Unfortunately, many young children and infants cannot withstand the rigors of the disease and fall victim to it. Dysentery is not as life threatening to adults as it is to the younger population.

The two most common types of dysentery are caused by bacteria (bacillary dysentery or *Shigellosis*) and protozoa (amebic dysentery or *Amebiasis*). The human serves as the reservoir of infection in both types.

There are several ways that the infection is transmitted, the most obvious of which is the ingestion of contaminated food and water. Transmission can also result by the hands coming in contact with sewage containing the cysts or by eating uncooked vegetables, berries, and fruits that have grown in soil that was fertilized with human feces.

Some cases of dysentery, particularly bacillary dysentery, are relatively mild. However, amebic dysentery is often prolonged and can be debilitating. This form of dysentery can be exhausting because of the number and frequency of stools and the resulting dehydration. The dysentery patient should drink large amounts of noncontaminated fluids to compensate for this dehydration. Warmth is also important in the treatment of dysentery.

As with tuberculosis, the best prevention against dysentery is a more sanitary living environment including the sanitary removal of human feces. Sanitary pits are being built as part of rural community development projects in Third World nations. Protection of human water supplies against human fecal material is also a necessity. People must be educated about personal hygiene.

Sexually Transmitted Diseases

There are at least twenty diseases that have been identified which are transmitted primarily by sexual contact. These are known as *sexually transmitted diseases (STDs)*. In the past, sexually transmitted diseases were referred to as venereal disease.

The term *venereal* comes from Venus, the Roman goddess of love. Venereal diseases were once associated with lovemaking, but since this classification does not necessarily involve lovemaking, today it now is felt that the term sexually transmitted better describes this group of diseases.

A number of infections can be classified as sexually transmitted diseases, with the most common being AIDS, chlamydia, genital herpes, gonorrhea, syphilis, and trichomoniasis.

Sexually transmitted diseases cause many physical and economical problems for millions of people each year. If left untreated, they can lead to serious complications and even debilitation, since damaged or destroyed body structures cannot be replaced. Reinfection is possible with new exposure since the body does not build up an immunity to these diseases. Some sexually transmitted diseases are incurable and may afflict one with pain and suffering throughout life.

The microorganisms that cause most of the sexually transmitted diseases have been identified. For the most part, it is relatively easy to diagnose the diseases, and all but herpes and AIDS are curable. Yet the National Institute of Allergy and Infectious Disease reports that one in twenty Americans is still affected by sexually transmitted diseases.

In spite of the fact that most sexually transmitted diseases can be identified and treated, the incidences continue to rise. Among teenagers and young adults this problem is viewed as a public health epidemic. There are several reasons for this continued increase in sexually transmitted diseases, but the primary reason is the greater number of sexually active individuals in our society. Sexual activity is particularly important in the fifteen-to-thirty-year age group. The sexually active individual runs the risk of becoming infected and spreading the sexually transmitted disease, particularly when sexual behavior is casual—with several different partners. Often one infected person can spread the disease to a multitude of contacts.

Despite the increased sexual activity, most people do not understand the dangers of sexually transmitted diseases. These diseases are a topic that many people find difficult to discuss because of taboos relating to historically negative attitudes toward sexual activity, particularly intercourse. Victims find their problem demeaning, as does society in general.

Some believe that a discussion of these diseases is unwarranted, particularly in the schools. They reason that any introduction to these diseases necessitates a discussion as to how they are spread, and as such is inappropriate for school-age children. Because people lack knowledge, our society continues to have a problem with these diseases.

In 1986, the Surgeon General, recognizing the dangerous lack of information about AIDS among the general population, called for the development of extensive school sex education programs. These programs should include instruction about AIDS. The Surgeon General recommended that such instructional programs should begin as early as the primary grades.

When infected, many young people do not seek medical care. This is often owing to the stigma placed upon them by their peers and also the fear of their parents' reactions. They fear that in the eyes of their peers they will be viewed as "pimps," "prostitutes," or other social outcasts. Many do not seek treatment because they do not know the symptoms. The infected individual may attempt to treat the problem with over-the-counter drugs, none of which is effective, or may even ignore the symptoms.

The question of whether the teenager's parents should be informed that their child is being treated at a public health clinic for a sexually transmitted disease is a difficult problem. In some jurisdictions, young people below the age of sixteen or eighteen are not treated in public clinics unless the parents are informed. But this policy discourages many young people from seeking badly needed help, since they do not wish to have their parents aware of the problem.

Many public health personnel who work with young people having sexually transmitted diseases feel that there should be no parent notification. The likelihood of the individual seeking early treatment is more probable if parents are not notified. Because of the importance of early diagnosis and treatment in protecting against permanent body organ damage, the issue is one of medical, legal, and social importance.

Health Effects of STDs

The sexually transmitted diseases cause many health problems. Generally, the initial symptoms are more easily noticed in males than in females, so the male usually seeks treatment earlier in the infectious stage than does the female. The female frequently has neither clinical signs nor other complaints during the first stages of the disease, though lesions and tissue damage may occur within the vagina or the cervix at this time.

One of the most serious problems is pelvic inflammatory disease (PID), which causes sterility in many women. Women who have PID are at increased risk for having an ectopic pregnancy, chronic pelvic pain, and tubal infertility. This condition results when microorganisms from the vagina and endocervix ascend to the endometrium, the fallopian tubes, and other reproductive organs. There are numerous ways in which such infection can occur. For example, use of the intrauterine device is a risk factor for the development of pelvic inflammatory disease. Since there may be different microorganisms involved in the infection, there is no single treatment of choice. Hospitalization is usually recommended in most cases of PID. Major surgery is sometimes required, often resulting in the removal of the reproductive organs.

Syphilis and Gonorrhea

Syphilis and gonorrhea are caused by bacterial organisms. Syphilis is caused by the spirochete bacterium (*Treponema pallidum*) and gonorrhea by the gonococcus bacterium (*Neisseria gonorrhoeae*). Gonorrhea is the most frequently reported communicable disease in the United States, with more than one-half million cases being reported annually, while more than 128 thousand cases of syphilis are reported each year.[21] It is not known how many unreported cases occur throughout the nation.

Syphilis

Nearly every organ of the body can be affected by syphilis. Its incubation period ranges from several days to as long as three months, but the normal span is about three weeks. The initial sign of syphilis is the presence of the chancre, a painless sore that develops at the site of the infection. It is oval in shape with hard edges. Within a few weeks the chancre disappears, regardless of whether or not the individual receives treatment. This stage is known as *primary syphilis,* when the disease can be cured by penicillin.

If the patient is not treated, the disease advances to the next stage, known as *secondary syphilis*. The signs and symptoms appear within about six months after the chancre disappears. The indications of secondary syphilis include a rash that covers different parts of the body, patches of hair loss, and the general symptoms of illness—fever, headache, and weakness.

During this stage the disease is highly infectious. This disease begins to damage the various organs and structures of the body. In time, the second stage's symptoms disappear and syphilis enters a *latent stage*. The latent stage may last for a lengthy period during which second-stage symptoms disappear and the individual appears healthy and is noninfectious. However, at some point in the future, possibly as long as ten to twenty years, the defenses of the body break down and the disease is reactivated. During this latent syphilis stage, the disease can still be cured, but whatever organ and tissue damage has occurred is permanent.

Early diagnosis of syphilis is necessary to prevent the more severe effects of the later stages. Diagnosis is made by examining tissue taken from a chancre and by blood testing. Syphilis is treated principally with penicillin. However, any physiological damage cannot be reversed, thus emphasizing the importance of early identification and treatment.

Gonorrhea

The incubation period of gonorrhea is normally about two to ten days. The first sign of infection in males is a discharge during urination of a thick, yellowish pus. A burning sensation often accompanies urination. These initial indications are usually of such a nature that males will seek some kind of treatment.

The situation is quite different for women. The initial symptoms may be an itching or burning in the genital area with a slight discharge. Often this is not enough indication to cause alarm. Consequently, the female often does not seek proper medical care during the early stage. Left untreated, the disease spreads to the upper organs of the reproductive system. Severe pain, pelvic inflammatory disease, and damage to the fallopian tubes often occur. If treatment is not sought in time, sterility results.

Penicillin has been particularly effective in treating gonorrhea. However, penicillin resistant strains of the bacteria have developed in recent years. In these situations other antibiotics must be used.

Gonorrhea is particularly dangerous if the woman is pregnant. As the infant passes through the birth canal, the bacteria can get into the baby's eyes and cause blindness. For this reason, drops of chemoprophylactic agents are put into the eyes of newborns.[22]

Genital Herpes

A particularly serious sexually transmitted disease, genital herpes is occurring more and more frequently. In the past two decades physician-patient consultations for this disease have increased fifteen-fold.[23] This increase has been about equal between males and females.

The disease is caused by the herpes simplex virus type 2. The initial symptom is the presence of small blisters on the genitalia of females or the glans penis in males. The prime reservoirs of infection are the cervix in females and the semen in males. The blisters of herpes tend to come and go; however, the virus is still present. For this reason one cannot consider that the individual is healed when the blisters go into remission. They are likely to return again.

These fluid-filled sores may burn and itch and are usually quite painful, as in urination. Many people with herpes get the burning, itching, and tingling symptoms just prior to the development of the lesions.

Acyclovir ointment is used in treating primary and recurrent cases of genital herpes. An oral form of this drug has been developed that is very effective. However, the long-term safety of oral acyclovir is still being studied. It must be noted that acyclovir is effective in managing genital herpes, but it does not kill the virus.

It is important to keep the sores clean and dry and not to scratch them. For an otherwise healthy person, genital herpes is usually not dangerous. However, if the virus comes in contact with the eyes and is left untreated, it can cause blindness. It can cause many problems during pregnancy such as spontaneous abortion and stillbirth. Pregnant women can transmit the disease to their babies if they have active lesions in the birth canal at the time of delivery. In the female, the infection may locate on the cervix and may cause cervical cancer. Women with genital herpes should get Pap smear tests annually.

Chlamydia

The most common sexually transmitted disease is *chlamydia,* with some three to four million cases being reported annually. It is caused by the bacterium *Chlamydia trachomatis.* This disease is transmitted only by sexual contact or from an infected mother to the infant at birth. Often chlamydia is without symptoms and is not diagnosed until complications develop.

Chlamydia is not a fatal disease and is curable. However, there are a number of complications that can be serious. In females, pelvic inflammatory disease sometimes leads to ectopic pregnancy—the fetus growing in a fallopian tube rather than in the uterus. Sterility may occur. Symptoms and signs in females include abnormal vaginal discharge, pelvic pain, nausea, fever, and pain upon urination.

Males with chlamydia may experience a number of genital infections. Infection of the tube between the testes and the penis—the epididymis—can occur. Some of the symptoms are similar to those of gonorrhea: painful, burning sensation upon urination and milky discharge from the urethra.

Antibiotics are very effective in halting this infection. Tetracycline and erythromycin are the antibiotics of choice at the present time. Penicillin, which is effective in treating several other STDs, is not effective against chlamydia.

Chlamydia is not a reportable disease. Therefore, many physicians do not report cases. The Centers for Disease Control and Prevention recommends that clinics specializing in the treatment of sexually transmitted diseases screen all patients for chlamydia. There are several diagnostic tests. The standard procedure is to culture a sample in tissue culture. This may take as long as a week, during which time the individual can infect others. Thus, the importance of prevention and education can be understood.

Prevention of STDs

Prevention must be emphasized in controlling sexually transmitted diseases. In order to reduce the possibility of contracting or spreading one of these diseases, sexually active males are advised to practice good genital hygiene and to use a condom during intercourse. Proper genital hygiene and medical examinations are precautions females should take.

The most important preventive measure is immediate treatment after infection. When a case of an STD is reported, it must be investigated. The infected individual must identify all previous sexual contacts to the public health sexually transmitted disease clinic or to other appropriate medical personnel. Only as these sexual partners are identified, contacted, examined, and treated will the epidemic proportions of STDs be reduced.

Ongoing research and development continue to supply more knowledge about the prevention and treatment of all sexually transmitted diseases. For example, attempts have been made to develop a vaccine to treat gonorrhea and to provide prolonged immunity against it. However, many suggest that the most important measure in reducing the incidences of STDs is providing information and knowledge that leads to behavioral change. The public must be aware of the dangers of not just the best-known STDs—chlamydia, syphilis, gonorrhea, and genital herpes—but also the numerous lesser-known diseases.

Lesser-Known STDs

Bacterial vaginosis—Common infection of the vagina characterized by a discharge. Not caused only by sexual activity.

Chancroid—Bacterial infection that begins with the appearance of painful open sores on the genitals.

Cytomegalovirus infections—Viral infection that infects many adults, usually without serious consequences. Virus is found in body fluids, such as saliva and urine, and is spread by various forms of physical contact. A risk of congenital disease in infants occurs when infection occurs during the pregnancy.

Genital mycoplasma infections—Infection caused by tiny bacteria found in the genital tracts of both males and females.

Granuloma inguinale—Progressive bacterial infection of the genitals that can cause serious complications if left untreated.

Group B streptococcal infections—Commonly found infections in the genitals of males and females in which the risk of infection increases with the level of sexual activity.

Pubic lice—Tiny mites that infest the pubic hair and feed on human blood. This itching disease is often spread by sexual contact.

Scabies—Highly contagious skin infestation that is spread primarily through sexual contact. This condition is characterized by intense itching.

Trichomoniasis—Protozoan-caused disease in which there is vaginal discharge, discomfort during sexual intercourse, and painful urination.

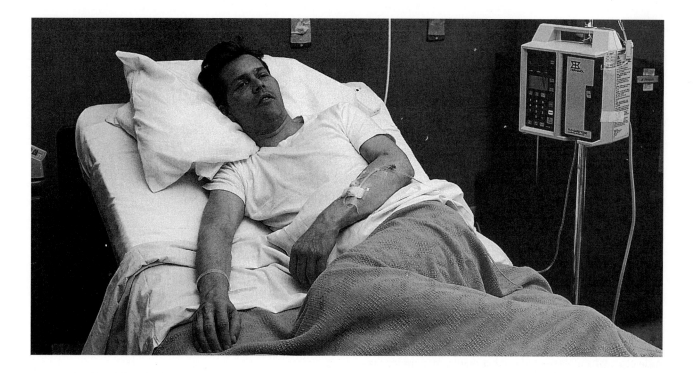

AIDS is a serious disease resulting in increased debilitation until death occurs.

Acquired Immunodeficiency Syndrome (AIDS)

The Disease

Possibly no human communicable disease in the twentieth century has caused as much fear, uncertainty, and emotional concern as has acquired immunodeficiency syndrome (AIDS). This disease is characterized by a breakdown of the immune mechanism, which combats certain infections. Since the first known cases of AIDS were reported in the United States, the number of cases has increased to more than 230,000 reported cases. Worldwide more than two million cases have been reported. The number of unreported cases is not known. Projections are that these numbers will more than double by the middle of the 1990s. In addition, the Centers for Disease Control and Prevention has estimated that there are between one and one-and-a-half million individuals who are infected with HIV (human immunodeficiency virus) in the United States. Worldwide there may be as many as five to ten

million infected individuals. By any estimate, numbers will increase dramatically in the 1990s. The Secretary of Health and Human Services predicted that more than a quarter million deaths from AIDS will be recorded in the early 1990s.

Cases have been reported in all fifty states, with nearly 90 percent being in the 20 to 49 age group. Nearly 90 percent of AIDS cases have been among males.[24] However, the number of cases among females has increased since the early 1990s. Most of these women contract AIDS as the result of IV drug use or heterosexual contact with IV drug users. Three-fourths of the females who have developed AIDS occur among the minority population. A concern that must be noted is that the HIV virus can be transmitted from an infected female to her fetus in utero and also during the birth process. This is leading to an increasing number of newborn infants with the HIV virus. Most cases have been found to be in urban metropolitan areas. However, an increasing number of AIDS cases are being noted in small cities and rural communities.

This disease was unknown until 1979 when it was noted in two individuals who died after receiving plasma for hemophilia. Since then more than 133 thousand people have died. So far there is no cure for AIDS, and it is estimated that none will be available until early in the twenty-first century. AIDS is 100 percent fatal, with death usually occurring within two to three years from the onset of the symptoms.

It is important to understand the development of this disease from the time that the HIV virus enters the human body. The Presidential Commission on the Human Immunodeficiency Virus (1988) suggested that the term HIV infection more correctly defines this disease than the term AIDS. The commission stated that it is necessary to direct the focus upon the entire spectrum of HIV disease, not just on the condition of AIDS itself.

When the HIV virus enters the human body the individual is said to have the HIV infection. It is at this time that HIV antibodies develop. For a period of several years the individual may present no symptoms. During this time the HIV attacks the immune system and begins to destroy white blood cells. As a result, fatigue, minor illnesses, and infections may cause the infected person increasing problems.

Usually it is not for five to ten years that the individual with HIV infection begins to develop the symptoms of AIDS. During this incubation period, when there are no symptomatic indications of AIDS, the individual is a carrier of the HIV virus. Obviously it is during these years that one can transmit the virus unknowingly to another person.

When AIDS first surfaced as a health problem, it was found mostly among homosexual males having numerous sexual partners. The greatest number of cases is still found among this population group. A second group at risk for AIDS is intravenous drug abusers sharing unsterile needles. Increasing numbers of AIDS victims can be found in the heterosexual population among persons having multiple sexual partners and among infants born to mothers carrying HIV. Some, particularly hemophiliacs, have reported contracting the disease by receiving blood transfusions. This population is at less risk since the development of a test in the mid-1980s that ascertains whether blood is HIV-positive before it is made available for transfusion.

The Cause of AIDS

The etiologic agent that causes AIDS is known as the human immunodeficiency virus (HIV). This virus was first identified in 1981 and is believed to have arisen in Africa. The virus was isolated and identified by researchers working separately at the National Cancer Institute in the United States and at the Pasteur Institute in Paris at about the same time. Research has shown that the virus attacks the T4 lymphocytes (a subgroup of white blood cells), which help defend the body against certain infections. It is believed that the virus enters the T cell and incorporates itself into the genetic material (DNA) in the nucleus. The virus reproduces itself and kills the T cell, which then releases new viruses that invade and kill other T cells. Because this destroys the defense function of the immune system, the infected person is unable to resist other pathogenic microorganisms.

The HIV virus is carried in body fluids: blood, semen, and saliva. It is transmitted by blood and semen into the bloodstream of a recipient. There is no proven transmission of the virus by saliva, tears, sweat, or urine. The virus is very fragile and does not survive outside of the body. It must reproduce inside human cells and is easily destroyed by soap and water and other cleansers. Medical authorities point out that it cannot be transmitted by casual contact such as touch or kissing.

Current screening tests cannot diagnose AIDS but can only detect antibodies in the blood. A test will not tell whether an individual will develop the disease; it is only an indicator that a person has at one time been infected by HIV. This means that the person is capable of transmitting the virus to another person by way of the blood and/or semen.

The most commonly used test is an enzyme-linked immunosorbent assay (elisa). This test is easy to conduct, relatively inexpensive, not technically difficult to do, and can be completed in about two or so hours. The elisa test identifies blood that contains antibodies to HIV. A problem with this test is that it sometimes produces false-positive readings in blood that does not contain the antibodies, so the elisa test alone is not a valid screening procedure.

Another more expensive, difficult, and complex test, the western blot, or immunoblot, is used to confirm a positive elisa test. This test is currently too expensive to

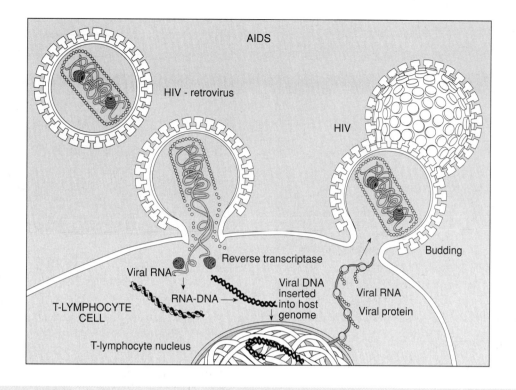

The AIDS life cycle.

Symptoms of the AIDS Patient

1. Early influenzalike symptoms (swollen lymph glands, night sweats, diarrhea) with recurrent respiratory and digestive infections
2. Recurrence of fungus infections
3. Development of purplish skin lesions (Kaposi's sarcoma)
4. Spread of Kaposi's resulting in bleeding from vital organs
5. Development of non-Hodgkin's lymphoma
6. Recurrent infections becoming more severe
7. Forgetfulness, impaired speech, tremors, seizures

be used as a primary test in large group screening efforts. Research is presently being conducted to develop more accurate, less expensive tests. If someone is found to be HIV positive using this test, the individual is assumed to be capable of infecting others.

Research and Education

There is no cure for AIDS, though current research is attempting to find one. More than fifty drugs are undergoing various tests to determine their effectiveness against HIV. Each of the institutes of the National Institutes of Health is involved in some aspect of AIDS research. The National Institute of Allergy and Infectious Diseases is specifically identified for coordinating, conducting, and supporting AIDS research. In 1989 the Division of AIDS within this institute was designated to manage research initiatives.

A number of clinical studies of promising AIDS therapies have been carried out by the National Institute of Allergy and Infectious Diseases. Investigations have been conducted on an international scale to ascertain the modes of disease transmission and the possible role of other factors such as diet, race, and genetics. The major aim of this institute and other research centers has been to

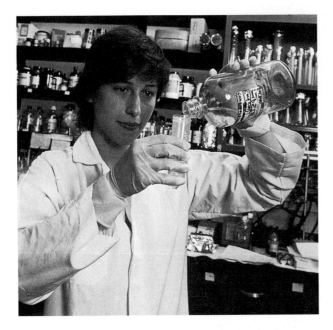

The Elisa Assay Test has been commonly used to identify HIV antibodies in blood.

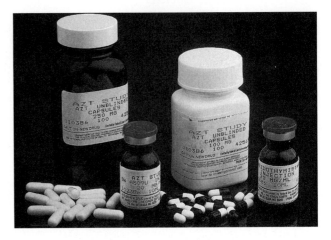

The drug azidothymidine (AZT) has been used widely to slow the progress of AIDS in some cases.

develop a vaccine that can prevent this disease. Currently there has been little success, and many project that a vaccine will not be available until into the next decade.

The antiviral drug azidothymidine (AZT) has been used in some AIDS cases. Research has shown that this drug slows the development of the disease in some cases. It cannot cure, but it has been effective in treating some AIDS-related symptoms.

Other research initiatives of the different National Institutes of Health have focused on the neurodevelopment of HIV-infected children, the transmission of HIV infection from mother to child, and the nursing needs of AIDS patients.

In the meantime, prevention is the most important community health measure that can be taken to fight AIDS. Educating the public about how the disease is spread, its potential danger, how to keep from getting the virus, and how to cope with and assist AIDS patients has become a major emphasis. In 1988 the office of the Surgeon General prepared a brochure entitled *Understanding AIDS*, which was mailed to every household in the United States. Its purpose was to inform the American public about the disease and eliminate much of the misinformation being spread about AIDS.

Educational initiatives must reach the population groups at risk, namely, the homosexual and bisexual population, IV drug users, and women. More schools are including AIDS instruction in their school curriculum, so children and adolescents should be better informed about this disease. Culturally sensitive information programs directed toward minority populations are needed.

In 1985 the Public Health Service published several life-style recommendations designed to reduce the risk of contracting AIDS.
1. Do not have sexual contact with persons known to have or suspected of having AIDS.
2. Do not have sex with multiple partners.
3. Do not use intravenous drugs.
4. Do not have sex with people who are known to inject drugs.
5. Avoid anal intercourse.
6. Protect yourself and your partner during sexual intercourse by using condoms and avoiding oral-genital contact, open-mouth kissing, and contact with body fluids (semen, blood, urine, and feces).

Social and Economic Factors

A number of social questions continue to confront medical personnel and public policymakers. The most significant issue is mandatory testing for HIV. A small minority of individuals has suggested that the entire population should be required to undergo testing for AIDS. A more

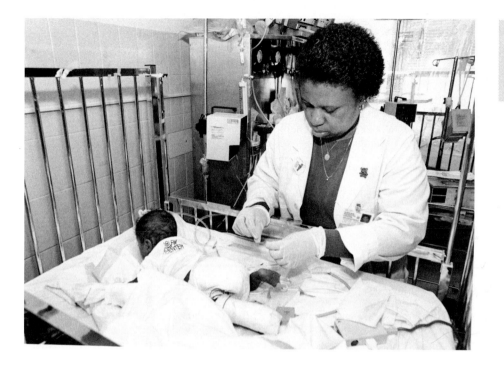

rational view is that individuals should be required to submit to AIDS testing as part of preemployment examinations or when applying for life and health insurance policies. However, this suggestion raises questions of infringement of individual rights and freedoms. It also creates a new issue: what is to be done with those who test positive for HIV/AIDS?

Increasingly, individuals who come into contact with human blood are taking precautionary measures. Physicians, dentists, nurses, dental hygienists, and other health care providers are wearing rubber gloves. Police authorities are wearing gloves when they come in contact with human blood. It has been reported that equipment managers for several professional football teams are now wearing rubber gloves when handling bloodied uniforms.

AIDS is a growing economic burden on the health care system as well as on individual families. With projections that the number of cases will escalate during the 1990s, the cost of caring for AIDS patients will add to the financial problems of a health care system that is already overextended. A study of the Agency for Health Care Policy and Research announced in 1992 that expenditures for AIDS treatment and care could rise 50 percent by the mid-1990s.[25] By 1995 the cost of treating people with AIDS could reach $15 billion, an annual cost of $38,000 per patient.

Basic patient care is usually long-term and thus very expensive. In addition, drugs such as AZT have been very costly. The problem is particularly acute for those health departments and hospitals that find it necessary to take high-risk patients—those who are drug users, homosexuals, or HIV-positive.

Governmental funding for AIDS, both federal and state, has increased significantly. Most federal funding has been applied to containing the spread of the disease and to research directed at finding a cure. Little funding has been directed at developing intervention strategies. Direct economic support for clinical services and the medical management of cases has been less. AIDS is projected to be a principal factor in the continuing escalation of health care expenditures throughout the 1990s.

Pediatric AIDS

The increasing number of AIDS cases among infants and children is a great concern. Until the latter part of the 1980s, there were relatively few cases among children. Nearly all were infected through blood transfusions

HIV/AIDS

Risk Reduction Objectives:

1. Reduce sexual intercourse among adolescents.
2. Increase use of condoms among sexually active, unmarried adults.
3. Increase involvement of intravenous drug abusers in drug abuse treatment programs.
4. Increase use of uncontaminated drug paraphernalia among intravenous drug abusers.

Source: Public Health Service. *Healthy People 2000: National Health Promotion and Disease Prevention Objectives.* Washington, D.C.: U.S. Government Printing Office, 1991, pp. 484–87.

Issue—Case Study
Control of AIDS

Today prevention of AIDS is receiving much attention. Educational initiatives have been designed for many different population groups: school-aged young people, business and industry employees, and at-risk populations, as well as senior citizens. Instruction in the use of condoms as an AIDS preventive measure has led to more openness about other means of birth control.

However, there are a number of social questions about public policy measures that should or should not be taken to control the spread of AIDS. The spread of HIV/AIDS must be managed within each individual community. What should be the role of the local health department in surveillance of AIDS cases?

A principal measure for controlling the spread of most sexually transmitted diseases has been to locate those individuals who have had sexual contact with anyone proved to have syphilis and/or gonorrhea. Some in America feel that partners who have been exposed to HIV should be located and informed of the potential danger they are facing. This could be accomplished either by having HIV/AIDS-infected persons directly notify their partners or by having health authorities do so. With this in mind, should health departments track down and locate those who have had sexual or needle contact with an AIDS-infected person? Should physicians be required, or expected, to inform the suspected sexual and/or needle contacts of their HIV/AIDS-positive patients?

including hemophiliacs. All these occurred before 1985 when blood testing was mandated.

The reason for the rising number of pediatric AIDS cases is illicit drug use. Children being born to women who are HIV-positive are being infected through perinatal transmission. It is now estimated that 80 percent of pediatric AIDS cases occur in this manner, with a majority being born to minority parents, Hispanics or African-Americans. The mothers are using many different drugs, but the crack-cocaine epidemic has been a major influence.

A problem related to pediatric AIDS is the difficulty of identifying infected infants immediately at birth. In addition, because of the drug-related problems with which the mother must cope, she often is not able or willing to care for the child. This has resulted in more babies with HIV infection needing foster care. Many foster parents are not interested in taking an HIV-infected infant.

Every day brings new developments in the biomedical, educational, social, and political arenas relating to HIV/AIDS. Until a cure is found and this disease is eradicated, the daily newspapers may be the most valuable source of current information and knowledge.

Lyme Disease

Not all diseases are pandemic, that is, worldwide, in scope. Some diseases tend to be restricted to smaller geographical locations. One disease that fell into this category during the 1980s was Lyme disease.

Lyme disease was unknown until 1975 when it was first recognized in Lyme, Connecticut. Since then there has been an increasing number of cases throughout the United States, with over 90 percent occurring in the northeastern and upper midwestern states.

Lyme disease is caused by a spiral-shaped bacterium that is spread by the bite of the deer tick, *Ixodes dammini*. This tick is very small and has a black head and an orange abdomen. Though part of the tick's life cycle is spent living off different kinds of animals, it has been noted particularly in locations with large deer populations. The prime habitat of the tick seems to be where grasslands meet the woods. Epidemiological studies have concluded that the tick attaches to people who are walking in grassy or wooded areas. For this reason, people who spend time in the woods during the summer or who live in rural or suburban locations with long grass and woods and the presence of deer are at risk. Early signs and indications include a number of influenzalike symptoms: headache, stiffness and aching of the joints and muscles, swollen lymph glands, nausea, fever, a spreading rash, and fatigue. The distinctive sign is a circular rash, which usually appears within a few days after the individual is bitten by an infected tick. This ring-shaped rash usually has a clearing in the center and appears at the site of the tick bite. Approximately 70 percent of those who contract Lyme disease develop this rash. Without treatment, these signs and symptoms may disappear. Several weeks later more serious complications involving the heart and/or nervous system develop. At this time the joints and muscles become painful. Arthritis is the most commonly noted long-term sign of Lyme disease. In some cases heart disease symptoms such as dizziness, shortness of breath, or an irregular heart beat have been noted. Meningitis and facial paralysis may also occur at this stage of the disease.

Antibiotics can cure the infection, but any damage done to the organs of the body prior to treatment cannot be corrected. Thus, it is important to avoid exposure and to take preventive measures to keep the ticks off the body. When in locations where ticks are likely to be present, one should wear long-sleeved shirts and pants. Wearing light colors makes it easier to spot ticks on the clothing. Socks and shoes must be worn, with socks pulled over the cuffs of the pants. The repellent DEET, which has been shown to be effective against the tick, may be applied to the skin and clothing.

Upon returning from the out-of-doors, the person should inspect the body for ticks. Because the tick is small and difficult to find on the human body, it often escapes attention unless very systematic and careful inspection is carried out. When found on the body, care must be taken in removing the tick. Because the tick may also be found on dogs and cats, it is necessary to examine pets upon their return to the house after being outside, particularly during the spring and summer.

Current research is directed at learning more about the life cycle of the tick. In addition, studies attempting to identify more effective antibiotics are under way. Epidemiological studies are providing more information about the geographical extent of the problem throughout the nation and the world.

Smallpox: Eradication of a Disease

Possibly the most dramatic disease eradication program in history was conducted during the 1970s. Smallpox, a viral disease transmitted from person to person, had been one of the most feared diseases through the centuries. Because it was so threatening, in 1967 the World Health Organization embarked upon a worldwide smallpox eradication program.

Smallpox had caused the deaths of hundreds of millions of people throughout history. Many cities, nations, and cultures were weakened or destroyed during epidemics of this disease. European explorers introduced smallpox to the Native Americans in both North and South America. Millions of these natives, who had no natural defenses against this disease, contracted smallpox and died. There is little doubt that smallpox contributed to the destruction of the great Inca and Aztec civilizations of South and Central America.

Edward Jenner discovered the vaccination process in the late eighteenth century. Through the years, science and medicine have worked to develop an effective measure to distribute the vaccination to people on mass

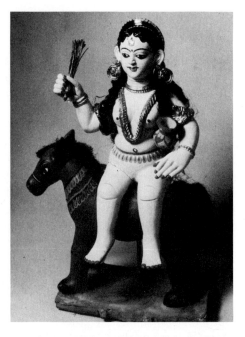

In order to eradicate smallpox, cultural beliefs had to be overcome. In India, Shitala Mata is worshiped as the goddess of smallpox. People had to be convinced that the disease was not a blessing from the goddess and that vaccination was vital to their health.

scales at low cost. It was not until the 1940s that smallpox was eradicated in the developed world—North America and Europe. However, it continued to be a serious health problem in many Third World nations. In 1967, when it was estimated that there were ten to fifteen million cases of smallpox in forty-four countries, the World Health Assembly established a policy of worldwide smallpox eradication.[26]

There was a great deal of doubt that such a goal was achievable. Many in the scientific community questioned the validity of such a program. Even the well-known authority René Dubos stated that such an attempt would be ". . . economically and humanly unwise."[27]

The World Health Organization program of smallpox eradication included mass vaccination. This was made possible by the development of a two-tiered needle that could be used by trained personnel. The needles could be sterilized and reused, and the training did not require a high level of skill. This had a profound effect on the cost of such a massive program.

An important strategy built into the smallpox eradication program was that of surveillance.[28] The practice of surveillance and containment involved moving directly into areas of smallpox outbreak and isolating known victims. In addition, everyone in the victims' communities was vaccinated. This procedure required several modes of transportation and the employment of many local people to aid the WHO medical teams.

In addition to mass immunization and surveillance, education and record keeping were employed. The educational efforts were designed to enlighten people about the disease so that they could report any suspected cases to the surveillance teams. Extensive efforts at collecting data about the presence of smallpox and the effect of the vaccine were important parts of the overall campaign.

Within eight years of the start of the program, smallpox had been eradicated from all but five countries. With concentrated efforts in these nations, any incidence of smallpox continued to be identified and eliminated. On October 26, 1979, the Director General of the World Health Organization declared that smallpox had been eradicated in all the world. The last known case was in 1979 in Somalia, in northern East Africa.[29]

As the result of this successful worldwide program of smallpox eradication, routine vaccination is no longer required. In the United States it is even impossible to obtain the vaccine in most communities. Some have questioned the future of a generation of children who have reached maturity without having smallpox vaccination. Is it possible that smallpox could reappear and create serious problems for an unvaccinated civilization? Scientists and medical professionals say this is most unlikely.

Summary

Communicable diseases were once the principal cause of sickness and death in the United States. Today, they are no longer a major threat to life. However, millions of people in America and elsewhere still suffer from one or more of these diseases annually. Therefore, communicable disease control is still an important responsibility of the public health department.

Living microorganisms are the causative agents of communicable diseases. The major pathogenic microorganisms are bacteria, viruses, fungi, protozoa, rickettsiae, and the multicellular metazoa. Communicable diseases are the result of these pathogenic microorganisms residing in a host and producing specific symptoms that lead to illness and debilitation.

When the microorganism enters a prospective host, certain defense mechanisms attempt to counter the disease. The human body has the ability to produce antibodies that can neutralize and destroy the pathogens. This ability is known as immunity. Naturally acquired immunity may be supplemented through the process of immunization.

The various communicable diseases affect many different body systems. A major focus of communicable disease control is directed at diseases of the respiratory system. All respiratory diseases follow a similar pattern. There are a number of different respiratory diseases, with the common cold, influenza, and pneumonia being the most widespread in the United States.

Tuberculosis has been the most feared respiratory disease throughout history. This disease, caused by the tubercle bacillus, has led to the death of millions. The incidence of tuberculosis has been greatly reduced in the United States, owing to improved hygiene, nutrition, and health care and effective screening procedures. However, this disease is still a widespread problem in many Third World nations and has shown an increase among the economically disadvantaged in the United States.

The number of sexually transmitted diseases is increasing in America. Ignorance, social restraints, and an increase in sexual activity have contributed to the upward swing in spite of the availability of diagnostic procedures and treatment measures. The sexually transmitted diseases are a problem particularly among teenagers and young adults in their twenties.

Gonorrhea and syphilis are probably the best known of the sexually transmitted diseases. Genital herpes is of particular concern as there is presently no effective treatment. The most prevalent sexually transmitted disease is chlamydia.

Since the early 1980s a new disease, acquired immunodeficiency syndrome (AIDS), has caused much concern and fear throughout the United States. This disease, for which there is presently no cure, is caused by the human immunodeficiency virus (HIV). It has been found principally among the homosexual population, intravenous drug users, and those who have received blood transfusions. Extensive research efforts are ongoing in an attempt to find a cure for this serious disease.

In the meantime prevention is the principal community health measure for protecting the public from AIDS. Educational initiatives have been designed for nearly all population groups. Help and understanding are very important for AIDS patients and their families. In many communities social programs have been designed to assist them.

Discussion Questions

1. What factors have led to the reduction in the past century of deaths caused by communicable diseases?

2. Explain the differences in the various pathogenic organisms that cause a majority of communicable diseases.

3. Describe the ways that pathogenic microorganisms are transmitted from a host reservoir to a new host.

4. Explain what is meant by immunity.

5. What role does the public health department play in immunization programs?

6. Be familiar with the recommended schedule for immunization of infants and children published by the Centers for Disease Control and Prevention.

7. Why is immunization for adults an important community health measure?

8. Identify those immunizations that are of particular concern to adults.

9. How do the common cold, influenza, and pneumonia differ?

10. What are the secondary factors that result in tuberculosis?

11. What are the two most effective measures available in the United States for identifying cases of tuberculosis?

12. Explain why the BCG vaccine is not widely used in the United States.

13. Identify several factors that have contributed to the increase of tuberculosis since the mid-1980s.

14. What population groups are particularly at risk for tuberculosis?

15. What measures might be most effective in reaching the goal of eliminating tuberculosis in the United States by the year 2010?

16. Identify the two most common types of dysentery.

17. Why is it difficult to control and reduce the incidences of sexually transmitted diseases?

18. What is pelvic inflammatory disease?

19. Explain the differences between syphilis and gonorrhea.

20. Why is genital herpes such a serious disease?

21. Explain the characteristics of chlamydia.

22. Discuss the preventive measures for sexually transmitted diseases.

23. What are some of the lesser-known STDs?

24. What is the incubation period for HIV?

25. Explain how the HIV virus affects the immune system.

26. Discuss the economic and political factors surrounding AIDS.

27. Identify the population groups at greater risk for HIV/AIDS.

28. Discuss the various ongoing research initiatives that are attempting to reduce the spread of AIDS.

29. Identify some of the preventive measures that have been suggested regarding AIDS.

30. In what ways is HIV/AIDS an economic factor in the health care system?

31. What are some of the factors associated with pediatric AIDS?

32. Discuss several of the recommendations identified by the federal government for coping with risk reduction for HIV/AIDS by the year 2000.

33. What are several of the characteristics associated with Lyme disease?

34. Explain factors related to treatment for Lyme disease.

35. Trace the development of the smallpox eradication program and describe its related activities.

36. Do you believe that it is a good policy to destroy or stop production of smallpox vaccine? Why or why not?

Suggested Readings

Cates, Willard, and Katherine M. Stone. "Family Planning, Sexually Transmitted Diseases and Contraceptive Choice: A Literature Update—Part I." *Family Planning Perspectives* 24, no. 2 (March/April 1992): 75–84.

Cates, Willard, and Katherine M. Stone. "Family Planning, Sexually Transmitted Diseases and Contraceptive Choice: A Literature Update—Part II." *Family Planning Perspectives* 24, no. 3 (May/June 1992): 122–28.

Centers for Disease Control. "A Strategic Plan for the Elimination of Tuberculosis in the United States." *Morbidity and Mortality Report* 38, no. S-3 (April 21, 1989—Suppl.): 25 pp.

Centers for Disease Control. "Interpretation and Use of the Western Blot Assay for Serodiagnosis of Human Immunodeficiency Virus Type 1 Infections." *Morbidity and Mortality Weekly Report* 38, no. S-7 (July 21, 1989): 7 pp.

Centers for Disease Control. "Prevention and Control of Influenza." *Morbidity and Mortality Weekly Report* 41, no. RR-9 (May 15, 1992): 4–5.

Centers for Disease Control. "Successful Strategies in Adult Immunization." *Morbidity and Mortality Weekly Report* 40, no. 41 (October 18, 1991): 700–709.

Centers for Disease Control and Prevention. "Update: Multistate Outbreak of Escherichia coli O157:H7 Infections from Hamburgers—Western United States, 1992–1993." *Morbidity and Mortality Weekly Report* 42, no. 14 (April 16, 1993): 258–63.

Department of Health and Human Services, Public Health Service, Centers for Disease Control. *AIDS Prevention Guide.* Rockville, Md.: National AIDS Information Clearinghouse, 1989.

"Emerging Viruses." *Medical World News* (June 26, 1989): 36–42.

Francis, Donald P. and James Chin. "The Prevention of Acquired Immunodeficiency Syndrome in the United States." *Journal of the American Medical Association* 257, no. 15 (April 17, 1987): 2039–42.

Guinan, Mary E., and Ann Hardy. "Epidemiology of AIDS in Women in the United States." *Journal of the American Medical Association* 275, no. 15 (April 17, 1987): 2039–42.

Henderson, Donald A. "Smallpox—Epitaph for a Killer?" *National Geographic Magazine* 154, no. 6 (December 1978): 797–805.

Henderson, Donald A. "Smallpox Eradication." *Public Health Reports* 95, no. 5 (September/October 1980): 422–26.

Mason, James O. "Addressing the Measles Epidemic." *Public Health Reports* 107, no. 3 (May–June, 1992): 241–42.

"Pelvic Inflammatory Disease: Guideline for Prevention and Management." *Morbidity and Mortality Weekly Report* 40, no. RR-5 (April 26, 1991): 1–25.

"Prevention and Control of Influenza: Recommendations of the Immunization Practices Advisory Committee (ACIP)." *Morbidity and Mortality Weekly Report* 41, no. RR-9, (May 15, 1992): 17 pp.

"Prevention and Control of Tuberculosis in U.S. Communities with At-Risk Minority Populations." *Morbidity and Mortality Weekly Report* 41, no. RR-5 (April 17, 1992): 1–11.

"Restrospective Assessment of Vaccination Coverage Among School-Aged Children—Selected U.S. Cities, 1991." *Morbidity and Mortality Weekly Report* 41, no. 6 (February 14, 1992): 103–7.

Schulte, Joann M., Frederick A. Martich, and George P. Schmid. "Chancroid in the United States, 1981–1991: Evidence for Underreporting of Cases." *Morbidity and Mortality Weekly Report* 41, no. SS-3 (May 29, 1992): 57–61.

Thomas, Patricia, "The Epidemic." *Medical World News* (July 24, 1989): 41–42.

U.S. Government. *Report of the Presidential Commission on the Human Immunodeficiency Virus Epidemic.* Washington, D.C.: U.S. Government Printing Office, 1988.

"Update: Acquired Immunodeficiency Syndrome—United States, 1991." *Morbidity and Mortality Weekly Report* 41, no. 26 (July 3, 1992): 463–68.

"Update: Influenza Activity—United States, 1991–1992 Season." *Morbidity and Mortality Weekly Report* 41, no. 4 (January 31, 1992): 63–65.

"Update on Adult Immunization: Recommendations of the Immunization Practices Advisory Committee (ACIP)." *Morbidity and Mortality Weekly Report* 40, no. RR-12 (November 15, 1991).

Woods, Diana R., and Dean D. Mason. "Six Areas Lead National Early Immunization Drive." *Public Health Reports* 107, no. 3 (May–June 1992): 252–56.

Endnotes

1. Public Health Service. *Healthy People 2000: National Health Promotion and Disease Prevention Objectives.* Washington, D.C.: U.S. Government Printing Office 1991, p. 3.

2. Beneson, Abram, S., ed. *Control of Communicable Diseases in Man,* 12th ed. Washington, D.C.: American Public Health Association, 1979, p. 354.

3. Centers for Disease Control. Annual Summary 1984. Reported Morbidity and Mortality in the United States. *Morbidity and Mortality Weekly Report* 33, no. 54 (March 1986): 61.

4. Centers for Disease Control. "Summary of Notifiable Diseases, United States, 1991." *Morbidity and Mortality Weekly Report* 40, no. 53 (October 2, 1992): 3.

5. Mason, James O. "Addressing the Measles Epidemic." *Public Health Reports* 107, no. 3 (May–June 1992): 241–42.

6. Centers for Disease Control. "Retrospective Assessment of Vaccination Coverage Among School-Aged Children—Selected U.S. Cities, 1991." *Morbidity and Mortality Weekly Report* 41, no. 6 (February 14, 1992): 103–7.

7. Report of Immunization Committee of the American College of Physicians reported in *The Nation's Health* (March 1985): 6.

8. Department of Health and Human Services. *Promoting Health, Preventing Disease: Objectives for the Nation.* Washington, D.C.: U.S. Government Printing Office, 1980, p. 57.

9. *Ibid.,* 57.

10. Carroll, Charles, and Dean F. Miller. *Health: The Science of Human Adaptation.* Dubuque, Iowa: Wm. C. Brown, 1991, p. 281.

11. Centers for Disease Control. "Prevention and Control of Influenza." *Morbidity and Mortality Weekly Report* 41, no. RR-9 (May 15, 1992): 4–5.

12. Centers for Disease Control, *Healthy People 2000,* 521.

13. *Ibid.,* 515.

14. *Ibid.,* 521.

15. National Institutes of Health, *NIAID Backgrounder* (May 1989).

16. Centers for Disease Control. "A Strategic Plan for the Elimination of Tuberculosis in the United States." *Morbidity and Mortality Weekly Report* 38, no. S-3 (April 21, 1989—Suppl.).

17. *Ibid.,* 1.

18. Reported in *The Nation's Health* (September 1989): 12.

19. Centers for Disease Control. "A Strategic Plan for the Elimination of Tuberculosis in the United States." *Morbidity and Mortality Weekly Report* 38, no. S-3 (April 21, 1989).

20. Blach, Alan B., and Dixie E. Snider. "How Much Tuberculosis in Children Must We Accept?" *American Journal of Public Health* 76, no. 1 (January 1986): 14–15.

21. Centers for Disease Control. "Summary of Notifiable Diseases, United States, 1991." *Morbidity and Mortality Weekly Report* (October 2, 1992): 3.

22. Abram S. Benenson, ed., *Control of Communicable Diseases in Man.* Washington, D.C.: American Public Health Association, 1979, p. 132.

23. Centers for Disease Control. "Genital Herpes Infection—United States, 1966–1984." *Morbidity and Mortality Weekly Report* 35, no. 24 (June 20, 1986): 402.

24. U.S. Department of Health and Human Services, Public Health Service, *Promoting Health/Preventing Diseases: Year 2000 Objectives for the Nation.* Washington, D.C.: U.S. Government Printing Office, September 1989.

25. Reported in *The Nation's Health* (September 1992): 3.

26. Henderson, Donald A. "Smallpox—Epitaph for a Killer?" *National Geographic Magazine* 154, no. 6 (December 1978): 803.

27. Dubos, Rene. *Man Adapting.* New Haven, Conn.: Yale Press, 1967.

28. Henderson, Donald A. "Smallpox Eradication." *Public Health Reports* 95, no. 5 (September/October 1980): 425.

29. Henderson, Donald A. "Smallpox—Epitaph for a Killer?" *National Geographic Magazine* 154, no. 6 (December 1978): 805.

CHAPTER ELEVEN

Chronic Diseases

Long-Term Problems with Few Cures

What Are Chronic Diseases?

Increased surveillance, expanded availability of immunization and vaccination, and continuing research have led to the elimination of many communicable diseases as major causes of death and debilitation in the United States. Whereas in the early part of the twentieth century the leading causes of death were communicable diseases, today five of the ten leading causes of death are chronic diseases: cardiovascular disease (heart attack), cancer, cerebrovascular disease (stroke), chronic obstructive pulmonary disease, and diabetes. Seventy-five percent of all deaths in the United States result from chronic diseases, accounting for more than a million-and-a-half deaths a year.

Chronic diseases are not caused by microorganisms. They tend to be long lasting and there is usually no complete cure. These conditions stem from a variety of primary as well as secondary factors. Often the causes are not known. However, the effectiveness of preventive measures for most are well documented. Many chronic diseases originate early in life with behavioral life-styles that place an individual at risk for the disease. For example, smoking,

diet, high blood pressure, and alcohol consumption play an important role in all the major chronic diseases.

Unfortunately, there is no medication that can "cure" most chronic diseases. Medication and health care procedures may bring relief and reduce the specific problem. However, damage to the body caused by the stroke, the malignancy, the diabetic condition, or the arthritis is unlikely to be repaired. Control of the risk factors, pharmacological intervention, and rehabilitation therapy are important in lessening the severity of chronic diseases.

Chronic diseases often cause debilitation. The various arthritic diseases result in crippling conditions. The inability to use the fingers and hands may limit the capacity to work or provide personal care. In the advanced stages of arthritic conditions, a person may not be able to function independently and need permanent, long-term nursing care.

Those with diabetes may also experience various stages of debilitation. After the initial diagnosis, people with diabetes must make major efforts to control their diet and insulin levels. The advanced stages of diabetes are linked to blindness and other crippling conditions needing long-term care. However, diabetics who control their condition have virtually the same risks as nondiabetics.

Chronic obstructive pulmonary lung disease, particularly emphysema and chronic bronchitis, causes very difficult breathing, which greatly reduces the patient's ability to function normally. As these diseases progress, the individual requires long-term, continuous nursing services and the assistance of breathing devices.

Cardiovascular Disease

The leading cause of death, debilitation, and health care expenditures in the United States are cardiovascular diseases: heart attack, stroke, and hypertension. These conditions involve the body's circulatory system—the heart and the blood vessels. It is estimated that over 930,000 deaths result each year from cardiovascular diseases. An estimated $117.4 billion were spent in one year for medical costs and disability related to these diseases.[1]

Coronary Heart Disease

When circulation of blood to and from the heart is obstructed, a heart attack ensues. Such a situation may occur because the major arteries supplying the heart muscle are narrowed by disease (arteriosclerosis), because the vessels are obstructed by a saclike bulging of the weakened arterial wall (aneurysm), or because an artery ruptures and blood is lost into the surrounding tissues.

Numerous factors may be linked to a heart attack. The underlying condition in most cardiovascular-related deaths is *atherosclerosis,* a slow, progressive narrowing of the arteries by fatty deposits called *plaques* that build up on the inner layer of the arterial walls. Eventually, the flow of blood is totally blocked.

When blood flow to the heart is reduced, *angina* may occur. An angina attack is characterized by pain in the chest. Atherosclerosis and hypertension—high blood pressure—tend to be major contributing factors to angina.

Cerebrovascular Disease

Cerebrovascular disease, or *stroke,* occurs when the blood supply to the brain cells is impaired by clots or hemorrhages. Different parts of the brain control different physical and mental functions. When an individual has a stroke, the symptoms vary according to which part of the brain is affected. Some people may experience paralysis of a limb, others a loss of speech or balance, and others difficulty in swallowing or impairments of mental functioning. Massive weakness or numbness of a part of the body may occur early in the episode. Sometimes the symptoms last only a few seconds or minutes; such TIAs (transient ischemic attacks) may be a warning sign.

Greater awareness of the dangers of hypertension and better screening along with changes in life-style and treatment have led to a decline in deaths due to stroke in recent years. However, death from stroke is still high among the African-American population. The Department of Health and Human Services has set an objective of reducing the deaths from stroke by the year 2000, with special attention given to program and research initiatives for reducing strokes among African-Americans. Factors needing specific emphasis have to do with dietary patterns, environmental living conditions, hypertension, and cigarette smoking.[2]

Hypertension

As blood is pumped through the cardiovascular system, pressure is exerted on the walls of the blood vessels. When this blood pressure is elevated, the risk of damage to the blood vessels and of developing stroke and coronary artery disorder is greater. Elevated blood pressure is known as *hypertension.* If identified early enough, hypertension can be kept under control with medical assistance. Prescribed antihypertensive drugs, weight control, reduction of sodium in the diet, and reduction and control of stress can all be important in reducing hypertension.

Though hypertension affects all racial groups and both sexes, it has been found to be more prevalent among African-Americans than among whites in the United States. It is the most common chronic disease among this population group. Hypertension is usually thought of as being a problem for middle-aged and elderly individuals. However, in the African-American population this condition has been shown to be a problem among young people. Some reasons that have been identified for this greater risk among African-Americans are possible genetic factors, greater rates of obesity among black females, and the tendency to high-sodium and high-fat diets.

Hypertension: A Major American Health Concern

Many people know that hypertension refers to high blood pressure, and they are aware that high blood pressure can be a problem. But what is blood pressure?

The first thing a nurse does in the doctor's office, at the health clinic, the hospital, or any place that one goes for health care is place a screening cuff around the arm and listen with the stethoscope. Blood pressure readings are taken today as part of some school health curriculum programs, hypertension programs are conducted for minority populations in churches, and many businesses and industries offer screening for hypertension. Despite all these activities, most people do not know what their blood pressure reading is.

Blood pressure involves two numbers: The first, and highest, number indicates the *systolic pressure*—the amount of force being exerted when the heart beats. The second number is the *diastolic pressure*—the pressure in the artery when the heart is at rest between the beats. This second number is usually of most concern to the doctor. The greater the number, the greater the force being exerted during what should be a period of rest.

One's personal physician determines the specific reading at which one needs attention. Usually treatment is suggested when the systolic pressure is 140 and the diastolic pressure is 90 or above (140/90).

What measures can be taken by schools, business and industry, and community health clinics to better educate the public about hypertension? Because hypertension is a particular problem for minorities, what programs and activities might be initiated to reduce the risk of high blood pressure among these groups? How often are hypertension screening costs covered by health insurance programs?

Prevention of Cardiovascular Disease

Extensive research into the causes and treatment of cardiovascular diseases has led to greater knowledge and more effective treatment.[3] Because of an increased interest in preventive medicine, it is now known that there are a number of risk factors for cardiovascular disease. An individual can take specific action to prevent or reduce the likelihood of developing cardiovascular heart disease. Diet plays an important role: reducing cholesterol and triglycerides, fats normally occurring in the blood, and saturated fats can be important in maintaining a healthy circulatory system.

As Americans become more aware of their cholesterol levels, the incidence of cardiovascular heart disease may be reduced. To assist in this endeavor, the National Cholesterol Education Program was started in 1985 with several goals for all adults:

All individuals over the age of twenty should have their blood cholesterol measured at least once every five years.

All adults should know their own cholesterol level. If the cholesterol level is elevated, steps should be initiated to lower it.[4]

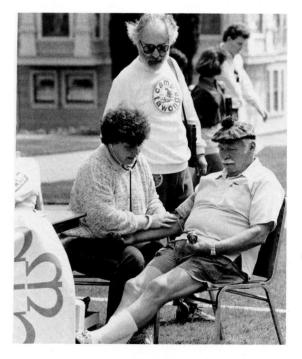

Blood pressure being taken at neighborhood health fair.

Along this same line, the Department of Health and Human Services has set as an objective by the year 2000 that at least 75 percent of all persons over the age of eighteen will have had their cholesterol checked within a preceding five-year period of time.[5] It was estimated that as of 1988, only about 60 percent of the population had *ever* had their cholesterol level checked.[6]

Sedentary individuals appear to have a significantly higher rate of death by heart attack than those who exercise regularly. Not only does exercise strengthen the heart muscle, but it also controls weight and reduces stress. Obesity and tension are identified risk factors for heart disease. The most effective exercise is aerobic activity.

Cigarette smoking is now known to be a major risk factor for cardiovascular diseases. The exact relationship has not been established, but nicotine and carbon monoxide probably play a part.

Heart disease affects millions of people throughout the United States, but the awareness of measures an individual can take to reduce the possibility of heart attack has increased. Changes in individual life-style such as reduced smoking, changes in diet, and increased physical activity have helped improve cardiovascular health in recent years.

Medical Technology

Nowhere in medicine have technological advances and developments been more apparent than in the treatment and prevention of cardiovascular disease. A decade or so ago an individual who had had a heart attack would have been kept quiet and told to limit activity for a lengthy period. Little could be recommended to counter the underlying causes of the attack.

Today a number of medical techniques can reduce the possibility of heart attack. Should an attack occur, a number of measures can help the patient recover.

Most hospitals now have coronary care units with sophisticated equipment and highly skilled personnel. Although costly, these units are credited with greatly reducing the rate of death from heart attack.

One effective method in the treatment of heart attack patients is the use of clot-dissolving drugs that are injected into the veins. These drugs are especially useful in dissolving the clots in the small blood vessels of the heart. Other drugs can prevent arrhythmias following a heart attack.

In the past, even if an individual survived a heart attack, little could be done to eliminate or reduce atherosclerotic plaque. It usually was only a matter of time until another blockage took place. Today there are several strategies to clear the small blocked arteries. One such technique is balloon angioplasty. A tiny balloon attached to catheters is passed through the blood vessels to the site of the plaque. The balloon is inflated and the deposit is broken up, opening the clogged artery. Angioplasty has been particularly effective with individuals having generally good cardiac function except for clogged cardiac arteries.[7]

Angiography is a procedure in which dye is injected into the arteries of an organ so that the circulatory patterns can be viewed by x-rays. Narrowing or tiny clots can be identified and clot-dissolving drugs or other techniques can then be used to open the arteries and restore blood flow.

In *heart bypass surgery,* blood vessels elsewhere in the body—often the legs—are surgically transplanted into the heart. They provide a channel for blood to flow around an area where there is blockage, or potential blockage. Bypass surgery is usually performed on people with symptoms of serious coronary (artery) disease diagnosed by exercise stress tests or angiography. It is most effective when only part of the blood vessel is blocked. Bypass surgery must be considered a preventive measure to protect against a heart attack. Balloon angioplasty is one alternative for patients with less severe blockage. Most individuals who undergo bypass surgery report feeling better than ever once they recover from the surgical procedure. Most are able to return to work and an active life-style several weeks after the surgery.

One can only imagine what developments in cardiac care will occur in future years. In all likelihood, microsurgical techniques will be used to clean away plaques from the arteries. Laser beams will be directed toward identified plaques in the blood vessels and remove them. It is possible that such techniques will make bypass surgery obsolete.

Cancer

The second leading cause of death in the United States is cancer. Over 22 percent of all deaths are caused by some form of cancer. This disease is one of the most dreaded afflictions; the very mention of cancer causes fear and

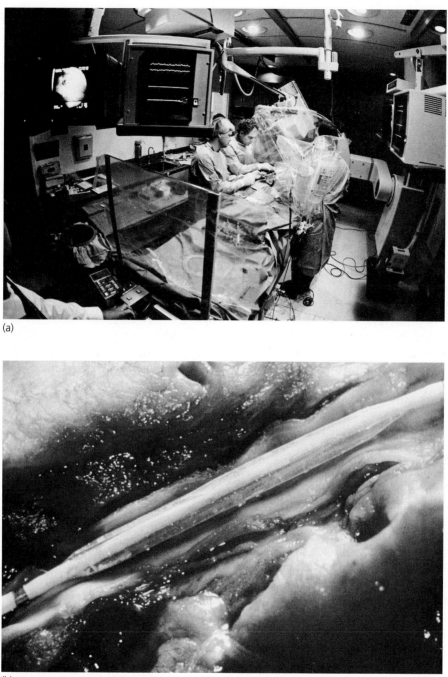

(a)

(b)

(a) Surgeons perform an angioplasty cardiovascular diagnostic operation in Mission Viejo, CA. Note computer data screens. (b) A balloon angioplasty catheter.

uncertainty for most people. However, improved treatments and earlier detection have increased survival rates for many cancer patients.

It is estimated that more than one million new cases of cancer are diagnosed each year, with nearly one-half million deaths annually. As many as one in three Americans will get cancer at some time in their lives. About half will die of the disease within five years of diagnosis—but half will survive for five years or more.

Cancer is not a single disease; each type of cancer presents specific problems. Diagnostic and screening procedures can identify some types of malignancy early. Other cancers are difficult to identify at an early stage of development. Specific treatments vary according to the site of the cancer.

For some malignancies, the survival rate is fairly high, assuming early diagnosis and proper treatment. For example, the survival rates for cancer of the thyroid and for testicular cancer are about 90 percent.[8] On the other hand, cancer of the pancreas is nearly 98 percent fatal,[9] and nearly 90 percent of lung cases are fatal. Among males the five leading cancer sites are the lungs, the colon and rectum, the prostate, the pancreas, and the blood (leukemia). Among females lung cancer is now the leading malignancy, having surpassed breast cancer. The next three leading types of cancer among women are cancer of the colon and rectum, pancreatic cancer, and cancer of the ovaries.

Biology of Cancer

Throughout the life cycle, new cells are being reproduced continuously, replacing old tissues, for example, in the repair of damaged tissue. The body is continuously replacing worn-out cells on the skin's surface. But cells sometimes reproduce in an uncontrolled way, leading to nonfunctional masses, or *tumors*. Unlike normal body tissues, tumors continue to grow. They lack the adhesiveness that is present in normal cells.

Some tumors remain localized and nonspreading, and for the most part are not life threatening. These are *benign* tumors. They are dangerous to the individual only when the growth harms nearby structures. On the other hand, some tumors spread into nearby tissues with claw-like protrusions and interfere with the function and nourishment of neighboring organs. These tumors are *malignant*, or *cancerous*. The process by which a normal cell is changed to an abnormal cell is known as *oncogenesis*.

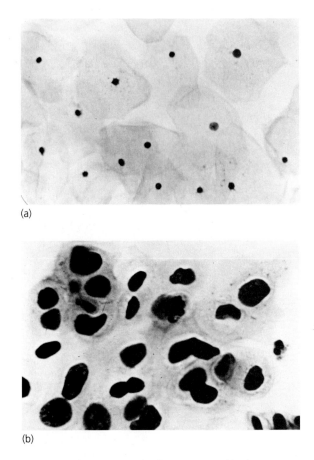

(a)

(b)

Normal and malignant cervical cells are compared in these photographs: (a) normal cells, (b) cancerous cells.

Cancerous cells have a distinctive microscopic appearance. For some unknown reason, these cells, unlike normal cells, do not stop growing and reproducing. They expand in a logarithmic progression, displacing normal tissue. The cancerous cells take over the blood supply of the normal tissue. In time malignant cells may separate from the tumor and spread to another location in the body. This process is known as *metastasis*. These cells can implant themselves in foreign cellular environments and continue to reproduce and grow.

Much research has been directed toward determining the factors that initiate the uncontrolled reproduction of cells. Some that have been identified include exposure to certain chemicals or to physical agents such as sunlight and x-rays. The role that diet plays in causing cancer cell development and growth is receiving more attention. Research has also focused on viruses. It is known that viruses do cause oncogenesis. However, there is no evidence directly linking any human cancer with a specific virus. Much still remains to be learned about what causes the initial development of cancer cells.

Risk Factors

The scientific community agrees that as much as 80 percent of all cancer is related to individual life-styles.[10] Smoking, diet, and environmental factors are currently receiving the most attention from scientists studying malignancies in the United States. Smoking is directly linked with several different types of cancer—lung cancer in particular as well as cancer of the mouth, esophagus, pancreas, and kidneys. It has been estimated that smoking accounts for 30 percent of all cancer deaths in the United States.[11]

The National Cancer Institute has estimated that as many as 35 percent of all cancer deaths may be associated with diet.[12] Findings of numerous studies cited by the National Cancer Institute that support this statement include the following:[13]

Populations that consume higher amounts of fiber have a lower rate of colon and rectal cancer.

Eating too much fat may increase the risk of getting cancer of the colon, breast, and prostate.

Obesity is linked with higher risks of developing colon, breast, prostate, gallbladder, and uterine cancer.

Heavy drinking of alcoholic beverages increases the risk of cancer of the mouth, throat, and liver.

The American Cancer Society notes that in parts of the world with large intake of salt-cured and smoked foods, greater amounts of cancer of the esophagus and stomach are reported.[14]

A number of factors have been identified that seem to be associated with an increased possibility of developing cancer at other selected sites. For example, excessive exposure to the sun is a major factor in the development of skin cancer. Heavy use of alcohol has been associated with cancers of the larynx, esophagus, throat, and liver. Exposure to high levels of radiation have been seen as risk factors for cancer, particularly lung cancer among individuals exposed to high levels of radon in their homes. Other risk factors include age and family history of cancer.

Early Warning Signs

Early identification of certain signs and indications is the best way to reduce fatality from cancer. There is no single sign, symptom, or test for cancer, but numerous signs and symptoms are considered important by physicians, including any unexplained weight loss or bleeding, anemia in adult males and in postmenopausal females, changes in elimination, digestion, or appetite, or pain, which may be due to the tumor enlarging or pushing on surrounding organs. Enlarged lymph nodes may also be indicative of cancerous growth. These are all indications that further examination for cancer is necessary.

The American Cancer Society has identified seven danger signals for cancer with which every person should be familiar:

1. Change in bowel or bladder habits
2. A sore that does not heal
3. Unusual bleeding or discharge
4. Thickening or lump in breast or elsewhere
5. Indigestion or difficulty in swallowing
6. Obvious change in wart or mole
7. Nagging cough or hoarseness

Several recommendations have been issued as preventive measures that should be encouraged for diagnosing as early as possible the development of cancer. The Pap test is a very effective early screening procedure for detecting cervical cancer among women. Current recommendations are that any woman who is sexually active or eighteen years of age or older should have an annual Pap test. It is now felt that these tests may be performed less frequently after a woman has three or more satisfactory normal annual examinations. Determination of the degree of test regularity should be at the decision of the woman's physician.

Other strong recommendations are now available for early detection of breast cancer and for colorectal cancer (cancer of the colon and rectum). These are discussed in the following section.

Selected Cancer Sites

Cancer may occur at several different locations throughout the human body. Actually, there are more than one hundred different diseases that have been identified in which uncontrolled cellular growth and spread of the abnormal cells takes place. The three leading causes of death from cancer are lung cancer, colorectal cancer, and breast cancer.[15] Among males lung cancer and colorectal cancer are the leading causes of death; among females it is lung cancer and breast cancer. Within the context of this chapter it is impossible to examine all types of malignancies, their locations, particular growth patterns, and treatment modalities. Presented will be the cancers resulting in the most fatalities among men and women: lung cancer, cancer of the colon and rectum, and breast cancer.

Lung Cancer

The leading cause of cancer death is cancer of the lungs. About 149,000 deaths occur annually from this malignancy. Several factors play a role in causing lung cancer. Without question, smoking cigarettes over a period of years is considered to be *the* major risk factor. Exposure to various industrial substances such as asbestos and coal dust are also risk factors. Exposure to second-hand smoke is also considered a risk factor.

Warning signs of lung cancer include a persistent cough or sputum that is streaked with blood. Chest pains and recurring pneumonia or bronchitis are often present. As with all types of cancer, early detection is imperative. Unfortunately, lung cancer is difficult to identify early; the signs and symptoms usually do not appear until the various structures of the lungs are damaged.

Lung cancer is diagnosed by chest x-rays. Fiberoptic bronchoscope and sputum cytology testing are also now being used. Treatment of lung cancer usually involves surgery, radiation therapy, and chemotherapy, alone or in combinations. The specific treatment depends on the type of the malignancy and the stage of development.

Cancer of the Colon and Rectum

Second to lung cancer as a cause of death is cancer of the colon and rectum, or colorectal cancer. Nearly sixty thousand deaths from this malignancy are reported annually. Colorectal cancer generally occurs among senior citizens. The risk increases with age. Early warning signals include bleeding from the rectum, blood in the stools, and any change in bowel habits.

Early detection of colorectal cancer has increased in recent years because of several recommended screening procedures. In one, digital rectal examination, the rectum is examined with the small finger, a procedure performed by a physician. Testing stool blood is also effective in identifying early colorectal cancer and is used by many physicians. This procedure is inexpensive and can detect malignancies at early stages. Sigmoidoscopy and colonoscopy have potential for detecting precancerous colorectal polyps as well as for earlier detection of cancerous cells. In proctosigmoidoscopy the rectum and lower colon are inspected with a lighted tube.

The American Cancer Society recommends that all adults over forty have annual digital rectal examinations. They also recommend an annual stool blood slide test examination, which shows if blood is in the feces, and a sigmoidoscopy examination every three to five years for individuals over the age of fifty. Sigmoidoscopy and stool blood screening should be done more frequently for individuals with a family history of colorectal cancer and for individuals with any of the symptoms of this malignancy.

Surgery is the principal means of treating colorectal cancer. It is often used in combination with radiation therapy.

Breast Cancer

Until the late 1980s, the leading cancer among women was breast cancer. This malignancy was the underlying cause of more than 46,000 deaths annually. Though currently surpassed by lung cancer, breast cancer is still extremely serious.

Breast cancer mortality increases with age, with a majority of deaths occurring in women over sixty-five years old.

Despite this high death rate, survival from breast cancer has improved in recent years because of earlier detection. More women are aware of the importance of breast self-examination and the use of mammography screening. The National Cancer Institute reports that the five-year survival rate is now 75 percent. Survival rates are lower among African–American women than among whites.

The exact cause of breast cancer is not known, but several factors have been identified. These are a family history of cancer, exposure to radiation, either early

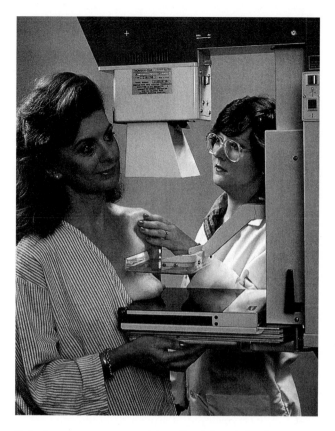

Today two mammograms are taken of each breast. One is a diagonal view low-dose x-ray; the other view is horizontal. The shield presses slightly down on the breast to get the best results.

age of forty. Between the ages of forty and forty-nine the screening should be conducted every one or two years; after the age of fifty it must be done annually. It has been estimated that one death in three from breast cancer could have been prevented if such screening procedures were carried out.

Despite the importance of screening, many women do not undergo the procedure. Many do not recognize its value. Others are mistakenly fearful that the procedure is painful, or that exposure to the radiation is harmful. Some women do not want to know if they have cancer and so refuse to be screened.

To increase the number of women who have mammogram screening, the Department of Health and Human Services has set the objective that by 2000 at least 60 percent of all women over fifty have the procedure annually. It was estimated that less than 25 percent had had mammogram screenings in 1987.[16] Special focus must be directed at minority women, particularly Hispanics and African-Americans. Women with less than a high school education and low-income women were also identified for special focus, as well as those over the age of seventy.

Cancer Treatment

Treatment for cancer includes three different procedures: (1) surgery, (2) chemotherapy, and (3) radiation. *Surgery* is used to remove the malignant tissue. This is a major surgical procedure and is most effective when there is reasonable assurance that the tumor is localized; that is, it has not spread beyond its original site. Surgery is most successful in treating cancer of the colon and rectum. Cancer of the breast is also treated primarily by surgery.

Chemotherapy, the use of drugs, is a procedure that is used separately or in conjunction with surgery. Hundreds of chemotherapeutic agents are used to treat cancer. The drug should kill the cancer cells but produce minimal harm to the surrounding normal tissue. This is not always easy to accomplish; often a chemotherapeutic agent that destroys malignant cells also damages noncancerous cells.

Chemotherapy may be given intermittently using several different drugs or be given on a continual, daily basis. Exposure to the drugs tends to cause a number of side effects. Many people who are given chemotherapy develop anemia. There can also be a drop in white blood cell count, which leads to problems with infections. In

menarche or late menopause, and childbearing at an older age. In addition, the consumption of alcohol and of animal fat and protein have been considered to be risk factors. The use of oral contraceptives has been investigated as a cause of breast cancer, though currently no known research proves a cause-and-effect relationship.

The most effective early detection measure for breast cancer is breast self-examination and regular examination of the breasts by mammography. Screening with mammography, a procedure that can detect tiny growths long before lumps form, reduces breast cancer mortality. Mammography has been improved in recent years, with less radiation now being used. At an early stage of development the cancer can be easily treated.

The National Cancer Institute and the American Cancer Society recommend that breast cancer screening be a part of any physical examination for women over the

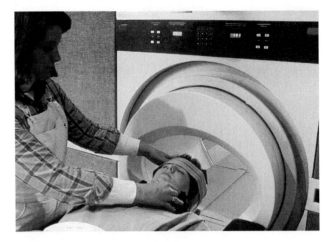

Magnetic resonance imaging (MRI) detects tumors by sensing vibrations of various atoms in the body.

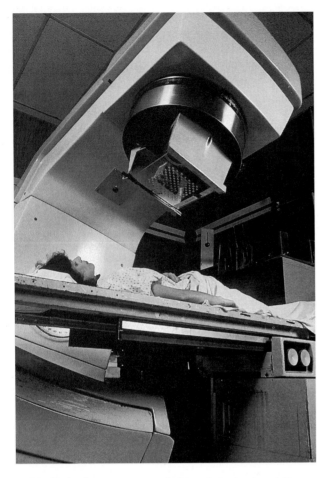

Various kinds of cancer are treated with radiation treatment. The rate of malignant cell growth is slowed by the x-rays and gamma rays.

addition, many individuals lose body hair. This mode of cancer treatment is most effective with the more serious malignancies. New chemical agents are constantly being tested for use in the treatment of cancer.

Radiation treatment, the use of x-rays and gamma rays, is effective for treating many kinds of cancer. About half of all cancer patients receive radiation either as the sole treatment modality or in combination with other therapy. Radiation slows down the cancer cell growth. Some tumors respond temporarily but are not cured. It is used for cancer of the oral cavity, bone, brain, prostate, testes, and skin. Radiation has been particularly successful in the treatment of Hodgkin's disease. Cure rates of nearly 80 percent are now being reported.[17]

Often the treatment for a malignancy will involve the combination of any two or all three of these modalities. For example, drugs and radiation are being used in conjunction with surgery for bone cancer. Dramatic improvements in survival rates have been reported.

Highly technical procedures are being developed to improve the chances of long-term cure for cancer. For example, in cryosurgery a stream of liquid nitrogen is directed into the cancer. Repeated freezing and thawing kills the malignant cells. Also heat, electrodesiccation, is useful in destroying malignant tissues in the early cases of skin cancer. Electrocoagulation, in which cells are destroyed by heat produced by electric current, is used in precancerous uterine malignancies.

Immunotherapy is designed to activate the body's immune system to destroy the cancer cells. Most immunotherapeutic agents are still in the early testing stages with humans.

The diagnosis of malignancies has been improved with highly technical procedures in recent years. Ultrasound, a procedure in which machines bounce sound waves off internal organs, is effective in locating tumors. Thermography, use of heat patterns, is also a technique for locating and destroying cancer cells. Research is attempting to ascertain whether hyperthermia, heat, can increase the effectiveness of radiation or chemotherapy in any way. Computerized x-rays provide three-dimensional pictures that facilitate cancer screening. Use has been made of magnetic resonance imaging (MRI), which detects tumors by sensing the vibrations of the different atoms in the body. Computerized tomography (CT scanning) is used to examine various parts of the body, including the brain.[18]

Greater knowledge about cancer has led to significantly improved chances for treatment and recovery. However, as for many other chronic diseases, prevention and early detection must be practiced by all individuals.

Chronic Obstructive Pulmonary Disease

The fourth leading cause of death in the United States is chronic obstructive pulmonary disease. Without adequate amounts of fresh, pure oxygen, humans cannot live for more than a few minutes. The lungs play an important role in the intake and exhalation of air. When functioning properly, the lungs are an efficient organ. However, when the bronchioles, or passages, become damaged and airflow is blocked, serious problems result.

Evidence suggests that there is a long latency period between exposure to the cause of chronic obstructive pulmonary disease and eventual incapacitation and death. This is demonstrated by the fact that the incidence of the disease has increased by 33 percent during the 1980s even though cigarette smoking has declined in this same time frame.[19] Death from chronic obstructive pulmonary disease is more prevalent among males and is 2.8 times higher in the white population than among minorities.[20]

Debilitation is an important factor that results from chronic obstructive pulmonary disease. Individuals affected with this condition often are disabled to the extent that they are unable to work productively. Many must take early disability retirement as the result of their condition. The federal government has recognized the seriousness of this disease by establishing an objective of slowing the rise in deaths from chronic obstructive pulmonary disease by the year 2000.[21]

Two common forms of chronic obstructive pulmonary disease are chronic bronchitis and emphysema. Though there are several risk factors associated with these conditions, the principal one associated with both is cigarette smoking, with an estimated 82 percent of deaths being attributed to smoking.[22]

An inflammation of the bronchial tubes, *chronic bronchitis,* is caused by prolonged irritation of the moist linings of the air passageways. The cilia present within these structures provide protection from outside dust and other particulate matter, but when they are damaged by environmental pollutants, cigarette smoke, disease, and allergens, the protective action is negated. As a result, excessive secretion of mucus or phlegm and shortness of breath develop. Coughing, which is nature's attempt to force up the mucous secretions, becomes progressively more violent, and wheezing occurs. Any type of physical exertion makes it difficult to breathe.

Chronic bronchitis usually is progressive and develops over a long period. Initial indications, such as coughing and spitting, are often ignored. Because the disease is progressive, damage to the bronchioles expands unless treatment is obtained. Without adequate treatment, prolonged disability occurs.

A second disease that is characteristic of chronic pulmonary disease is emphysema. This condition gradually destroys the alveoli of the lungs. These small air sacs lose their elasticity and tear apart, and thus air spaces are formed within the lungs. A person with emphysema finds it increasingly difficult to breathe because exchange of oxygen for carbon dioxide is impaired. As a result, breathing becomes more rapid.

Treatment of emphysema includes taking measures to relieve the inflammation of the respiratory tract. Drugs that assist the opening of the air passages are often helpful. Portable oxygen devices and intermittent positive-pressure breathing apparatus are employed to reduce severe breathing distress in victims. Some individuals adapt to some extent by practicing breathing exercises. However, breathing capacity has been reduced, and little can be done to reverse the damage that has been done to the alveoli.

Diabetes

The seventh leading cause of death in the United States is diabetes, accounting for about thirty-seven thousand deaths annually. Because the person with diabetes often experiences a number of other problems related to the diabetic condition, it is estimated that diabetes may be the contributory cause of death for as many as four times that number, if one counts individuals whose primary cause of death is recorded as something else.

It is estimated that more than 650,000 new cases are diagnosed each year.[23] The costs associated with this chronic disease are in the range of $20 billion.[24]

Diabetes is a chronic disease that affects the way that food is used. In normal physiological functioning, sugars, starches, and other foods are changed to glucose. Glucose is carried in the bloodstream to the body cells where, with the help of *insulin,* a hormone formed in the pancreas, it is used to produce energy. Insulin is made by the beta cells of the pancreas and is the basic factor in regulating the transformation of food to energy. The healthy pancreas continually adjusts to the needs of the body and produces the needed insulin as the body takes in food or uses energy.

Problems arise when the amount of insulin produced by the pancreas is inadequate or when the insulin cannot be used effectively. This condition is diabetes, a chronic disease affecting people of all ages and races.

Types of Diabetes

There are two principal types of diabetes: type I and type II.

Type I (insulin-dependent or juvenile-onset) diabetes is the more severe. With this type of diabetes the pancreas does not produce adequate insulin and serious problems develop. This condition often begins early in life, during childhood or adolescence. Onset is often rather sudden. People with this type of diabetes must have daily insulin injections in order to live.

Type II diabetes (noninsulin-dependent or maturity-onset) is more common and is less severe. It usually does not present itself until middle age. With this type of diabetes, insulin is produced by the pancreas, but it cannot be used effectively. Type II diabetes may go undetected for years before it comes to the individual's attention. It can be controlled by proper activity, medication, and diet—the individual will need to eat less sugar. Drugs are available that assist the body in using the insulin that is produced.

Several risk factors have been associated with diabetes. The probability of getting diabetes increases with body weight. Obesity is found to be a problem of many diabetics. It is also known that controlling smoking and hypertension decreases morbidity and mortality among diabetics. Diabetes tends to be present within families. This suggests that the cause may be related to an inherited chemical defect. Another risk factor associated with type II diabetes is age.

Warning Signs of Diabetes	
Type 1	**Type 2**
Abnormal thirst	Blurred vision
Frequent urination	Drowsiness
Nausea and vomiting	Excess weight
Unusual hunger	Skin infections
Weakness and fatigue	Tingling, numbness in hands and feet
Weight loss	Slow healing of cuts

Source: American Diabetes Association, 2 Park Avenue, New York, New York 10016.

Treatment

Since the discovery of insulin in 1921, diabetics have been able to receive successful treatment for their condition. A person with diabetes must be taught how and when to inject the needed insulin. Although treatment can effectively control diabetes, it does not cure the disease. Dietary management in conjunction with regular exercise is an important part of treatment for most diabetics.

Recent developments have improved the lives of diabetic people. Home blood glucose monitoring provides accurate readings. Diabetics can know their exact blood glucose level and take appropriate measures in regard to food intake and activity. Improved forms of insulin and better syringes continue to help diabetics perform self-care. Diabetes is different than other chronic diseases in that the diabetic must be taught to provide for his or her own daily medical needs. This presents a major need for education for both the patient and, in the case of children, for parents.

Complications Associated with Diabetes

A number of complications are associated with diabetes. It is a major cause of kidney failure. Many diabetics eventually require kidney dialysis or transplantation. As many as 40 percent of patients with type I diabetes develop kidney disease.

The diabetic is also at risk for foot problems. Nerve damage often leads to a loss of normal sensation, so that the individual may be unaware of cuts, blisters, ingrown toenails, improperly fitting shoes, or infection. Infection may spread, leading to gangrene and bone damage, sometimes necessitating amputation. Because of poor circulation, a diabetic is seventeen times as likely as a nondiabetic to have gangrene.[25] As many as 50 percent of nontraumatic amputations in the United States are performed on diabetics. Diabetic persons must take particular care of their feet by wearing properly fitting shoes, inspecting their feet daily, exercising to improve circulation, and seeing a podiatrist as soon as any problem is noticed.[26]

Diabetes is a leading cause of blindness, with about six thousand people becoming blind annually.[27] Elevated blood sugar levels damage the blood vessels of the retina and cause a condition known as diabetic retinopathy, which impairs vision and may lead to blindness. Just how high blood sugar damages the retina is not yet known. However, research is ongoing to learn more about these relationships.

Diabetes is also associated with cardiovascular disease. Diabetics are twice as likely to have coronary artery disease as is the general public.

Research Developments

Research has provided many answers about the biology of this chronic disease, and methods of care have improved. The Juvenile Diabetic Foundation, a major voluntary health organization dedicated to improving life for those with diabetes, has targeted the 1990s as the "Decade for the Cure."

Today research interests are investigating why the pancreas cannot produce insulin and what role genetic and environmental factors play in the development of this chronic disease. They are also working on more effective treatments. One interesting development is an implanted glucose monitor that continuously reads blood sugar levels and signals an implanted pump to send insulin when appropriate.[28] Research has also examined the relationship between diabetes and kidney disease. Measures have been examined to find ways to stop the damage to the kidney before it progresses to a serious stage.

Cirrhosis of the Liver

The liver, the largest internal organ of the human body, serves a number of important functions. It produces proteins that assist in blood clotting, is involved in carbohydrate metabolism that converts glucose to glycogen, and plays a role in cleansing toxic chemicals and wastes from the body. The liver is also the location where bile is produced.

This organ, unlike most others of the body, is capable of functioning with as much as 80 percent of its mass removed.[29] However, in the case of cirrhosis of the liver, actual structures of the organ are destroyed. As a result, the many necessary actions of the liver cease. Cirrhosis is characterized by a shriveling and hardening of the liver. Regular cells are replaced by scar tissue. Though several causes have been identified, the major risk factor is chronic alcohol abuse. The risk of this disease increases with the amount and duration of alcohol consumption.

Cirrhosis is another leading cause of death in the United States. The majority of these cases are related to heavy alcohol consumption. Currently research is attempting to ascertain the predisposing and precipitating factors related to the disease.

The Department of Health and Human Services has recognized the importance of reducing the incidence of cirrhosis in the United States. It has set an objective reducing deaths caused by cirrhosis of the liver by the year 2000.[30] Special concern has been expressed about the high mortality rates from cirrhosis among minorities, particularly African-American males and Native Americans.

Arthritis

The place within the human body where two or more bones meet is known as a joint. Fluid, efficient movement occurs at joints, permitting humans to carry out thousands of different activities daily. Bones are covered by cartilage,

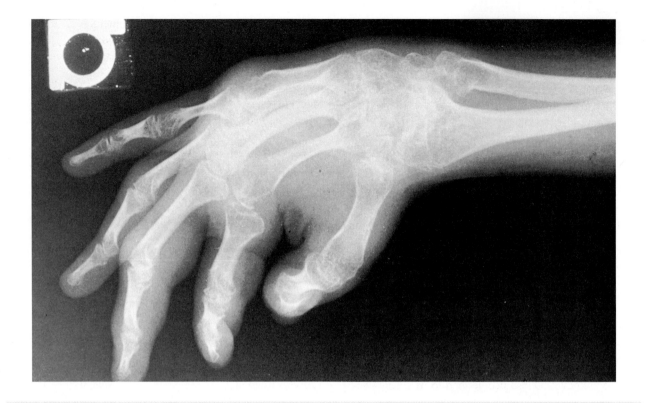

Arthritic joint.

which keeps their ends from rubbing against each other. The joint is enclosed in a capsule known as the synovial membrane. This membrane releases a fluid into the space between the bones that nourishes the cartilage and keeps the joint lubricated. This facilitates good movement.

If the joint is injured or if it becomes inflamed, a condition known as *arthritis* develops. Individuals with arthritis experience swelling, redness, pain, and loss of motion. Arthritis is not a single disease, but a family of over one hundred different diseases. Osteoarthritis is the most common; others include rheumatoid arthritis, gout, juvenile rheumatoid arthritis, and tendinitis.

Though not one of the ten major causes of death in the United States, arthritis is a chronic condition that affects more than thirty-seven million Americans. It is estimated that more than a million people a year learn that they have some type of arthritic condition. This disease is progressive and long lasting, with no known cure for most forms. Pain and debilitation are present in most cases.

The cost of arthritis in the United States exceeds $13 billion.[31] This accounts for direct costs of medical care as well as those associated with loss of earnings due to debilitation and early death. Unfortunately, over a billion dollars a year are spent by arthritis sufferers on questionable medications and cures.[32]

The prolonged nature of arthritic conditions places significant pressure on health care resources. During a visit to most nursing homes one is likely to notice that a majority of the residents have some type of arthritis. Arthritis is a difficult condition for the medical profession to treat. This can lead to depression and frustration as well as other physical and emotional problems.

Cause

The exact cause of arthritis is not known. However, research has provided some clues about the causes of certain types of arthritis. In some cases the disease onset is triggered by viruses. Another possibility is genetic, or inherited, susceptibility. Osteoarthritis is often the result of injury or overuse of certain joints.

Types of Arthritis

Though more than a hundred different diseases are identified under the umbrella of arthritis, three of the most common will be examined. The most common of the arthritic conditions, affecting as many as fifteen million Americans, is *osteoarthritis*. This disease, which is the result of degeneration of the cartilage and bone at the joints, is most common as one grows older. It is estimated that most elderly people over the age of sixty have this condition to some degree, and it gets worse with advancing years. Osteoarthritis is most commonly found in the hip, the knees, and the fingers.

Pain in the joint is the principal indication of osteoarthritis. It is noticed after extensive, stressful use of the joint or at times when the joint has not been active for a time, as upon awakening in the morning. Loss of mobility also occurs.

For many individuals the cause of osteoarthritis may be unknown. Obese people tend to be susceptible to this type of arthritis. People who put abnormal stress on a joint often develop osteoarthritis. This is common among baseball pitchers' elbows and shoulders. Knee injuries to football players usually lead to some degree of osteoarthritis. Ballet dancers often experience osteoarthritis of the ankles. Coal miners and construction workers often have osteoarthritis.

The role that heredity plays in this type of arthritis is receiving greater attention. One's basic anatomical and physiological structure is inherited, and the way one walks, moves, or functions may place particular stress on the joints and thus lead to osteoarthritis. The role of hormones has also been implicated by some because three times more women than men have osteoarthritis, and the condition often appears after menopause.[33] This type of arthritis cannot be cured. Treatment usually involves the use of drugs, heat and cold, exercise regimens, and rest. Surgical procedures can repair damaged joints and provide some relief from the pain and loss of motion. Physical therapy, which strengthens muscles and helps improve flexibility, assists the individual in adapting to this condition.

Aches and severe pain are two major indications of *rheumatoid arthritis,* a condition of inflammation of the joint. The inflammation usually begins in the synovial membrane; it then may spread to other tissues that make up the joint. In time the joint may become deformed from damage caused by the inflammation. Deformity to the fingers and toes can leave an individual paralyzed or incapable of carrying out normal activities.

Initial indications of rheumatoid arthritis may be fatigue, aches, and stiffness. In time swelling and stiffness develop, making for painful and difficult movement. The hands and feet are commonly affected. However, the larger joints such as the knee may also become inflamed.

An interesting characteristic of rheumatoid arthritis is that one often experiences remissions and exacerbations. The aches and pains may go away for certain periods, often leading people to believe that they are improving. Unfortunately, there is no cure, and the arthritic sufferers must not be misled into thinking that some unproven treatment has in fact healed them.

Although there is no cure for this chronic condition, pain can be relieved by heat treatments, physical therapy, regular exercise, and aspirin. Aspirin is particularly helpful in that it reduces the joint inflammation. The Food and Drug Administration has approved several medications that provide relief to the rheumatoid arthritis sufferer. A number of anti-inflammatory medications are recommended.

The third most common arthritic condition among the U.S. population is *gout,* a painful swelling of the toe. Gout results from an abnormal buildup of uric acid, a substance that circulates in the blood until passed through the kidneys into the urine. For some reason, metabolism of uric acid becomes impeded, and needlelike crystals of uric acid appear in the joint. Irritation occurs, followed by inflammation. Even though gout can affect any number of joints, it chiefly affects the joints of the big toe.

As with other arthritic conditions, there is pain, tenderness, and swelling at the joint. The individual may experience fever and body chills due to the inflammation. In time, deformity, along with the formation of subcutaneous nodules at the place of inflammation, can result. Gout can be controlled by medication. In addition, diet can help control the painful episodes.

Signs and Indications

As with all chronic diseases, early identification is important so that proper medical attention can be obtained. A number of signs and symptoms serve as warning signals for arthritis. The Arthritis Foundation has suggested that individuals should consult medical personnel if any of the following are present.[34]

Swelling in one or more of the joints

Stiffness upon arising in the morning

Any recurring pain or tenderness in a joint

Loss of the ability to have normal movement at a joint

Redness and warmth in a joint

Any unexplained weight loss, fever, or weakness combined with joint pain

Research Activities

Much research is being carried out to learn more about arthritis. Though a great deal has been learned about the biology of this disease, medical scientists still need to know more about the role of the body's immune system as it relates to inflammation of the joints. The major thrust of many research programs is to identify the causes, including the genetic factors that predispose individuals to arthritis. Research is also attempting to develop new drugs that can provide relief from the pain associated with this disease. A number of anti-inflammatory drugs provide some relief for most types of arthritis.

Chronic Diseases and Community Health

The nature of most chronic diseases requires long-term, individual treatment and care. In some respects the direct care of those suffering from these diseases is not a community concern. Treatment is usually obtained from one's individual physician. Little care is obtained from community health agencies. In fact, less than 3 percent of state health expenditures are allocated to the major chronic diseases.[35]

On the other hand, today many community agencies are carrying out initiatives to reduce the risk of chronic disease by encouraging early detection. These include blood pressure screening, referral, and follow-up

programs. Smoking cessation programs and support for exercise activities are other examples.

Major research to better understand the nature of these diseases and to find cures is being carried out by the initiatives of governmental agencies, in particular the National Institutes of Health.[36] Additionally, supporting research is an important emphasis of the various voluntary health organizations.[37] Funding from these organizations is made available to scientific researchers in medical care facilities, universities, private medical research centers, and other scientific research programs.

A major focus of chronic disease programming is prevention. Today much is known about preventable risk factors for the various chronic diseases. Cigarette smoking, overweight, high cholesterol, high blood pressure, a sedentary life-style, and heavy alcohol consumption play major roles in causing several of the chronic diseases. Various initiatives focus on preventing these diseases. However, very little state and federal money is allocated for prevention of chronic diseases. It has been estimated that the mean annual per capita expenditure by states for such prevention is about sixty-six cents.[38]

Educating the public about chronic diseases is crucial. Many different community organizations and agencies plan and present instructional initiatives. This is an important focus of the voluntary health organizations. For example, the American Cancer Society has targeted nutrition, lowered tobacco use, and breast health as major priorities for public education regarding cancer. Their *Smart Move, Special Delivery* program is aimed at pregnant women who smoke. The American Heart Association has established programs to encourage people to eat low-fat, low-cholesterol diets, and to help people modify their diets in order to help prevent cardiovascular disease.

Most state and local health departments and many businesses and industries have educational programs designed to help reduce the risk factors associated with chronic diseases. The *Heart at Work Program* is an American Heart Association program in cooperation with businesses which helps employees to take measures that will reduce the risk of cardiovascular disease.

Coalitions of organizations and agencies have come together to provide programs to reduce specific chronic disease. For example, the National Cancer Institute has initiated two research and demonstration programs designed to reduce cigarette smoking. These community-based programs, the Community Intervention Trial for Smoking Cessation and the American Stop Smoking Intervention Study, are bringing the resources of the American Cancer Society and state and local health departments together with the National Cancer Institute.

The Centers for Disease Control and Prevention under authority of federal legislation initiated a National Breast and Cervical Cancer Early Detection Program in 1991. CDC makes funds available to state health agencies to provide screening for breast and cervical cancer among low-income females. In addition, programs are supported to help elderly women and ethnic minority females with these cancers. Several services are included in this program: Pap tests, pelvic examinations, mammography screening, and clinical breast examinations.[39]

The Centers for Disease Control and Prevention also cooperates in chronic disease prevention programs with individual state agencies. For example, the Colorado Cardiovascular Disease Prevention Coalition is a five year project designed to teach and encourage implementation of strategies for preventing and controlling cardiovascular disease.

Summary

The leading causes of death and debilitation among the U.S. population in the 1990s are chronic diseases. These diseases are not caused by microorganisms but are related to a variety of different factors.

Chronic diseases include the cardiovascular diseases, cancer, chronic pulmonary disease, cirrhosis of the liver, arthritic diseases, and others. Many life-style patterns present risk factors for these diseases. For example, smoking has been linked with cardiovascular diseases, pulmonary diseases, and cancer. Diet patterns are linked with several of the chronic diseases. Because these diseases are usually long-term and may become debilitating, many problems arise for the caretakers as well as for the patients.

Though there are no cures for the chronic diseases, treatment can provide relief from the symptoms of many. The patient must be under the care of a physician to know the appropriate medication needed. The diabetic needs insulin. The sufferer of arthritis needs to take certain medication for relief from pain.

Prevention is an important factor related to chronic diseases. Though in many cases it may be impossible to totally eliminate these diseases, individuals may practice certain life-style patterns to reduce the risk of contracting some of the diseases.

Research has played an important part in better understanding the causes and treatment of chronic diseases. More is known today than at any time in the past. With more research, it must be hoped that improvements will continue to occur, and that cures may even be found.

Discussion Questions

1. In what ways do the chronic diseases differ from communicable diseases?
2. Describe and differentiate the types of cardiovascular disease.
3. What is hypertension?
4. Identify some of the risk factors associated with cardiovascular disease.
5. In what ways has medical technology had an impact on the treatment of individuals with cardiovascular disease?
6. Biologically, what is a cancerous cell?
7. Explain the process of metastasis.
8. What are some early danger signs of cancer?
9. Explain some of the screening procedures used today to detect colorectal cancer.

10. Why do many women fail to have mammogram screening for breast cancer?

11. Explain and compare the different types of cancer treatment.

12. Discuss some of the characteristics of chronic obstructive pulmonary disease.

13. What are some problems faced by the person with emphysema?

14. What are some of the differences between type I and type II diabetes?

15. In what ways is diabetes a related factor to other health problems?

16. What is cirrhosis of the liver?

17. What is arthritis?

18. Differentiate between osteoarthritis and rheumatoid arthritis.

19. What impact have research developments on arthritis had in the past decade?

20. What are the roles of economics and politics in chronic disease programming?

Suggested Readings

Bankhead, Charles D. "Americans Are Having as Many Strokes, but Fewer Prove Fatal." *Medical World News* 30, no. 5 (March 13, 1989): 15.

———. "Options and Optimism Growing: Type II Diabetes." *Medical World News* 30, no. 19 (October 9, 1989): 35–40.

Bild, Diane, and Steven M. Teutsch. "The Control of Hypertension in Persons with Diabetes: A Public Health Approach." *Public Health Reports* 102, no. 5 (September/October 1987): 522–29.

Blalock, Susan J. "Coping with Rheumatoid Arthritis: Is One Problem the Same as Another?" *Health Education Quarterly* 20, no. 1 (Spring 1993): 199–232.

Centers for Disease Control. "Chronic Disease Reports: Deaths from Lung Cancer—United States, 1986." *Morbidity and Mortality Weekly Report* 38, no. 29 (July 28, 1989): 505–13.

Centers for Disease Control. "Deaths and Hospitalizations from Chronic Liver Disease and Cirrhosis—United States, 1980–1989." *Morbidity and Mortality Weekly Report* 41, no. 52/53 (January 8, 1993): 969–73.

Centers for Disease Control. "Trends in Colorectal Cancer Incidence—United States, 1973–1986." *Morbidity and Mortality Weekly Report* 38, no. 42 (October 27, 1989): 728–31.

Centers for Disease Control. "Update: National Breast and Cervical Cancer Early Detection Program, July 1991–July 1992." *Morbidity and Mortality Weekly Report* 41, no. 40 (October 9, 1992): 739–43.

Davidson, John K. "Teaming Up Against Diabetes." *Health Aims* 4, no. 1 (Spring 1988): 41–43.

Dylak, Sandy. "Diabetes Education: Helping Kids Manage Their Own Diabetes." *J.D.F. International Countdown* 14, no. 2 (Spring 1993): 14–18.

Manson, JoAnn E., and others. "A Prospective Study of Obesity and Risk of Coronary Heart Disease in Women." *The New England Journal of Medicine* 322, no. 13 (March 29, 1990): 882–89.

Middaugh, John P. "Cardiovascular Deaths among Alaskan Natives, 1980–1986." *American Journal of Public Health* 80, no. 3 (March 1990): 282–85.

Sherman, Gary. "Foot Care and the Diabetic." *Diabetes Countdown* 6, no. 1 (Winter 1985): 18–20.

Tanne, Janice Hopkins. "New Insights on Diabetic Eye Disease." *Diabetes Countdown* 10, no. 2 (Spring 1989): 20–24.

Taplin, Stephen, and others. "Breast Cancer Risk and Participation in Mammographic Screening." *American Journal of Public Health* 79, no. 11 (November 1989): 1494–98.

Thompson, Grey B., and others. "Breast Cancer Screening Legislation in the United States: A Commentary." *American Journal of Public Health* 79, no. 11 (November 1989): 1541–43.

Wysowski, Diane K., and others. "Prescribed Use of Cholesterol-Lowering Drugs in the United States, 1978 through 1988." *Journal of the American Medical Association* 263, no. 16 (April 25, 1990): 2185–88.

Zapka, Jane G., and others. "Breast Cancer Screening by Mammography: Utilization and Associated Factors." *American Journal of Public Health* 79, no. 11 (November 1989): 1499–1502.

Endnotes

1. Information provided by American Heart Association, 7272 Greenville Avenue, Dallas, Texas 75321.

2. Department of Health and Human Services. *Healthy People 2000: National Health Promotion and Disease Prevention Objectives,* Washington, D.C.: U.S. Government Printing Office, 1991, p. 396.

3. Discussion of research relating to cardiovascular disease is discussed in chapter 2.

4. Centers for Disease Control. "State-Specific Changes in Cholesterol Screening and Awareness—United States, 1987–1988." *Morbidity and Mortality Weekly Report* 39, no. 18 (May 11, 1990): 304–14.

5. Department of Health and Human Services, *Healthy People 2000,* 405.

6. *Ibid.,* 405.

7. Agency for Health Care Policy and Research. *Research Activities* no. 158 (November 1992): 1.

8. American Cancer Society. *Cancer Facts and Figures—1993.* Atlanta, Ga.: American Cancer Society, 1992, p. 15.

9. *Ibid.*

10. National Cancer Institute. *Cancer Facts* (May 1986): 1.

11. American Cancer Society, *Cancer Facts and Figures—1993,* 19.

12. National Cancer Institute, *Cancer Facts,* 1992, p. 1.

13. *Ibid.,* 2.

14. American Cancer Society, *Cancer Facts and Figures—1992,* 20.

15. Department of Health and Human Services, *Healthy People 2000,* 418.

16. *Ibid.,* 428.

17. American Cancer Society, *Cancer Facts and Figures—1992,* 15.

18. American Cancer Society. *Cancer Facts and Figures—1988.* New York: N.Y.: American Cancer Society, 1988, p. 4.

19. Centers for Disease Control. "Chronic Disease Reports: Chronic Obstructive Pulmonary Disease Mortality—United States, 1986." *Morbidity and Mortality Weekly Report* 38, no. 32 (August 18, 1989): 552.

20. *Ibid.,* 549.

21. Department of Health and Human Services, *Healthy People 2000,* 138–39.

22. Centers for Disease Control, "Chronic Disease Reports," 552.

23. Department of Health and Human Services, *Healthy People 2000,* 460.

24. United States Department of Health and Human Services. *Promoting Health/Preventing Disease: Year 2000 Objectives for the Nation.* Washington, D.C.: U.S. Government Printing Office, 1989, p. 17–1.

25. Wechsler, Rob. "Foot Notes." *JDF International Countdown* (Spring 1990): 18.

26. Sherman, Gary. "Foot Care and the Diabetic." *Diabetes Countdown* 6, no. 1 (Winter 1985): 20.

27. Department of Health and Human Services, *Promoting Health/Preventing Disease,* 17–10.

28. Ryan, Margaret. "The Rewards of Research." *Diabetes Countdown* 11, no. 1 (Winter 1990): 34–35.

29. Van DeGraaff, Kent M., and Stuart Ira Fox. *Concepts of Human Anatomy and Physiology.* Dubuque, Iowa: Wm. C. Brown Publishers, 1986, p. 845.

30. Department of Health and Human Services, *Healthy People 2000,* 167.

31. Arthritis Foundation. *Arthritis: Basic Facts, Answers to Your Questions.* Atlanta, Ga.: Arthritis Foundation, p. 3. (pamphlet).

32. "Living with Arthritis." *Newsweek* (March 20, 1989): 65.

33. *Ibid.,* 67.

34. Arthritis Foundation, 3400 Peachtree Rd., N.E., Atlanta, Ga. 30326.

35. Centers for Disease Control. "Chronic Disease Prevention and Control Activities—United States, 1989." *Morbidity and Mortality Weekly Report* 40, no. 41 (October 18, 1991): 697.

36. Research programs of the National Institutes of Health are discussed in chapter 2.

37. Work of the voluntary health organizations is discussed in chapter 5.

38. Centers for Disease Control. "Chronic Disease Reports: Deaths from Nine Chronic Diseases—United States, 1986." *Morbidity and Mortality Weekly Report* 39, no. 2 (January 19, 1990): 19.

39. Centers for Disease Control. "Update: National Breast and Cervical Cancer Early Detection Program, July 1991–July 1992." *Morbidity and Mortality Weekly Report* 41, no. 40 (October 9, 1992): 739–43.

CHAPTER **TWELVE**

The Environment

More than a Search for the Cause of Disease

Since the mid-nineteenth century, environmental health has been a vital component of public health activity. Classics in the field of public health literature have focused attention on the importance of improving the sanitary environment.[1] Sanitary concerns as they affect the health of the public have become important aspects of public health programming.

Numerous communicable diseases have resulted from unsanitary conditions throughout recorded history. During much of the nineteenth century, the causes of sickness and ill health were thought to be impure atmospheric and environmental conditions. The germ theory of disease was then unknown. As a result, sanitary programs were developed to create and maintain a clean environment. These were the beginnings of many local public health departments in the United States.

Throughout the first half of the twentieth century, local and state environmental sanitarians focused on such problems as food sanitation, public building sanitation, housing, rodent control, and prevention of air and water pollution. But efforts to improve environmental conditions seem to have peaked in recent years. There have been numerous projects, programs, and activities devoted to providing a better ecosystem for humanity. Concern over the despoiling of the environment was highlighted in April 1970 with the national observance of Earth Day. Hundreds of thousands of people demonstrated throughout the country for improved environmental conditions and effective government environmental policies. Throughout the 1970s citizen involvement in the environmental movement led to an increased environmental awareness and the subsequent passage of legislation.

In the United States a number of federal legislative acts were passed that provided impetus for environmental health programming. Environmental Protection Agencies were legislated at the national level and in many states. Today the responsibility for managing environmental health programs is found in a number of different agencies, although the basic governmental unit having environmental program responsibility is the state health department. Other departments with programming for the environment are the state agricultural department and the departments of water resources, human resources, and natural resources.

In the more than two decades since Earth Day, 1970, the problems related to environmental destruction have escalated. Some of the worst environmental accidents in history have occurred, including Chernobyl, thousands of oil spills each year such as that which occurred in Alaskan waters when the tanker *Exxon Valdez* ran aground, and increased pollution of groundwater by toxic wastes. Problems of the environment have increasingly become global in nature. For example, the depletion of the ozone layer in the atmosphere has many people very concerned. Acid rain damage cuts across the borders of many nations. Many scientists believe that air pollution is resulting in a worldwide warming trend. Destruction of tropical rainforests affects the whole world.

The growth of most of the large cities throughout the world, with accompanying smog and air pollution, is an escalating concern. With greater industrial development and numbers of people, the need for waste disposal is expanding at a time when land available for sanitary landfills is disappearing.

Many people feel that between now and the year 2000 will be a time of continuing serious environmental problems. The worst scenarios project that by the early part of the twenty-first century the conditions on planet Earth will be intolerable for humans. Only if individuals take action with such measures as recycling and energy conservation and if business and industry focus on environmental improvement rather than economic expansion will this scenario be prevented. The life-style of every person must change by the year 2000 if the environment is to be preserved.

A Safe Water Supply

How safe is the water you drink, the water with which you shower and bathe? Is the water that flows in the rivers and streams in your community contaminated with pesticide residues, with toxic substances, or other invisible substances? Water pollution has become a matter of great concern in community health in recent years. Today, once-pure sources of water are contaminated by a variety of pollutants. Increased population, additional sewage and industrial wastes, and the dumping of other contaminants have been major contributors to water pollution.

Americans use an enormous amount of water each day. It is estimated that the average person uses one hundred gallons of water daily. A shower may use between twenty-five and fifty gallons. Approximately seven gallons are used to flush a toilet, two gallons to brush the teeth. Thousands of gallons of water are used when washing the car, watering the lawn, washing the sidewalk, and performing numerous other activities.

In the United States, citizens assume that the drinking water is pure. Little thought is given to the quality of water from a tap in the office building, the glass of water served in the restaurant, or the water obtained from a park drinking fountain. This complete trust in the purity of drinking water is due in part to the activities of public health departments.

There is little incidence of waterborne disease today in the United States. Many of the water-related problems common in other parts of the world have been nearly eliminated in our country. For example, such widespread diseases as typhoid and cholera are rarely seen. But illness does result from water contamination, usually gastrointestinal illness. The Centers for Disease Control

and Prevention has estimated that there are four thousand cases of waterborne illnesses reported every year. It is probable that many more cases of illness associated with the ingestion of contaminated water go unreported or are assumed to be linked to other causes. Waterborne outbreaks are primarily caused by overflow or seepage of sewage from septic tanks, chemical contamination of water supplies, and surface runoff contamination.[2]

In spite of the fact that there is no widespread epidemic of waterborne disease in the United States today, it is important to be concerned about the safety of the water supply of our communities. Episodes of acute illness resulting from water contamination are easily traced, but prolonged exposure at very low levels to contaminants such as cadmium, lead, mercury, and pesticides may have long-term negative health effects. There is speculation that such exposure may eventually cause cancer, heart disease, and other chronic diseases, plus a host of other health problems.

Concern must be expressed about contamination of groundwater. Possibly as much as 90 percent of the drinking water supply comes from underground water sources. Groundwater is the source of water for many households, agricultural enterprises, and some municipal water systems, as well as for businesses and industries. Groundwater originates as rain or melted snow. It enters layers of earth below the surface known as aquifers. Water collects in holes, cracks, and spaces in the ground. Though groundwater may contain dissolved mineral particles, it rarely in nature contains disease-causing organisms.

Numerous chemicals have been found in groundwater that have been shown to have adverse effects on human and animal health. Particular concern has been expressed regarding long-term, low-level exposure to

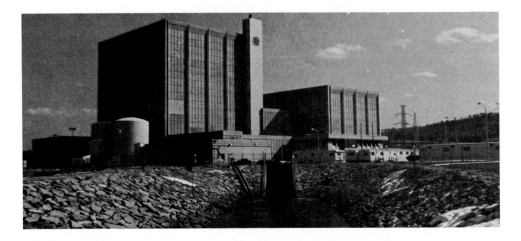

Water pollution is often the result of such industrial processes as energy production. When the water used to generate electricity is returned to its source, it is usually polluted and is often warmer, causing an ecological disruption.

drinking water containing toxic chemicals from waste disposal landfills. Leakage of underground chemical storage tanks is contributing to these problems of water pollution.

A variety of different industries have been implicated in water contamination. Even the high-tech electronics industry has been responsible for contaminating water resources. The industry's toxic chemicals have been linked to a rate of miscarriages and birth defects two to three times the national average.[3]

In congressional testimony it was reported that "no community in the country is free from . . . sources of groundwater contamination."[4] Testimony indicated that there is no data currently available to reveal the true extent of the problem.

Runoff of pesticides from farms and lawns contributes to contamination of underground water sources. In addition, runoff from streets—oil, grease, and other pollutants—can be expected to have an effect on these drinking water sources.

Rivers and lakes are sources of water for many communities. There is increasing concern about contamination of these sources of water.

Two Major Sources of Water Pollution

Industrial and agricultural operations are the major users of water and so are responsible for much of the water pollution in our nation. Industry uses water in the manufacturing process to cool equipment and also converts it to steam to provide heat and generate electrical power. Many chemicals are dumped into rivers, streams, and lakes as the result of industrial processes. Runoff of pesticides

used in agriculture contributes significantly to the pollution of groundwater, rivers, and lakes.

Industry

Water is used as a machinery coolant in many industrial settings. Over 80 percent of water used by industry is used for cooling.[5] The water is usually taken from a stream, river, or lake and poured over the heated equipment. When the water is returned to its source, it is warmer than normal, thus raising the temperature of the principal water supply. Warmer water absorbs less oxygen, which results in a retarded decomposition of organic matter. This problem, termed *thermal pollution,* is of particular concern with regards to power-generating plants, especially nuclear power plants.

Fish cannot adjust to abnormal changes in water temperature, though their life cycle is closely related to normal changes in water temperature. Some fish, for example, spawn when water temperatures drop in the fall; others spawn when temperatures rise in the spring. Imagine, then, how artificially induced changes in temperature can affect this delicate system. In other instances, fish have adjusted to the higher water temperature caused by a manufacturing process or by a nuclear power plant. But when the plant closes down for repairs or for other reasons, the fish cannot readjust to the cooler water and so die.

Agriculture

Agriculture is the largest user of water in America. Not only is water consumed by cattle and other livestock, but it is necessary for growing all crops. It has been estimated that one bushel of wheat requires fifteen thousand gallons of water from the time the seeds are planted until the wheat is eaten as bread. Irrigation, which makes agriculture possible on land that would otherwise be useless for growing purposes, requires tremendous amounts of water.

Agriculture's abundant use of water leads to water pollution. Besides water, crops require nutrients and so are fertilized. It is estimated that each year 22.3 billion pounds of nitrogen fertilizers and 850 million pounds of pesticides are used on crops in the United States. Up to one-fourth of these inorganic fertilizers are lost in surface runoff before the plants can use them. They are carried to the stream or river and become part of the downstream town's water supply. The Environmental Protection Agency reported that forty-six different pesticides used in normal agricultural practices have been found in groundwater.[6]

Siltation from erosion creates a very similar problem. As the soil is plowed, it is exposed to erosion. Erosion, as well as damaging the terrain and removing badly needed topsoil, carries the nutrients from the eroded areas. The soil and nutrients end up in streams and rivers, polluting the water.

Animal wastes present another water pollution problem. Animal feedlots, where cattle are brought for fattening, have created a particular problem. A feedlot holding ten thousand head of cattle produces as much waste as a community of 160,000 people. Runoff from these feedlots obviously creates serious water pollution problems.

Municipal Water Systems

There are at least fifty-eight thousand municipal community water supply systems in the United States.[7] Owing to the growing urban population, water pollution control has focused on the reduction of pollution of these water resources. The Clean Water Act has provided federal support to communities for modernizing their sewage control systems. Some $50 billion has been authorized for improving community water quality.[8] In 1987 this federal legislation was reauthorized over the veto of the president. It provided funds for the construction of local sewage treatment systems and helped individual states tighten controls on discharges of toxic substances into community water sources.

Municipal water purification systems should contain primary and secondary treatment processes. Primary sewage treatment is the process of screening and sedimentation. Water is placed in a tank where the large impurities, such as sand, trash, and other suspended solids, settle. There is also a filtration process that removes large objects as the water passes through a series of screens. About one-third of the communities in the United States are served by systems providing only this primary treatment of water prior to returning it to the original source. After this treatment the water does not look bad, but it still contains microorganisms and organic nutrients.

The secondary sewage treatment process is important because it is in this stage that microorganisms and organic nutrients are removed. For particles too small to filter, a coagulation process is used. Small particles are made larger through coagulation so that they will settle or can be filtrated.

During this secondary process, the water is sprayed over a bed of stones. While it is trickling around the stones, the nutrients are reduced by bacterial action, thus biologically purifying the water. Aerobic bacteria, air, and sunlight help oxidize and purify the water. The final step in the secondary process involves disinfection of microorganisms by chlorination. This process reduces the bacterial content and is considered by most public health officials to be the safest technique in providing safe drinking water. Many major cities do not have effective secondary treatment systems.

Tanker Spills

Waste, garbage, and litter have been discharged into the waterways of the world since the beginning of humankind. In the past such pollutants were absorbed by the oceans, lakes, and rivers, and natural regeneration reduced the need for worry. However, in the twentieth century many more people and larger vessels are using the world's waterways, and the problem has become increasingly serious.

Today huge tankers carry garbage, chemicals, and oil in all parts of the world. Dumping, either purposefully or accidentally, of such pollutants can have long-term destructive effects on life within the water and in the surrounding environment. It is estimated that there

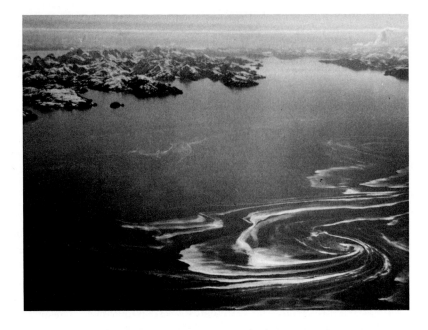

The oil slick in Prince William Sound, 50 miles from the *Exxon Valdez* tanker.

are as many as ten thousand spills of pollutants into the waters of the world annually.

One of the worst spills in history occurred when the *Exxon Valdez* ran aground in Prince William Sound in March 1989. Eleven million gallons of oil were spilled into these waters. Within a month oil had spread some four hundred miles from the site of the accident. More than twelve hundred miles of Alaskan coastline was despoiled. Thousands of birds, including more than a hundred bald eagles, and sea life, including fish and otters, were killed.

How this spill will affect the environment in the long term remains to be seen. With larger numbers of supertankers carrying oil and other potentially damaging substances, it is likely that more spills will happen in the future. Measures, legislative and regulatory, must be developed to reduce the possibility of these occurrences, which cause catastrophic damage to the environment.

Legislation for Clean Water

In 1914 the first federal drinking water standards were developed.[9] These early standards applied only to water provided by interstate carriers—in those days, trains. Until the 1950s, this and other federal water pollution control programs were designed to prevent the spread of communicable diseases.

The Water Pollution Control Act of 1956, amended in 1965 and again in 1972, was the first legislation to establish water quality standards. In the 1972 reauthorization of this legislation Congress established a national system of permits aimed at controlling discharges of pollutants by industries, municipalities, and agriculture. Pollution control equipment had to be installed by those agencies and by industries discharging effluents into navigable waters. This legislation also provided large sums of money for building municipal sewage treatment facilities. This legislation has been reauthorized several times since 1972, with Congress overriding the veto of the president in 1987.

In the more than two decades that have passed since 1972, more than $84 billion has been spent for water pollution control. Some successes have been reported along with a number of failures.[10] Controlling runoff of pesticides and fertilizers is still a problem. In this period of time many acres of the nation's wetlands have been lost to development and to pollution. It is the feeling of many concerned about the quality of water that protection of wetlands must occur, that effective municipal wastewater treatment procedures must be a high priority, and that toxic chemicals must be controlled and not reach the sources of water for people and animals.

Other legislation implemented in 1977, the Clean Water Act, provided monies to build water treatment plants and prohibited the discharge of harmful waste materials into navigable waters. There is little doubt that the funding provided by this legislation has had beneficial effects in many localities. For example, since the early 1970s billions of dollars have been spent to clean up the Great Lakes. Today they look and smell better. Fishing, once prohibited in Lake Erie, is now a profitable occupation. Other lakes, rivers, and streams throughout the nation have been improved.

However, problems still occur. The Clean Water Act does not require pollution controls on storm sewers. Rainwater runs into street drains, then into sewers, often carrying gas, oil, fertilizers, and other substances. From the storm sewers it often drains into nearby lakes, rivers, and other bodies of water that serve as community water supplies. Toxic substances may also work their way into the water sources. Despite improvement, over four hundred toxic chemicals have been found in the Great Lakes. Often they are in only minute levels, but as one goes upward in the food chain the level increases. Reducing the amount of toxic chemicals is very difficult. The Clean Water Act is due for reauthorization in the mid-1990s. Changes and modifications to be made remain to be seen.

Another federal law, the Safe Drinking Water Act of 1974, directed the Environmental Protection Agency to establish drinking water standards. These standards would ensure that drinking water contaminants, such as cadmium, fluoride, mercury, and other elements, did not exceed a specified limit, thus meeting purity standards. Noncommunity settings, such as trailer parks, camping sites, and roadside motels with their own water supplies, also must meet the standards.

The establishment of such standards is no easy task. There are more than three hundred organic chemicals that have been identified in drinking water in the United States. Little or no testing has been done on most of these to ascertain the specific cause-and-effect relationships on health. The Safe Drinking Water Act was strengthened and reauthorized in 1986.

Air Pollution

Life on earth cannot exist without oxygen, the most vital component of air. Air is limited and must be reused, and if polluted, it can cause a variety of health problems.

There has always been limited pollution of the air. Fires, wind erosion, and dirt particles have naturally contaminated the air. However, nature solves this problem too: wind, snow, and rainfall clean the air. In settings not disturbed by humans and modern technology, the air is relatively pure and does not contribute to health problems.

Industrialization, the development and expanded use of the motor vehicle, increased human population, and growth of urban communities have significantly aggravated the problem of air pollution. As a result, the quality of the air today in many parts of the world, including America, is poor. The major sources of air pollution in the United States are the burning of fossil fuels, the internal combustion engine in motor vehicles, fuel furnaces used to generate electricity, and industrial processes.

The effect of some types of air pollution on humans is easily observable. During hot weather air pollution in many cities becomes dangerous for people with respiratory problems, the elderly, and those who must work and play outside. According to the Environmental Protection Agency, the summer of 1988 was the worst ever recorded for smog pollution in the United States.[11] Smog conditions are a concern not only in America but worldwide.

Air quality in Mexico City is considered to be as bad as any other city in the world. By late morning the air is so filled with pollutants that it is usually impossible to see the sun clearly. Unfortunately, smog and air pollution seem to be getting worse in many of the nations of the developing world. For example, in such Asian metropolitan areas as Jakarta, Hong Kong, Taipei, and Seoul, hundreds of thousands of people are exposed every day to levels of air pollution that can have negative effects on health. The same could be said about several African, Latin American, and European cities.

Many indirect, nonobservable effects of air pollution are a concern to scientists, medical professionals, and public health personnel. Long-term exposure to only traces of air contaminants has a very detrimental effect on people's respiratory systems.

Pollutants

Many of the more than three hundred air pollutants identified by the Environmental Protection Agency have known adverse effects on human health. They have the potential for causing illness, debilitation, and even death.

Under provisions of the Clean Air Act of 1970 the Environmental Protection Agency was directed to develop regulations for restricting these pollutants. By 1990 regulatory standards had been established for only seven: (1) carbon monoxide, (2) hydrocarbons, (3) lead, (4) nitrogen oxide, (5) ozone, (6) particulate matter, and (7) sulfur oxide.

Carbon Monoxide

Produced by the incomplete combustion of organic materials, carbon monoxide's major source is the internal combustion engine of the automobile. This gas is breathed into the lungs and enters the red blood cells where it combines with hemoglobin, which normally carries oxygen to the body cells. Because of hemoglobin's affinity for carbon monoxide, normal oxygen supply is replaced by carbon monoxide. This causes a reduction in oxygen supply to the various body cells.

Carbon monoxide in the body can cause death if too much oxygen is replaced, particularly in the brain cells. As many as one thousand deaths occur each year from accidental carbon monoxide poisoning. Exposure to this pollutant over a lengthy period has a detrimental effect on respiratory functioning and the cardiovascular system, as well as alertness and perception.

Hydrocarbons

Compounds containing both carbon and hydrogen, hydrocarbons are the products of incomplete combustion of gasoline and the evaporation of petroleum fuels and industrial solvents. The main sources of hydrocarbons are motor vehicles, refineries, and petroleum-processing facilities.

Hydrocarbons have been shown to have a negative effect on people with upper respiratory problems. Hydrocarbons are also a concern because they are a major component in the reaction that forms ozone and other photochemical oxidants.

Lead

This substance enters the atmosphere principally from automobile exhaust and from industries that process this metal. Most airborne lead is created by automobiles, so all new automobiles must now use lead-free gasoline. However, many older cars still use leaded gasoline.

Lead is injurious to several body systems since it is absorbed into the blood and accumulates in several locations, chiefly the bones. Concern has been expressed regarding the effect of lead on young children, who are particularly susceptible to lead poisoning.

Nitrogen Oxides

These are highly toxic gases that are the result of high-temperature combustion of such energy sources as coal, oil, and gasoline. The major outlets of nitrogen oxides are electric utilities, industrial boilers, and motor vehicles.

Exposure to high levels of nitrogen oxides can be fatal. The general public usually is exposed to low levels, which can irritate the lungs and the eyes and compound the causes of certain lung diseases. Nitrogen dioxide in combination with water vapor in the air produces nitric acid, which can corrode metal surfaces and damage vegetation.

Ozone

Produced by chemical reactions that occur when hydrocarbons and nitrogen oxides are exposed to sunlight, ozone is a photochemical oxidant. Hydrocarbons and nitrogen oxide compounds are broken up, and oxygen atoms are released. These oxygen atoms join other oxygen atoms already in the atmosphere to form ozone. Ozone acts as an irritant to the respiratory system, causing coughing, tightness of the chest, and difficult breathing. Long-term exposure can lead to permanent damage of lung tissues. Ozone also irritates the eyes. It has been shown to cause damage to plants also.

Children are more vulnerable to ozone than are adults owing to their cellular immaturity and ongoing growth processes. For example, children's airways are narrower than are those of adults, so swelling of the airways can be dangerous in some children.

Particulate Matter

Airborne particles of solid or liquid substances are particulate matter. Soot, dirt, dust, and fly ash are examples of particulate matter found in the air. Particulate matter is the result of many industrial processes. For example, steel plants, electric generating plants, cement factories, and other similar industrial processes put wastes into the ambient air.

Particulate matter damages the protective cilia of the respiratory system. The damaged or destroyed cilia are likely to be a factor in disease and infection. In addition, toxic chemical substances may be carried into the respiratory system by particulate matter or may cause serious eye irritation.

Sulfur Oxide

The combustion of fuels that contain sulfur results in the production of sulfur oxides. Coal burning accounts for the major portion of sulfur oxides in the air. In addition to coal, the burning of residual oil, paper, rubber, and other solid wastes contributes sulfur dioxide to the air.

The major health effect of the various sulfur oxides is irritation of the respiratory system, so it is especially detrimental to victims of bronchitis, emphysema, and asthma. Children and the elderly are particularly susceptible to sulfur oxides. In addition to contributing to respiratory problems, sulfur oxides cause corrosion and damage vegetation.

Legislative Action

The increased awareness of health problems, particularly of respiratory and cardiovascular disease, and the exposure to air pollutants have provoked action to improve the quality of air. This action has taken several different directions. Some actions have been directed at individual behaviors, such as prohibiting the burning of leaves in the fall. Others have been directed at industrial sources of air pollution, requiring emission control devices on smokestacks. Since the motor vehicle is a major contributor to air pollution, changes in the exhaust system have been mandated by the federal government.

Unfortunately, measures designed to clean the air are costly. These costs have been passed on both directly and indirectly to the consumer, to the industrial manufacturer, and to the government. All too often the costs to industry and to government are then passed along to the individual. For example, air pollution emission regulations mandate the installation of exhaust devices on all cars, an expense that is passed along to the buyer in the purchase price of the automobile, hence contributing to the higher prices of automobiles.

Many industries, corporations, and individuals feel that current air pollution laws and regulations are inflationary and should be reduced or eliminated. This issue has resulted in one of the major political debates of recent years. For instance, the automotive industry would like to see reductions in the regulatory requirements of the Clean Air Act. On the other hand, many environmental groups and public health organizations are opposed to any weakening of such standards.

The Clean Air Act

The federal government took legislative action in 1955[12] and in 1963[13] to deal with the problems of air pollution. These legislative actions provided funds for research and financial assistance to local agencies. In 1970, Congress enlarged the role of the federal government by passing the Clean Air Amendments of 1970 (PL 91–604), legislation that gave the Environmental Protection Agency the responsibility to establish standards for all major air pollutants. This legislation gave cities and states five years to meet standards for selected "priority" pollutants.

Since 1970, the Environmental Protection Agency has set standards for seven major pollutants. In addition, strict emission standards for the manufacture of new automobiles and the building of power plants and factories were established. Compliance timetables were set, revised, and extended in many instances. Through the 1970s, the Clean Air Act was the principal legislation for improving the quality of air in the United States.

Authorization by Congress of the act expired in 1982. Though the act itself was not reauthorized, the provisions of the law were extended annually until 1990. During this period of time little was done either to pass any new clean air legislation or to reduce such air pollution as acid rain or toxic chemicals.

After much debate and discussion, a reauthorization of the Clean Air Act was passed in 1990. This legislation, though broad in effect, had three basic goals: (1) Smog in urban localities is to be reduced by requiring the automotive industry to manufacture and sell cars that give off less nitrogen oxide and hydrocarbons. (2) New acid rain controls are to be enforced. Acid rain is to be reduced by lowering sulfur dioxide emissions. This is likely to have an impact on the coal-mining industry, as many utility plants burn coal. Coal-burning utility plants will be required to install pollution-reducing scrubbers or switch to low-sulfur coal. (3) Cancer-causing toxins are

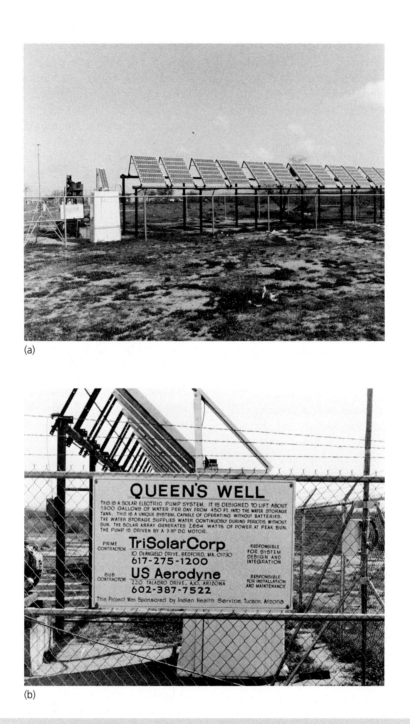

(a)

QUEEN'S WELL

THIS IS A SOLAR ELECTRIC PUMP SYSTEM. IT IS DESIGNED TO LIFT ABOUT
5900 GALLONS OF WATER PER DAY FROM 450 FT. INTO THE WATER STORAGE
TANK. THIS IS A UNIQUE SYSTEM, CAPABLE OF OPERATING WITHOUT BATTERIES.
THE WATER STORAGE SUPPLIES WATER CONTINUOSLY DURING PERIODS WITHOUT
SUN. THE SOLAR ARRAY GENERATES 2664 WATTS OF POWER AT PEAK SUN.
THE PUMP IS DRIVEN BY A 3 HP DC MOTOR.

PRIME
CONTRACTOR **TriSolarCorp**
10 DeANGELO DRIVE, BEDFORD, MA. 01730
617-275-1200

RESPONSIBLE
FOR SYSTEM
DESIGN AND
INTEGRATION

SUB
CONTRACTOR **US Aerodyne**
220 TALADRO DRIVE, AJO, ARIZONA
602-387-7522

RESPONSIBLE
FOR INSTALLATION
AND MAINTENANCE

This Project Was Sponsored by Indian Health Service, Tucson, Arizona.

(b)

Effective, clean, and reasonably priced energy sources must be developed in the 1990s. Though solar energy is not widespread in its current use, many people believe that the sun can be a major provider of energy. This may be most effective in parts of the nation with a lot of sunshine. (a) Solar panels provide an environmentally appropriate energy source for an Indian Health Service Hospital in Arizona. (b) A solar electric pump supplies several thousand gallons of water daily.

to be eliminated from the air. Industry must reduce emissions of carcinogenic air pollutants by 90 percent by the year 2000.

After some initial improvement when the original legislation was passed in the 1970s, the problem of air pollution now appears to be getting worse. Today as many as 60 percent of the U.S. population lives in cities with unhealthy air.

In 1991 the Environmental Protection Agency reported that ninety-eight urban areas did not attain acceptable ozone standards under provisions of the National Ambient Air Quality Standards.[14] In addition, the EPA indicated that 76 percent had not attained carbon monoxide standards, 70 percent had not attained standards for particulate matter, 50 percent had not met standards for sulfur dioxide, and 11 percent had not met standards for lead.

The future of the Clean Air Act is on shaky ground. Officials in industry, business, and government are opposed to the strict standards and compliance timetables. They question the way these federal standards have been established. For most pollutants, there is little clear evidence to indicate the level at which a pollutant can be considered safe, so it has been difficult to develop acceptable threshold levels. For these reasons, those opposed to the Clean Air Act suggest that current standards cannot be justified and therefore must either be compromised or totally eliminated.

Opponents also contend that it is too costly to enforce and to meet standards. Such standards interfere with the concept of free enterprise and create governmental interference. This position was supported in 1990 by President George Bush when he stated that no clean air legislation should be passed that would restrict economic growth and cause unemployment.

Environmental and health advocates have argued strongly that the Clean Air Act should not be weakened, but in fact strengthened. They contend that any action that would extend compliance deadlines, weaken implementation requirements, or raise already established standards would only add to air pollution.

Those who support new clean air legislation believe that action must be taken to reduce the emission of gases that cause acid rain. They would also pass regulations to control the release of toxic industrial chemicals into the atmosphere—some 2.7 billion pounds per year are put into the air annually. In addition, realistic but firm compliance schedules for meeting standards must be established and met.

The Environmental Protection Agency has the responsibility to develop guidelines and establish licensing fee procedures for industry. There is little doubt that this legislation will have a variety of economic impacts. Utility rates will increase, particularly in those parts of the country that rely heavily on coal. The cost of all motor vehicles will rise. Both industry and consumers will experience higher costs.

It seems logical to suggest that major research and development must occur in the motor vehicle industry, since motor vehicles are the single largest source of urban air pollution. Development of "cleaner" gasoline must become a central focus if clean air is to be achieved in the United States. Several options have been suggested; however, major efforts have not been employed by the motor vehicle industry to develop and manufacture vehicles using these types of gasolines.

The options include development of methanol gasoline from natural gas, coal, and wood. Up to 50 percent less hydrocarbons and 10 percent less carbon dioxide would be produced by the use of methanol. Another alternative to gasoline is the development of ethanol. Ethanol is made from coal or sugar. If ethanol were mixed with gasoline, the carbon monoxide and smog could be reduced significantly. Less hydrocarbons, carbon monoxide, and carbon dioxide would result from use of compressed natural gas. Also, the development of electricity-operated motor vehicles needs further attention. Electricity-operated vehicles would significantly eliminate many emissions of concern.

Global Concerns

Every environmental problem has worldwide implications. However, some do not seem as close and pertinent as others. Three global problems concern scientists and environmentalists today. Only recently has the general public become interested and knowledgeable about these issues: (1) acid rain, (2) the global warming trend, and (3) depletion of the ozone layer in the stratosphere.

Acid Rain

Not only are lakes, rivers, streams, and underground water tables often polluted, but there is evidence that even rainfall is polluted. This is a condition known as *acid rain* and results when the oxides of sulfur and nitrogen are released into the air from tall industrial smokestacks. These pollutants react with water vapor in the clouds and form acids. The clouds become acidic, so when rain and snow fall from them, acid falls to the earth and affects the flora, water, fish, and probably humans and animals.

Acid rain has developed into a significant problem—especially since the early 1970s, when industries began building taller smokestacks. Today many smokestacks are more than five hundred feet high and some are even taller than one thousand feet. These smokestacks emit nitrogen and sulfur oxides high into the atmosphere; as a result, the upper-level winds carry the oxides a great distance from their source, resulting in serious pollution problems several hundred miles downwind.

In the United States, environmentalists have become particularly concerned about fish kills in the Adirondack Lakes region of upstate New York. It is believed that the sources of this lethal acid rain are industrial plants along the Great Lakes.

Acid rain has also become an international problem. In 1981 the Ontario, Canada, government attempted to persuade the United States Environmental Protection Agency to maintain its air pollution standards. Acid rain, a by-product of mid-western industries, was killing fish in Ontario lakes. Since tourism in Ontario depends on the lakes, this problem has serious economic consequences as well as environmental ramifications.

Although acid rain has proved toxic to fish, its effects on vegetation and wildlife are still uncertain.[15] Although no direct cause-and-effect relationship with human health has been documented, acid rain must be considered a possible health hazard. It is probable that increased exposure to acid in the environment will in some way be detrimental to human well-being.

Efforts to control acid rain have encountered roadblocks. One Environmental Protection Agency regulation allows each state to regulate its own output of sulfur and nitrogen oxides. Hence the level of acceptable emissions differs from one state to another. As a result of this variance, states with strong emission control

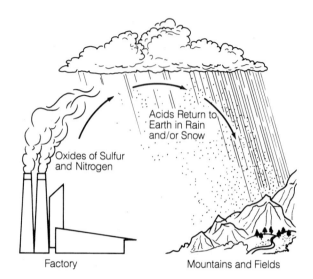

Acid rain results when the oxides of sulfur and nitrogen are poured into the air from tall industrial smokestacks. These pollutants react with water vapor in the clouds and form acids. These acids fall to the earth some distance away in the form of rain or snow.

regulations may be affected by acid rain originating in distant states having less stringent regulation standards.

The cost of implementing a solution to the acid rain issue has proved to be another stumbling block. It is costly to place scrubbers in the smokestacks of all industries. In spite of this, Japan has shown that not only is such action possible, it can be effective and economical, too.[16] Emissions were decreased by 50 percent in that nation after strong sulfur oxide regulations were implemented in 1968. Today there are six times more scrubbers in Japan than in the United States.[17]

Politically there have been few agreements about what measures need to be taken to alleviate the problem of acid rain. Because of the international scope of the problem, nations must come together to work to solve it. Unfortunately, little international cooperation has occurred. With more than 160 million tons a year of sulfur dioxide being poured into the atmosphere, it seems only logical that measures must be adopted to decrease such production. The United States government has recommended that sulfur dioxide be reduced by at least half by placing controls on smokestacks and encouraging the burning of cleaner coal.

Global Warming

The 1980s had six of the ten warmest years on record. This trend has continued into the 1990s. During the latter part of the 1980s much of North America experienced prolonged heat and drought. These facts gave significant support to the idea that the Earth is getting warmer.

For years scientists have been concerned about the effects of air pollutants on the Earth's temperatures, particularly the increasing concentrations of carbon dioxide. In the presence of carbon dioxide, heat energy radiation is absorbed. As precipitation cycles are affected, average temperatures are higher and climates drier. This phenomenon has been referred to as the "greenhouse effect." It has been theorized that global surface temperatures could increase between three and nine degrees Fahrenheit in the next century, causing a number of major environmental changes. The likelihood of drought would increase. This would affect agricultural patterns, with less land available for raising needed food supplies.

Another possibility is that the levels of oceans and seas would change owing to the melting of polar ice caps. As large blocks of ice break off and melt, they would cause extensive flooding along low-lying land in many nations of the world, such as Bangladesh and India. Not only would hundreds of thousands of people be displaced in already overcrowded nations, but farmland would be destroyed as well.

Except for several scientific and political conferences focusing on the "greenhouse effect," there have been no clear-cut initiatives established as yet. In 1989 representatives from more than seventy nations gathered in the Netherlands to discuss the problem. It was generally agreed that carbon dioxide emissions must be stabilized. Many nations agreed to cut emission levels by the year 2000. The United States and several other of the industrialized nations asked for more time to study the problem.

This matter cannot await much more discussion and theoretical debate. Some may be right in suggesting that we are already into a "warming" trend that has little chance for reversal unless major changes are instituted immediately to curtail air pollution worldwide.

One factor related to this problem that has received increasing attention has been the destruction of the rainforests. Forests help regulate precipitation cycles and provide oxygen to balance the gases in the atmosphere. In recent years thousands of square miles of rainforests have been destroyed. The trees are cut down for farming and resettlement, and are sold for lumber. The method of clearing the forests, that is, by burning, adds great amounts of carbon dioxide to the atmosphere, compounding the warming trend.

Numerous health problems are created by these actions. Tropical diseases increase as the ecology of the forests are disturbed and insects and pests populate areas. As land becomes exposed there is greater runoff of soil into the rivers and streams, greatly contributing to the pollution of the water that people use for drinking and eating. Food shortages are affected as useful and productive land becomes denuded and destroyed.

This issue presents an interesting paradox. The developing nations see the destruction of the rainforests as necessary for expansion and development of their nations and their economies. The developed nations plead with these countries to stop destroying the environment. However, little notice is given to the destruction of the North American forests in the 1700s and 1800s. Measures must be instituted throughout the world to encourage the growth of forests. Planting trees is an activity that has positive long-range environmental effects.

Depletion of the Ozone Layer

In the stratosphere some ten to twenty-five miles above the earth there is ozone. This gas, made up of oxygen atoms, acts as a shield that screens out the ultraviolet radiation from the sun.

In 1984 scientists discovered that there was a large hole in the ozone shield over Antarctica. It has since been found that the ozone layer is being destroyed by chemicals called chlorofluorocarbons (CFCs), which contain chlorine, fluorine, and carbon. The chlorine atoms destroy ozone molecules.

Chlorofluorocarbons are being used in an increasing number of consumer products—as coolants in air conditioners and motor vehicles and in refrigerators. CFCs are also used in foam insulation for packaging, in pillows, car seats, and carpet padding. They are used in cleaning solvents for manufacturing machinery and in dry-cleaning procedures.

Halons, chemicals used in fire extinguishers, have been found to be a more potent ozone depleter than CFCs. They leave no residue, so they are also used in procedures to protect valuable papers and books.

Destruction of this layer in the stratosphere could lead to major health problems. Most medical scientists believe that there will be an increase in certain cancers, particularly skin cancer. Additionally, exposure of the lens of the eyes to ultraviolet light contributes to cataracts; the vision of thousands of people could be harmed.

Several actions have been taken to stop the damage being done to the ozone layer. In 1987 at a meeting in Montreal the need for international agreement and cooperation in controlling the manufacture and use of certain chemicals was recognized. It was agreed that nations would work toward a 50 percent reduction in CFC production and a freeze on halons. Recognizing the need for even greater controls, in 1989 eighty-one nations and the European Economic Community agreed to a total ban of all chemicals that deplete the ozone layer by the year 2000 at a conference in Helsinki, Finland.

Even though governments have sought to place restrictions on the use of CFCs, phasing them out is not easily accomplished. They are inexpensive and used in many everyday consumer products. Until recently industry has not supported these restrictive measures. As more evidence is being presented, some companies have announced plans to cut back on manufacture and use of CFCs.

The depletion of the ozone layer is not a scientific theory for researchers to calculate with their computers. It is a very real problem that could have a major impact on life on Earth. Major steps must be taken to eliminate the use of chemicals that damage ozone in the atmosphere.

United Nations Conference on the Environment and Development, 1992

A major international conference on the environment was held in Rio de Janeiro, Brazil, in 1992. One hundred and seventy-eight nations sent representatives to this conference. There were one hundred fifteen heads of state along with more than 30,000 participants. The participants included a broad range of individuals representing government, nongovernmental agencies, and religious, corporate, and private organizations. This conference received major worldwide media attention.

Many issues were discussed at this conference; the three major problems that received consideration were depletion of the ozone layer, global warming, and transboundary air pollution. Also, the importance of management of water resources and the provision of safe drinking water were highlighted. The conference attempted to establish a balance between environmental and development concerns.

Several agreements were reached. It was concluded that there are many environmental problems needing attention. Several agreements created new international institutions. For example, new bodies for providing scientific and technical advice regarding climatic change are to be established. Governments will be required to report their efforts to monitor and control emissions that contribute to global warming. It was agreed that a need exists for communication and exchange of information worldwide to curb continuing environmental destruction.

Many feel that the Rio conference provided opportunity for improvement of worldwide environmental standards. The need to integrate environmental factors into public policy was emphasized. It will not be easy to identify ways in which environmental improvement and economic development can both occur. However, the Rio conference was seen by many as the beginning of a long process that cannot be ignored.

Solid Wastes

Billions of tons of solid waste are produced annually in the United States. More than two hundred million tons of garbage alone is generated annually by Americans—nearly six pounds daily for every man, woman, and child.

Solid waste includes paper, foodstuffs, glass, metals, plastics, pesticide containers, paint cans, tires, batteries, old cars, disposable diapers, and a number of other items found in every household. Permanent disposal of these materials is an ever increasing problem in the world.

The question of solid waste removal has been amplified in recent years because the population in the world, the manufacture of consumer products, and the manufacture and use of materials that do not burn or decay have all increased. For example, the use of plastic containers, which are very difficult to burn and do not decay, has increased extensively in recent years.

In addition, a number of products are being manufactured that present special difficulties, for example, disposable diapers. It is estimated that 85 percent of diaper changes in the United States involve disposable diapers today. Sixteen billion are sold annually. This has created an extremely large amount of solid waste. As much as three million tons a year adds mass to already overstretched waste disposal sites.

Though individuals who use these diapers are instructed to empty feces into the toilet before placing in the waste can, often this does not happen. This creates a potential for health risks from viruses known to be in human feces. Some people have raised the question of whether it is even possible to develop a diaper that is recyclable.

Solid waste removal is not just a problem in cities and towns, but also in rural communities. Agricultural wastes, including animal manure and orchard prunings, account for much of the solid wastes produced each year. Two billion metric tons of animal waste are produced annually, half generated by livestock and poultry.

Methods of Disposal

The disposal of solid wastes is achieved in several different ways. Dumping is a time-honored measure, and sanitary landfills are widely used today. Incineration and recycling, though not as widely used, are also found in many localities.

Dumping

Probably the oldest and most traditional method of solid waste disposal is *dumping*. Waste material is brought to a specified location and thrown away. No effort is made to cover the waste, and it is usually burned to reduce the bulk. In these settings, the wind scatters the paper and other light objects, rodents and other scavengers search for food, and mosquitoes and flies reproduce in the open garbage.

Many dumps are situated where they drain into the groundwater supply. This drainage results in contamination of drinking water and may create many health problems.

Open dumps not only hold a potential for disease but are also an eyesore in any community. They contribute to environmental problems, such as air pollution, water contamination, and the rodent population. Burning, either purposeful or spontaneous, almost always occurs in dumps. Organic matter that is not consumed by insects, rodents, and other animals is slowly reduced by decomposition.

Today open dumping and burning is prohibited in much of the United States. The sanitary landfill has replaced open, uncontrolled dumping as the procedure for elimination of solid wastes.

Sanitary Landfill

A much more effective procedure for the removal of solid wastes is an adequate, well-designed, and well-engineered sanitary landfill. At a properly operated sanitary landfill, the waste material is compacted when dumped, then covered with dirt. After a time, during which the landfill area is covered with dirt each day, the site is compressed and smoothed by large bulldozers.

A major advantage of a sanitary landfill is that the waste material is buried each day. Thus, burning and blowing of material is kept to a minimum and rodents are few. Land that is of little other use may be reclaimed by the fill and then developed into a park, recreation site, golf course, or housing area.

Many problems result from an improperly engineered and operated sanitary landfill. Anaerobic decay of the buried wastes may lead to continuous settling of the land for many years. As a result, it becomes difficult to utilize the reclaimed area until the settling is minimized. It is also extremely important that the landfill area be planned and operated to protect against possible contamination of water supplies. Numerous geological considerations are important in site selection. Water table levels are crucial since areas with high levels are potential runoff sites and so are not satisfactory as landfill locations.

Methane gas is a by-product of the compaction at a sanitary landfill. Landfill methane gas, when mixed with air in a 5 to 15 percent concentration, is flammable.[18] Because of the methane, vegetation has been destroyed, fires have resulted, and on the site of a New Jersey landfill, two individuals were killed by a methane explosion.[19] These dangers can be reduced by proper venting of the sanitary landfill.

It is increasingly difficult to find suitable locations for the sanitary landfills. Residents are usually opposed to a sanitary landfill in their neighborhood. It is also politically unpopular to be responsible for a policy decision that establishes a sanitary landfill in a given location.

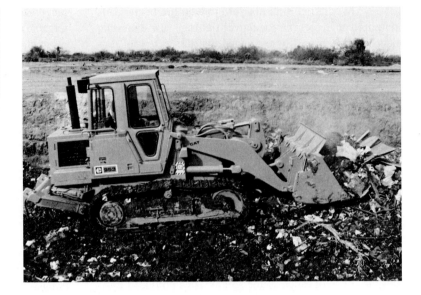

Disposal of solid wastes is an increasing problem in the United States. Sanitary landfills have been the principal means of disposal, but as they are filled to capacity and closed, communities are faced with serious questions about what can be done with solid wastes.

Each year a number of landfills close because they are at capacity. It is projected that increasing numbers of sanitary landfills will not be available to receive solid wastes by the turn of the century. This will compound an already serious problem. It is estimated that by the mid part of the 1990s some states will be out of land that can be used for new landfills. Most of these states are highly populated, and some are already transporting their garbage to other states with operating landfills. This often leads to resentment and opposition among citizens in communities located near the receiving landfills.

Not only do some communities send their wastes to other states, some even ship it to other countries. One of the classic occurrences appeared in newspapers in 1987 when a barge loaded with more than three thousand tons of rotting garbage left New York in search of a place to dump the load. Attempts were made to unload the garbage along the eastern coast of the United States and in several countries in the Caribbean. The barge traveled more than six thousand miles in 164 days. No one wanted this rotting garbage.

Currently some communities are reporting that they have no place to take garbage. For example, in 1990 one Michigan community had to stop picking up garbage from homes because all the landfills within many miles were filled and no others were available. Serious questions will face our nation as this problem gets worse during the 1990s.

Hauling trash to distant locations results in rising costs. Communities, as well as individuals, will be forced to pay greater amounts of money for trash removal. People will be forced to either allocate more of their budget for solid waste removal or seek alternatives.

Incineration

The burning of solid wastes has probably been practiced since the beginning of humanity. Today, incinerators are still operated by municipalities and in private homes, apartment complexes, and industries. Incineration is useful because it destroys solid substances and in the process reduces the volume of solid waste. It is estimated that 10 percent of solid wastes are incinerated. As localities have run out of landfill space, interest has grown in incineration. The Environmental Protection Agency says that there are about 140 incinerators now operating with more than 200 under construction. But construction of some facilities has been canceled because of controversy.

A number of environmental concerns have been expressed by those opposed to incineration. Burning of solid wastes releases soot, smoke, and particulate matter into the air, adding to air pollution. Another major concern is exposure to the dioxin, which is toxic, emitted by some garbage burners.

Incineration is also expensive. Not only is the cost of building an incinerator high, but the operation of

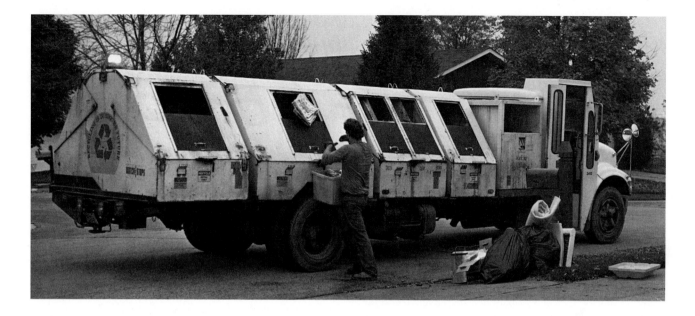

As communities pass ordinances that require the separation of food, glass, cans, and other items, vehicles that have compartments for each must be available. People will have to learn to separate their trash more thoroughly.

community incinerators is more than twice as costly as using a sanitary landfill. The installation of scrubbers to help reduce air pollution, which is mandated by regulations, is another major cost. It has been estimated that the cost of incinerating solid waste could run as high as one hundred dollars per ton to recoup the manufacturing and production costs of the facility.

Incineration could be used to generate heat and energy if properly constructed. This process has had rather limited application in the United States, but some European cities do use the heat and energy generated by incineration, often for residences and apartments. Despite some advantages and interest in incineration as a procedure to reduce the bulk of waste in our communities, it is likely that recycling will have greater value and appeal in the next decade.

Recycling

There is growing interest in the United States regarding recycling. This is due in part to the reduction of land available for landfills and the rising costs of hauling trash. As landfills become full, communities will be forced to recycle.

Historically Americans, oriented to throwing away all waste products, have not been too receptive to the need to separate their waste for recycling. Only in the past decade have significant numbers of people begun to practice recycling. Often this has been forced upon them by state and local legislation.

Several states and communities now require separation of food, glass, and cans. In cities with mandatory programs of waste separation, residents are fined if their trash is not separated. There will most likely be more legislation in the years ahead to reduce the amount of solid wastes taken to dumps and landfills.

Some communities are developing economic incentives to encourage recycling. In some cities waste haulers are paid for recycled materials by the municipal government. Some communities now give residents credit on their trash removal bills if items are separated. In other communities the collection of recyclables is free, whereas garbage disposal fees are being increased for nonrecyclable items.

In the past it was not economical to recycle, and the availability of resources made recycling unnecessary. Today, however, many products can be recycled, for

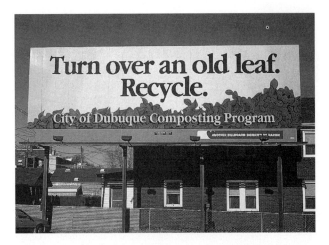

A number of strategies must be used to inform the public about recycling. This billboard provides an opportunity for education.

example, paper. Old newspapers can be recycled into tar paper for roofing, cardboard cartons, and numerous other items. Metals, including copper, lead, and zinc, are other resources that can be recycled.

Glass, too, can be recycled effectively and completely. One out of every fifteen bottles and jars currently produced in the United States is recycled into new bottles and jars.[20] Through the process of grinding, glass can be reduced to particles that can then be used as soil conditioners in compost or for road surfacing.

The goal of the Environmental Protection Agency is that 25 percent of all garbage be recycled. The federal government has set as a health promotion objective that recycling programs be in place in at least 75 percent of all counties by the year 2000.[21]

Future technology will develop new and more economical uses for recycled solid wastes in our society. It is important that people become conscious of the importance of recycling solid wastes and discontinue their "throw-away" habits. Recycling must become the norm for all citizens in the 1990s.

Toxic Wastes

The disposal of toxic wastes creates many serious problems and concerns. American industry generates as much as seven billion pounds of toxic chemicals annually. Included are numerous chemicals, such as dioxin, PCB, PBB, vinyl chloride, mercury, arsenic, and lead, that are potentially hazardous to human health. The Environmental Protection Agency has reported that the six most common chemicals released into the environment in terms of quantity are aluminum oxide, ammonium sulfate, hydrochloric acid, ammonia, phosphoric acid, and sulfuric acid. These threaten to contaminate groundwater, kill vegetation, birds, and animals, and emit toxic fumes. They are toxic when inhaled and when they come in contact with the skin and eyes. In some cases they may be fatal upon internal exposure.

Storage of chemical wastes has also created serious problems. Usually chemical wastes are deposited in dumps and sanitary landfills in steel drums. Solid waste disposal sites vary in geological, hydrological, physical, chemical, and ecological nature. For example, clay soils retard leakage and absorb many chemicals, whereas sand and gravel do not provide good containment of chemicals.

As time passes and rust develops, poisons seep from the drums into the soil and eventually work their way into the groundwater. The Environmental Protection Agency estimates that a frightening 90 percent of all industrial wastes are improperly disposed.[22]

In addition to concern over leakage from old and improperly managed dumps and landfills, accidental spills and illegal dumping of toxic substances occur all too often. Transportation of toxic wastes is a particularly dangerous action. Spills of highly toxic chemical wastes have occurred on the nation's transportation arteries: roads and expressways, rivers and streams, and railroads.

Often toxic wastes are transported by rail. One of the most serious rail accidents involving chemical wastes occurred in Louisiana in 1982. Freight cars carrying chemicals such as vinyl chloride and phosphoric acid derailed, causing serious explosions and fires. Nearby residents were forced to evacuate their homes for more than a week until the danger had subsided.

Almost weekly an accident involving the transport of chemicals is reported somewhere in the nation, either on the rails or highways. Many times people living in the immediate area must be evacuated temporarily. Often fire accompanies the accident. Occasionally people in the vicinity need emergency and medical care.

In 1976, Congress passed the Resources Conservation and Recovery Act, which established safety regulations for landfills. The Environmental Protection Agency was assigned the responsibility of establishing regulatory standards for landfills and of monitoring and enforcing these standards. The law, in spite of its good intentions, provided exemptions for many businesses and industries. For example, any business that produces less than one ton of toxic wastes each month is exempt. Other loopholes in the law have permitted unsafe disposal of many toxic wastes without penalty or punishment of any kind.

One of the most toxic chemicals that has received attention is dioxin. This chemical has caused the forced evacuation of towns in Missouri and Michigan. In Times Beach, Missouri, more than two thousand people were forced to relocate. In 1972, chemical sludge combined with waste oil was used as a sealant on the roads of this rural community. The sludge contained dioxin. For the next decade there was no concern. However, in 1982, following a widespread flood, residents of the city became aware of the dangerous situation in their town. After the flood the residents were warned that they should not return owing to the toxic danger. Today Times Beach is a vacant town; nearly all of its home owners had to relocate.

Another classic case relating to toxic waste is the case of Love Canal at Niagara Falls, New York. In the latter 1970s residents were suffering from an unusual amount of skin ailments, respiratory problems, headaches, epileptic seizures, and hair loss. It was also noted that the rate of miscarriage and birth defects was higher among residents of this area than for those in surrounding communities. Several years previously a chemical company had deposited some twenty-one thousand tons of hazardous toxic chemicals in an area dump site. By 1978 a national emergency was declared at Love Canal and over six hundred families had to be evacuated. Since 1978 scientists have identified over 240 different toxic chemicals in this area, and in 1985 dangerous levels of dioxin were still being reported in the area by the Environmental Protection Agency.

Though much is not known about the long-term effects of dioxin on human health, it is known that it causes hair and weight loss, headaches, tingling of the extremities, and may well be a cause of cancer. It has been shown to cause birth defects, miscarriage, and death in laboratory animals. It can adversely affect immunosystem response and liver function in humans.[23]

High levels of DDT, PCBs, and other toxic chemicals have been reported in a number of America's waterways along the East Coast, including Chesapeake Bay, New York Harbor, and Boston Harbor.[24] Although DDT has been banned for sale and use in the United States since the early 1970s, it is still being found in the coastal waterways. DDT and PCBs are long-lasting chemicals and tend to remain in the ecosystem for long periods, contaminating fish and marine life.

Superfund

Efforts to clean up toxic wastes have been minimal. With as many as ten thousand hazardous waste sites in the United States, the cost of cleaning up would possibly run into the hundreds of billions of dollars. Obviously, the expense would be enormous.

In 1980 Congress created a $1.6 billion, five-year program under the authority of the Comprehensive Environmental Response, Compensation and Liability Act, which provided funding and authority for cleaning up hazardous waste sites. This program was established to clean up thousands of dumps that were leaking toxic wastes into underground water sources. Funds came from taxes on petroleum and certain chemicals as well as from general federal appropriations. The program came to be referred to as the Superfund program.

The Environmental Protection Agency has identified more than 1,300 sites as having priority for cleanup. More than 70 percent of these may cause pollution of groundwater.

The Superfund program has seen its share of controversy. By 1985 when the law expired the money was gone, and little impact had been made on the problem of solid waste contamination. Only six sites were reported to have been cleaned up.[25] Even then many questions were raised as to whether the cleaning of these sites had been successful. It has been pointed out that the cleaning of these sites has only transported the problem elsewhere. For example, in one case, soil contaminated by PBB, PCB, and DDT was removed from a golf course developed next to an old chemical dump and was deposited at another location.

Much political debate, argument, and controversy between Congress, the president, and the Environmental Protection Agency undercut any chance of this program being effective. The lack of funds to perform these measures, the reduced funding and staff of the Environmental Protection Agency to oversee the corrective measures, and the reluctance of industry and the general public to comply with the orders have all contributed to less than successful cleanup results.

There is difference of opinion as to how much it would cost to effectively clean up priority sites. In 1984 the Environmental Protection Agency estimated that as much as $22.7 billion would be needed to clean up all priority sites. Other estimates run into the hundreds of billions of dollars. According to a House of Representatives Appropriations Committee, the average cost of cleaning up one waste site may run between $21 and $30 million. Congress asked for over $10 billion and finally in 1986 settled on an appropriation of $9 billion for continuation of the Superfund Program. Unfortunately, it is still cheaper to dump, and only when the dangers of toxic wastes affect the population directly, as at the time of a spill, a fire, or contamination of a water supply, do people become concerned enough to demand action.

Radiation

When atoms are split, energy and radiation are released. This release of radiation is known as *radioactivity,* which has been shown to have a major effect upon the health and well-being of people. Radiation at certain high levels can kill outright or may linger in the body for years. Exposure to radiation injures human tissue and causes a number of health problems. When a person is exposed to 25 to 50 roentgens (r), the white blood cells may be affected. Radiation sickness, a condition resulting in nausea, fatigue, anemia, diarrhea, and loss of hair, occurs as the result of exposure to 100 to 200 roentgens of radiation. Exposure to 350 to 500 roentgens will usually be fatal.

More subtle, but just as much of a concern, is the effect of exposure to low levels of radiation over a long period of time. Such exposures often occur in occupational settings, in various community settings, and as has been reported recently in the case of radon, in our own homes. We do not know as much as we would like about long-term effects of continuous or intermittent exposure to low levels of radiation. There is evidence that certain kinds of cancer—skin, bone, skeletal, leukemia, and lung—can be caused by such exposure.

Increasing concern has also been expressed about the damage that may be done to reproductive cells over a long period of time. This exposure may result in damage to or alteration of human genes—chromosomes—and the long-term effects may not be revealed until future generations are born. The exact effect of radiation on a person depends on the body part exposed, the potency of the dose, and the rate at which it is received.

Humans have been exposed to small amounts of radiation in nature since the beginning of time. Radioactive gases are released by soil and rock formations as uranium. Cosmic radiation is given off in outer space and is measurable on earth in small amounts. Radioactive agents in the atmosphere result from sunflares, which give off solar particle beams. People are exposed to an average of 175 millirems a year of natural radiation.[26]

Radon Gas

Since the mid-1980s there has been increasing concern about the levels of radon in homes. In 1988 the Surgeon General declared radon to be a serious public health hazard in the United States. The Environmental Protection Agency first became aware of this problem in the early 1980s in Pennsylvania. It now estimates that radon causes more cancer deaths per year than any other pollutant under its jurisdiction; reports of incidence run as high as twenty thousand lung cancer deaths a year.[27] Until the 1980s radon was considered to be primarily a health hazard for mine workers. Studies of miners have shown a relationship between lung cancer and radon exposure.[28]

Radon is an odorless, colorless, tasteless radioactive gas that is produced naturally in the ground. It is the product of underground uranium decay. High radon levels are found in areas with granitic bedrock, lower levels in localities with sedimentary rock.

In the out-of-doors the threat to personal health is minimal because radon is diluted to very low, nondangerous levels. The problem arises indoors, where the radon can build up. The Environmental Protection Agency has indicated that as many as 12 percent of American homes may have radon levels above the EPA recommended standard for safe exposure.

The problem expanded during the 1980s as new houses were built with increased amounts of insulation for energy savings. This energy-efficient construction has tended to keep radon inside. In addition, central air conditioning, which is being installed in many homes in much of the country, results in less ventilation from the outside.

Radon seeps through soil and rock and enters homes through cracks in the foundation and house floors and around loose-fitting pipes, floor drains, and sump pumps. It is also released into the atmosphere when water is heated, as in showering or when washing clothes. The radioactive particles become airborne, attach themselves to dust, and are breathed in. This natural radioactive gas, which decays into four radioactive elements, can become lodged in the lungs and cause damage to the lung cells.

The Environmental Protection Agency has announced that homes in areas with potential for radon gas should have ventilation systems constructed that can help in removing the radon from the interior of the house.

The Environmental Protection Agency has set guidelines for indoor exposure to radon. The level of radon is measured in terms of *picocuries per liter*. Four picocuries per liter of air has established as the safe level for houses.[29]

Testing is simple, effective, and inexpensive. Most health departments have personnel trained in the procedures for measuring radon. In some communities the law requires that before a home can be sold the potential buyer must be provided with information about the radon level. For this reason many real estate firms have personnel capable of measuring radon levels.

A number of measures can be taken to lower or remove radon from a house. Protective barriers may be constructed under and around concrete basements. Sealing around pipes and cracks will help prevent radon from coming into the house. In addition, proper ventilation and air movement throughout the home is beneficial.

Commercial Sources of Radiation

Since the atom was first split in 1942 at the University of Chicago, thus ushering in the nuclear age, many new sources of radiation have been introduced into the environment. The development, testing, and use of nuclear weapons have contributed to this increased radiation. In addition, many domestic uses of radioactive rays have been found. For example, some home appliances emit small amounts of radiation. X-rays used in medicine and dentistry account for much radiation exposure.

There has been increasing concern about possible links between human cancer and low-frequency electromagnetic fields. Electric and magnetic fields are created when electricity is present. A major source of exposure is believed to result from the presence of electric power transmission lines. Studies have suggested that certain human cancers, particularly leukemia, are more prevalent among electrical line workers and individuals whose homes are located in close proximity to high-tension electrical power lines. It is difficult to ascertain a cause and effect relationship and to identify certain amounts of exposure at which malignancies occur. Much uncertainty still exists, with some suggesting that exposure to commercial products in the home may also be a risk factor. Future research must be conducted before definitive risk relationships can be safely ascertained.[30]

Nuclear Power

The world's need for and consumption of energy have resulted in the development of nuclear energy power plants. Nuclear energy creates heat that is used for steam-generated electricity. This production of electricity is the most important use of nuclear power today. The nuclear power plant contains a core of nuclear fuel, chiefly uranium. The energy potential in uranium, the primary ingredient of nuclear power, is exceptional. One pound of this fuel contains nearly three million times the energy found in a pound of coal.[31] Uranium does not burn like the fossil fuels—oil, coal, and wood. Heat is produced in the nuclear reactor by a process known as *fission.* During this process uranium atoms in the reactor are split and energy in the form of heat is released. The heat from fission turns water into steam, and steam spins the turbine generators.

About two decades ago, many people felt that the eventual solution to the world's energy shortage rested in nuclear power. The first nuclear power plant in the United States began operation in 1957 in Shippingport, Pennsylvania, on the Ohio River. This plant was shut down in 1982, and decommissioning of it was a five-year $100 million project. Since 1957 more than a hundred plants have been licensed for operation in the United States. Worldwide there are more than three hundred licensed nuclear power plants in twenty-five nations.

The future use and development of nuclear power are clouded in controversy since many oppose both the development and expansion of nuclear energy. These opponents are concerned about the safety of this energy source. For many, their questions have not been satisfactorily answered.

Small amounts of radiation are released from the reactors of nuclear power plants. It is not known how much of this radiation humans can withstand before health is affected. Although there are claims that the amount released is infinitesimal and of no danger, the long-term risks of exposure are not known.

The disposal of nuclear wastes presents another serious environmental problem. The wastes must be buried in isolated locations, and every measure must be taken to assure that the radiation does not escape. Since nuclear wastes are radioactive for years after their burial, opponents are concerned that future contamination could result from an accident, a natural occurrence such as an earthquake, or damage to the burial vaults. In spite of assurances by the nuclear power industry that these disposal procedures are safe, many opponents of nuclear energy remain unconvinced.

The announcement that a certain area is to be the site of a nuclear dump brings out extensive civic and political opposition. Even the possibility of potential radiation is feared by most citizens. The economic effects are many: land values fall, new companies and industries refuse to move into the area, and land for agricultural purposes may be lost. Many health-related concerns are expressed at these times.

Nuclear energy can best be developed near large sources of water, as large amounts of water are needed to cool the reactors. Many nuclear power plants use millions of gallons of water per minute in this cooling process. It is important that the used water be kept in a holding lake or pond before being returned to its original source. Even then, care must be taken not to upset the ecological balance of a lake or river by returning water that is warmer than the natural temperature.

In 1979 the attention of the entire United States was focused on Three Mile Island near Harrisburg, Pennsylvania. A nuclear accident caused many people to question the safety of nuclear power plants. The accident was kept under control, yet small amounts of radioactivity were measured in the air around the site. Fortunately, meltdown did not occur.

Meltdown occurs if the water that cools the heat-producing nuclear reactor core is shut down. This action would result in the melting of the nuclear core. The liquefied uranium core would then drop through the protective shielding. Without this shielding, the uranium would spread radiation into the air and the ground, causing serious consequences to the environment and to human life. The potential for large-scale destruction by nuclear accident was exemplified at Three Mile Island.

The most serious nuclear accident in history occurred in 1986 in Chernobyl, USSR. An explosion followed by fire in one of the four nuclear reactors led to the release of a cloud of radiation into the air that spread far beyond the Soviet Union throughout Eastern Europe and into Scandinavia. This was the largest release of radioactive material ever in an accident. The release measured millions of *curies*, the radioactive decay rate of one gram of radium. By contrast, Three Mile Island is reported to have released fifteen curies.[32]

The radioactive cloud spread northwest over Poland, into the Scandinavian countries, then two days later it spread west-southwest, over Europe, as far as England, Germany, and Holland. Some three hundred to four hundred million people in fifteen nations were placed at risk.[33] Several hundred people died, and thousands were hospitalized with radiation sickness. Many of the hospitalized victims were treated with bone marrow transplants.

Since the breakup of the former Soviet Union in 1991, increasing information has come forth about the long-term, continuing impact of this incident. There continues to be a significant number of children with

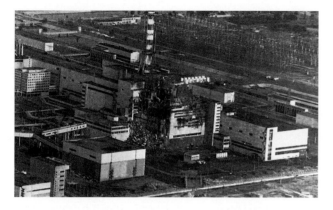

The most serious nuclear accident in history occurred in 1986 at Chernobyl, USSR. Millions of people throughout Europe were placed at risk by this accident, hundreds died, and thousands were hospitalized.

leukemia and thyroid cancers in the children's hospitals in and around Chernobyl. Childhood thyroid cancer has increased in Belarus, the republic that is situated downwind from Chernobyl.

In Gomel, which was the community first hit by radiation, the rate of cancer of the thyroid among children is eighty times greater than what would be considered normal. This seems logical in that iodine concentrates in the thyroid gland, and radioactive iodine was released during the Chernobyl meltdown. Radiation is known to cause thyroid cancer, and children are especially susceptible. Unfortunately, it is unknown how many people, children and adults, continue to be affected by the tragedy of this nuclear accident.

This tragic incident showed that there was no adequate international warning system to alert governments and people of impending nuclear danger. Nor have any international standards for nuclear safety been developed and implemented.[34]

Problems with the design and operation of some nuclear plants have caused shutdowns until repairs or appropriate corrections could be made. The corrosion of the steam generators that carry hot radioactive water has caused several plants to stop operation until repairs could be made. The Nuclear Regulatory Commission has warned a number of nuclear plants that radiation was making the steel shell that surrounds the uranium core susceptible to cracks and possible meltdown.

The future of nuclear energy is dependent upon the answers to many questions. The development and construction of new nuclear power plants have been greatly curtailed since the Three Mile Island incident. The accident at Chernobyl only heightened the fear and concern of many about the future development and use of nuclear power.

Yet nuclear power is still a major energy producer in many parts of the United States, particularly in New England and the Great Lakes region. If nuclear power is to continue as a means of providing energy in the world, it must be proved that radiation can be controlled and the environment kept safe for all humanity.

Nuclear Weapons

In spite of concern over radiation and nuclear wastes from nuclear power plants, by far the greatest generation of nuclear wastes has resulted from military nuclear weapons systems programs. The United States weapons programs have generated seven million cubic feet of waste, which is seven hundred times more than that generated by nuclear power plants.[35] Concern obviously needs to be directed toward the many problems of nuclear weapons deployment and potential use.

It can only be hoped that the decrease in political tension between the world's nuclear superpowers as seen in the early 1990s will lead to a de-escalation of the nuclear arms race. With agreements being reached to reduce, or eliminate, certain nuclear missile systems, it would seem that the potential for environmental damage should be lessened. However, while the world's major nuclear powers seem to be on the course of reducing nuclear arms, several smaller, developing nations have been reported to be devising nuclear armaments. This should cause great concern to people throughout the world.

Lead Poisoning

Lead poisoning is an environmental concern that affects thousands of individuals, particularly young children. Also at risk are individuals who are plumbers, welders, and painters, and those employed in automotive repair. Gun handlers have been found to be at risk for increased lead in the body.

Exposure to lead can occur from a variety of sources. One of the most common sources is older homes located in economically depressed urban communities. When these homes were constructed, lead-based paint was commonly applied throughout the building. It has been estimated that 74 percent of houses built before 1980 contain some lead paint. In 1978 the federal government banned the use of lead-based paints. However, this has not solved the problems for people residing in older houses.

Another source of lead is the lead pipes used in building construction, particularly prior to 1930. Lead soldered joints in copper water pipes were used until banned by the Safe Drinking Water Act of 1986. At times lead pipes were used to connect water systems in the street to the house.

Lead has also been found to be present in public drinking water systems. The Environmental Protection Agency has stated that one in five public water supply systems has high lead levels in its drinking water. In 1991 the Environmental Protection Agency adopted a ruling that any water system serving more than 50,000 people must begin measures to reduce the amount of lead in the water.

The use of imported ceramic dishes and the storing of liquids in lead crystal can also cause an increase in lead among users.

Lead is a toxic, heavy metal that causes a number of serious health problems. It has no known purpose in the human body. It is considered to be the most serious environmental problem affecting children between the ages of six months and six years. It has also been shown to affect a developing fetus. The National Institutes of Health estimate that one out of six children under seven have some degree of lead poisoning.

The body does not totally and adequately rid itself of lead. It is ingested and absorbed in soluble form into the bloodstream and is eliminated from the body through the feces and urine and by means of perspiration. However, some lead accumulates in the body and over an extended period of time dangerously high concentrations of lead can accumulate.

Lead can harm every body system. It settles in bones, blood, and soft tissues and is particularly harmful to the developing nervous system and the brain. The body mistakes lead for calcium and disruption of enzymes essential to brain functioning occurs. Since lead does not decompose, it is absorbed into an exposed child's brain forever.

As a result of lead absorption, intelligence and behavior are affected. Behavior is affected by low levels of lead. As the level of lead increases, performance on IQ and developmental tests tends to become lower. A number of nonspecific symptoms, such as hyperactivity, irritability, aggressive behavior, and in some cases lethargy have been associated with lead exposure. Children with high levels of lead exposure are six times more likely to have reading disabilities.[36]

Lead poisoning in the early stages produces signs of anemia. With increased moderate exposure the individual experiences headaches, weakness, fatigue, stomach ache, weight loss, constipation, and general pain. The kidneys can be affected, and nephritis often occurs. The nervous system may become affected. If the person is left untreated, blindness, seizures, paralysis, coma, and death can result.

How much exposure to lead is safe? The answer to this question is uncertain. For years the Centers for Disease Control and Prevention had established 25 micrograms per deciliter as the level considered to be safe. However, following much research and epidemiological study, CDC has replaced the former guidelines with a measurement of 10 micrograms per deciliter as the level at which attention must be given to an individual. This change was brought about as there has been increasing awareness that a low to moderate level of lead exposure is dangerous to the human body. Evidence of impairment of cognitive developmental and behavioral difficulties were reported where there were readings of between 10 and 25 micrograms per deciliter.[37]

Damage to the body from exposure to lead is usually irreversible. However, it is possible to remove some lead from the blood. A procedure known as chelation has been developed that is able to cleanse blood of lead. This is a rather painful treatment procedure.

As with many other human diseases, early prevention can greatly reduce the occurrence of lead poisoning. Many public health agencies recommend that all children be tested for lead poisoning at the age of one year. This would seem to be particularly a beneficial practice for children of lower socioeconomic status living in older homes. It is important for adults to understand that any disturbing of lead-based paint by such measures as sanding, stripping, or other renovation activities can expose individuals to dangerously high lead levels. A child may become ill by simply touching a windowsill or staircase with paint dust or by sucking a thumb that has dust on it.

Test kits are available to test the level of lead in rooms of older homes. One should always have a house tested for lead paint prior to purchasing the home. Also, there is a need to test lead contaminated soil around houses and schools and on playgrounds where children play.

The federal government recommends that by the year 2000 at least 50 percent of all homes built before 1950 should be tested for lead-based paint.[38] It has also recommended that states require prospective buyers be informed of the presence of lead-based paint.[39] Unfortunately, lead paint removal procedures can be a rather costly activity. Discussion of mandated measures to be taken to remove this environmental hazard from homes and how such procedures will be paid for continues.

Noise Pollution

Sounds move through the air in waves similar to the movement of water upon an ocean beach. When these waves make contact with the eardrum, sound is heard. These sound waves are then transmitted to and interpreted by the human brain. Human beings communicate by sound: we relax to the sound of music, the sound of an infant's cry tells us that the baby has some need, and most of our contact with the environment takes place by way of sound.

When sound is unwanted, it is termed noise. A sound that is tolerable for one person, however, may be noise to another. For example, the sound of trucks passing in front of a house on the expressway is tolerated by the truck driver because a livelihood is involved. But to the person attempting to sleep, the trucks are making noise. Thus, sound is subject to individual interpretations. It is termed sound or noise depending on the experiences and background of each person.

Sound has three characteristics: (1) pitch, (2) volume, and (3) timbre. Pitch and volume, especially, are of concern to health. Timbre is the quality of sound. Pitch is the height or depth of the sound, and is measured in units based upon the cycles per second (c.p.s.), called *hertz*. The human ear can detect sound as low as twenty hertz and as high as twenty thousand hertz. Volume is recorded in units called decibels (dBs). Zero decibel is the weakest sound level that can be detected by the human ear.

Decibels are logarithmic, not linear, units of measurement. For this reason, there is a sharp increase in the loudness of sound with each decibel increase. For example, ten decibels of sound is ten times more intense than one decibel. However, twenty decibels is one hundred times more intense than one decibel. Thirty decibels is one thousand times as intense as one decibel. Continuing this progression, one hundred decibels is ten billion times as intense as one decibel of sound.

Most sound that humans encounter ranges between fifty and ninety decibels. The level at which most people begin to feel pain is about 120 decibels. The sound level of a two-person conversation is usually around sixty decibels, and traffic noise in a city ranges from seventy to over ninety decibels. If you have ever been on the ground near a jet airliner when it is taxiing for takeoff, you will recall the ear-shattering noise. The sound level being generated by that plane is near 140 decibels.

The principal and most obvious health-related problem of noise pollution is the loss of hearing. It has been estimated that over twenty million Americans are exposed daily to noise that may permanently damage their hearing.[40] People may not be aware of the danger of noise exposure for a period of several years. Loss of hearing results from progressive destruction of sensory cells in the ear.

A number of early warning signals indicate possible hearing loss. The inability to hear high-pitched or soft sounds is one indication. Difficulty in understanding normal conversation may also be noted. Hearing ability is being affected when there is prolonged ringing or roaring in the ears or when hearing no longer returns after exposure to high levels of sound.

In addition to this hearing loss, exposure to noise causes a number of other physiological effects. Noise causes an increase in adrenaline output, dilation of blood vessels in the brain, an increase in heart rate, and a rise in blood pressure. All these physiological reactions are related to cardiovascular disease. Though there has been no proof of a direct relationship between noise pollution and heart disease, it is a possibility considering the physiological changes that result from exposure to noise.

Noise also contributes to the level of stress in people. The physiological effects of noise on the human body create the same problems associated with other stress-related problems: headaches, tension, and sleep disruption.

Noise pollution is found in many environmental settings. All forms of transportation and construction equipment are major sources of noise pollution in our society. Though noise pollution is generally an urban problem, machinery in rural localities is also a source of noise. Studies have shown that farmers and other agricultural workers use equipment that generates noise levels between eighty and ninety decibels.

Concern has been expressed about the high levels of sound young people are exposed to when listening to highly amplified sound systems. For over a decade most young people have listened to sound systems through earplugs. Music that demands excessive amplification to be acceptable is now popular. Pickup trucks contain sound systems that literally shake surrounding building windows as they cruise the campus. Excessive noise can cause serious damage to hearing and permanent hearing loss, so it is the opinion of many that in the years ahead this problem may become a major health concern of adolescents and young adults.

In the home, appliances produce high noise levels. Garbage disposals, blenders, dishwashers, power tools, and stereos cause noise levels that have been found to exceed ninety to 100 decibels.

Some people are exposed daily to high sound levels at their place of employment. There is little doubt that this exposure to both continuous and intermittent sound levels over an extended period of time is injurious to hearing.

Since many industrial processes in the workplace produce noise levels above 100 decibels, the Occupational Safety and Health Act required the establishment of standards for noise exposure in the occupational setting. The standards that have been established by the Occupational Safety and Health Administration allow up to ninety decibels of exposure for an eight-hour day. Industry is now required by law to reduce the sound levels at the source of the noise generation or to provide protective equipment for all employees. The federal government has set as a goal the reduction of exposure to noise levels *above 85 decibels* in the workplace.[41]

Summary

Efforts to provide a safe and healthful environment have been a major focus of community health programming. Activities in the latter part of the 1800s were designed to control communicable diseases. Today, however, a greater number of environmental problems necessitates a wider range of environmental program emphases.

The provisions of a safe water supply and the presence of pure air are two important emphases of an environmental health program. In spite of the fact that waterborne diseases do not reach epidemic proportions in the United States today, water pollution remains a problem. Many municipal water systems are not providing the purest water for residents. Various chemicals dumped into the lakes and rivers, industrial processing measures, and agriculture are major sources of water pollution.

Likewise there are many sources of air pollution. Most air pollution in this country is the result of emissions from the internal combustion engine of motor vehicles, the burning of fossil fuels, and other industrial processes. These produce many different pollutants. The Environmental Protection Agency has established standards to control several of these pollutants, including carbon monoxide, hydrocarbons, lead, nitrogen oxide, ozone, particulate matter, and sulfur oxide.

Three major problems related to air and water pollution have become apparent: acid rain, the global warming trend, and depletion of the ozone layer in the stratosphere. All these matters have global ramifications and demand the cooperative efforts of government, industry, and citizens if improvements are to be made.

Throughout the United States the amount of solid waste is increasing at the same time that useful sanitary landfills are reaching capacity. With fewer places to dump solid wastes, communities must develop alternatives. Recycling has become more important.

The disposal of toxic chemical wastes has created a number of serious problems. The presence of toxic chemicals in groundwater is an increasing concern in many localities. The presence of chemical dumps and the use of chemical agents for a variety of uses have led to the necessity to evacuate two cities in the United States. The long-term effects of toxic wastes are not totally known.

Increasing concern about radiation has been noted in recent years. The nuclear power plant accidents at Three Mile Island and Chernobyl have caused concern about the potential for catastrophic dangers of nuclear power. Humans are exposed to radiation in a variety of different localities: radon in their homes, radiation from natural sources, and radiation emitted from scientific and military uses.

Though not considered by many to be environmental problems, lead poisoning and noise pollution cause serious health problems for thousands of Americans. Lead poisoning is the major environmental problem for children of preschool age. Exposure to both lead and noise need to be dealt with through the implementation of various preventive initiatives.

Discussion Questions

1. What are some significant problems of the environment that have surfaced since Earth Day 1970?

2. What are some of the major causes of water pollution?

3. What is thermal pollution?

4. In what ways is groundwater being affected by chemical dumping today?

5. Explain why agriculture is a major contributor to water pollution.

6. What are some of the basic provisions of the Clean Water Act?

7. What were some of the impacts of the oil spill of the *Exxon Valdez* in Alaska?

8. How is human health affected by carbon monoxide, hydrocarbons, nitrogen oxides, and ozone?

9. Do you feel that the Clean Air Act should be changed, modified, or rescinded? Explain your answer.

10. How successful has the nation been in improving the air under provisions of the Clean Air Act?

11. What are some issues discussed in the debate over development of "cleaner" gasoline?

12. What is acid rain, and what are its effects on humans, animals, and vegetation?

13. What has been considered to be the major cause of depletion of the ozone layer in the stratosphere?

14. What are the various uses for chlorofluorocarbons?

15. Discuss ways in which destruction of the ozone layer can affect human health.

16. Discuss the significance of the outcomes of the United Nations Conference on the Environment and Development in Rio in 1992.

17. What is the difference between a dump and a sanitary landfill?

18. Why is incineration not acceptable to many environmentalists?

19. What changes will individuals need to make before more recycling can take place?

20. What measures have you taken to practice recycling?

21. Why have the problems associated with toxic wastes become a serious concern in the United States?

22. What is the Superfund?

23. Identify some of the controversy surrounding the Superfund program.

24. What are some of the problems associated with radon gas?

25. What are measures that can be taken to protect against radon leakage into homes?

26. Discuss the significance of the concerns about the relationships between electromagnetic fields and human cancers.

27. Explain some of the concerns about nuclear power plants in the United States.

28. What is the significance of Chernobyl and Three Mile Island?

29. What has been learned in recent years about the extent of health problems now experienced by individuals living in the area near Chernobyl?

30. Do you support further development of nuclear power? If so, why? If not, why not?

31. Explain what lead does physiologically to the human body.

32. Discuss the issues centering on establishing a level of safe exposure to lead.

33. What are some preventive measures that could be incorporated that would reduce the risk of lead poisoning?

34. Identify some of the health problems associated with noise pollution.

35. What population groups are at greatest risk to loss of hearing due to noise pollution?

Suggested Readings

Bacon, J. Maichle, and William A. Gleckno. "Groundwater Contamination: A National Problem with Implications for State and Local Environmental Health Personnel." *Journal of Environmental Health* 48, no. 3 (November/December 1985): 116–21.

Bierma, Thomas J. "Radon Risk Factors." *Journal of Environmental Health* 51, no. 5 (May/June 1989): 277–81.

Browne, Sally de la Rue. "Food Irradiation: A Challenge to Public Health." *Journal of Environmental Health* 51, no. 5 (May/June 1989): 269–70.

"Can We Repair the Sky?" *Consumer Reports* 54, no. 5 (May 1989): 322–26.

Cortese, Anthony D. "Acid Rain Control: The Policy Dilemma." *Journal of Environmental Health* 41, no. 2 (September/October 1986): 90–95.

Davis, Trenton G. "Chernobyl: The Aftermath." *Journal of Environmental Health* 51, no. 4 (March/April 1989): 184–90.

Dowling, Michael. "Defining and Classifying Hazardous Wastes." *Environment* 27, no. 3 (April 1985): 18–20, 36–41.

Environmental Protection Agency. *Unfinished Business: A Comparative Assessment of Environmental Problems.* Washington, D.C.: U.S. Government Printing Office, 1987.

Gellert, George A. "New Directions in Environmental Health and Old Ties to Public Health." *Journal of Environmental Health* 55, no. 4 (January/February 1993): 38–40.

Gerusky, Thomas M. "The Pennsylvania Radon Story." *Journal of Environmental Health* 49, no. 4 (January/February 1987): 197–200.

Goodman, Patricia G., and C. Edwin Vaughan. "The Implications of Times Beach." *Journal of Environmental Health* 51, no. 1 (September/October 1988): 19–21.

Greenberg, Michael. "Local Health Officers' Views on Hazardous Waste Remediation." *American Journal of Public Health* 83, no. 5 (May 1993): 752–54.

Haas, Peter M., and others. "Appraising the Earth Summit: How Should We Judge UNCED's Success?" *Environment* 34, no. 8 (October 1992): 6–11, 26–33.

"Health Aspects of Hazardous Waste Disposal." *Environment* 28, no. 3 (April 1986): 38–45.

Heil, Jeffrey, and James Van Blarcom. "Superfund: The Search for Consistency." *Environment* 28, no. 3 (April 1986): 6–9.

Hesse, John L., and others. "Problems and Responsibilities Associated with Hazardous Waste at the State Level." *Journal of Environmental Health* 48, no. 4 (January/February 1986): 186–89.

Hester, Gordon L. "Electric and Magnetic Fields: Managing an Uncertain Risk." *Environment* 34, no. 1 (January/February 1992): 7–11, 25–32.

Hodgson, Bryan. "Alaska's Big Spill: Can the Wilderness Heal?" *National Geographic Magazine* 177, no. 1 (January 1990): 5–43.

"Indoor Air Pollution." *Consumer Reports* (October 1985): 600.

Knopman, Debra S., and Richard A. Smith. "20 Years of the Clean Water Act: Has U.S. Water Quality Improved?" *Environment* 35, no. 1 (January 1993): 16–20, 34–41.

Koorse, Steven J. "Toxics Regulations Take Hold." *Water Environment and Technology* 5, no. 1 (January 1993): 36–40.

Kreisel, Wilfred. "Affecting Change: Environmental Health in the 1990s." *Journal of Environmental Health.* (Spring 1990—Special Issue): 18–24.

Leaf, Alexander. "Potential Health Effects of Global Climatic and Environmental Changes." *The New England Journal of Medicine* 321, no. 23 (December 7, 1989): 1577–83.

Martin, Danny. "Lead Poisoning in Children. *Journal of Environmental Health* 54, no. 1 (July/August 1991): 18–19.

National Geographic Society. *Energy: A Special Report in the Public Interest.* Washington, D.C.: The Society (February 1981).

National Research Council. *Health Risks of Radon and Other Internally Deposited Alpha-Emitters.* Washington, D.C.: National Academy Press, 1988.

Neufeld, William P. "Five Potential Crises: The Greenhouse Effect." *The Futurist* 18, no. 2 (April 1984): 9–10.

Nichols, Alan B. "It's Clear, U.S. Waters Have Improved." *Water Environment and Technology* 4, no. 10 (October 1992): 44–50.

Parker, Jonathan, and Chris Hope. "The State of the Environment." *Environment* 34, no. 1 (January/February 1992): 18–20, 39–44.

Popkin, Roy. "Hazardous Waste Cleanup and Disaster Management." *Environment* 28, no. 3 (April 1986): 2–5.

Report from the United Nations Environment Programme and the World Health Organization. "Monitoring the Global Environment: An Assessment of Urban Air Quality." *Environment* 31, no. 8 (October 1989): 6–13, 26–37.

Russell, Milton, and others. "The U.S. Hazardous Waste Legacy." *Environment* 34, no. 6 (July/August 1992): 12–15, 34–39.

Sanderson, George F. "Climate Change: The Threat to Human Health." *Futurist* 26, no. 2 (1992): 34–38.

Sciarillo, William G., and others. "Lead Exposure and Child Behavior." *American Journal of Public Health* 82, no. 10 (October 1992): 1356–60.

Wade, Richard. "The *Exxon Valdez* Oil Spill." *Journal of Environmental Health* 52, no. 4 (January/February 1990): 213–15.

Waldman, Steven. "Lead and Your Kids." *Newsweek* (July 15, 1991): 42–48.

Walker, Bailus, Jr. "The Future of Public Health: An Analysis of the NAS Report and Its Implications for Environmental Health." *Journal of Environmental Health* 51, no. 3 (January/February 1989): 133–35.

Walker, Bailus, and Vicien Li. "The Development of State Policies and Systems for Toxic Substance Management." *Journal of Environmental Health* 49, no. 4 (January/February 1987): 202–6.

Wolf, Frederick. "Superfund." *Journal of Environmental Health* 54, no. 4 (January/February 1992): 18–22.

Woods, Frank W. "The Acid Rain Question." *The Futurist* 21, no. 1 (January/February 1987): 34–37.

Young, John, and others. "A Survey of State Asbestos Programs." *Journal of Environmental Health* 48, no. 6 (May/June 1986): 332–35.

Endnotes

1. Carson, Rachel. *Silent Spring.* Boston: Houghton-Mifflin, 1962; Dubos, Rene. *Man Adapting.* New Haven: Yale University Press, 1965; Ehrlich, Paul R. *The Population Bomb.* New York: Ballantine Books, 1971.
2. Craun, Gunther. "A Summary of Waterborne Illness Transmitted through Contaminated Groundwater." *Journal of Environmental Health* 48, no. 3 (November/December 1985): 122–27.
3. Reported in the *Wall Street Journal,* January 17, 1985.
4. LaVeen, E. Phillip. "Protecting the Nation's Groundwater from Contamination." *Environment* 27, no. 4 (May 1985): 26.
5. Wagner, Richard H. *Environment and Man.* New York: W. W. Norton and Company, 1971, p. 133.
6. United States Environmental Protection Agency. *Pesticides in Ground Water Data Base, 1988 Interim Report.* Washington, D.C.: The Environmental Protection Agency, December 1988.
7. Public Health Service. *Healthy People 2000: National Health Promotion and Disease Prevention Objectives.* Washington, D.C.: U.S. Government Printing Office, 1991, p. 326.
8. Easterbrook, Gregg. "Special Report: Cleaning Up." *Newsweek* (July 24, 1989): 35.
9. Oleckno, William A. "The National Interim Primary Drinking Water Regulations." *Journal of Environmental Health* 44, no. 5 (March/April 1982): 236.
10. Nichols, Alan B. "It's Clear, U.S. Waters Have Improved." *Water Environment and Technology* 4, no. 10 (October 1992): 44–50.
11. American Association for World Health. *Our Planet, Our Health: Think Globally, Act Locally.* Washington, D.C.: The Association for World Health, January 1990, p. 5.
12. Public Law 84–159, passed July 15, 1955.
13. Public Law 88–206, the Clean Air Act, passed December 17, 1963.
14. U.S. Environmental Protection Agency. "Air Quality Designation of Classifications: Final Rule." *Federal Register* 56 (1991): 56694.
15. La Bastille, Anne. "Acid Rain, How Great a Menace?" *National Geographic* 160, no. 5 (November 1981): 673.
16. *Ibid.,* 680.
17. *Ibid.,* 680.

18. White, Peter T. "The Fascinating World of Trash." *National Geographic* 163, no. 4 (April 1983): 440.

19. *Ibid.*

20. *Ibid.,* 450.

21. Public Health Service, *Healthy People 2000,* 331.

22. "The Toxic Waste Crisis." *Newsweek* (March 7, 1983): 20.

23. News release, American Medical Association, April 17, 1986.

24. "Don't Go Near the Water." *Newsweek* (August 1, 1988): 42–47.

25. "A Problem That Cannot be Buried." *Newsweek* (October 14, 1985): 77.

26. Plant, Robert. "The Dangerous Atom." *World Health* (January 1969): 17.

27. Public Health Service, *Healthy People 2000,* 332.

28. National Research Council. *Health Risks of Radon and Other Internally Deposited Alpha-Emitters.* Washington, D.C.: National Academy Press, 1988.

29. United States Environmental Protection Agency. *A Citizens Guide to Radon.* Washington, D.C.: U.S. Government Printing Office, August 1986, p. 1.

30. Hester, Gordon L. "Electric and Magnetic Fields: Managing an Uncertain Risk." *Environment* 34, no. 2 (January/February 1992): 7–11, 25–32.

31. National Geographic Society. *Energy: A Special Report in the Public Interest.* Washington, D.C.: The National Geographic Society, 1981, p. 67.

32. Hohenemser, C. "Chernobyl: An Early Report." *Environment* 28, no. 5 (June 1986): 6.

33. *Ibid.,* 39.

34. *Ibid.,* 40.

35. "Nuclear Power: Answers to Your Questions." Edison Electric Institute, Publication no. 78–24, p. 24.

36. Waldman, Steven. "Lead and Your Kids." *Newsweek* (July 15, 1991): 42.

37. Sciarillo, William G., and others. "Lead Exposure and Child Behavior." *American Journal of Public Health* 82, no. 11 (October 1992): 1356–60.

38. Public Health Service. *Healthy People 2000,* 328–29.

39. *Ibid.,* 329.

40. *You Make the Difference.* Pamphlet. Washington, D.C.: U.S. Government Printing Office, n.d., VII–10.

41. Public Health Service, *Healthy People 2000,* 302–3.

CHAPTER **THIRTEEN**

Injury Prevention and Control

The Importance of Safe Living

What would happen in the United States if a communicable disease caused nearly one hundred thousand deaths and some nine million injuries in the next twelve months? In all likelihood a major national disaster would be declared. Millions of dollars would be put into research to find a "cure" for the disease. All kinds of governmental, as well as private, initiatives would be instituted to assist those affected by this national tragedy. There would be television, radio, and other mass media events to publicize, examine, and analyze the situation. Educational measures would be designed to protect people from the deadly disease.

In the United States this very situation has been taking place for many years with little notice from the press, the general population, or governmental agencies. The fifth leading cause of death in America is unintentional injuries. For the population group between ages one and forty-four, unintentional injuries are the leading cause of death.[1] Among teenagers and young adults aged fifteen to twenty-four, these injuries claim more lives than all the other causes of death combined. It is estimated that about eighty-three thousand individuals die from all types of unintentional injuries yearly. Nearly half these fatalities occur as the result of motor vehicle accidents.

Not only do unintentional injury events lead to fatalities, but they also cause nearly 17.1 million disabling injuries annually. These circumstances cost more than $399 billion annually, including the cost of medical care, insurance, property damage, loss of wages, and the operation of such public agencies as the police and fire departments.

Why, considering these data, is there no major national outcry about unintentional injury events and safety? Have we become so complacent about this matter that little concern is expressed? Do most people simply accept them as an unavoidable part of life?

For far too long most people have considered an accident as an act of chance or fate, an unavoidable circumstance. The concept of accident implies that not much can be done to protect oneself. Thus, little public policy and individual and organized community action have been directed at reducing fatalities and injury-producing situations.

However, "accidents" can be understood, studied, and prevented. The basic principles of epidemiology can be applied to reducing the incidence of injuries. In 1987 at the Conference on Injury in America, it was concluded that if injury research and control programs were given more emphasis, injuries could be prevented and reduced.[2] It was concluded at this conference that for better understanding and program support to occur, the word "accident" should be eliminated and the use of the concept of injury should become the norm. This would then direct emphasis upon injury prevention and control. Rather than focusing upon accident prevention, which is often misunderstood, the thinking has been since the issuance of this conference report that the focus should be upon unintentional injury events.

Today, the federal government and many state and local agencies develop programs for reducing injuries. At the federal government level, the National Center for Injury Prevention and Control has been established within the Centers for Disease Control and Prevention, and funding, programming, and research in injury prevention and control have been increased. Collaboration between various community agencies is crucial for effective injury prevention programs. This includes the resources and activities of state and local health departments, traffic safety personnel, law enforcement departments, the medical community, emergency medical service personnel, and public policymakers, as well as the mass media.

Home Safety

As a person sits at home reading the newspaper, watching television, or doing any number of other tasks, the possibility of injury seems remote. Nearly everyone considers the home a place of safety. Yet many unintentional injuries, minor and major, happen in and around the home.

It is estimated that more than twenty thousand fatalities and three million disabling injuries occur annually from home accidents. The two age groups most affected by home accidents are the elderly and preschool children. For these two population groups, the home is the principal focus of their activities.

Fatalities and injuries from fires and falls are the major home safety problems. Falls are the leading cause of all home fatalities for those over the age of sixty-five; injuries resulting from fires are the leading cause among preschool children.

Falls

Falls cause over a million injuries each year in the United States. They are the leading cause of nonfatal injury and the second leading cause of injury-related death in the United States. The year 2000 Health Objectives for the Nation initiative has set an objective of reducing fatalities from falls and fall-related injuries to no more than 2.3 per 100,000 by 2000. Baseline datum in the 1980s was 2.7.[3]

The risk of falls increases with age. People over eighty-five years old are at greatest risk for a number of reasons.[4] As people age, their senses, including vision, deteriorate, and coordination and balance are reduced. Because of this, good lighting must be provided in rooms and stairways. Loose rugs and other items that can cause a stumble or fall must be kept off floors. Nonskid mats should be placed in showers and bathtubs, and on bathroom floors.

Most of what is known about falls has been learned from an analysis of the effects of falls on people. Less is known about the causes of falls that result in injury and/or death. For this reason research is being conducted examining the various risk factors for falls. For example, studies of the effects of the use of prescription and over-the-counter drugs and of sleeping pills are being conducted with the purpose of attempting to learn about their relation to falls among the elderly. Also research is being conducted attempting to learn more about physiological factors that result in balance abnormality.[5]

For the elderly, experiencing a fracture is a major danger of falling. Hip fracture is particularly serious. Half of all elderly people who have hip fractures have difficulty walking normally again.

Fires

Injury and death are often caused by fire. Home fires account for as many as four thousand deaths a year. Many of these fatalities are children. Home fires have many causes. Playing with matches is common among children. Abandoned or carelessly disposed of smoking materials ignite upholstery, sofas, mattresses, and bedding. Another leading cause of home fire injury, particularly among children, is cooking equipment. Children are often burned by spilling hot grease, water, or other liquids from cooking pans on the stove. More than one-fifth of all home fire-related injuries

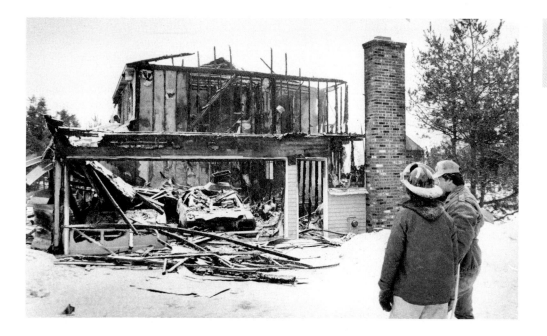

are from cooking fires, ovens, and stoves. Deaths from fires have increased during the past decade with the greater use of portable heaters and wood-burning stoves.

Smoke detectors play a major role in reducing the likelihood of injury from residential fires. They are inexpensive and very reliable in warning of fire in the home. The number of smoke detectors in homes increased significantly during the 1980s from only 5 percent in the early 1970s to about 75 percent today. This is owing to increased public awareness about their value and to their affordability, as well as to mandated public policy. Legislation in many communities now requires the installation of smoke detectors in homes. It is the objective of the Department of Health and Human Services that by the year 2000 every residential dwelling will have a functional smoke detector on all floors.[6]

Smoke detectors should be located near the bedrooms and at the top of stairways, as well as in basements. Fire safety personnel recommend that smoke detectors be checked once a month to ensure they are working and that batteries be replaced annually.

Another important fire safety feature that should be available in every home is a fire extinguisher. Every individual should know how to operate the extinguisher and be aware of the type of fire for which it is most effective.

Consumer Products

In and around our homes, apartments, and college dormitories there are a multitude of consumer products that cause injury and, in all too many cases, death—for example, engine-operated equipment such as lawn mowers, snowblowers, and rug sweepers. In some instances the product itself may be hazardous. It may be toxic, like many household cleansers and flammable liquids kept in the closet, basement, or garage. Some products may not be thought of as being dangerous, but certain parts can cause injury, for example, many children's toys.

Injury and fatality from home consumer products may be caused through misuse or product failure. Though product failure does occur, misuse is more common, so knowing and following instructions must be emphasized. In addition, proper care must be taken of all consumer products.

In 1972 the federal government passed the Consumer Product Safety Act, which created the Consumer Product Safety Commission (CPSC). This regulatory agency is assigned the task of ensuring that products are safe and reliable.

The commission works with industry to develop and enforce voluntary safety standards. Research is carried out to identify and analyze potential hazards in consumer products. To ensure that manufacturing firms comply with laws, regulations, and standards, the commission carries out a compliance and enforcement program. Programs are conducted to inform Americans of potential dangers. The commission has the authority to recall products that do not comply with standards and to ban products that are considered particularly dangerous.

For example, in 1988 the Consumer Product Safety Commission banned recreational lawn darts. These heavy metal darts, which are tossed at a ring on the ground, were reported to have caused several thousand injuries and several deaths. Another well-known action of the CPSC is their ban on the sale of three-wheel all-terrain vehicles (ATVs). ATVs have been blamed for nearly a thousand deaths and hundreds of thousands of injuries.

The Consumer Product Safety Commission is responsible for carrying out and enforcing the Flammable Fabrics Act, the Federal Hazardous Substance Act, the Poison Prevention Packaging Act, and the Refrigerator Safety Act. The Flammable Fabrics Act includes standards to ensure that the clothing we wear, particularly children's night wear, is flame-retardant.

A number of consumer products are regulated by the Federal Hazardous Substance Act. For example, many toys for young children have the potential to injure. Some of these either have been banned by the CPSC or must carry warning labels on their boxes. Toys with sharp edges and points, those with electrical components, and those that can serve as projectiles are particularly a concern. The CPSC has the authority to ban any toys that present mechanical, thermal, or electrical hazards.

Many injuries and some deaths are caused each year as the result of accidentally ingesting poisonous substances. Many products and medicines around our homes are poisonous, such as antifreeze, lighter fluid, turpentine, furniture polish, and cleansers. Children of preschool age are particularly susceptible to poisoning from household products because they touch and taste whatever is within their reach. CPSC regulations protect the public, particularly young children, from these substances. For example, most prescription and over-the-counter medications must now be sold in child-resistant containers.

Individuals must make sure that poisonous substances are stored out of reach of children. These products must also have appropriate labels so that adults will not come into contact with them accidentally.

Every adult should know basic first aid measures to be taken when a poisoning occurs. Poison control centers have been established throughout the nation to provide sources of information about countermeasures for every poisonous substance. Information about the composition of the poison, measures that need to be taken to neutralize the toxic effect, and other appropriate information is available. Most poison control centers provide twenty-four-hour-a-day service.

Motor Vehicle Safety

In 1899 in New York a man stepped off a streetcar and was struck by an automobile. He was pronounced dead shortly thereafter. This was the first recorded automobile fatality in the United States.[7]

Today about 158 million Americans are licensed to drive motor vehicles. It is estimated that annually one in eight experiences a crash.

More than 40,000 fatalities and about 2.2 million disabling injuries occur annually as the result of motor vehicle accidents. The National Safety Council estimates that the annual cost of motor vehicle accidents exceeds $156 billion. Though all age groups are involved, the majority of fatalities are teenagers and young adults.

Several measures can be taken to reduce the carnage from motor vehicle accidents. These measures relate to the vehicle, the driving environment, and the human element.[8]

A number of engineering and manufacturing improvements have made vehicles safer over the years. Money spent on research and safety modifications should be seen as an investment rather than a cost, because injuries and fatalities can be lowered. Better braking systems, padded dashboards, and energy-absorbing steering systems have saved lives and reduced injuries since their introduction nearly twenty years ago. Motor vehicle tires are much safer today than those manufactured in the past.

High-penetration resistant windshields have reduced injuries to the face. Putting a layer of plastic on the inner surface of the windshield prevents serious face and scalp lacerations when a crash occurs. The roadway environment has been improved in a number of ways in recent years. For example, during the 1980s some $1.2 billion of federal money was spent on railroad crossing modifications,

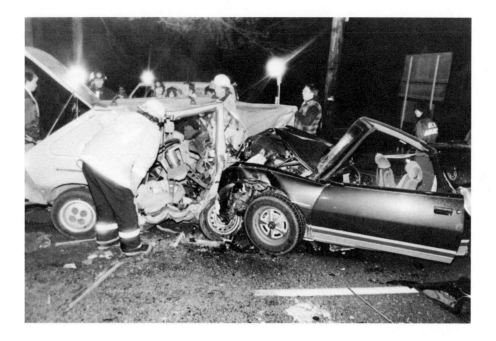

Motor vehicle crashes result in nearly 50,000 fatalities a year. There are a variety of factors, individual and environmental, that cause such crashes.

saving an estimated twenty-five hundred lives annually and reducing nonfatal injuries. This has saved $5 billion in lost wages and other costs nationwide.[9]

Several issues have been the focus of safety programs directed at the human element—the driver and vehicle occupants. Education has had an important role in motor vehicle safety. Most states require driver education before an individual can be licensed. Driver education programs are considered valuable in countering traffic accidents. Though studies have challenged whether these programs contribute to roadway safety, they are still popular and mandated in many localities.[10]

The two most important factors in reducing fatalities and injuries from motor vehicle accidents are greater use of passive restraints (air bags and seat belts) and less alcohol consumption with driving.

Seat Belt Use

Possibly the most important measure an individual can take to protect against a fatality or injury at the time of a motor vehicle crash is wearing a seat belt. Passenger restraint belts were first introduced in the mid-1950s. At that time they were considered an "extra" with the purchase of a new vehicle. Not until 1964 did belts become

standard equipment. Since then a series of federal regulations have required that all vehicles be equipped with belts. In 1984 the Department of Transportation ruled that all new cars have passive restraints—air bags or safety belts—by 1990. Until the late 1980s most regulations were directed only toward the front seats. The National Highway Safety Administration ruled that by 1990 all cars had to have lap and shoulder safety belts for two riders in the back seat. Vans, small trucks, and utility vehicles were exempted from this regulation.

Obviously safety belts are useless unless they are worn by the vehicle occupants. Despite research indicating that wearing belts provides much protection, a majority of Americans do not use them. To encourage wider use of vehicle restraints, thirty-seven states and the District of Columbia have implemented laws declaring seat belt use mandatory. New York, in 1985, was the first state to pass a law involving safety belt use. Fatalities and serious injuries dropped to the lowest level ever the first year the law was in effect. The objective for the nation for the year 2000 is that safety belt use be mandated in all fifty states.[11]

Despite laws, many people still do not "buckle up" when riding in a motor vehicle. The normal pattern is an initial surge in belt use after passage of the law. This is followed by a drop in use due to less publicity about the law and a perceived lack of enforcement. Many feel it is a bother to put the belt in place. Others suggest that it is an infringement on individual rights and that the government should not be involved. In most states enforcement procedures have been rather ineffective.

Small children are at special risk when riding in a motor vehicle at the time of a crash. They can be thrown into the windshield or the dashboard or tossed about the vehicle. All fifty states now require that small children ride in child restraints. After becoming the first state, in 1978, to pass such a requirement, Tennessee reported that injury rates had dropped 30 percent and fatality rates over 50 percent for children under the age of four.

In spite of the mandatory laws in every state, many adults do not place children in the child restraint seats. Some oppose mandatory regulations, others suggest that they cannot afford the seats, and in some cases it is the desire of the parents to hold their child on their lap while riding in the car. Holding a child on the lap is particularly dangerous in that upon collision the child can be thrown about the car or the adult may be thrust forward and crush the child against the dash and/or the window.

Airbags

The use of airbags in motor vehicles has been very controversial. The airbag inflates upon an initial impact of collision. The forward momentum of the occupants is absorbed by the airbag. This protects the individual from being thrust into the steering wheel, the window, or being thrown about in the interior of the vehicle.

Since the introduction of airbags in the 1950s the automotive industry has been opposed to federal mandates that would require the inclusion of these passive restraints in motor vehicles. Among several reasons given is that of cost. It is estimated that the inclusion of airbags can add nearly a thousand dollars to the cost of a motor vehicle.

Whether airbags will be standard items in motor vehicles by the year 2000 is open to discussion. There is some question as to whether the public desires to have airbags. Further research and development in the improvement of airbags will be necessary if they are to become standard equipment in the near future.

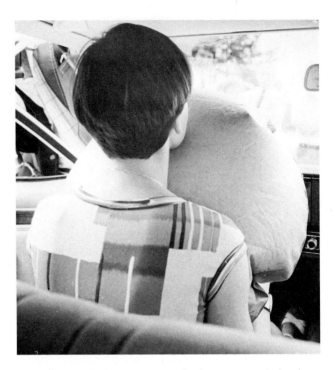

Research continues in an attempt to develop an economical and effective passive restraint system. The airbag has received the most attention and interest.

Drinking and Driving

The carnage on the highways caused by drunken driving has been a particular concern since the 1980s. Approximately 50 percent of motor vehicle–related fatalities stem from this cause, which accounts for more than twenty thousand deaths annually. Drunken driving is a particular problem among teenagers and young adults. It is reported that 90 percent of teenage automobile accidents involve alcohol.[12] Males drive and drink three times more often than women.

The problems related to teenage drinking and driving are compounded by the fact that it is illegal for alcoholic beverages to be sold to anyone under the age of twenty-one. Prior to the mid-1980s many states had minimum drinking ages of eighteen and nineteen. The federal government passed the Uniform Minimum Drinking Age Law in 1984. This legislation required the United States Department of Transportation to withhold federal highway funds to any states that did not raise the minimum

Issue—Case Study
Teenagers Drinking and Driving

The young woman was a senior in her local high school, eighteen years of age, and would graduate in two weeks. Her classmates realized that shortly they would all be going their separate ways, so they planned a party at the young woman's home at the edge of town.

Some fifty to sixty teenagers came to the party in fifteen to twenty cars. They were talking, listening to music, playing volleyball—drinking. Nearly every one of the teens was drinking. All were between the ages of sixteen and nineteen—friends and schoolmates of the young woman sponsoring the party.

Considering that the minimal drinking age in every state today is twenty-one and that drunken teenagers are a major cause of motor vehicle accidents, the activities of this party bring up some serious questions that many people are not willing to confront.

Because the party was out-of-doors, any neighbor or passerby could see what was happening. If you were a neighbor concerned about driving and alcohol consumption, would you report the teenagers to the police? You may feel this is not a matter for you to become involved in. But would your opinion change if one of these teenagers crashed into a close friend or relative later in the evening, causing death or disabling injuries?

What are the responsibilities of the young woman's parents? Do you feel their permitting the party on their property is appropriate, or should they be held responsible for the actions of the party goers? Along the same line, to what degree should the store who sold them the liquor be held accountable for injuries occurring after the party?

---

drinking age to twenty-one. In 1988 Wyoming became the last state to comply. Many people were opposed to this action. Some viewed it as political blackmail. The Supreme Court refused to support an appeal declaring this federal legislation illegal.

Numerous studies have been conducted on the effects of raising the legal drinking age. Some evidence indicates a slight drop in drunken driving fatalities and liquor sales to those between the ages of eighteen and twenty-one. Generally, the authors of these studies conclude that fatal accidents among the affected age group have been reduced.[13] Nevertheless, all do not agree—debate continues, and thousands of accidents involving this population group still occur weekly.

Another controversial issue related to drunken driving has been the establishment of police sobriety checkpoints. Drivers are randomly stopped by law enforcement officers and their level of alcohol consumption evaluated. If suspected of being intoxicated, the driver can be required to take a blood alcohol test. Sobriety checkpoints have been found to be very effective deterrents for drunken driving.[14] Controversy surrounds the use of sobriety checkpoints; opponents believe that stopping any citizen without due cause is an infringement of privacy

and thus unconstitutional. However, the United States Supreme Court in 1990 ruled that sobriety checkpoints are not an infringement of individual rights. As a result, they are used in most states. Opponents also question whether sobriety checkpoints actually deter drunken driving.

A movement to curtail drunken driving has been initiated in recent years. These efforts have led to a variety of state and local regulations and legislation. The catalyst for this movement has been voluntary groups such as Mothers Against Drunk Driving (MADD) and Students Against Drunk Driving (SADD). The concept of a "designated driver," one who abstains from alcohol to drive others home after parties and other activities, has been widely advertised and strongly encouraged.

In a number of states fines and other penalties for driving while under the influence of alcohol have been stiffened. In addition, many local ordinances now hold those who provide minors with alcoholic beverages liable. Some evidence supports the position that legal changes lead to a decline in alcohol-related traffic fatalities.[15]

Federal and state courts have extended the liability for drunken driving. In 1984 the New Jersey Supreme Court ruled that a host could be held liable if he or she served liquor to a guest who subsequently caused injuries to others in a motor vehicle accident. Other courts have extended liability to employers who provide alcoholic beverages at a party or picnic, to bartenders and tavern owners, and to wholesale vendors. The number of civil suits with jury verdicts placing responsibility on third-party providers of alcohol has increased.

To help employees in the restaurant business cope with their responsibilities relating to consumption of alcoholic beverages, the Educational Institute of the American Hotel and Motel Association has developed a program entitled *Serving Alcohol with Care*.[16] Concern about alcohol-related traffic accidents was the basic motive behind the development of this program. The program informs the student about liability laws that apply to servers of alcoholic beverages and provides suggestions to help prevent intoxication.

A number of states have established third-party liability, referred to as *Dram Shop Acts*. These laws hold that the proprietor of an establishment that serves alcohol to a person who commits an alcohol-related offense may be prosecuted and held liable for damages incurred by that person. In some cases liability extends to a host serving alcohol in a private setting.

The amount of alcohol in the bloodstream is known as the blood alcohol level or the blood alcohol concentration (BAC). The greater the BAC level, the greater the level of functional impairment. Impairment begins when BAC levels reach 0.10 percent. Historically anyone with a 0.10 percent BAC was considered legally intoxicated. However, four states have now lowered this to 0.08 percent. One state has a BAC level of 0.12 percent; all others are 0.10 percent. Many suggest that drunken driving could be significantly reduced if BAC levels were lowered to 0.08 percent in all states.

To focus national attention on the problem of drunken driving, the Surgeon General in 1988 held a workshop that developed several recommendations for national and local public policy action. The workshop called for an all-out attack on alcohol consumption and driving.[17] It was felt that increasing liquor taxes and placing strict curbs on advertising would reduce the misuse of alcohol. Banning advertising of alcoholic products on college campuses was strongly recommended. As the minimum drinking age is twenty-one throughout the nation, it seems illogical and inappropriate to permit such advertising on campuses where the majority of students are under this age.

The Surgeon General's Workshop on Drunk Driving also called for the end of sponsorship of athletic events and youth-oriented musical concerts by alcoholic beverage companies. Another recommendation would require antialcohol advertising to counter beer and wine commercials. The workshop urged that penalties for those found to be driving under the influence of alcohol should be stiffened.

The goal set by the Year 2000 Health Objectives for the Nation is that all states mandate driver's license suspension and/or revocation and establish programs for people guilty of driving under the influence of alcohol.[18]

During the 1980s more than four hundred drunken driving laws were passed throughout the nation. Penalties have been stiffened, laws leading to conviction have been strengthened, and suspension of the driver's license is now mandatory upon first conviction in some states. License suspension has been determined to be an effective measure for reducing motor vehicle crashes. However, courts tend to be hesitant about suspending a license when it can cause economic hardship for the operator.

No one measure has significantly impacted the problem of drunken driving.[19] Although more laws have been passed and penalties stiffened, many times enforcement is minimal. All too often judges are reluctant to convict and police are reluctant to arrest. Consistent enforcement, effective educational measures, and active concern by the American public are needed before alcohol-related fatalities and injuries are reduced significantly in motor vehicle accidents.

Safety in the Rural Setting

The apparent serenity of hundreds of acres of corn on a Midwest farm, of fields of golden wheat as far as the eye can see in the Great Plains, or of a forest of timber in the Pacific Northwest is all too often broken by death or serious injury. Farming, including ranching, forestry, and commercial fishing, is one of the most dangerous occupations in America. Though the number of fatalities in the construction industry is greater according to the National Safety Council, the ratio of deaths to workers is higher in agriculture.

Nearly one thousand fatalities a year occur among agricultural workers, with as many as one hundred thousand disabling injuries. Data indicate the importance of developing measures to make the rural occupational setting safer. Most farm worker fatalities and injuries are the result of accidents involving tractors, machinery and equipment with fast-moving parts, and problems associated with grain storage, and of exposure to chemicals, particularly pesticides.

Most farmers, ranchers, and rural agricultural workers are quite independent. A vast majority live on their farms or ranches and often work alone in the fields. When an accident occurs, it may be some time before anyone realizes that the individual is in trouble. For this reason, appropriate and early emergency care for the injured farmer may be delayed.

In addition to working alone, farmers usually perform their own maintenance on the many pieces of equipment used during the farming season. Sometimes these repairs are inappropriate and result in injuries. Young people may lack experience and training. Farmers may become careless during harvest season when they fall behind schedule owing to bad weather or other factors. Working hours are stretched, and the potential for injury increases.

The part-time farmer has also contributed to rising injuries. This individual may work full-time in the city but buys some acreage, purchases some used equipment, and works on the farm weekends and evenings. Usually this person has had little experience with farming equipment, and used equipment often does not have all the needed safety features. These factors, combined with the likelihood that the individual has already put in a full day of work elsewhere and may be fatigued, make for a dangerous situation.

Most farmers and ranchers operate as self-contained small family businesses. As such, any disabling injury can mean serious economic setbacks. Farmers often resent the intrusion of safety regulations as mandated by governmental agencies. They are unable to pass on the costs of safety features or newer equipment to the consumer.

Causes of Agricultural Injuries

Probably the most commonly used piece of equipment on farms and ranches is the tractor. Nearly half of all farm-related fatalities stem from tractor rollovers. In these situations the driver is often pinned under the tractor, unable to escape, or is caught in the power take-off, the engine drive shaft that operates the equipment. There are two types of tractor rollovers: side and rear overturns.

Side overturns occur when the tractor is crossing a slope or is driven too close to a ditch. It is particularly dangerous to drive a tractor on a slope greater than 25 percent. Depressions in the land and rocks and other obstacles can tip the tractor over, as can taking a turn too quickly. Tractors are used to pull many types of machinery, wagons, and equipment. Rear overturns occur because the hitch is positioned at a point too high on the rear of the tractor. Then when the rear wheels become bound in the mud or when the tractor accelerates too rapidly, it overturns.

There are two measures that can provide protection for the tractor operator: the rollover protection system (ROPS), designed to prevent the tractor from turning upside down and crushing the driver, and seat belts. Farm safety professionals feel that if every person using a tractor had these two objects, many fatalities and injuries would be eliminated. Many farmers oppose the use of seat belts on tractors. They feel that it is a nuisance to buckle the belts every time they get on. Research has established the value of seat belts in saving lives and protecting from serious injury in tractors, just as it has in cars. Seat belts are a stabilizing factor and keep the operator from being thrown from the vehicle.

Farmers use a great deal of high-speed machinery. Shields have been placed on these pieces of equipment to prevent injury. Unfortunately, many times the person using the equipment removes the protective pieces, either to repair the machine or simply because the individual does not care to have them. Thus, serious accidents often occur. Protective shields should always be in place any time that the machinery is in operation.

Another source of injury and fatality is grain elevators and silos. When grain stored in these facilities begins to move, there is danger to anyone working in the area. Moving grain can entrap an individual very easily, much like quicksand, and unless someone is present to rescue the trapped person, suffocation may occur.

Fires are a serious threat around grain elevators and silos. Grain moving through the pipes in a storage bin can create static electricity. Dust explosion may occur whenever grain dust, oxygen, and a source of energy are present. The spark from the static electricity when combined with dust in the silo can cause an explosion that may destroy the entire building and even surrounding structures. Keeping the grain storage bin clean and well ventilated will protect against these dangers.

Many herbicides, fungicides, insecticides, and fertilizers contain ingredients suspected of causing cancer. Others can cause chronic bronchitis, skin disorders, poisoning, and general illness. Some fertilizers, such as anhydrous ammonia, can cause coughing spasms, asphyxiation, and skin burns. Because many of these are toxic on direct contact, farm workers must be familiar with proper handling procedures to avoid misuse.

It is important that the individual wear appropriate personal protective clothing when working with such substances. They must be properly stored, and empty containers should be thrown away. Application instructions must be followed. Everyone working with farm chemicals should be aware of appropriate first aid measures to be taken at time of exposure.

Injury occurs from a number of other circumstances in the rural setting. Though the occurrence is not widespread, animals may bite, kick, or fall on people and cause injury. The ratio of serious injury from horseback riding is greater than those for motorcycle riding as well as automobile racing.[20] Electrocution kills and injures many individuals; for example, equipment such as aluminum ladders and tall farm machinery may come in contact with overhead electrical lines.

More effective safety regulation of farm workers is needed. Federal regulations relating to agricultural workers do exist under provisions of the Occupational Safety and Health Act. However, farms with ten or fewer workers are exempted from these regulations. In addition, research must be conducted and data collected on rural farm injuries and fatalities to determine measures for creating a safer agricultural environment.

Emergency Medical Service Systems (EMS)

Historically, the provision of emergency medical care service systems has been less than effective. For example, in many communities there were inadequate vehicles to take injured individuals to the hospital. In some rural towns the only organization with a vehicle large enough to carry injured people was the local funeral home—in their hearse.

Also, little care was rendered to the injured before their arrival at the hospital emergency room.

In 1973 the Emergency Medical Service Systems Act was passed by Congress to assist individual communities in developing comprehensive regional emergency medical service systems. The act defined an emergency medical system as ". . . a system which provides for arrangement of personnel, facilities, and equipment for the effective and coordinated delivery . . . of health care services under emergency conditions."[21] As a result, today much of the U.S. population has access to emergency medical care. The objective of the Department of Health and Human Services is that by the year 2000 emergency medical service systems be in place in all fifty states.[22] The establishment of regional EMS systems has reduced loss of life and serious injury.

Personnel providing emergency care in EMS systems are very highly trained, far better than prior to the federal legislation. Emergency medical technicians (EMTs) must undergo over a hundred hours of training to be qualified to work in an EMS unit; paramedics receive more than a thousand hours of training.

The EMS systems are implementing procedures to better integrate the prehospital care provided by the EMTs and paramedics with the hospital care. This is accomplished by a well-designed communications system that links the various personnel of the hospital facilities and the emergency rescue teams. The emergency vehicle at the scene of the accident or fire must be able to communicate with the medical specialists at the clinic or hospital.

Emergency system transportation equipment has been standardized in recent years. Today's emergency rescue vehicle must have two separate compartments, one for the driver and one for the injured. There must be space in the patient compartment to apply life-support measures while enroute to the hospital. Regional EMS system plans integrate air and water vehicles where appropriate. Aircraft, particularly helicopters, have been particularly effective in getting injured individuals from rural, isolated locations to hospital facilities. In addition, aircraft have been used to transfer patients from smaller, general hospitals to larger, urban hospitals for specialized care.

The regional emergency medical service systems have been integrated with other community services. Planning is important when transferring patients to facilities for follow-up care and rehabilitation or when carrying out emergency care in a catastrophe, such as a

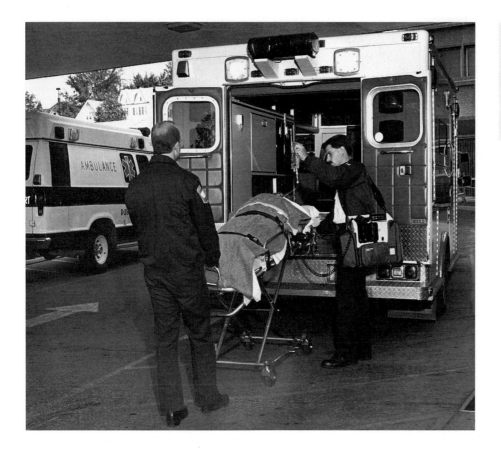

Emergency medical vehicles and the skills of the EMTs are standardized throughout the nation. As a result injured persons begin to receive needed emergency care from the moment they are met by the EMTs, not upon arrival at the hospital.

tornado or hurricane or an explosion or fire. Some communities have developed plans for community agencies to follow in the event of an airplane accident at a nearby urban airport.

Recreational Safety

Recreation in America is a big business. The majority of Americans participate in at least one and many in several recreational activities. Interest in golfing and tennis is at an all-time high. Water sports, including swimming, boating, fishing, waterskiing, and surfing, have become major recreational outlets. Some are as low key as walking in the woods, playing croquet in the backyard, or pitching horseshoes at a family reunion. Others involve high-speed machines, such as snowmobiling or running an all-terrain vehicle (ATV) out across the desert sands of the Southwest. Recreational activities often require skill to be safe. This is true in downhill and cross-country skiing, mountain climbing, and waterskiing.

Every type of recreational activity involves some possibility of fatality and injury. No one would suggest that, because of these risks, we should not be involved. But measures must be taken to prevent accidents.

Before participating in a recreational activity, the individual should be familiar with the necessary safety measures. These measures must be practiced at all times. Developing skills is important in preventing serious injury. Before one enters the water, it is essential that swimming skills be mastered. Snow skiers must be aware of their skill level before selecting and negotiating a ski run.

Many injuries and fatalities result from improper use of equipment. Machine-operated recreational vehicles should be in safe operating condition, and all equipment, both new and used, examined regularly to assure safe operation.

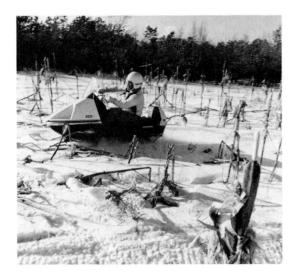
Care is needed in the operation of snowmobiles to protect the rider from injury-causing circumstances.

Water Safety

Possibly the most popular recreational activities involve water. Swimming, boating, fishing, and a host of related activities are practiced by most Americans at some time in their lives. For most, these recreational pursuits lead to relaxation, excitement, and the simple stimulation of being in and around water. However, for between five and six thousand Americans annually, water activity ends in drowning.

Drowning is the second leading cause of unintentional injuries resulting in death. The highest incidence occurs in children under the age of five. Two other population groups at high risk for drowning are males in the fifteen-to-thirty-four age group and African-American males.[23]

Many factors contribute to drowning, including inability to swim, failure to use personal flotation devices, and improper operation of boats. Educational programs about risks associated with water activity must be expanded. All people pursuing water recreational activities should be able to swim and possess basic skills in rescuing others in the water.

The single most important factor related to drownings is alcohol consumption. In fact, an estimated 50 percent of teen and adult drownings are alcohol related. Visit any marina on a hot summer weekend, and many individuals will be seen on their boats drinking alcoholic beverages. The combination of alcohol, heat, relaxation, and boat engine power can be deadly. Alcohol impairs a person's ability to operate a boat safely as well as the ability to swim. It shortens cold water survival time, compounds the effect of wind, sun, and fatigue, and slows reaction time and coordination. An estimated twelve hundred deaths each year are due to boating accidents, half alcohol related.

A number of states have passed alcohol and boat operation laws. It is the goal of the National Transportation Safety Board that all states have such statutes. Many in the public are calling to restrict the sale and consumption of alcoholic beverages around boating areas. Enforcement of alcohol regulations by the United States Coast Guard is increasing. Some states now routinely check boaters for alcohol. In jurisdictions where there are such laws, boating deaths have been reduced. Several states have implied consent laws: refusal to take sobriety tests can be used against the boater in court. Many feel imposing stiff penalties and sanctions on drunken boat operators is a must.

Boating safety instruction classes are provided in many communities by the Coast Guard Auxiliary and local Power Squadrons. Anyone operating a boat must know how to handle it in all weather conditions. All necessary safety gear, such as life jackets, flares, foghorn, paddles, cushions, and first aid kits, must be on board. All too often boat owners have only the required minimum amount of safety gear on board. For example, on a sixteen-to-twenty-five-foot powerboat, only one fire extinguisher is required by law in most jurisdictions. Yet one needs more than the protection of a single fire extinguisher. The same could be said of other safety equipment.

The majority of drownings among children under five years of age occur in home pools, bathtubs, and unmarked and unprotected areas of lakes and streams. All pools should be surrounded by barriers to keep children from wandering into the area. Careful, watchful supervision around any water is necessary to keep small children from drowning.

Motorized Vehicles

Riding motorized vehicles such as snowmobiles and all-terrain vehicles (ATVs) is a popular recreational activity. Injuries and fatalities associated with both vehicles have increased dramatically in recent years for numerous reasons. Studies have indicated that one major risk factor in ATV injuries and fatalities is the failure to wear helmets.

In 1988 sale of the three-wheel ATV was banned in the United States. The safety and stability of this vehicle were felt to be inadequate. Unfortunately, all three-wheel vehicles currently owned by individuals can still be operated. Many of these have been purchased by parents for their children, who are often too young and inexperienced to operate such a vehicle safely. Today only four-wheel ATVs, which are more stable, can be sold.

Snowmobiles, motorized vehicles that move on a pair of metal skis combined with a rubber belt tread, can travel at speeds greater than eighty miles per hour. The snowmobile is capable of taking people into localities where one cannot usually go because of snow. In spite of their popularity in regions of the nation having significant amounts of snow, many injuries and fatalities occur from operating these vehicles. Snowmobile collisions are particularly dangerous because seat belt restraints are not on most vehicles and an individual can easily be thrown into other vehicles, trees, or other objects.

Several states have implemented regulations to control the operation of snowmobiles and to enhance safety. For example, several states prohibit their operation on public roads. Driver regulations, particularly for teenagers, have been established for operation of these vehicles. Regardless of regulatory efforts, measures need to be taken to reduce the numbers of injuries and deaths that occur every year from the operation of these vehicles.

Operating either the snowmobile or the ATV demands appropriate dress. Care must be taken when driving the vehicles onto ice-covered bodies of water. Laws and local ordinances must be known and obeyed, and drivers must refrain from alcohol use.

Cycle Operation—The Need for Helmets

Operation of two-wheel cycles—the motorcycle and the bicycle—results in numerous fatalities and injuries. Bicycle riding has become an increasingly popular recreational pursuit since the 1980s. Whereas bicycles were operated principally by children and young people in the past, today many adults purchase and use bicycles. Most are used for recreational purposes; however, in some cases adults ride their bicycles to work.

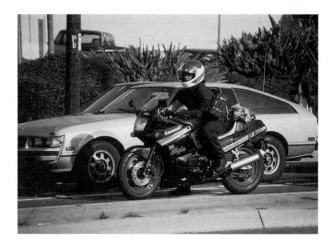

Research indicates that many fatalities and serious injuries are reduced when motorcycle riders wear a helmet.

Conditions are not always conducive to safe riding. In most urban localities bicyclists must share busy streets with motor vehicles, so they must be alert and ride defensively. The bicycle is no competitor for a motor vehicle.

Bicycle injuries account for the greatest number of recreational injuries requiring hospital emergency care. Nearly half a million emergency room visits stem from bicycling. Eighty-five percent of fatalities and two-thirds of hospital admissions from bicycling are the result of head injuries.[24] Many bicyclists do not wear a helmet. Very few children and young people are ever seen wearing head protection. Adults offer many excuses—they are only going for a short ride, or the helmet is uncomfortable.

It is estimated that there are more than four million motorcycles in the United States that travel an estimated 8.8 billion miles each year. These motorized cycles come in many different sizes, shapes, and styles. Unfortunately, more than 66,000 riders and passengers are injured annually, and nearly 2,700 fatalities associated with motorcycle riding occur each year.[25]

The issue of requiring motorcyclists to wear helmets has been an area of controversy for many years. By the mid-1970s all but three states had laws requiring that motorcycle drivers and passengers must wear safety helmets. Owing to litigation, court decision, and state legislatures repealing actions, a number of states withdrew the mandates. Today motorcycle riders are required to wear helmets in fewer than half the states.

Should motorcyclists be mandated to wear helmets? Those opposed to such laws suggest that adults should be permitted to make their own decisions; it should be a voluntary decision. On the other hand, proponents point out that such mandates benefit society. For one thing, when a person is injured, police, fire, and ambulance costs are often paid by the public. Recognizing that head injuries are the leading cause of death in motorcycle crashes and that helmets are effective in preventing fatalities, it would seem that motorcycle helmet laws are a worthwhile injury prevention measure. The federal government health promotion initiative has set an objective of at least 80 percent use of helmets by the year 2000.[26]

Summary

The fifth leading cause of death in the United States is unintentional injury. In addition to fatalities, many disabling injuries occur, with an annual cost of more than $399 billion. The causes of accidents have been studied for years. Injury control and prevention programs involve the cooperation and interaction of numerous community agencies.

A number of fatalities and injuries stem from accidents in and around the home. Falls are the leading cause of home fatalities, affecting principally the elderly. Fires also pose a serious risk.

In every home numerous products used every day have the potential for injury. The Consumer Product Safety Commission, a regulatory agency of the federal government, is responsible for assuring the safety of many consumer products.

The leading cause of unintentional injury and death in the United States is motor vehicle accidents: more than 40 thousand fatalities and 2.2 million disabling injuries occur annually. Modifying the structure of the motor vehicle and improving the roadway environment have been important injury reduction initiatives.

Occupants of vehicles have been encouraged to use safety restraints and to reduce the incidence of drunken driving. Research supports the view that fatalities and disabling injuries are reduced when individuals involved in vehicular crashes are wearing safety belts. The problems of driving while under the influence of alcohol are extremely difficult to deal with, but numerous measures have been designed to reduce this major cause of motor vehicle accidents.

Though safety is important in any setting, the rural setting is of particular concern. Agriculture is one of the most dangerous occupations in America. A variety of causes, including tractor rollover and operation of high-speed farm machinery, lead to death and injury. Grain elevators and silos pose the threat of explosion, fire, and suffocation. Handling hundreds of different chemicals presents dangers to agricultural workers.

Throughout the 1980s significant improvement in regional emergency medical service systems took place. Today emergency workers are more highly trained than ever before. EMS transportation units are better equipped than in the past, having direct communication with the hospital emergency facilities. As a result, emergency care can be given to an injured person before they reach the hospital.

Americans spend hundreds of hours in many recreational pursuits, all of which have the potential for injury and death. Whether involved in water sports, driving a motorized vehicle, or playing individual or team sports, care must be taken to protect against injury.

Discussion Questions

1. Discuss data relating to fatalities and injuries stemming from accidents.

2. In your opinion does the term "accident" seem inappropriate? Explain the reason for your response.

3. Why are falls a particular concern to the elderly population?

4. Discuss some of the major causes of fire in the home.

5. Where should smoke detectors be placed in the home?

6. What kinds of services and information can be obtained from Poison Control Centers?

7. What are some initiatives for reducing the number of motor vehicle crashes that focus upon the vehicle?

8. Discuss some of the issues that center on the mandating of individuals to wear safety belts.

9. What is the present status of requiring the installation of airbags in motor vehicles?

10. Do you agree with the position of the United States Supreme Court regarding the legal status of sobriety checkpoints? Defend your response.

11. What was the motivation that was used to get all states to raise the legal drinking age to twenty-one?

12. Discuss your position on requiring a legal drinking age of twenty-one.

13. What is your opinion of some of the recommendations that came out of the Surgeon General's Workshop on Drunk Driving?

14. Why is the rural setting a particularly dangerous environment?

15. Identify some of the dangers associated with grain elevators and silos.

16. Discuss some of the benefits of EMS systems.

17. In what ways do EMS systems bring about the integration of several different community agencies?

18. What are some of the factors related to drowning being the second leading cause of unintentional injuries resulting in death?

19. What can be done to reduce the problems of drunken operation of boats on the waterways?

20. How can fatalities and injuries from the operation of snowmobiles be reduced?

21. Why have three-wheel all-terrain vehicles been banned for manufacture and sale in the United States?

22. Should motorcycle riders be required to wear helmets when riding the cycle? Discuss this issue.

Suggested Readings

Fisher, Leslie. "Childhood Injuries—Causes, Preventive Theories and Case Studies." *Journal of Environmental Health* 50, no. 6 (May/June 1988): 355–60.

Foss, Robert D. "Evaluation of a Community-Wide Incentive Program to Promote Safety Restraint Use." *American Journal of Public Health* 79, no. 3 (March 1989): 304–6.

Gulaid, Jama A., Richard W. Sattin, and Richard J. Waxweiler. "Deaths from Residential Fires, 1978–1984." *Morbidity and Mortality Weekly Report* 37, no. SS-1 (February 1988): 39–45.

Hingston, Ralph W., and others. "Effects of Legislative Reform to Reduce Drunken Driving and Alcohol-Related Traffic Fatalities," *Public Health Reports* 103, no. 6 (November/December 1988): 659–67.

Holden, Janet A., and Tom Christoffel. "Preparing and Presenting an Introductory Course on Motor Vehicle Injury." *Public Health Reports* 103, no. 2 (March/April 1988): 153–61.

Howland, Jonathan, and Ralph Hingson. "Alcohol as a Risk Factor for Injuries or Death Due to Fires and Burns: Review of the Literature." *Public Health Reports* 102, no. 5 (September/October 1987): 475–82.

Lambert, Deborah A., and Richard W. Sattin. "Deaths from Falls, 1978–1984." *Morbidity and Mortality Weekly Report* 37, no. SS-1 (February 1988): 21–26.

Maghsoodloo, Saeed, David B. Brown and Perry A. Greathouse. "Impact of the Revision of DUI Legislation in Alabama." *American Journal of Drug and Alcohol Abuse* 14, no. 1 (1988): 97–108.

Miller, Barrett C. "Falls: A Cast of Thousands Cost of Millions." *Safety and Health* 137, no. 2 (February 1988): 22–26.

National Committee for Injury Prevention and Control and Education Development Center, Inc. *Injury Prevention, Meeting the Challenge: A Summary.* Report to the Bureau of Maternal and Child Health and Resources Development, 1989.

Overend, Robert B. "Safety on Two Wheels." *Safety and Health* 139, no. 4 (April 1989): 59–60.

Pollock, Daniel A., Daniel L. McGee, and Juan G. Rodriquez. "Deaths Due to Injury in the Home among Persons under 15 Years of Age, 1970–1984." *Morbidity and Mortality Weekly Report* 37, no. SS-1 (February 1988): 13–20.

"Recognizing the Common Problem of Child Automobile Restraint Misuse." *Pediatrics* 81, no. 5 (1988): 717–20.

Robertson, Leon S. "Risk of Fatal Rollover in Utility Vehicles Relative to Static Stability." *American Journal of Public Health* 79, no. 3 (March 1989): 300–303.

Robertson, Leon S. "Roadway Modifications." *Public Health Reports* 102, no. 6 (November/December 1987): 671–74.

Rook, Martin. "ROPS: No Tractor Should Be without One." *Ohio Monitor* 60, no. 11 (November 1987): 14–15.

Rosenberg, Mark L. "1987 Conference on Injury in America: A Summary." *Public Health Reports* 102, no. 6 (November/December 1987): 577–81.

Runyan, Carol W. "Progress and Potential in Injury Control." *American Journal of Public Health* 83, no. 5 (May 1993): 637–39.

Russ, Nason W., and E. Scott Geller. "Training Bar Personnel to Prevent Drunken Driving: A Field Evaluation." *American Journal of Public Health* 77, no. 8 (August 1987): 952–54.

Shaw, Kathy N., and others. "Correlates of Reported Smoke Detector Usage in an Inner-City Population: Participants in a Smoke Detector Give-Away Program." *American Journal of Public Health* 78, no. 6 (June 1988): 650–53.

Stoskopf, Carleen H., and Jonathan Venn. "Farm Accidents and Injuries: A Review and Ideas for Prevention." *Journal of Environmental Health* 47, no. 5 (March/April 1985): 250–52.

United States Department of Health and Human Services. *Surgeon General's Workshop on Drunk Driving: Proceedings.* Washington, D.C.: Public Health Service, 1989.

Waller, Anna E. "Childhood Injury Deaths: National Analysis and Geographic Variations" *American Journal of Public Health* 79, no. 3 (March 1989): 310–15.

Wasserman, Richard C., and others. "Bicyclists, Helmets and Head Injuries: A Rider-Based Study of Helmet Use and Effectiveness." *American Journal of Public Health* 78, no. 9 (September 1988): 1220–21.

Wells-Parker, Elisabeth, and Pamela J. Cosby. "Behavioral and Employment Consequences of Driver's License Suspension for Drinking Driving Offenders." *Journal of Safety Research* 19, no. 1 (September 1988): 5–20.

Zador, Paul L., and Michael A. Ciccone. "Automobile Driver Fatalities in Frontal Impacts: Air Bags Compared with Manual Belts." *American Journal of Public Health* 83, no. 5 (May 1993): 661–66.

Endnotes

1. National Safety Council. *Accident Facts, 1993.* Chicago, Ill. National Safety Council, 1993, p. 7. Data presented in this chapter are from *Accident Facts, 1993* unless otherwise noted.

2. Rosenberg, Mark L. "1987 Conference on Injury in America; A Summary." *Public Health Reports* 102, no. 6 (November/December 1987): 577.

3. United States Department of Health and Human Services. *Healthy People 2000: National Health Promotion and Disease Prevention Objectives.* Washington, D.C.: U.S. Government Printing Office, 1991, p. 276.

4. Lambert, Deborah A., and Richard W. Sattin. "Deaths from Falls, 1978–1984." *Morbidity and Mortality Weekly Report* 37, no. SS-1 (February 1988): 21–26.

5. Ertas, A. "Design and Development of a Fall Arresting System." *Journal of Safety Research* 21, no. 3 (Fall 1990): 97–102.

6. Department of Health and Human Services, *Healthy People 2000,* p. 285.

7. "First Auto Crash Victim Died Seventy-two Years Ago Today." *Journal of the American Medical Association* 217, no. 11 (September 13, 1971): 1461.

8. Dugoff, Howard J. "A Research Administrator's Perspective." *Public Health Reports* 102, no. 6 (November/December 1987): 686.

9. Robertson, Leon S. "Roadway Modifications." *Public Health Reports* 102, no. 6 (November/December 1987): 671.

10. Potvin, Louise, Francois Champagne, and Claire Laberge-Nadeau. "Mandatory Driver Training and Road Safety: The Quebec Experience." *American Journal of Public Health* 78, no. 9 (September 1988): 1206–9.

11. Department of Health and Human Services, *Healthy People 2000,* p. 284.

12. United States Department of Health and Human Services. *Surgeon General's Workshop on Drunk Driving: Proceedings.* Washington, D.C.: Public Health Service 1989, p. 10.

13. Hoskin, Alan F., and others. "The Effect of Raising the Legal Minimum Drinking Age on Fatal Crashes in Ten States." *Journal of Safety Research* 17, no. 3 (Fall 1986): 117–28.

14. McGuire, Frederick L. "The Accuracy of Estimating the Sobriety of Drinking Drivers." *Journal of Safety Research* 17, no. 2 (Summer 1986): 81–85.

15. Hingston, Ralph W., and others. "Effects of Legislative Reform to Reduce Drunken Driving and Alcohol-Related Traffic Fatalities." *Public Health Reports* 103, no. 6 (November/December 1988): 660.

16. Educational Institute of the American Hotel and Motel Association. *Serving Alcohol with Care: A Manual for Servers.* East Lansing, Mich.: The Educational Institute, 1985, p. 3.

17. Department of Health and Human Services, *Surgeon General's Workshop on Drunk Driving,* 10.

18. Department of Health and Human Services, *Healthy People 2000,* 175.

19. Maghsoodloo, Saeed, David B. Brown, and Perry A. Greathouse. "Impact of the Revision of DUI Legislation in Alabama." *American Journal of Drug and Alcohol Abuse* 14, no. 1 (1988): 105.

20. Centers for Disease Control. "Injuries Associated with Horseback Riding—United States, 1987 and 1988." *Morbidity and Mortality Weekly Report* 39, no. 20 (May 25, 1990): 329.

21. P.L. 93–154, 93rd Congress, Emergency Medical Service Systems Act of 1973.

22. Department of Health and Human Services, *Healthy People 2000,* 287.

23. *Ibid,* 277.

24. Wasserman, Richard C., and others. "Bicyclists, Helmets and Head Injuries: A Rider-Based Study of Helmet Use and Effectiveness." *American Journal of Public Health* 78, no. 9 (September 1988): 1220–21.

25. National Safety Council, *Accident Facts, 1993,* 68.

26. Department of Health and Human Services, *Healthy People 2000,* 283.

CHAPTER FOURTEEN

Community Nutrition

Developing Healthy Eating Patterns

" . . . the eating patterns of this century represent as critical a public health concern as any now before us."

Senator George McGovern, Chairman, Select Committee on Nutrition and Human Needs, U.S. Senate, 1977.

Health problems related to nutrition are prevalent throughout the world, though they vary significantly from person to person, from community to community, and from culture to culture. The problems of hunger, starvation, and malnutrition are grave concerns worldwide. These conditions, affecting millions of people, occur principally in the poorest of the Third World nations and in those localities where political and natural tragedies have uprooted large populations.

Hunger and starvation, for the most part, are not characteristic of the developed world. In fact, a major health problem in the United States and many other industrial nations is *overconsumption* of food. Excessive intake of food, accompanied by a relatively sedentary life-style, results in obesity and an increased risk for major health problems.

Medical science has recorded an association between eating patterns and many of the chronic degenerative diseases.

Hypertension, heart disease, and other chronic conditions are related to excessive intake of certain nutrients.

In recent years people have responded to these findings and have altered their life-style, making weight loss and good nutrition priorities. This concern about obesity and overconsumption of food is demonstrated by the number of books dealing with the subject, the opening of more natural food stores, and the interest in fitness programs. However, many issues related to diet and weight control are controversial. Not all the books provide nutritionally sound advice. Many emphasize a particular item or dietary approach to the exclusion of all others, and do not consider an overall well-balanced diet. Also, many products sold in natural food stores are of questionable nutritional value.

Though food overconsumption and limited activity is the principal nutritional problem in America today, malnutrition does exist. It is found in various degrees among certain segments of the U.S. population. A physicians' task force studying hunger in America in 1984 found evidence of hunger and malnutrition.[1] The task force estimated that twenty million people are hungry at some time each month. This condition was found to be present basically among the economically disadvantaged, who encounter numerous health problems that are caused by malnutrition.

This population group includes many single-parent women, jobless minorities, unemployed blue-collar workers in times of depressed economic conditions, poor elderly, Native Americans, and migrant workers. In comparison to the relationships between chronic diseases and overconsumption, a different set of factors is associated with malnutrition. These factors are communicable diseases, developmental retardation, and reduced nutrient intake.

Poor nutrition is a problem for many pregnant teenagers, infants and school children, and the elderly. Local, state, and federal community health programs have been developed to meet the nutritional problems of these individuals.

Community nutrition programs have to deal with both malnutrition and overconsumption. Not only must programs be designed to provide foodstuffs, calories, and nutrients for the hungry and malnourished, but some guidance about eating patterns for weight reduction must also be available.

What to Believe?

The American consumer makes decisions about what to eat based on a variety of information. This information is often confusing and conflicting. Not only are the food advertisements that are developed by marketing specialists biased, misleading, and sometimes difficult to understand, but the recommendations of national boards and commissions often differ.

Standardization of nutrient and energy requirements is an inexact science. These standards, established by committees of experts, are published for the public. These are estimates of the proper nutrient intake for the good health of the average consumer.

Recommended Dietary Allowances (RDAs)

In the United States, the Recommended Dietary Allowances (RDAs), published by the Food and Nutrition Board of the National Research Council, have been the standards by which many dietitians, nutritionists, and physicians identify adequate nutritional intake. The Food and Nutrition Board published its first listing of RDAs in 1943 and has updated the chart periodically. The RDAs update is based on newly acquired nutritional knowledge and research findings.

The tenth edition of the Recommended Dietary Allowances (RDAs) was scheduled to be released in 1985. However, controversy kept these guidelines from being accepted and published. The basic conflict centered on RDA values for vitamins A and C.

The committee that was appointed to submit the 1985 RDAs recommended reducing RDA values for vitamin A and vitamin C by about one-third. The National Academy of Science rejected these recommendations.

They wanted these RDA values retained at the same levels as in the 1980 edition. Agreement could not be reached and, as a result, the academy rejected the entire report.

Debate among nutritionists continued for more than four years. Finally, in 1989 the tenth edition of the RDAs was published, with the RDA for both vitamins A and C at the same level as in the previous edition. One change was the recommendation extending the period of elevated calcium consumption from the age of eighteen to the age of twenty-four in the hope of preventing osteoporosis as one grows older.

It is important to understand that RDAs are not standards of minimum requirements, but indications of nutrient and caloric levels that should provide adequate nourishment for most consumers.[2] They establish guidelines for planning diets for public assistance programs, for nutrition education programs, and for other community nutrition activities.[3] The RDA listings as defined by the Food and Nutrition Board are ". . . levels of intake of essential nutrients considered . . . to be adequate to meet the known needs of practically all healthy persons."[4]

Dietary Food Guide

Another set of guidelines, the Dietary Food Guide, was published by the U.S. Department of Agriculture and Harvard University's Department of Nutrition. These guidelines have had the support of the American Medical Association.[5] They identify four different food groups: (1) milk and milk products; (2) meats, fish, poultry, dry beans, and other protein sources; (3) vegetables and fruits; and (4) breads and cereals. The guidelines recommend a moderate daily consumption of foods from each of the four food groups.

Dietary Goals for the United States

In 1977, the Senate Select Committee on Nutrition and Human Needs prepared a report that has received widespread attention.[6] The principal outcome of this report was the identification of six basic nutritional goals for the United States.

In addition to establishing the dietary goals, the committee set a number of buying guidelines for the American consumer. It was believed that by following these guidelines, the dietary goals could be met.

The buying guidelines recommended an increased consumption of fruits, vegetables, poultry, fish, and whole grains. These foods are important sources of vitamins and minerals yet are relatively low in fats, particularly saturated fat and cholesterol. Foods high in cholesterol, sugars, salt, and alcohol are directly related to six of the ten leading causes of death in America—heart disease, cancer, cerebrovascular disease, arteriosclerosis, diabetes, and cirrhosis of the liver.[7]

The subcommittee reported that the average American consumes 125 pounds of fat and one hundred pounds of sugar per year. Together, these two comprised 60 percent of the average diet.[8] Since two dietary goals called for the reduction of consumption of saturated fat and cholesterol, it was recommended that the American consumer decrease the amount of meat and other foods high in fat content. Americans were also advised to lower their intake of butterfat and eggs, and to substitute nonfat milk for whole milk.

The committee also strongly recommended a decrease in the consumption of sugar and salt. Soft drinks are a major source of sugar in the diet. In 1960, the average American consumed 13.6 gallons of soft drinks per year. By 1976, at the time of the subcommittee report, this amount had more than doubled to 27.6 gallons per year.[9] Not only has this contributed to a number of health problems because the sugar replaces necessary complex carbohydrates, but it has also reduced milk consumption, an excellent source of nutrition.

The American public uses salt, which is primarily sodium, for many purposes, including food preservation, food preparation, and general seasoning. The human body needs about one gram of salt a day to maintain body homeostasis, but the average American consumes between ten and twenty grams per day. Obviously, this is far too much.

Dietary Goals for the United States

1. Increase carbohydrate consumption to account for 55 to 60 percent of caloric intake
2. Reduce fat consumption from 40 to 30 percent of caloric intake
3. Reduce saturated fat consumption to account for about 10 percent of caloric intake
4. Reduce cholesterol consumption to about three hundred milligrams a day
5. Reduce sugar consumption by about 40 percent
6. Reduce salt consumption by about 50 to 85 percent to approximately three grams per day

Source: Select Committee on Nutrition and Human Needs, U.S. Senate. *Dietary Goals for the United States.* Washington, D.C.: U.S. Government Printing Office, 1977.

Too much sodium in the diet increases the risk of high blood pressure. It has been shown that individuals who live in areas where salt intake is high are much more likely to have hypertension than those who reside in localities with little sodium in the diet. Thus, a reduction in salt intake lowers the probability of hypertension.

Opinion about what is an appropriate level of sodium consumption differs. Scientific and medical recommendations suggest a range of 1.1 to 3.3 grams per day.[10] The average per capita sodium intake in the United States ranges from four to six grams per day. An individual following a salt-restricted diet, which is often recommended for those who have hypertension or who are at risk for this condition, may take in 3 grams per day.

Most people have little idea of how much sodium they ingest each day. To educate the public about the potential health danger of sodium, it seems reasonable to have warning labels on food products. Individuals at risk for hypertension could then avoid purchasing these foods. This would have not only a preventive effect but could also result in a long-range economic benefit. In congressional testimony, it was reported that the benefits of sodium labeling on all processed foods would lower the incidence of high blood pressure and save over one billion dollars in health care costs.

The Senate subcommittee, in addition to identifying dietary goals, advised that nutrition education programs be presented in the schools. It also recommended that improved food-processing methods be developed. The importance of food labeling for all foods was

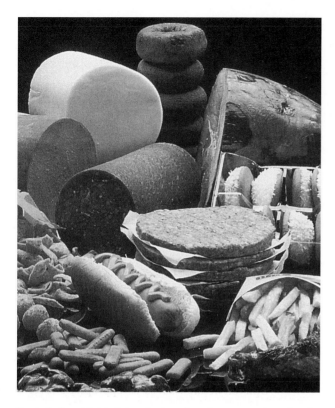

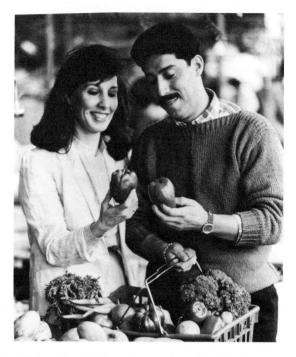

Healthful nutrition includes eating a variety of fruits and vegetables daily.

Foods that are high in fat content are favorites among many people. The dietary goals for the United States include a recommendation to reduce fat consumption from 40 percent to 30 percent of caloric intake.

addressed in this report. Realizing that there are many questions yet unanswered regarding human nutrition, the subcommittee also called for increased research.

The dietary goals have received widespread attention. As a result, they have encountered opposition from various groups. A frequently expressed concern is that the goals were set by political personnel after hearing hand-selected testimony. The food industry, such as the United Egg Producers, strongly opposes the recommendations that Americans cut back egg and meat consumption. They argue instead that their products contribute to good health.

Dietary Guidelines for Americans

In early 1980 the federal departments of Agriculture and of Health and Human Services issued the report *Dietary Guidelines for Americans*. This report, like the Food and Nutrition Board report, recommended that Americans eat

a variety of foods, avoid excess sodium, take alcohol only moderately, and maintain an ideal body weight. However, these two reports differed significantly on the role of fat, cholesterol, and carbohydrates in the diet.

The Department of Agriculture (USDA) and Health and Human Services (HHS) guidelines recommend that Americans avoid excessive fat, cholesterol, and sugar in the diet. It suggested that most Americans should increase the consumption of complex carbohydrates. On the other hand, the Food and Nutrition Board report suggested that only people at risk for heart disease need be concerned about cholesterol intake, and only obese individuals and those at risk for heart disease need be concerned about too much fat.

In 1985 the United States Department of Agriculture and the Department of Health and Human Services issued a second edition of the federal dietary guidelines. The original guidelines were slightly modified. The 1985 document stated that the diet of most Americans is adequate. It recommended that large-dose nutrient supplements be avoided. This report noted the usefulness of salt as a food preservative and stated that sodium is but one

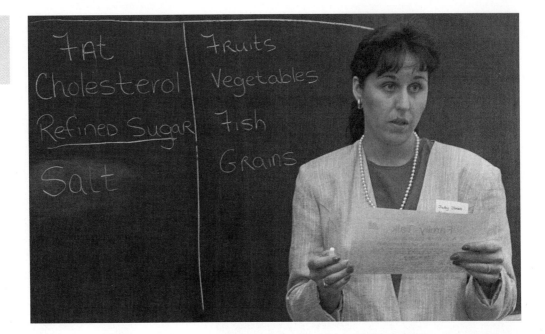

The need for decreasing sodium, fat, and sugar in the diet is noted by the nutrition expert.

factor known to affect hypertension. The guidelines included a strong caution warning of the dangers of drinking alcoholic beverages and driving. The public was instructed that if they drink, they should not drive.

In 1990 an updated statement was issued which was designed to make the guidelines more understandable and easier to implement. The responsibility for choices was placed more directly on the consumer by use of the words "choose" and "use." These revised guidelines incorporated the findings reported in the *Surgeon General's Report on Nutrition and Health of 1988* and the report of the National Research Council of the National Academy of Sciences, *Diet and Health: Implications for Reducing Chronic Disease Risk*, published in 1989.

The Surgeon General's Report on Nutrition and Health

The Surgeon General of the United States issued a report in 1988 on nutrition and health.[11] The main conclusion was that overconsumption of certain dietary components is now a major problem. Among the U.S. population there is a disproportionate consumption of foods high in fats at the expense of foods high in complex carbohydrates and fiber.

Dietary Guidelines for the United States 1990

1. Eat a variety of foods.
2. Maintain a healthy weight.
3. Choose a diet with plenty of vegetables, fruits, and grain products.
4. Choose a diet low in fat, saturated fat, and cholesterol.
5. Use sugars only in moderation.
6. Use salt and sodium only in moderation.
7. If you drink alcoholic beverages, do so in moderation. Moderation means no more than one drink a day for women and two drinks a day for men.

The report recommended that individuals eat vegetables, fruits, whole-grain products, fish, poultry without skin, lean meats, and low-fat dairy products. Thus the intake of complex carbohydrates and fiber would be increased and the intake of calories, fats, and cholesterol reduced.

The report spoke out against taking nutrient supplements. More than $2.7 billion is spent annually on supplemental vitamins, minerals, and other dietary substances that have no known value for healthy people. Therefore, many Americans are spending money on needless substances.

Usually nutritional supplements are safe for human consumption. However, taken in large quantities they have been shown to be harmful.

Food Guide Pyramid

In 1992, after more than a year of development, research, study, and evaluation, the United States Department of Agriculture introduced a new guide for nutrition, the Food Guide Pyramid. This pyramid was designed as a nutrition education graphic to replace the "Food Wheel" depicting the four basic food groups that had served for many years as a food guide for the American public. The Food Guide Pyramid has been designed to communicate the recommendations and health messages presented in the Dietary Guidelines for Americans.

Numerous pictographs were developed and evaluated. For example, blocks in a row, blocks in a circle, an inverted pyramid, a bowl, and even a shopping cart in pictograph presentation were analyzed.[12] Finally after testing and evaluating numerous variations of each design, the pyramid was selected.

The pyramid design indicates that the foundation of a nutritious diet should be six to eleven servings daily from the bread, cereal, rice, and pasta group. At the second level of the pyramid are the vegetable and fruit groups. An individual should have three to five servings daily of vegetables and two to four servings of fruit. Two to three servings daily from the milk, yogurt, and cheese group and also from the meat, poultry, fish, eggs, and nuts group are depicted in the pyramid. At the apex of the Food Guide Pyramid it is recommended that fats, oils, and sweets should be used sparingly.

These findings and recommendations by such prestigious groups have raised questions in the minds of many Americans about proper nutrition. Who is correct? Is fat a danger? How does cholesterol relate to health problems? It is the responsibility of those involved in community nutrition to provide accurate information without bias. Currently, much nutrition information is false or misleading, and the average individual must sort this out in order to develop a healthy diet.

Community nutrition has an important goal: the improved health of all people within the society. In a society where the average life-style results in obesity, heart disease, and numerous other diet-related health problems, this goal is most important. Not only is it difficult to cope with measures to control weight problems, but there are many conflicting opinions about what is good nutrition and adequate diet, and appropriate governmental responsibility in nutritional programming.

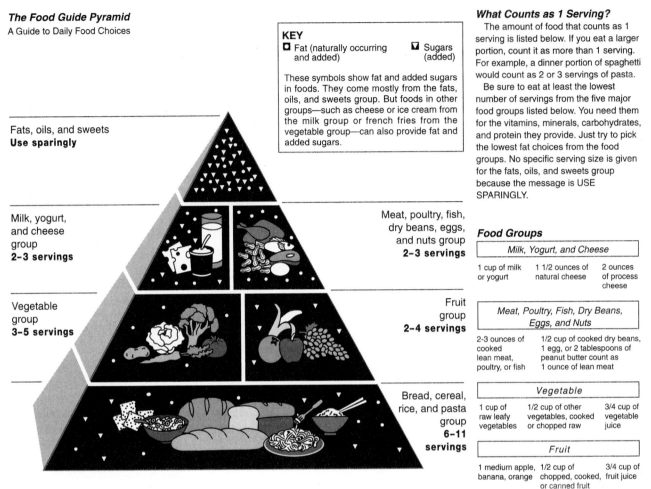

The Food Guide Pyramid
A Guide to Daily Food Choices

Fats, oils, and sweets
Use sparingly

Milk, yogurt,
and cheese
group
2–3 servings

Vegetable
group
3–5 servings

Meat, poultry, fish,
dry beans, eggs,
and nuts group
2–3 servings

Fruit
group
2–4 servings

Bread, cereal,
rice, and pasta
group
**6–11
servings**

KEY
☐ Fat (naturally occurring   ☑ Sugars
and added)   (added)

These symbols show fat and added sugars
in foods. They come mostly from the fats,
oils, and sweets group. But foods in other
groups—such as cheese or ice cream from
the milk group or french fries from the
vegetable group—can also provide fat and
added sugars.

What Counts as 1 Serving?

The amount of food that counts as 1
serving is listed below. If you eat a larger
portion, count it as more than 1 serving.
For example, a dinner portion of spaghetti
would count as 2 or 3 servings of pasta.

Be sure to eat at least the lowest
number of servings from the five major
food groups listed below. You need them
for the vitamins, minerals, carbohydrates,
and protein they provide. Just try to pick
the lowest fat choices from the food
groups. No specific serving size is given
for the fats, oils, and sweets group
because the message is USE
SPARINGLY.

Food Groups

Milk, Yogurt, and Cheese		
1 cup of milk or yogurt	1 1/2 ounces of natural cheese	2 ounces of process cheese

Meat, Poultry, Fish, Dry Beans, Eggs, and Nuts		
2-3 ounces of cooked lean meat, poultry, or fish	1/2 cup of cooked dry beans, 1 egg, or 2 tablespoons of peanut butter count as 1 ounce of lean meat	

Vegetable		
1 cup of raw leafy vegetables	1/2 cup of other vegetables, cooked or chopped raw	3/4 cup of vegetable juice

Fruit		
1 medium apple, banana, orange	1/2 cup of chopped, cooked, or canned fruit	3/4 cup of fruit juice

Looking at the Pieces of the Pyramid

The Food Guide Pyramid emphasizes foods from the five major food groups shown in the three lower
sections of the Pyramid. Each of these food groups provides some, but not all, of the nutrients you
need. Foods in one group can't replace those in another. No one of these major food groups is more
important than another—for good health, you need them all.

Nutrition Programs

Child Nutrition

Nutrition affects the health and well-being of all age
groups, races, and populations. Special concern should
be focused on the problems of malnutrition and obesity
in infant and child development. Malnutrition increases
the likelihood that exposure to infection will lead to disease. Also, it retards cognitive and social development.

Malnutrition has been shown to impair brain development in the early years of life, whereas good nutrition
among pregnant and lactating women has an important
positive influence on the health of newborn babies.

On the other hand, obesity among children has
increased in recent years. One in four obese children becomes an obese adult who experiences an increased risk
of such chronic conditions as heart disease, hypertension,
susceptibility to certain cancers, and arthritis. Obesity in
childhood also causes a number of psychological effects

on children. For example, low self-esteem, rejection by peers, and social isolation are often noted among obese children. Parents need to become better informed concerning proper nutrition for children to reduce the likelihood of obesity occurring. Reduction of fat in the diet is one of several important steps that can help to reduce this problem.

Because of the significant problems caused by malnutrition and obesity in infants and pregnant women, a number of child nutrition programs have been established in the United States. Child care food programs provide meals and food supplements for children in daycare centers and other similar facilities. The Head Start Program supplies food for economically disadvantaged children enrolled in the program. Another important program that provides food supplements to mothers and children is the Special Supplemental Food Program for Women, Infants, and Children (WIC). Many children receive at least one-third of the recommended dietary allowance (RDA) for nutrition through the School Lunch Program.[13]

Head Start Program

Though not designed primarily for nutrition, the federal Head Start Program has an important nutrition component. The basic purpose of Head Start is to provide children from low-income families with services that will enhance their personal development. Since many are physically, socially, and emotionally disadvantaged, this program provides opportunities and services that will help the young children to function adequately once they enter school.

Another important component of Head Start is the health program, in which the physical and mental health of each child is developed. Assessment activities include medical examinations and screening. Immunizations for common childhood diseases are provided. Improvement of the children's nutrition is an important aspect of the overall health program.

Meals are served to children enrolled in the Head Start Program. Breakfasts, lunches, dinners, and snacks are provided. The specific meals that each child receives are determined by the child's individual needs and the length of time the child is in the Head Start facility each day.

Not only do children enrolled in the Head Start Program receive nutritious meals, but parents are sometimes included in aspects of the programming. The parents become involved in the planning and preparation of the meals. This part of the program educates the parents. As they become involved in the process of creating good, nutritious meals for their children in the program, they are, in turn, learning to do the same at home for their families.

Special Supplemental Food Program for Women, Infants, and Children (WIC)

A major federal program designed to improve the nutrition of women and children is the WIC program. Known officially as the Special Supplemental Food Program for Women, Infants, and Children, it was started in 1972 as a pilot program. It has since expanded both in focus and emphasis. The WIC program provides nutritional assessment, counseling, free nutritious foods, nutrition education, access to health services, and supplemental foods to certain high-risk population groups in terms of nutrition-related health problems. Four groups were designated as recipients of the aid: (1) pregnant women, (2) new mothers, (3) infants, and (4) children under five years of age.

In order to qualify for the WIC program, the individual must be certified as "low income" by the state, a physician must indicate that there is a nutritional risk to the individual's health, and the individual must live in the geographical area in which the WIC program is located. State and local agencies do not always use the same criteria to establish risk. Only one risk factor is necessary for eligibility. The most common nutritional risks by participant category are:[14]

Infants
  Mother on WIC during pregnancy
  Inadequate nutrition intake
  History or presence of anemia
Children
  Inadequate nutrition intake
  History or presence of anemia
  Low height for age
  Low weight for height
  High weight for height
Pregnant Women
  Inadequate pregnancy weight gain
  History or presence of anemia
  Teenage pregnancy
  Inadequate nutrient intake
  Excessive pregnancy weight gain

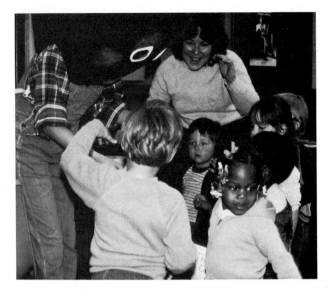

The Special Supplemental Food Program for Women, Infants, and Children (WIC) includes education. Here, "Fredwick" discusses good foods with the children to encourage proper eating patterns.

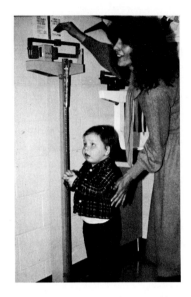

Participation in the WIC Program includes record keeping of the children's growth patterns. Each child weighs in to ascertain the growth that has taken place.

Postpartum Women
    Inadequate nutrient intake
    Teenage mother
    History of anemia
    High weight for height

The supplemental food received under this program contains nutrients that are often lacking in the diets of the populations at risk. The foods are high in protein, calcium, iron, and vitamins A and C. Infant formula, milk, juice, and other nutritious foodstuffs are made available.

Those who participate in the WIC program do not have to pay for the food because the program is funded by the United States Department of Agriculture. Funds are channeled through local agencies who certify the eligibility of participants. Local agencies providing direct services for WIC programs are city and/or county health departments, hospitals, and nonprofit organizations serving health and welfare needs. The state health department is the state agency responsible for this program; funds are channeled through this agency from the federal government. The state agency manages the program and sets standards for its operation.

A component built into the WIC program is nutrition education. Not only are food supplements available, but participants in the program receive instruction in nutrition. They are taught to read and understand food labels as well as how to prepare nutritious meals. The purpose of this is to improve the eating patterns of the participants. Nutrition education is also seen as an important preventive health measure.

The WIC program has been a very effective nutritional program because it affects the health status of many women and children.[15] Studies have reported that WIC participants eat more nutritious food than do non-WIC, low-income individuals. Nutrient quality of the diet continues to be better for WIC participants.[16] Not only does it have the positive effect of providing needed nutrients, but other health-related benefits have been identified. For example, WIC participants have increased their use of medical services in the community.[17] It is estimated that for every dollar spent on WIC, three dollars are saved in future health care costs.[18]

The federal government has exempted the WIC program from inclusion in the block-grant funding programs. Federal support for this program has remained

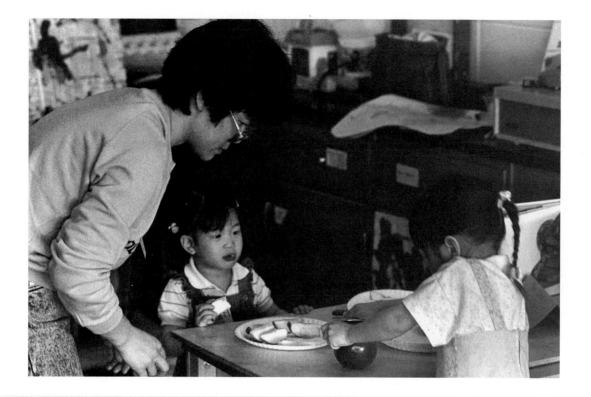

Teaching young children about good eating patterns is an important component of the WIC Program. During these early years lifetime eating habits are formed.

constant while reductions have occurred in other child nutrition programs. Because of increased needs and the relative stability of funding, there has been a reduction in the number of individuals being served in this program. In some localities, this has meant that many women and infants in need of nutritional assistance cannot obtain that help any longer. Often those who are just above the poverty level may not be eligible for the WIC program. It is to be hoped that this very effective program will continue to be operational in the years ahead.

Infant Breast-Feeding

Breast-feeding versus bottle-feeding has become a nutritional issue in many parts of the world, including the United States. Throughout many parts of the world, as economic development occurs, modern procedures are adopted. This has been the case in the way that mothers feed their infants.

Of course the natural way for an infant to be fed is from the mother's breast. Nutrient absorption, particularly of fat and iron, is greater with breast milk. Also, there are immunologic advantages to breast-feeding. The American Medical Association supports breast-feeding unless there are medical reasons for not doing so.[19] The only disadvantage of breast-feeding is in those few cases where insufficient milk can deprive the infant of necessary nutrients.

As countries develop and as mothers become more involved in working outside the home, infants are more often fed infant formula from the bottle, replacing breast-feeding. Unfortunately, a number of health problems have been identified with formula-feeding, particularly in the Third World. These problems include increased diarrhea, sickness, respiratory illness, allergic reactions to the formula, and stomach ailments. Without

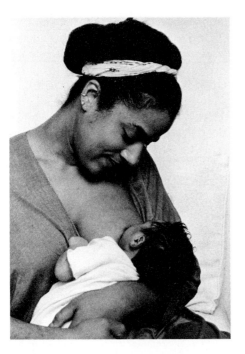

There are numerous health advantages to breast-feeding a newborn child. A mother's milk contains all the nutrients that a baby needs. Also, protection against certain childhood diseases is obtained from the mother's antibodies.

any question, breast milk is more nutritional and is a major contribution to the improved health and survival of infants.

All too often in Third World settings there are inadequate facilities to wash a used bottle before it is reused. Also, because of low economic status and a lack of knowledge, many mothers dilute the amount of formula with larger than required amounts of water. Usually this water has not been purified and, as a result, many waterborne illnesses are contracted by the infant.

In 1981 the United Nations passed a nonbinding code—a statement of principle, which had no enforcement mechanism—restricting the marketing of infant formula in the world. One hundred and nineteen nations supported this action; only the United States opposed it. The American government stated that the code unfairly restricted commerce.

The pressures of corporate industry were more influential than the health of children throughout the world. This unfortunate action of the presidential administration was soundly opposed by most public health personnel, agencies, and organizations. Interestingly, both houses of Congress passed resolutions that condemned the stand taken by the United States government. An action as important to the overall health of children as breast-feeding must not be negatively affected by political determinates.

Breast-feeding is a concern not only in developing nations but also in the United States. In the United States there has been a downward trend in the percentage of mothers who breast-feed their newborn babies. Older women, women with higher levels of education, and professional women are most likely to breast-feed, while teenage mothers, women of low socioeconomic status, and minorities are least likely.[20]

Reports state that African-American mothers are one-third as likely to breast-feed as Caucasian mothers. Breast-feeding by Hispanic mothers dropped by nearly one-half in the United States during the 1970s. In the case of Indochinese refugees, the incidence of breast-feeding drops to 25 percent from nearly 100 percent within six months of their arrival in America.[21]

The importance of promoting breast-feeding has been noted in the Year 2000 National Health Objectives. An objective of 75 percent of mothers who breast-feed with 50 percent continuing to breast-feed for the first five or six months has been established. The accompanying box illustrates the significant difference between the goal and the percentage of women, particularly minority females, who breast-feed their infants.

Programs have been developed to promote breast-feeding among low socioeconomic working women. These programs include education to inform the women of the importance of breast-feeding and to encourage employers to establish policies that will assist the new mothers. Many local health departments have developed programs in liaison with other community agencies to promote breast-feeding.

Nutrition education programs need to be designed to encourage all mothers to breast-feed their infants. Business and industry must establish maternal leave policies that would permit women to breast-feed. Only as people understand the long-term health values and benefits of breast-feeding will the health status of children improve. Women who cannot breast-feed will not necessarily have children with lower health status if they use infant formula as directed.

Year 2000 Objectives—Breast-feeding		
	1988	**Objective–2000**
Proportion of All Mothers Who Breast-feed	54.3%	75%
Low-Income Mothers	32%	75%
African-American Mothers	25%	75%
American Indian Mothers	47%	75%
Hispanic Mothers	51%	75%
Mothers Who Breast-feed for Five to Six Months	22%	50%

Source: Department of Health and Human Services. *Healthy People 2000: National Health Promotion and Disease Prevention Objectives.* Washington, D.C.: U.S. Government Printing Office, 1991, Obj. 2.11, p. 123.

Food Stamp Program

A federal program that has helped to meet the nutritional needs of many U.S. citizens is the Food Stamp Program. This program, in its present form, was started in 1961 as a pilot project in several selected localities. With the passage of the Food Stamp Act of 1964, the program was established nationwide.[22]

The basic purpose of the Food Stamp Program is to provide the means for the economically disadvantaged to obtain needed foodstuffs. The population served by food stamps includes households with incomes below the federal poverty level, with eligibility based on income and other financial resources. The head of the household must apply to receive food stamps, and then local offices evaluate the application to approve eligibility for involvement in the program.

Those who are qualified and registered to receive food stamps receive them on a regular basis through the mail. The stamps are used to purchase groceries through the normal food-marketing channels, and food stores redeem the stamps at face value. An individual may purchase any food item with the stamps. Nonfood items, such as paper products, alcoholic beverages, pet food, soap, and cleaning products, cannot be purchased with the stamps.

The Food Stamp Program was established principally to improve the nutrition of the poor in America. Malnutrition and hunger affect the elderly, infants and children of the poor, Native Americans, migrants, and pregnant teenagers. It is these populations that have benefited the most from this federal program.

Another purpose of the Food Stamp Program, as noted by Congress, is to strengthen the agricultural economy.[23] When people are able to purchase more foodstuffs, the demand for these foodstuffs increases and the agricultural industry is able to sell more products, thus stimulating the agricultural economy.

The effectiveness of the Food Stamp Program is questionable because of the numerous problems associated with it. One problem has been nonparticipation by many who are qualified.[24] Many people who are qualified to receive food stamps do not do so because they do not understand the program, because of bureaucratic problems associated with registering and qualifying, or because of personal pride. On the other hand, a significant problem is involvement in the Food Stamp Program by individuals who do not qualify or for whom the program was not principally designed.

In spite of the problems associated with the Food Stamp Program, it must be recognized that over twenty-five million people a year benefit who otherwise would not have been able to obtain adequate nutrition. More than half of these people are children and adolescents under eighteen years of age. The importance of good nutrition for infants, children, and the elderly, in particular, makes this program seem most worthwhile, despite its abuses.

Since 1981, governmental regulations have reduced the number of people eligible to receive food stamps. These regulations have placed greater financial responsibility for this program on the individual states. Certain population groups who could receive food stamps in the past are no longer eligible. Unfortunately, many people who need the assistance, especially the borderline poor, may not qualify.

Food Information Labeling

What we eat has a direct relationship to disease and to the quality of our personal health. Failure to obtain certain essential nutrients can result in specific diseases or health problems. In addition, excessive intake of certain nutrients contributes to health problems.

In order to be able to make intelligent food selections, people should have information about the nutrients found in food. Therefore, the public should be provided with as much information about the food they eat as is possible. This means that nutritional labeling should be a part of the marketing of all foods. This labeling must be informative and meaningful to the average consumer.

Food information labeling was introduced in 1973. Three federal agencies are responsible for governing food labeling in the United States. The labeling of all foods except meat, poultry, and egg products is administered by the Food and Drug Administration. The United States Department of Agriculture (USDA) regulates meat, poultry, and egg products. Food advertising is governed by the Federal Trade Commission.

The Food and Drug Administration requires that all packaged foods display the name of the product and the manufacturer. Any food to which a nutrient has been added or that makes a nutritional claim must have a label. The list of ingredients included in the food must also be indicated.

Labeling is helpful in the selection of foods. It is helpful for those individuals who are counting calories or for people on special diets recommended by their physicians. Reading labels is also helpful in comparing the costs of two similar products.

In 1990 Congress passed the Nutrition Labeling and Education Act. This legislation was designed to require that food labels be developed that the public could understand and that would be useful to all individuals in helping to make healthy food choices. It is the responsibility of the Food and Drug Administration todevelop labels that give information regarding food in the context of the total diet. Food manufacturers were required to comply with the new labeling requirements by mid-1994.

Uniform information regarding cholesterol, saturated fats, calories, complex carbohydrates, sugars, fibers, and protein must be provided for all processed foods. Consumers are now able to compare these nutrients found in a given food product with their overall daily dietary needs. The serving size is to be the basis for reporting the nutrient content of food. Serving sizes under provision of the new labeling regulations will be more uniform and reflect the amount that people actually eat at one time.

In addition, it is now necessary that there be a commonality in the use of terms such as: "free," "low," "light," "less," "high," "source of," "more," "fresh," and "reduced." When such terms are used by a food or beverage

Examples of Acceptable Nutrient Descriptors on Food Labels

"Free"—product contains no, or negligible, amounts of fat, saturated fat, cholesterol, sodium, sugars, and calories.

"Low"—term used when the foods can be eaten frequently without exceeding dietary guidelines. For example, "low fat" signifies three grams or less per serving.

"Less"—the food contains 25 percent less of a nutrient or calories than the reference food.

"Light"—the product contains one-third fewer calories or half the fat of the reference food.

Source: *FDA Backgrounder*, BG 92–4 (December 10, 1992).

manufacturer, there must be a measurable frame of reference used for all consumers to understand.

Under provisions of this legislation, labeling requirements do not apply to fresh meat, fish, poultry, and produce products. Also, food served in restaurants, on airplanes, and in hospital cafeterias is exempt from nutrition labeling. Food served by food service vendors and in bakeries and delicatessens is also exempt.

The food labels now include information as to the percent of the Daily Value of the particular food. The Daily Values tell the nutritional content based on a 2,000-calorie-per-day diet. In other words, for each nutrient the amount of the particular food will be presented as a percentage of what would be the Daily Value for that particular nutrient.

The regulations permit a statement on the food label describing the relationship between a nutrient and the risk of a particular disease for seven different conditions. These include the relationship between the following:[25]

1. Calcium intake and osteoporosis for individuals in certain population groups.

2. A low-fat diet and the reducing of some types of cancer.

3. Foods low in saturated fat and cholesterol and reducing the likelihood of coronary heart disease.

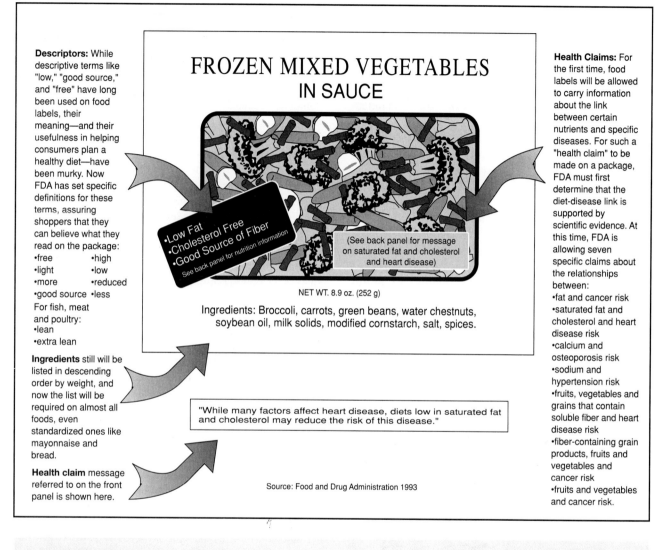

Descriptors: While descriptive terms like "low," "good source," and "free" have long been used on food labels, their meaning—and their usefulness in helping consumers plan a healthy diet—have been murky. Now FDA has set specific definitions for these terms, assuring shoppers that they can believe what they read on the package:
- free
- light
- more
- good source
- high
- low
- reduced
- less

For fish, meat and poultry:
- lean
- extra lean

Ingredients still will be listed in descending order by weight, and now the list will be required on almost all foods, even standardized ones like mayonnaise and bread.

Health claim message referred to on the front panel is shown here.

FROZEN MIXED VEGETABLES IN SAUCE

- Low Fat
- Cholesterol Free
- Good Source of Fiber

See back panel for nutrition information

(See back panel for message on saturated fat and cholesterol and heart disease)

NET WT. 8.9 oz. (252 g)

Ingredients: Broccoli, carrots, green beans, water chestnuts, soybean oil, milk solids, modified cornstarch, salt, spices.

"While many factors affect heart disease, diets low in saturated fat and cholesterol may reduce the risk of this disease."

Source: Food and Drug Administration 1993

Health Claims: For the first time, food labels will be allowed to carry information about the link between certain nutrients and specific diseases. For such a "health claim" to be made on a package, FDA must first determine that the diet-disease link is supported by scientific evidence. At this time, FDA is allowing seven specific claims about the relationships between:
- fat and cancer risk
- saturated fat and cholesterol and heart disease risk
- calcium and osteoporosis risk
- sodium and hypertension risk
- fruits, vegetables and grains that contain soluble fiber and heart disease risk
- fiber-containing grain products, fruits and vegetables and cancer risk
- fruits and vegetables and cancer risk.

The new food label at a glance.

4. Foods high in fiber and reducing certain types of cancer.

5. Foods high in fiber and reducing the risk of heart disease.

6. Foods low in sodium and preventing the development of high blood pressure.

7. Fruits and vegetables and reducing the risk of cancer.

It is now the responsibility of the individual states to enforce labeling regulations. In spite of much opposition from the food industry, it is the position of the federal government that the cost of implementing this labeling initiative will be cost effective. It is estimated that the cost to implement the nutrition labeling program will be $1.7 billion. However, between $4 and $20 billion will be saved in reduced health care costs, deaths, and improved quality of life over a period of time.[26]

The federal government, in its objectives for the nation, stated that by the year 2000 at least 85 percent of all adults should be reading food labels to assist in their food selections.[27] Since the mid-1980s the demand for regulation of health-related or disease prevention claims on food labels has risen. But there is controversy about the kind of scientific evidence necessary to substantiate the claims.

Not everyone agrees that nutrition labeling, required by both federal and state governments, is needed. As expected, many in the food industry have been opposed to the regulations; they do not believe the government should regulate private enterprise. In addition, they point out that food labeling increases production costs, which are then passed on to the consumers. Other opponents suggest that most Americans do not read or understand the warning labels. Nevertheless, as consumers become more knowledgeable and concerned about cholesterol, fat, and sodium intake, they have a right to be provided with as much information as possible to assist in their food selection.

Food Additives

Much of the food and drink Americans ingest contains added chemicals. Over thirteen hundred additives have been approved by the Food and Drug Administration (FDA) for use in foods for human consumption. Only about a third of these are actually used as food additives, and these are used for a variety of purposes.

For centuries people have added substances to their food. Over 90 percent of all processed food sold today contains additives. They are used as preservatives, thickeners, and emulsifiers to improve texture, and for flavor and color.

Before the advent of refrigeration, meat was salted, smoked, and sun dried in order to preserve it. Some food additives serve other useful purposes. Without preservatives to prevent the formation of mold and bacteria, many foods would spoil and could not be shipped great distances, which would lead to geographical limitations on the availability of foods. In particular, the vast assortment of foods in urban areas would be greatly reduced.

Humectants are added to food to retain texture by preventing and retarding moisture loss. These additives are found in marshmallows as well as in many tobacco products. Many food additives serve as artificial flavorings, for example, monosodium glutamate. Although this additive is considered to be safe for human consumption, some individuals are sensitive to it and experience nausea, headache, and chest pains after ingesting it.

Concern has been expressed in recent years about the increased use of food additives. These concerns have developed over the uncertainty of the amounts that are safe for human consumption, the quality of testing by the Food and Drug Administration, and the possible connection between certain additives and cancer, cardiovascular diseases, and hyperactivity.

Having food additives in our diet is a topic of great debate. Some additives are felt to be useful only as marketing ploys. For example, artificial coloring and flavoring have no nutritive value. Their sole purpose is to make food appear more appealing to the consumer. Artificial flavoring is used in a variety of foods, particularly in soft drinks.

Artificial coloring gives the consumer the impression that the product has a greater content of a given ingredient than is really present. For example, artificial coloring is used in flavored ice cream to give the impression that there is more lime, raspberry, or cherry than is really in the product. Artificial coloring, the most controversial of food additives, is suspected of being carcinogenic. But little is actually known about the effects of using these chemicals over a long period of time.

It must be noted that most chemicals used as food additives are safe. However, the Food and Drug Administration has banned over twenty-five additives known to be toxic to humans or animals. Over half have been coal tar dyes known as "artificial colors."[28]

When combined in the digestive system with other chemicals, certain food additives may be dangerous. For example, nitrites that are used in meat to make it look fresh and attractive have been associated with cancer. Research has shown that nitrite, even by itself, might cause cancer.[29] Approved since 1925, it has been used for years as a meat preservative because it inhibits the growth of bacterial spores that cause botulism. In the 1960s, scientists discovered that, in combination with other substances, nitrite produces a family of chemicals called nitrosamines. Some of these chemicals have caused cancer in laboratory animals. This has caused great concern in the meat industry because one-tenth of the nation's food supply is dependent upon this single food additive.[30]

Calcium cyclamate was a widely used artificial sweetener, but it was banned in the early 1980s when it was linked with testicular atrophy, chromosome damage, and bladder cancer.

How strict should federal regulations be in controlling the amount of additives in food that is sold in our stores? Should food additives that contain even a small portion of a possible cancer-causing agent be banned? These questions and similar issues have caused serious debate, differences of opinion, and legislative action.

Under provisions of the food and drug laws known as the Delaney Amendment[31] any substance found to be carcinogenic in either animals or humans cannot be approved as a food additive. This legislation has been the source of much controversy. Critics say it is inflexible and confusing. For example, the law does not apply to many additives introduced before 1958, the year it became effective. They also argue that in some situations, additives in trace amounts are essential for human nutrition, but in large doses may be carcinogenic. Advocates of the Delaney Amendment suggest that to permit the use of certain additives that may be carcinogenic will "open the door" for other cancer-causing agents.

Several food additives have been declared unsafe for human consumption. In some instances, particularly in the case of saccharin, many people have questioned the efficacy of such a ruling. Under the Delaney Amendment, saccharin would have been banned; however, Congress ruled that this could not occur.

It is the position of many, particularly the food-marketing industry, that no food additive can be declared absolutely safe. They argue that food additives should be allowed if the risk to humans is not significant.

The quality of additive testing by the Food and Drug Administration has been questioned by consumer groups. A time lapse of as much as five years may occur between the declaration that a substance is dangerous and the actual outlawing of that additive. Consumer

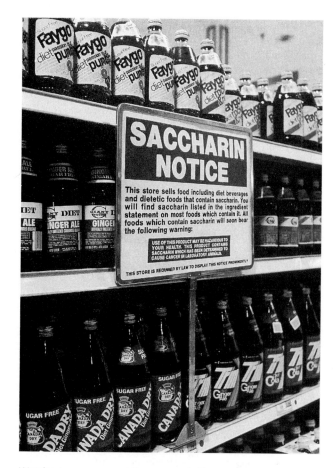

Warning to consumers at the grocery shelf.

groups maintain that the Food and Drug Administration acts too slowly in warning the public and then permits the public to consume the substance while it is still being investigated.

As can be seen, there are many questions about the use of food additives in the American diet. Admittedly, some additives are necessary, but there are potential dangers in others. A definitive response to this issue will not appear in the immediate future. In the meantime, the consumer should learn to eat food that does not contain excessive amounts of additives. Eating fresh fruit and vegetables, fresh meat, and whole-grain products is most important in order to protect ourselves from additives.

Learning to read the labels on food will also be useful in reducing the amount of nonnutritious food additives ingested.

Chemicals, Pesticides, and Foods

Several thousand pesticides are manufactured and used in the agricultural industry today to control weeds, fungi, and insects, and to facilitate the growth of fruits and vegetables. People are becoming increasingly concerned about the effect of these chemicals on human health. Evidence indicates that long-term exposure to some of these chemicals through the food we eat can cause disease. The Environmental Protection Agency has concluded that the risk for cancer linked to pesticides in food is surpassed only by occupational exposure to chemicals and indoor radon.[32]

Many different pesticides are used by farmers on most vegetables, including spinach, lettuce, and celery. Some fifty pesticides are permitted to be used in broccoli production.[33] Particular concern has been expressed about parathion, which is considered a possible human carcinogen.

The matter of Alar and apples brought the matter to a head. Since the 1960s apples in many parts of the country have been sprayed with deminozide, a chemical used to prevent apples from dropping from trees before they are ripe. Apples treated with this chemical have better color and are firmer. However, it has been shown that the chemical penetrates the apple so that it cannot be washed off, or removed by peeling the apple. Neither can it be destroyed by cooking.

When heated, Alar breaks down into UDMH, which may cause cancer. The level in the human body at which this chemical causes cancer is not known. In fact, it is not known whether UDMH is carcinogenic. However, nutritionists, scientists, and oncologists are suggesting that those who eat large amounts of apples and drink a lot of apple juice may be at greater risk for cancer.

In 1989 nationwide attention was brought to the problem of Alar in apples. Many individuals refrained from buying apples and apple products, and some schools banned apples from their menus. The issue confused many people, and confidence in the safety of apples was undermined.

Strong public action forced apple producers to stop using Alar, and the manufacturer agreed to voluntarily remove it from production and use. By the end of 1989, public confidence in apples had been restored. Sales were reported up 10 to 30 percent from the previous year.[34]

The food-processing and retail industries have been very opposed to similar bans on other chemicals used in food growth and production. Agricultural managers also have been very upset at such initiatives because they want to be able to use chemicals to enhance the growth of their crops and thus get better economic returns.

Beef and fish present other concerns. Hormone implants are used in steers to stimulate the growth of lean muscle. Because these hormones remain in the animal, they are taken into the human body when one eats beef. No danger to human health has been proved at this time. However, little research has investigated the long-term effects. Fish taken from lakes, particularly the Great Lakes, contain toxins. For example, salmon and coho have been shown to contain PCBs, dieldrin, and increased levels of DDT.

Under provisions of the Federal Insecticide, Fungicide, and Rodenticide Act, the Environmental Protection Agency has the responsibility for regulating chemicals used in food production, but it has not been able to conduct research and set levels for thousands of these products manufactured in the United States. In addition, this federal agency does not have the work force to sample the food supply of the entire nation. The Environmental Protection Agency is not responsible for monitoring meat and poultry products. This is the responsibility of the United States Department of Agriculture.

With the American public consuming greater amounts of chicken, concern has been expressed about recent outbreaks of salmonella. Salmonella is a bacterial organism that causes serious food poisoning. The United States Department of Agriculture reported increasing numbers of cases of chickens being contaminated with salmonella. The Centers for Disease Control have reported a significant increase in food poisoning from the consumption of fresh eggs. The use of raw eggs in such items as eggnog presents the danger of contracting this disease.

Mass Media Influence

Much of the public's knowledge and information about foods is obtained through the mass media. Advertisements on radio, television, and in newspapers, books, and journals entice the consumer to eat a range of appetizingly packaged foods. Little is said about the nutrient values of these products. Many times marketing and sale of the food—not the product's health value to individuals—are the prime goals.

Children are encouraged by entertaining advertisements to eat sugar-coated cereals, creamy candy bars, and other foods high in sugar. Numerous sales approaches are used to interest growing children in eating foods that contain little or no nutrient value. Adults are presented with similar advertisements for soft drinks and other foods high in sugar, salt, and saturated fat.

It is doubtful that society can expect the corporate food industry to highlight the inherent dangers of excessive sugars, high levels of sodium, and increased fat and cholesterol in their marketing promotions. Some consumer and nutrition groups have advocated federal regulations to control media advertising, particularly in television. It is unlikely, though, in a time of increased opposition to federal regulatory activities, that such restrictions will become a reality.

It is increasingly important that public nutrition education programs focus upon these dangers so that the consumer is better prepared to buy intelligently. Food product advertising in the mass media should be countered by effective and accurate nutrition messages informing the population of healthful diets. This would probably be more effective than the regulation of advertising in the mass media.

Eating Behavior

Dietary Factors

The American public displays a significant interest in diet. What we eat, how much we eat, and other factors in our life-style associated with eating are of great importance to many people. Some people spend a lot of time reading food labels, listening to those selling special diets, talking about eating, and taking classes in diet control.

Every year a number of new diets with various claims and promises gain attention. Some diets promise to solve a particular problem, while others indicate that the diet will contribute to weight control and good health. The weight loss diets seem to be the most popular. Anything that promises quick weight loss has much appeal to many people. Other diets, particularly high-fiber diets, promise protection against certain diseases.

Certainly how and what we eat does contribute to health and wellness. For example, certain relationships between diet and headache have been established. It has been shown that certain foods which contain tyramine, cheeses for example, can dilate and constrict blood vessels and bring on headaches. Chemical imbalance resulting from diet also contributes to headaches.

In recent years there has been an increased consciousness regarding what we eat and how it affects one's health. Awareness that meats such as pork, lamb, and beef are rich in fat has led to a reduction in consumption of these products. In 1976 beef consumption was a little over ninety-four pounds per person; by the start of 1990 it had dropped to sixty-seven pounds per person. In contrast, the per capita consumption of chicken rose from forty-three to sixty-nine pounds during this same period. In the early 1990s Americans are eating more chicken than beef.

The meat-growing industry is changing its product to address these new concerns of the American public. Both pigs (pork) and cattle (beef) are being bred leaner. Pork is now allowed about half the amount of fat it had twenty-five years ago, and the meat-packing industry is making efforts to trim fat from the product in the marketplace. Cattle are spending less time in feedlots, where they are fattened for market. Leaner cattle from abroad have been imported for mating in an effort to produce a less-fattened product.[35]

Restaurants are providing options on their menus for people wishing diets low in fatty foods and in calories. Today one finds more salad bars and more fish and chicken dishes on the menus of most restaurants. Juices, fruit, decaffeinated coffee, and diet soft drinks now experience widespread popularity. The interest in healthier dietary patterns is highlighted by the fact that schools that train chefs now include instruction in nutrition.

One of the nation's health promotion/disease prevention objectives is that 90 percent of all restaurants should offer low-fat, low-calorie food choices by the year 2000. This is particularly important when one realizes that on a normal day in the United States as many as one-fifth of the population eat in a food establishment.[36]

Margarine, which contains less saturated fat than butter and little cholesterol, is found in many restaurants. In 1986 the McDonald Corporation announced that Chicken McNuggets and Filet of Fish would be cooked in 100 percent vegetable oil only. This popular fast-food chain also indicated that they would no longer serve whole milk; only 2% milk or nonfat milk is available.

The American Heart Association, working in cooperation with restaurants throughout the nation, has developed menus that are low in cholesterol and other elements that are risk factors for cardiovascular disease. The association has set certain guidelines and criteria that the restaurant must meet in order to advertise that their menu is acceptable for positive cardiovascular health. Any restaurant or restaurant chain that wishes to indicate to their customers that items on their menu meet American Heart Association guidelines may do so. This program is known as the *Creative Cuisine* program.

Combined with this increased concern about how and what we eat has been interest in a number of other factors related to weight control and good health. The emphasis on physical activity along with diet in disease prevention has also become an interest of thousands. In addition, the relationships of food intake and chronic diseases and the role of genetics in obesity are being investigated by those involved in community nutrition programs.

Eating Disorders

Two eating disorders have received increased attention in recent years: (1) *anorexia nervosa* and (2) *bulimia*. The incidence of these two different but interrelated disorders is increasing dramatically in our society, particularly among young women in their teens and early twenties.

Anorexia nervosa is not a new disorder. Documented cases can be traced back to at least the thirteenth century; however, it was about a hundred years ago in England when the disorder was given the description we

---

Diagnostic Criteria for Anorexia Nervosa

1. Intense fear of becoming obese
2. Disturbance of body image, claiming to "feel fat"
3. Weight loss of at least 24 percent of original body weight
4. Refusal to maintain body weight over a minimal normal weight for age and height
5. No known physical illness that would account for weight loss

Source: Northwest Ohio Center for Eating Disorders, St. Vincent Hospital, Toledo, Ohio.

---

know today as anorexia nervosa.[37] This disorder is characterized by a refusal to eat and a fear of weight gain.

Concern about weight gain reaches such magnitude that the individual develops an obsession with weight loss, actually resulting in a fear of weight gain. Excessive dieting reaching starvation levels produces a number of serious physiological and psychological problems. The desired body image is usually extreme thinness. The individual seems to enjoy losing weight. The refusal to eat is a pleasurable indulgence.

A second eating disorder is bulimia. The term means "ox hunger" or "voracious appetite." In this disorder the individuals may stuff themselves with food, then take laxatives or force themselves to vomit in order to eliminate the food. This practice, often referred to as the "binge-purge" syndrome, leads to dehydration, possible damage to the esophagus, and dental decay. Laxative abuse may result in damage to certain digestive organs.

Bulimia is not an incapacitating condition. However, the individual tends to spend time eating alone. After eating the individual feels fat and fears getting fatter; this results in the purging.

Treatment centers have been established in a number of medical facilities throughout the nation. Hospital inpatient care is one part of the program. During this phase of the treatment program a nutritional assessment is usually conducted. Therapy is provided to help the individual recover lost nutrients. Supplementary feedings and other nutrient disturbances accompany the return to normal eating patterns. While hospitalized, the person participates in a number of activities designed to help him or her overcome the psychological problems associated with the eating disorder.

Diagnostic Criteria for Bulimia

1. Recurrent episodes of binge eating
2. At least three of the following:
   A. Consumption of high-caloric, easily ingested food
   B. Inconspicuous eating during a binge
   C. Termination of eating episode by abdominal pain, sleep, or self-induced vomiting
   D. Repeated attempts to lose weight
   E. Frequent weight fluctuations greater than ten pounds
3. Awareness that eating pattern is abnormal
4. Fear of not being able to stop eating voluntarily
5. Depressed mood and self-deprecating thoughts following binges
6. Bulimic episodes not due to any known physical disorder

Source: Northwest Ohio Center for Eating Disorders, St. Vincent Hospital, Toledo, Ohio.

Relaxation therapy designed to teach body awareness, physiotherapy, individual psychotherapy, and group therapy have all been used to treat those with eating disorders. Behavior modification strategies have also been used.[38]

Both eating disorders require several years of active treatment once the person is released from the hospital. This requires involvement of family, friends, and others who are important in the life of the patient. Self-help groups have been established in many communities to provide supportive assistance. The goal of all treatment programs, both inpatient and outpatient, is to positively influence eating patterns and to develop a more appropriate and positive self-image.

Summary

A variety of health problems that involve nutritional patterns afflict humanity. In the United States overconsumption of food results in obesity and an increased risk for a number of different chronic diseases. On the other end of the spectrum, malnutrition is found among certain segments of the American population, particularly the economically disadvantaged.

A wealth of nutritional information, recommendations, and guidelines is available to the American consumer. For years the Recommended Daily Allowances (RDAs) have served as guidelines for adequate nutrition. The Dietary Guidelines for Americans, first published in 1980 and revised and updated in 1985 and 1990, now serve as guidelines for nutritional food intake. Based upon these guidelines the Food Guide Pyramid has been developed to serve as a pictograph to provide guidance to Americans about good nutrition.

Even though nutritional status affects the health of people in all age groups, several federal programs have been developed with the goal of improving the diets of pregnant women, newborn infants, and children. The Head Start Program provides meals for economically disadvantaged children. The Supplemental Food Program for Women, Infants, and Children (WIC) provides food supplements for mothers and children. These programs, along with others, have been effective in improving the nutritional status of women, infants, and children.

Another federal program, the Food Stamp Program, allows the economically disadvantaged to obtain needed foodstuffs. The food stamps are used to purchase groceries and so improve the nutritional status of many poor people in America.

In order to make intelligent decisions in food selection, people need information about the nutrients in the food that is purchased. In order to be better informed, people need labeling on all packaged foods. Labeling should inform the consumer of the nutrients and additives in the food. Many foods contain additives that are not nutritious, and some may even be harmful.

A number of different chemicals are used by the agricultural industry to facilitate growth of crops. Concern about the effects of these chemicals on humans has grown in recent years. This concern was highlighted in 1989 by the problem of Alar in apples and apple products. Measures must be taken and research conducted to reduce the potential dangers of these chemicals.

There is an increasing interest in weight control and disease prevention as it relates to eating patterns among many Americans. This has led to greater intake of such products as chicken and fish, and less consumption of beef, pork, and lamb. Restaurants, the food-marketing industry, and agriculture have all been influenced by these changing American eating patterns.

Two eating disorders are noted among many people of high school and college age, particularly women. These eating disorders are anorexia nervosa and bulimia. Anorexia is a condition wherein the individual develops an unrealistic body image and fails to eat adequate amounts of food. As a result there is not only weight loss but also serious nutrient depletions. In bulimia the individual overeats, then purges the food by vomiting. Both eating disorders usually require the help of medical personnel and self-help therapies to overcome the problems.

Discussion Questions

1. Which is the greater problem in America, overconsumption of food or malnutrition? Explain your answer.

2. How are the Recommended Dietary Allowances (RDAs) designed to be used?

3. Discuss the dietary goals for the United States as stated by the Senate Select Committee on Nutrition and Human Needs.

4. Do you support the dietary goals of the senate subcommittee? Why or why not?

5. Explain which health problems are caused by excessive intake of sodium.

6. Discuss the dietary guidelines for Americans as published in 1990.

7. Identify several of the recommendations highlighted in the Surgeon General's Report on Nutrition and Health (1988).

8. Explain the purpose for development of the Food Guide Pyramid.

9. What provisions for improved nutrition are part of the Head Start Program?

10. Explain the various components and objectives of the Special Supplemental Food Program for Women, Infants, and Children (WIC).

11. Discuss the impact that the WIC program has had on the health status of women and children.

12. What issues were involved in the United States' position taken in 1981 at the United Nations regarding infant formula?

13. Discuss the national health objective for the year 2000 as it relates to infant breast-feeding.

14. Explain the various components of the Food Stamp Program.

15. Do you believe that all foods should have complete information labeling? Defend your answer.

16. What information is to be included on food labels under mandate of the Nutrition Labeling and Education Act?

17. What are some of the purposes of food additives?

18. Should food additives that contain a small portion of a carcinogenic agent be marketed for human consumption?

19. What were the issues in the controversy surrounding Alar and apples?

20. Should press and mass media food advertisements be regulated? Defend your answer.

21. Discuss some of the measures being taken by the food-marketing industry and restaurants to accommodate the concern of many people over diet and health.

22. Explain some of the differences between bulimia and anorexia nervosa.

23. Discuss some of the diagnostic criteria for anorexia and bulimia.

24. What are some of the treatment modalities followed in care for those with eating disorders?

Suggested Readings

"An End to Label Hype?" *Consumers Report* 57, no. 1 (January 1992): 32–33.

Bailey, Sue. "Diagnosing Bulimia." *American Family Physician* 29, no. 5 (May 1984): 161–64.

Blumenthal, Dale. "A New Look at Food Labeling." *FDA Consumer* 23, no. 9 (November 1989): 14–17.

Department of Health and Human Services, Public Health Service. *Report of the Surgeon General's Workshop on Breastfeeding and Human Lactation.* Washington, D.C.: National Maternal and Child Health Clearinghouse, 1984.

Department of Health and Human Services, Public Health Service. *The Surgeon General's Report on Nutrition and Health: Summary and Recommendations.* DHHS Publication no. (PHS) 88–50211 (1988): 78 pp.

Hadigan, Colleen M., and others. "Patterns of Food Selection During Meals in Women with Bulimia." *American Journal of Clinical Nutrition* 50, no. 4 (October 1989): 759–66.

Hunter, Beatrice Trum. "What's Wrong with Nutrition Labeling?" *Consumer's Research* 76, no. 2 (February 1993): 10–14.

Kahler, Lucinda R., and others. "Factors Associated with Rates of Participation in WIC by Eligible Pregnant Women." *Public Health Reports* 107, no. 1 (1992): 60–65.

Kalina, Barbara B., and others. "The NET Program: A Ten-Year Perspective." *Journal of Nutrition Education* 21, no. 1 (February 1989): 38–42.

Ku, Leighton. "Factors Influencing Early Prenatal Enrollment in the WIC Program." *Public Health Reports* 104, no. 3 (May/June 1989): 301–6.

Kurinv, Natalie, Patricia H. Shiono, Sandi F. Ezrine, and George G. Rhoads. "Does Maternal Employment Affect Breast-Feeding?" *American Journal of Public Health* 79, no. 9 (September 1989): 1247–50.

McNutt, Kristen. "$3.6 to $21 Billion Benefit from New Labeling Regulations." *Nutrition Today* 27, no. 2 (March/April 1992): 39–43.

McSherry, James A. "The Diagnostic Challenge of Anorexia Nervosa." *American Family Physician* 29, no. 2 (February 1984): 141–45.

Miller, Virginia, Sheldon Swaney, and Amos Deinard. "Impact of the WIC Program on the Iron Status of Infants." *Pediatrics* 75 (1985): 100–105.

National Dairy Council. "Nutrition and Modern Lifestyles." *Dairy Council Digest* 59, no. 5 (September/October 1988): 25–30.

"Pass the Pesticides." *Nutrition Action* 16, no. 3 (April 1989): 5–7.

"Pesticides in Foods Could Harm Children." *Nutrition Week* 19, no. 11 (March 16, 1989): 4–5.

Potts, Nicki Lee. "Eating Disorders: The Secret Pattern of Binge/Purge." *American Journal of Nursing* 84, no. 1 (January 1984): 32–35.

"RDA Revision Ends Vitamin Row." *Medical World News* 30, no. 22 (November 27, 1989): 28–31.

Regan, Claire. "Promoting Nutrition in Commercial Food Establishments." *Journal of the American Dietetic Association* 87, no. 4 (1987): 486–88.

Rose, Andy N. "1990 Dietary Guidelines: Implications for Health Educators." *Journal of Health Education* 23, no. 5 (July/August 1992): 293–95.

Rudd, Joel. "Consumer Response to Calorie Base Variations on the Graphical Nutrient Density Food Label." *Journal of Nutrition Education* 21, no. 6 (December 1989): 259–64.

Rush, David. "National WIC Evaluation." *Public Health Currents* (1986): 17–20.

Select Committee on Nutrition and Human Needs, U.S. Senate. *Dietary Goals for the United States.* Washington, D.C.: U.S. Government Printing Office, 1977.

Slattery, Marty. "Developing a Community-Based Program." *The Community Nutritionist* 1, no. 1 (January/February 1982): 9–11.

Sweet, Cheryl A. "Rethinking Eating Out." *FDA Consumer* 23, no. 9 (November 1989): 8–13.

Vaden, Allene G. "Child Nutrition Programs: Past, Present, Future." *Nutritionist* 13, no. 1 (Winter 1981): 7–10.

Welsh, Susan, Carole Davis, and Anne Shaw. "A Brief History of Food Guides in the United States." *Nutrition Today* 27, no. 6 (November/December 1992): 6–11.

Welsh, Susan, Carole Davis, and Anne Shaw. "Development of the Food Guide Pyramid." *Nutrition Today* 27, no. 6 (November/December 1992): 12–23.

White, Philip L. "Setting New Diet and Health Directions." *Nutrition Today* 21, no. 4 (July/August 1986): 4–6.

Zarkin, Gary A., and others. "Potential Health Benefits of Nutrition Label Changes." *American Journal of Public Health* 83, no. 5 (May 1993): 717–24.

Endnotes

1. American Public Health Association. *The Nation's Health* (April 1985): 20.

2. Council on Scientific Affairs. "American Medical Association Concepts of Nutrition and Health." *Journal of the American Medical Association* 242, no. 21 (November 23, 1979): 2335.

3. "Recommended Dietary Allowances Revised 1980." *Dairy Council Digest* 51, no. 2 (March/April 1980): 10.

4. Food and Nutrition Board. *Recommended Dietary Allowances, 9th Ed.* Washington, D.C.: National Academy of Sciences, National Research Council, 1980.

5. Council on Scientific Affairs, "Concepts of Nutrition and Health," 2335.

6. Select Committee on Nutrition and Human Needs, U.S. Senate. *Dietary Goals For the United States.* Washington, D.C.: U.S. Government Printing Office, 1977.

7. *Ibid.*

8. *Ibid.,* 9.

9. *Ibid.,* 46.

10. Department of Health and Human Services, Public Health Service. *The Surgeon General's Report on Nutrition and Health: Summary and Recommendations.* DHHS Publication no. (PHS) 88–50211 (1988).

11. *Ibid.*

12. Welsh, Susan, Carole Davis, and Anne Shaw. "Development of the Food Guide Pyramid." *Nutrition Today* 27, no. 6 (November/December 1992): 12–23.

13. The School Lunch Program is discussed in chapter 16.

14. U.S. Department of Agriculture, Food and Nutrition Service. *Study of WIC Participant and Program Characteristics.* Washington, D.C.: U.S. Government Printing Office, 1986, p. 23.

15. Testimony before U.S. Senate Subcommittee on Agriculture, Nutrition, and Forestry. Washington, D.C.: U.S. Government Printing Office, April 12, 1978.

16. Rush, David. "National WIC Evaluation." *Public Health Currents* (1986): 19–20.

17. Benedick, M., I. H. Campbell, D. S. Bowden, and M. Jones. *Towards Efficiency and Effectiveness in the WIC Delivery Service.* Washington, D.C.: The Urban Institute, 1976.

18. "Child Nutrition Programs Update." *Dairy Council Digest* 53, no. 6 (November/December 1982): 35.

19. Council on Scientific Affairs, "Concepts of Nutrition and Health," 2336.

20. Department of Health and Human Services, Office of Maternal and Child Health. *Child Health USA 1989.* Washington, D.C.: U.S. Government Printing Office, October 1989, p. 19.

21. "Infant Formula Promotion a Domestic Threat, Too." *Nutrition Action* (August 1981).

22. Food Stamp Act of 1964, Public Law 88–525, August 31, 1964.

23. *Ibid.*

24. Caliendo, Mary Alice. *Nutrition and Preventive Health Care.* New York: Macmillan Publishing Co., 1981, p. 594.

25. Food and Drug Administration. "The New Food Label." *FDA Backgrounder* BG 92–4 (December 10, 1992): 5.

26. McNutt, Kristen. "$3.6 to $21 Billion Benefit from New Labeling Regulations." *Nutrition Today* 27, no. 2 (March/April 1992): 39–43.

27. *Ibid.,* 124.

28. Hausman, Patricia. "The Cancers of Affluence." *Nutrition Action* (December 1981): 7–11.

29. Select Committee on Nutrition and Human Needs, *Dietary Goals,* 46.

30. *FDA and the 96th Congress.* Washington, D.C.: U.S. Government Printing Office, 1981, p. 86.

31. Food Additives Amendment, Public Law 85–929, passed by Congress, 1958.

32. "Pass the Pesticides." *Nutrition Action* 16, no. 3 (April 1989): 5–7.

33. "Warning: Your Food, Nutritious and Delicious, May Be Hazardous to Your Health." *Newsweek* (March 27, 1989): 17.

34. "EPA Bans Fungicides for Agricultural Uses: Delays Action for Eighteen Months." *Nutrition Week* 19, no. 48 (December 7, 1989): 2.

35. Mayer, Jean, and Jeanne Goldberg. "Nutrition" syndicated column, December 23, 1986.

36. Department of Health and Human Services. *Healthy People 2000: National Health Promotion and Disease Prevention Objectives.* Washington, D.C.: U.S. Government Printing Office, 1991, Obj. 2.16, p. 125.

37. National Dairy Council. "Eating Disorders." *Dairy Council Digest* 56, no. 1 (January/February 1985): 1.

38. Ching, Chwee Lye. "Anorexia Nervosa: Why Do Some People Starve Themselves?" *Journal of School Health* 53, no. 1 (January 1983): 22–26.

CHAPTER **FIFTEEN**

Community Mental Health

From Sad Past toward a Dynamic Future

". . . even at its best state hospital care is bad for many patients; . . . mental hospitals can be valuable social institutions only if they are restricted to caring for patients they do not harm . . . alternatives to hospital care and methods of redistributing patients must be devised—and quickly."[1]

As recently as two decades ago this statement might have summarized the major mental health need in the United States. By the mid-twentieth century, people should have developed more effective, positive outlooks regarding the care, treatment, and rehabilitation of the mentally ill. Yet in spite of significant programs, governmental funding, community mental health centers, public education, and extensive research on the dynamics of mental illness, this statement is still relevant in the latter part of the twentieth century.

Mental Illness in America

The extent and nature of mental and emotional problems in the United States are difficult to ascertain. In some measure, this is owing to the fact that there is little agreement on what constitutes a mental disorder. Some people think of mental illness as only severe depression, schizophrenia, and suicide. Yet a number of psychiatric disorders, including anxiety disorders, sleeping and eating dysfunctions, many forms of dementia, and a variety of childhood disorders, present themselves.

It is estimated that twenty-three million American adults experience major mental illness of some kind.[2] Also, it is estimated that 10 to 12 percent of all children and adolescents experience some mental disorders.[3] One family in three is affected by mental illness, and one person in ten is hospitalized for mental or emotional disorders at some point in life.

The cost of psychiatric disorders in the United States has been estimated at over $73 billion a year, including expenditures for clinical care and lost productivity.[4] These data must be considered when dealing with the various issues of community mental health.

More than two million Americans experience schizophrenia, a condition in which perception, emotions, relationships, and sensation are affected. Individuals tend to lose touch with the real world and exhibit a variety of unnatural behaviors. Though this disorder can affect people at all ages, it often has its initial impact in adolescence and early adulthood. Patients with schizophrenia occupy more than 20 percent of the beds in mental hospitals.[5] Since 1986 the National Institute of Mental Health has made schizophrenia its first priority for research and programming.[6] In doing so the agency noted that today there are opportunities to alleviate this major community health problem.

Other mental disorders are also the focus of medical and community health attention. However, instead of concentrating primarily on the illness, as was the case in the past, there has been an increased emphasis on maintaining and restoring mental and emotional well-being. Efforts to prevent mental illness and emotional problems are receiving greater attention. In spite of these new directions in understanding mental health, there are still many misunderstandings and misconceptions about mental health.

Learning to cope with mental problems is a significant community health concern. People who experience emotional and mental disorders must receive care. This care is time-consuming and costly in terms of both money and stress on the family. As a result, mental illness does not involve only the patient, but also the family and, in turn, the community at large. Because the community often misunderstands those experiencing mental problems, these people are often denied a very vital support framework.

Owing to this misunderstanding, a major goal of any mental health program is to educate the public about mental illness and positive mental health. With such educational efforts, mental health and mental illness can be better understood and a healthier emotional climate result.

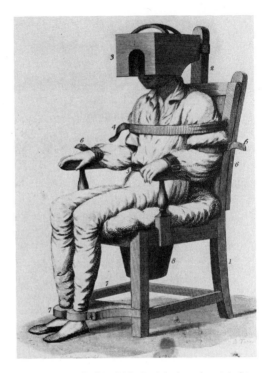

In the 1700s, a mentally ill individual might have been tied to a chair, with feet locked and head tightly restrained. Such inhumane action left no opportunity for treatment, rehabilitation, or improvement in conditions.

History of Mental Health Care

Care of the world's mentally ill has not been a "bright" chapter in the history of humanity. The mentally ill were often neglected or were the recipients of cold, harsh, impersonal care. They were kept in jails or poorhouses, known as almshouses, along with convicted criminals. They were placed in these environments because, like the criminals, they had behaved in a manner considered improper by the community. In most almshouses no medical care was provided, no effort was made to rehabilitate the patient, and only basic sustenance was provided.

Inhumane treatment of the mentally ill was common in the past. Stories of torture and brutality are frequent and disgustingly true. The mentally ill were often kept in iron cages with no heat and little or no light. In many parts of Europe in the seventeenth and eighteenth centuries, the mentally ill were shackled with irons and chains. There were times these individuals were exhibited in towns, fairs, and circuses for the amusement of the general population. They were called "lunatics," a term used because of the belief that the moon affected the mind.

The practices of "muffling" and "forcing" were commonly used. Pieces of cloth were bound tightly over the mouth and nostrils of screaming patients, hence the term "muffling." Also patients who refused to eat were tied to a bed, their teeth were forced open, and food was forced down their throats. This practice often resulted in broken teeth, damage to the palate of the mouth, as well as choking and suffocation.

The mentally ill were also considered to be possessed by evil spirits. They were tortured in order to exorcise the evil spirits from the individuals and the community. These patients were burned, flogged, and forced to endure other inhumane treatment in efforts to "purify" the community.

Historically, the care of the mentally ill in the United States did not reflect any great enlightenment either. Adequate care was never provided for these unfortunate people. Often those in need of care for mental and emotional problems were placed in large, impersonal, public institutions. The type, quality, and effectiveness of care in these settings left much to be desired. Usually, however, patient care was primarily custodial and little effort was made to rehabilitate the patient.

By the end of the eighteenth century, reforms in the treatment and care of the mentally ill occurred in parts of Europe. During the 1790s, Philippe Pinel worked for the reform of the treatment of the mentally ill in France. Pinel felt that these patients should not be kept in chains but should be cared for in hospitals. He worked for the placement of patients in dry, sunlit rooms rather than in dungeons. He also did away with violent treatment, bleeding, and purging. Pinel encouraged talking with patients and listening to their problems. He began to use case histories by keeping records of patients. Pinel's theories and practices were highly unpopular among the public, who had no understanding of the true nature of mental illness and emotional disorders. Even Pinel's fellow physicians opposed his ideas.

During the nineteenth century, care of the mentally ill in the United States gradually became the responsibility of the individual states. The work of Dorothea Lynde Dix in the mid-1800s established the insane as "wards of the state." Thus, it became the state government's responsibility to care for the mentally ill. This resulted in state-operated mental hospitals. However, care received in these institutions was still custodial in nature, and only a few treatment programs were made available. The consensus in the late 1800s and early 1900s was that the mental patient needed to be isolated from society and the family. As a result, many government mental hospitals were located some distance from cities.

The poor condition of state mental hospitals disturbed many people in the early twentieth century. Clifford Beers's 1906 book, *A Mind That Found Itself,* has become a classic on the sad state of affairs in mental hospitals.[7] Beers told of his experiences during the three years he was a patient in several mental health institutions. His experiences convinced him of the need for change in the nation's mental health system, and he called for reform of care for the mentally ill. He also emphasized the need for better understanding of the nature of mental health and mental illness. As an outgrowth of this book and other efforts led by Beers, the Connecticut Society for Mental Hygiene was founded in May 1908. This organization was the first state association in the Untied States established for mental health.

Other individuals worked to improve the condition of mental health care during the early twentieth century. Though well-meaning and effective in some settings, none of these efforts had a major national impact.[8]

Later efforts were designed to cure the mentally ill. Insulin shock treatment and electric shock therapy were introduced during the 1930s. Psychosurgery was also performed on some mental patients during these years. These and other procedures created some controversy.

Until World War II little substantive change occurred in the care and treatment of the mentally ill. The war, however, highlighted the serious state of mental health in the United States, especially the lack of effective treatment and rehabilitative services. Over a million men were rejected for military duty because of neuropsychiatric disorders.[9] Three out of every five beds in Veterans Administration hospitals following the war were occupied by individuals with mental disorders.[10]

Many military personnel returned from combat in need of psychological care and treatment. The sheer numbers of those needing treatment encouraged the improvement of mental health programs. In spite of the need, mental health personnel were still inadequately trained and treatment facilities remained overcrowded.

This state of affairs, which occurred despite good intentions, generated some discussion about the inhumane care of those isolated in state mental health institutions. A well-received book written in 1948 proved that, indeed, there were tragic problems in the state institutions. Albert Deutsch, in *The Shame of the States,* enlightened readers about the plight of the institutions' patients.[11]

Change was accelerated by the passage of federal legislation designed to improve the care and treatment of mental health patients. In 1943, vocational rehabilitation legislation (the Barden-LaFollette Act) was amended so that mental as well as physical rehabilitation was funded. For the first time, vocational counseling and training for the mentally ill were made possible.

Another major legislative breakthrough occurred in 1946 with the passage of the National Mental Health Act. This established the National Institute of Mental Health and supported programs to train professionals for work in the mental health fields. It also made monies available to states for development of community mental health clinics. Even more significantly, the act funded research into the cause, diagnosis, and treatment of mental disorders. The National Institute of Mental Health was also charged with developing demonstration projects, experiments, and studies to find improved and effective ways to rehabilitate the mentally ill.

Mental Disorders and Illnesses

A system for classifying abnormal behavior has been established and published by the American Psychiatric Association. This document, the *Diagnostic and Statistical Manual (DSM) of Mental Disorders,* lists various psychopathologies by groups of disorders based on symptoms and observable signs. Some disorders result in severely disrupted behavior necessitating recurring and long-term care. Others are less debilitating; they are controllable by medication and therapy, and provide sufferers with the opportunity to overcome their mental illness.

Those disorders in which there are related physiological factors are known as *organic mental disorders.* A group of symptoms in which there is a decline in intellectual functioning due to degeneration of brain cells is termed dementia. Alzheimer's disease, which mostly affects the elderly, is one of the organic mental disorders receiving much concern, attention, and research today. Many of these types of disorders result from the use of psychoactive substances such as cocaine, alcohol, and amphetamines.

Schizophrenia is the most common psychopathology and is characterized by disorganization of the thought processes. Various types of behavior are reported by patients with schizophrenia, such as disturbances in motor behavior, paranoia, withdrawal from the external world, and delusions of grandeur. Disturbances in motor behavior are seen as patients may remain motionless or assume unusual body postures for long periods of time.

Functional disorders produce behaviors that are related to psychological stressors. Severe depression, caused by a number of possible stressors, is a common functional disorder. Mood changes, such as hyperactivity, inability to sleep, or fear about many things, are functional mental disorders.

The importance of the fact that people with major depressive disorders should obtain treatment has been highlighted by the national disease prevention objectives.[12] An objective has been established that by the year 2000 an increase by 50 percent of people with major depressive disorders should obtain treatment.

Another classification of mental disorders is *anxiety disorders.* Fear, distress, and a variety of phobias are common occurrences in this classification of mental disorders. One example of anxiety disorders is the obsessive-compulsive disorders, such as obsessions with thoughts, actions, or factors impacting one's life. For example, an individual may display a compulsion to wash one's hands repeatedly and excessively, may continually check the windows or doors to assure that they are locked, secure, and safe, or may carry out numerous other repetitive actions. Generally, irritability, tension, sweating, and increased heart and breath functioning are identified among people with anxiety disorders.

A number of behavioral patterns occur in situations where there are *personality disorders*. There may be mood changes, difficulty in establishing positive interpersonal relationships, and unpredictable actions. Certain behaviors of individuals with personality disorders are marked by serious antisocial actions. Violent behavior resulting in homicide or injury to others may occur, and there is an inability of the individual to feel any type of guilt for the actions taken. Other personality disorders include: histrionic disorders—exuberant display of the overly dramatic; narcissistic disorders—an exaggeration of self-importance and need for attention; and paranoid disorders—envy, jealousy, and unwarranted suspicion.[13]

Another category of mental disorders is the *somatoform disorders*. These disorders are characterized by unfounded or unsubstantiated physical complaints when there is no observed or identifiable physiological cause for the individual's symptoms. Hypochondria, a preoccupation with one's body and fear of presumed disease, may result in complaints of physical illness. In an attempt to maintain perceived bodily function the hypochondriac may overdose with multiple vitamins or food supplements for the purpose of remedying supposed health problems.

Disturbing memories, thoughts, and feelings associated with severe stress are examples of *dissociative disorders*. With this type of disorder it is not unusual for development of multiple personality traits to occur in the same individual. Many people who are experiencing stress fail to obtain help to control or reduce this problem. The health objectives for the nation have recommended that initiatives need to be instituted to decrease the number of adults who experience stress in their lives and do not take steps to correct the situation.[14] Particular focus was noted of the role of providing stress management programs by business and industry to reduce employee stress.[15]

Mental Health Facilities

The mentally ill and emotionally disturbed are cared for in a number of different facilities. Historically, the mental health movement existed within the confines of the institutional setting. Today, more admissions for psychiatric treatment and service take place on an outpatient basis than that which occurs as inpatient or residential treatment.[16]

Most mental health care and treatment are provided in one of the following types of facilities:

1. State and county public psychiatric hospitals—Inpatient care and treatment of the mentally ill are provided. Not all public psychiatric hospitals are state operated; some are operated as private psychiatric facilities. State and county hospitals are often referred to as public psychiatric hospitals.

2. Veterans Administration (VA) psychiatric services—One hundred and thirty VA medical centers have psychiatric bed services.[17] In addition, drug dependence treatment programs and mental hygiene clinics are available for individuals qualified for veterans' benefits.

3. Community hospital psychiatric services—Usually a separate psychiatric unit operates within the general hospital setting.

4. Community mental health centers—Centers are established in many localities to provide a broad range of mental health care within the community setting.

5. Residential treatment centers—Treatment is available to those who are diagnosed as moderately disturbed. The patient usually resides in these settings under supervision.

6. Outpatient psychiatric clinics—The patient receives care and treatment on an outpatient basis within the community.

7. Psychiatric day/night facilities—The patient spends part of the twenty-four-hour day in these settings. Planned therapy and treatment are provided during this period. For the remainder of the day the patient returns to the community.

State Mental Hospitals

The first hospital in the United States specifically for the mentally ill was established in Williamsburg, Virginia, in 1773.[18] Since then, psychiatric care has been considered a responsibility of the state.[19] Large state-operated mental hospitals have been the states' response to this onus. The individual in need of mental health professional services went or was taken there to receive proper care. Although state mental hospitals vary in size, organization, and program effectiveness, their basic function is, and has been, to provide custodial care for the mentally ill. For a majority of patients the hospital stay may exceed a year. Organic disorders and schizophrenia are the predominant conditions necessitating long-term care.

The quality of care given to a mental patient varies. There have been questions raised about the adequacy of care and attention given in state mental institutions. Reports have called attention to inadequate diets, poor living conditions, overuse and improper use of drugs, and personal abuse of the patients. The fact that as many as 80 percent of admissions to state public psychiatric facilities are readmissions demonstrates that these institutions or the community have failed to provide rehabilitative care.

In many states, the professional personnel are inadequate both in number and in training to cope with the many problems presented by the patients. Often the available staff members are ill prepared to meet the needs of the patients. Overcrowding of facilities and budget deficiencies have also led to serious problems.

As a result of these conditions, long-term placement in mental institutions often does not help the psychiatric patient. Such placement can further contribute to stress and related problems. Nor are many rehabilitative measures followed in mental hospitals. An institutionalized patient is usually isolated from family and familiar surroundings, lacks exposure to normal role models, and is unable to develop meaningful personal relationships. This traditional approach to the treatment and institutionalization of the mentally ill has recently received negative publicity.

Little change occurred in the mental health care provided in mental hospitals until the end of World War II. In 1955, a congressional committee on mental health studied national mental health problems. A number of recommendations that served as the foundation for governmental support in the 1960s were made by this commission.

The resident population in state mental hospitals increased annually until 1955, when it reached a total of 558,922 in the United States.[20] In 1956, the number of patients declined and continued to drop annually. By the early 1990s slightly over 90,000 resident patients were reported to be in these institutions.[21]

In 1955, one-half of all mental health care was provided in state mental hospitals; today less than 10 percent takes place in these facilities. In 1955, less than one-fourth of all care was on an out-patient basis; currently, three-fourths of all mental health care is provided by outpatient psychiatric services or in community mental health centers. Today more people are seeking help for emotional disorders, but they are relying less on the mental hospitals.

According to federal government data, there are 266 state and local mental hospitals currently in operation, with a little more than 98,000 beds. This is some eighty hospitals fewer than were in operation in the mid-1970s, with a reduction in state mental hospital beds of over 200,000 since the beginning of deinstitutionalization.[22] Today state mental hospitals are focusing their services on long-term care for the chronically ill, such as schizophrenics, and on care for the criminally insane.

A number of major changes in the operation of the state mental health hospitals have taken place. In addition to the reduction of inpatient services since 1954, different types of services are often available. Many state facilities provide acute short-term care. Outpatient care, day-care programs, and special service programs for the elderly and children are also available.

The opportunity to obtain professional help on an outpatient basis, in nursing homes, in community mental health centers, or in halfway houses, rather than in the institutional setting, has resulted in major changes in mental health care. A number of factors have contributed to this development. During the latter part of the 1950s, psychotropic drugs for treating the mentally ill were introduced. These drugs and tranquilizers were used to help control two major psychoses that led to many cases of institutionalization: depression and schizophrenia.

In 1954, New York became the first state to enact a community mental health services act.[23] Within the next decade, nineteen other states passed similar legislation. Most states now have legislation that encourages the use of community services in the care of mental patients.

Another factor in the reduction of admissions to state mental hospitals is the change in the basic care of the elderly. There has been an increase in elderly placement in nursing homes. Prior to the mid-1960s these patients were often sent to the state mental hospitals. This change, however, now permits the elderly patient to be near family and familiar surroundings.

Political and economic considerations have also influenced the reduction of state mental hospital use. Maintaining such large and crowded facilities became costly. Long-term hospital care is very expensive. Many state governments encourage the community mental health service concept to reduce the financial burden of maintaining the hospital system.

Several pieces of federal legislation passed in the 1960s contributed to the decreased patient number in state hospitals. In 1963 Congress passed the Community Mental Health Services Act. This provided funds to local communities for the construction and staffing of mental health facilities. The Mental Retardation Facilities and Community Mental Health Centers Construction Act, also passed in 1963, supported the development of programs in which care of the mentally ill is moved from state hospitals to community facilities. The passage of Medicare and Medicaid also provided funding for mental health services within local communities.

Deinstitutionalization

In order for deinstitutionalization of the chronically mentally ill patient to work, there must be appropriate living arrangements for the individual upon returning to the community. There must also be adequate support services. Unfortunately, the growth of facilities in the community has not kept up with the need. As a result, many chronically mentally ill individuals are now being placed in facilities such as nursing homes or boarding homes, which cannot provide appropriate services to meet their needs. Numerous problems have resulted; homelessness is one of the most apparent.

Has deinstitutionalizing the mental patient been effective? Some view it as a failure. Patients have been removed from mental hospitals and placed in the community where they often cannot find employment. Many times they commit crimes, are imprisoned, or simply live on the streets of the big cities. These individuals find it most difficult to adjust to and be accepted by society. All too often, the patient enters the "revolving door"; unable to adjust to the community, the patient returns to the facility. But the facility fails to rehabilitate and prepare these people for reentering community life.

Many others feel that deinstitutionalization has been successful. They hold that it is better than keeping the mental patient in an isolated state hospital removed from family, friends, and familiar surroundings. Treatment and rehabilitation near family and friends are felt to be more effective.

General Hospital Psychiatric Services

An important factor in the treatment of mental illness in recent years has been the expanded role of general hospital psychiatry. During the 1980s psychiatric admissions to general hospitals increased. Both inpatient and outpatient psychiatric services are offered in this setting. Today more admissions for inpatient and residential treatment of the emotionally disturbed are provided in nongovernmental, general hospital psychiatric units than in any other type of psychiatric facility. Also, nearly 40 percent of outpatient services are provided in general hospitals and free-standing psychiatric patient clinics.[24] Inpatient psychiatric treatment, for those in need of twenty-four-hour services, is the most expensive mode of care in the hospital.

The general hospitals have become involved in psychiatric care in the effort to "deinstitutionalize" the mentally ill and because of the recent emphasis on community-based care. The general hospital is geographically accessible to the majority of the population in any given community. In addition, the general hospital offers comprehensive, collaborating medical services for treatment of the psychiatric patient. Many patients with psychiatric needs have accompanying medical problems that can also be cared for in the hospital.

The general hospital has an accessible psychiatric emergency care facility. When a person needs immediate care, as during a breakdown or when under stress, effectively trained personnel are usually available to treat the person. Round-the-clock emergency psychiatric services extended by the general hospital include walk-in clinics, suicide prevention centers, home visitation programs, and crisis intervention centers, as well as psychiatric emergency room care.

Both public and private general hospitals have psychiatric departments. However, the type of patient usually admitted differs. Private hospitals admit a greater number of patients with depressive disorders, while public general hospitals admit the more severely disabled who have schizophrenic disorders.[25] The general hospital has become the focus for mental health care in communities throughout the United States during the past decade.

Community Mental Health Centers

Legislation in the 1960s and subsequent developments in community mental health focused on involving the community in care of the mentally ill. The typical community mental health center is staffed by a multidisciplinary team of mental health workers. The Community Mental Health Services Act identified several priority populations to whom the community health program must be directed. The first group includes the chronically mentally ill who leave the state mental institution and return to the local community. Once back in that community, they need adequate and effective support services.

A second priority population includes disturbed children and adolescents. Many stressful and emotional events occur in the formative years. Communities need to establish and strengthen community services, outreach, and education that assist children with emotional problems. Such programs can be conducted by schools, churches, and families, as well as by other community agencies. Children at high risk for emotional disorders are those who experience family separation, conflict between parents, the loss of parents through death or divorce, difficulty in school, or those with teenage parents. Other children who are more likely to have mental problems are those having multiple stressors in life or whose parents are mentally ill or drug or alcohol abusers.[26]

The elderly constitute the third priority group. For some people emotional problems develop with age, retirement, and the loss of loved ones and close friends. Adjustment to such circumstances merits emphasis. Supportive measures, treatment, and care need to be provided in the community setting. Recently mental health services have been available to mentally impaired and emotionally distressed senior citizens in nursing homes.

Because the community mental health center has developed as an alternative to the state mental hospital, a number of changes have occurred in program direction:[27]

1. Increased emphasis on community-based services
2. Emphasis on prevention of mental illness
3. Emphasis on a mental health "system" with effective community planning
4. Emphasis on the short-term therapeutic approach to mental health
5. Emphasis on indirect services (educational, consultative)
6. Emphasis on an expanded use of nonprofessionals in the provision of mental health services

Since passage of the Community Mental Health Services Act in 1963, over seven hundred community mental health centers have been funded. The first center began operating in 1966. Federal funding supported the construction of the center and its staffing and operation. As the result of federal assistance, community mental health centers were established in all fifty states. Federal funding of community mental health centers was discontinued in 1981 when the block-grant funding programs were established. This resulted in funding decisions relating to mental health being transferred to the states. Funding, both federal and state, has been significantly reduced, leading to cutbacks in programs and personnel in many localities.

The National Institute of Mental Health estimates that only about 55 percent of the national population lives within reasonable distance to such services. Since these facilities are basically located in urban population centers, people living in rural areas are usually underserved.

Since the passage of the original legislation supporting these centers, there have been several important amendments. The 1968 amendment included coverage for alcoholics and narcotics addicts. Services for drug abuse were added in 1970. A significant change occurred in 1981 with the passage of the Omnibus Budget Reconciliation Act. This legislation consolidated all federal programs related to mental health, alcoholism, alcohol abuse, and drug abuse into a block grant. This action in effect repealed the original 1963 Community Mental Health Centers Act.

Services are provided in the community mental health centers on both an inpatient and outpatient basis. Community mental health centers provide inpatient care in one of three different administrative patterns.[28] (1) Some operate their own inpatient units. In these the patient is not hospitalized but kept at the center. (2) Other community mental health centers develop affiliate relationships with a hospital so their patients have access to inpatient facilities. These centers contract with a hospital for use of beds when needed. (3) The third pattern is one in which the community mental health center is based at the hospital. The hospital operates the center in these situations.

The duration of treatment varies from several weeks to a few months on an inpatient basis. Short-term accommodations are available for those who need help for a relatively short period. Numerous outpatient services are provided, including group therapy, which has been found to be very effective.

The increasing incidence of AIDS has had a significant impact on community mental health centers. It is estimated that over half of these centers serve people diagnosed with AIDS. Many of these individuals experience emotional health problems. Feelings of helplessness, hopelessness, guilt, and isolation are common, as well as depression and anxiety. In addition, the families and close friends of AIDS patients, who often have the burden for caring for them, feel guilt, anger, and confusion.

The community mental health center also provides emergency care. These services are needed in situations of panic, personal disorganization, destructive outburst, or in times of stress. For instance, personnel are trained to assist potential suicide victims. They frequently operate telephone crisis and other forms of emergency intervention centers.

Both education and consultation are available at these centers. The educational objective is to inform the patient, the family, and the public about mental illness and to encourage measures to cope with such a condition. These activities are also intended to stimulate principles of good mental health. Consultation is provided for a variety of emotional problems.

Residential Treatment Services

In the past decade the community residential treatment approach has expanded to become an effective alternative to institutionalization. A variety of approaches can be used to help rehabilitate the patient in such settings.

The most common community residential treatment program is the halfway house. The halfway house serves as a bridge between hospitalization and the community. While living in a halfway house, the patient continues to receive treatment but is also mobile in the community. The resident may be on medication, but this is often unsupervised; the patient is responsible for this aspect of rehabilitation. There is usually twenty-four-hour staff support, and some halfway houses even hire a live-in staff.

The cooperative apartment type of community residential treatment differs from the halfway house in that there are fewer residents. The staff is available "on call." A reasonable amount of independent living is permitted, and the residents determine many of the program activities.

Another approach to community residential treatment involves family homes and foster homes. This approach places the patient in a private home where activities are family oriented. The patient becomes involved in shopping, house maintenance, gardening, and socializing. Of great importance in the rehabilitative process is the support given by the host family and close neighbors.

There are several other variations of community residential treatment services. Boardinghouses, group homes, foster communities, and nursing homes offer these services, too.[29]

Respite Care

The shift from hospital institutionalization of the chronically mentally ill back to the community has increased the burden on families. Two out of every three patients in mental health facilities are released to relatives,[30] and many end up living with family members. Most community mental health and social service programs tend to focus on the needs and care of the patient. All too often the needs of the primary care givers go unnoticed.

Communities must develop programs to provide information about the disease for family and care givers, including information on how to cope with the condition and how to obtain appropriate medical assistance for the patient.

The care givers must often make a number of emotional adjustments as they experience many pressures. Locating appropriate care for the patient can be stressful. Additionally, many do not understand the behavioral patterns of the emotionally sick individual.

The need for respite care in our communities is becoming increasingly recognized. *Respite care* is the provision of temporary relief for primary care givers of

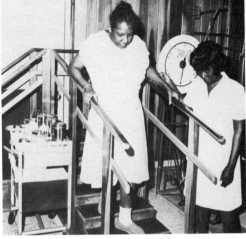
(a)

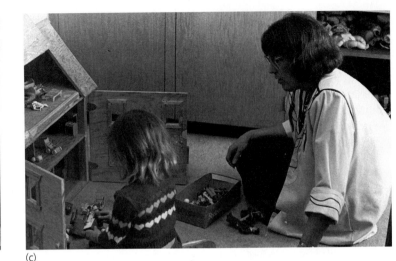
(c)

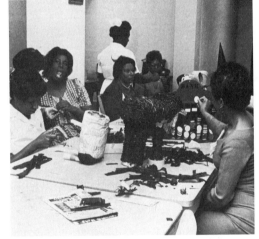
(b)

the disabled, the elderly, and the mentally ill. Residential alternatives must also be developed as part of respite services to ensure continuity of care for the ill. These services are provided on a short-term basis, which allows the care giver to rest, do personal errands, or have a time of relaxation and leisure. This role is usually filled by home health nurses or volunteer workers, or by placing the individual in some facility outside the home.

Daycare services, sometimes referred to as *day hospital, day treatment centers* or *day/night programs,* are furnished for those who do not need twenty-four-hour hospitalization, yet for whom normal outpatient care is inadequate. These facilities provide some respite for the care givers and help meet the ongoing needs of the patient.

Mental Health Personnel

There continues to be an increased need for professional personnel in the mental health field. This need has resulted in an increase in the number of psychiatrists, psychologists, psychiatric social workers, and psychiatric nurses. These are the "core" professionals who serve those in need of mental health care. These professionals work in all of the community settings previously discussed.

The difference between psychiatrists and psychologists is often misunderstood by the general public. The psychiatrist is a medical doctor whose specialty training lies in the prevention, diagnosis, treatment, and care of individuals with mental disorders. The psychiatrist usually needs three years of training beyond basic medical education in the treatment of the mentally ill in order to become certified. Psychiatrists use a variety of skills. In addition to talking (counseling) with the patient, the psychiatrist can prescribe drug treatment and other medical therapy modalities.

On the other hand, the psychologist studies the nonmedical science of human behavior for the purpose of diagnosing, treating, and preventing mental illness. These professionals cannot prescribe drug therapy. They use the techniques of case study, experimental research, surveys, and observation in their work. The emphasis of psychology is upon human behavior.

Paraprofessionals have become increasingly involved in mental health services. People with various degrees of training now work in crisis centers, suicide prevention centers, and support groups. They have been very effective in dealing with drug addicts, alcoholics, and the economically disadvantaged. The paraprofessional offers a number of skills in mental health patient care, including diagnosis, counseling, and supervision of medication. In addition, patient support, education, referral, admission, and case recording are paraprofessional tasks. They also staff halfway houses and provide child care.

Training of community mental health paraprofessionals varies. Sometimes it involves a preservice orientation followed by in-service continuing education sessions including group discussions, seminars, and sensitivity training. More recently, college preparations for such positions has become the norm. A two-year Associate Degree program for the paraprofessional mental health worker is now available in many localities.

Several different tasks performed by the paraprofessional have been identified:[31]

1. Intervene in critical treatment situations
2. Provide psychiatric help for those who could not otherwise receive such assistance
3. Provide needed care where a shortage of mental health professionals exists
4. Mobilize community resources
5. Interpret client needs to a professional
6. Serve as a role model to clients

These tasks, combined with many services provided by mental health "core" professionals, are significant parts of mental health treatment and rehabilitation. Each person, professional and paraprofessional, has an important, specific role to play in caring for the mentally ill, assisting the emotionally distraught individual, and setting goals and conducting programs for preventive mental health.

National Institute of Mental Health

The federal agency concerned with mental health program development is the National Institute of Mental Health (NIMH). NIMH was founded in 1946 with the passage of the National Mental Health Act by Congress. Through the years, the National Institute of Mental Health has developed, conducted, and supported programs directed at mental illness and emotional disturbance. Among the most visible has been its role in mental health research.

NIMH Research

Research has played an important role in improving the care, treatment, and understanding of the mentally ill. The National Institute of Mental Health has supported research into the causes, treatment, and prevention of a number of mental and emotional disorders, including schizophrenia, severe depression, anxiety disorders, and manic-depressive illnesses. Specific problems such as the mental health of children, minorities, the aging, criminals, delinquents, and the elderly have been important research areas.

Although the primary purpose of mental health research is the improvement of treatment for individuals with mental illness and emotional problems, there are other specific goals, too. Extensive efforts have been directed at learning more about the underlying causes of mental illness. Such efforts involve learning more about how the mind works, about the relationship between the body and the brain, and the adjustment into society of the emotionally troubled individual. The biological basis of memory and learning and various physiological and chemical influences on human behavior are also researched.

An important discovery made by biomedical researchers was that information is transmitted through the central nervous system by chemicals in the brain called *neurotransmitters*. Neurotransmitters are essential for normal mental functioning. One of the neurotransmitters, norepinephrine, is considered crucial in the parts of the brain that govern emotions.

Since 1986 research on schizophrenia has been a scientific priority of NIMH. Research has shown that heredity is a factor in schizophrenia. The specific relationship and the measures that would reduce the individual's susceptibility are current areas of research. The role heredity plays in other mental illnesses is under investigation.

Drug therapy for mental illness has resulted in the study and development of many drugs that affect human behavior. For example, tranquilizers and antidepressive medication are effective in helping hospitalized mental patients. Tranquilizers are useful in treatment of patients with schizophrenia. Antidepressive drugs can improve the condition of individuals experiencing various states of depression. Treatment combination studies are being conducted. These studies look at factors involved in the use of medication and psychotherapy.

Behavioral research has investigated behavior in a variety of situations. This includes individual behavior as well as interactions in group settings. Studies of sociocultural influences on behaviors that result in emotional disturbances or in alcohol and drug abuse, as well as studies into child development, have led to better understanding of how to care for the patient. The issue of hyperactive behavior among children has been an important research initiative of NIMH.

In a study reported in 1993, the National Institute of Mental Health suggested that primary care physicians need to be better trained in mental health concerns. It stated that many people with mental disorders are undertreated. Those individuals most likely to seek help were persons with more severe problems.[32]

Depression is experienced by millions of Americans. NIMH initiatives are attempting to identify new medications for individuals with this condition. Some research is aimed at understanding what, if any, genetic factors are associated with depressive disorders.[33] Also, computer-analyzed brain activity measurements are providing new information about depression.

NIMH has supported research examining treatment for narcolepsy. Particular emphasis has focused on the effects of various drugs and therapy on this sleep disorder.

Epidemiological research looks at the extent of mental illness, stress, and emotional disability in the country. This data, however, is often hard to obtain since many families are reluctant to report that a family member is experiencing a problem. Often the data available is based only on those who are treated in public facilities. However, accurate data is needed in order to ascertain the extent of specific mental health problems in a given community and to assist in appropriate program planning.

The National Institute of Mental Health has supported research to learn more about mental disorders of the elderly. Special attention has been given to Alzheimer's disease—its causes and treatment, as well as possible prevention. Other initiatives have investigated the effects of family and other support systems on the care of senior citizens with mental disorders.

National Institute of Mental Health research has been looking at problems related to stress. Not only has such research attempted to learn more about the dynamics of stress on human lives but also how to encourage health-promoting behaviors.

Related NIMH Tasks

Though research is important and consumes a major portion of the efforts and financial support of the National Institute of Mental Health, this federal agency also conducts a number of other activities designed to improve the mental health of the country as a whole. A demand for professional and paraprofessional personnel in the mental health field has necessitated educational programs. Many training programs, in-service sessions, and financial fellowship programs are funded by NIMH.

A number of mental health services are either provided by NIMH or coordinated by this agency. The national institute supports innovative mental health services in community settings, such as day-care centers, schools, hospitals, and the community mental health facilities. The National Institute of Mental Health operates the St. Elizabeth Hospital in Maryland, where staff members provide treatment and rehabilitation for psychiatric patients. A model community mental health center is operated within this hospital.

The institute also distributes public and professional literature and information about mental health and related concerns. Monographs, pamphlets, and other publications update the general public and mental health professionals about effective programs and techniques for the treatment of mental illness and emotional disturbances.

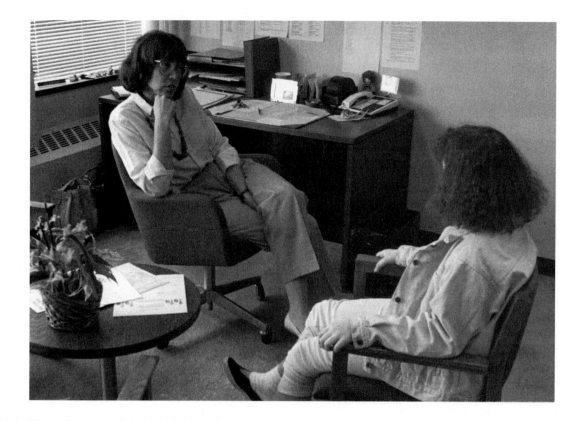

Social workers provide counseling to young people with emotional problems.

Initiatives and Support

Support for community health programming comes from a variety of different sources. Some communities have created integrated community-based programs. For example, the Robert Wood Johnson Foundation has supported a multisite child mental health initiative designed to expand services of support to children and their families. Several agencies within the community, including the schools, are a part of this program.

Another foundation has supported the establishment of a child mental health program for economically disadvantaged inner-city children. Prevention services of early intervention as well as treatment are provided. This program has sought to link schools with community social agencies providing help to children and families needing assistance with emotional health problems.

As plans are developed for national health care coverage, it is important that mental health services be included. This should include alcoholism, drug abuse, and mental health treatment. Coverage should be provided for diagnostic, treatment, and rehabilitative services for everyone. The same policies should be put in force for mental health services as for physical health care.

Mental health services tend to require long-term attention, hence resulting in high costs. However, it has been shown that when individuals receive comprehensive community-based mental health care, health care costs will drop. Conversely, when treatment is not obtained there is an accompanying rise in health care costs.

Summary

Mental illness of some type affects many Americans. Such illnesses may take the form of severe depression, schizophrenia, or a number of other psychiatric disorders. Mental and emotional disorders require the attention and services of community health and medical care personnel and facilities.

The mentally ill have been treated inhumanely in the past. Mental patients were treated little better than animals; they were chained, imprisoned, tortured, given only subsistence food supplies, and exhibited as human "freaks." Little effort was made to treat or rehabilitate the mentally ill. Isolated attempts in parts of Europe to improve mental health care met with little acceptance, but in the early twentieth century, the work of Clifford Beers initiated a more positive approach to mental health.

Mental patients seeking treatment were institutionalized in state hospitals in the early part of this century. The quality of care they received here was often poor, as no major developments in better understanding of the patients or in rehabilitation had occurred.

Since 1955 the number of patients in state mental hospitals has been reduced by about 60 percent. This is due to a number of reasons. The development of drug therapy meant that many mental patients could often be treated on an outpatient basis. Another new concept in the treatment of the mentally ill was the care of the patient in the community—not in an isolated, impersonal state hospital. This led to the Community Mental Health Services Act, legislation that created a community mental health center system. Today a majority of the American population seeking mental health services contacts such facilities.

Other community-based facilities provide both outpatient and inpatient mental health services along with emergency care. These facilities include general community hospitals, residential therapy services, and private psychiatric services.

Deinstitutionalization has increased the burden on families and care givers of former patients. This has led to a need for short-term care for mentally ill individuals to provide relief for the care givers. This service is known as respite care.

The National Institute of Mental Health was established by federal legislation in the 1940s. It has supported major research efforts to learn more about mental illness and the emotionally disturbed. Biomedical research has focused on the physiological and chemical aspects of mental disorders. Research has also investigated the hereditary, socioeconomic, and epidemiologic dynamics of mental health.

In addition to research, NIMH supports mental health education and training programs, publishes both public and professional material about mental health, and supports and coordinates the mental health services in local communities.

Discussion Questions

1. How extensive is the problem of emotional illness in the United States?

2. Describe some of the abuses that have been reported in the history of treatment of the mentally ill.

3. Identify and compare some of the contributions to the mental health movement made by Philippe Pinel, Clifford Beers, and Dorothea Lynde Dix.

4. Following the Second World War, what role did the federal government play in improving mental health care in the United States?

5. What are the organic mental disorders?

6. Identify some of the types of behavior exhibited by schizophrenics.

7. What are the somatoform disorders?

8. What are some of the contributing factors in the reduction of the number of patients in state mental hospitals since 1956?

9. Explain what is meant by deinstitutionalization.

10. In your state, how many state mental psychiatric hospitals are in operation and what services do they provide?

11. How does a general hospital psychiatric department differ from a state mental hospital?

12. Identify some of the characteristics of the community mental health centers.

13. Discuss the question: has deinstitutionalization been as successful as hoped in the 1960s and 1970s?

14. How has the increase of AIDS had an impact on community mental health centers?

15. Explain the organization and services of residential treatment centers.

16. What is meant by daycare services in the field of mental illness?

17. Identify some of the problems faced by families and care givers of the chronically mentally ill due to deinstitutionalization.

18. What are the basic tasks carried out by mental health "core" professionals?

19. Explain the difference between a psychologist and a psychiatrist.

20. How has drug therapy changed the care and treatment of the mentally ill?

21. Identify some of the functions of the National Institute of Mental Health.

22. Why is payment for mental health care often not provided by health insurance programs?

Suggested Readings

Bachrach, Leona L. "The Effects of Deinstitutionalization on General Hospital Psychiatry." *Hospital and Community Psychiatry* 32, no. 11 (November 1981): 786–90.

———. "Progress in Community Mental Health." *Community Mental Health Journal* 24, no. 1 (Spring 1988): 3–6.

Beers, Clifford W. *A Mind That Found Itself.* New York: Doubleday and Company, Inc., 1906.

Grob, Gerald N. "Mental Health Policy in America: Myths and Realities." *Health Affairs* 11, no. 3 (Fall 1992): 7–23.

Knox, Michael D. "Community Mental Health's Role in the AIDS Crisis." *Community Mental Health Journal* 25, no. 3 (Fall 1989): 185–96.

Lefley, Harriet, and David Cutler. "Training Professionals to Work with the Chronically Mentally Ill." *Community Mental Health Journal* 24, no. 4 (Winter 1988): 253–57.

Linn, Margaret W., and others. "Effects of Unemployment on Mental and Physical Health." *American Journal of Public Health* 75, no. 5 (May 1985): 502–06.

National Institute of Mental Health. *Approaching the Twenty-first Century: Opportunities or NIMH Neuroscience Research.* DHHS Publication no. (ADM) 89–1580 (1989).

National Institute of Mental Health. *Caring for People with Severe Mental Disorders: A National Plan of Research to Improve Care.* Rockville, Md.: NIMH, 1990.

National Institute of Mental Health. *National Leadership Workshop on the Homeless Mentally Ill. Proceedings of the Workshop.* Rockville, Md.: NIMH, 1985.

Neighbors, Harold W. "Seeking Professional Help for Personal Problems: Black Americans' Use of Health and Mental Health Services." *Community Mental Health Journal* 21, no. 3 (Fall 1985): 156–66.

Parker, Zoe H. "The Chronically Ill, Will the Community Accept Them?" *Hygie* 5, no. 3 (1986): 13–16.

Pollack, David A., and David L. Cutler. "Psychiatry in Community Mental Health Centers: Everyone Can Win." *Community Mental Health Journal* 28, no. 3 (June 1992): 259–67.

Ridenour, Nina. *Mental Health in the United States: A Fifty-Year History.* Cambridge, Mass.: Harvard University Press, 1961.

Snowden, Lonnie R., and others. "Low-Income Blacks in Community Mental Health: Forming a Treatment Relationship." *Community Mental Health Journal* 25, no. 1 (Spring 1989): 51–59.

Sommers, Ira. "Geographic Location and Mental Health Services Utilization among the Chronically Mentally Ill." *Community Mental Health Journal* 25, no. 2 (Summer 1989): 132–44.

Stetzer, Edward. "Bringing Sanity to Mental Health Costs." *Business and Health* 10, no. 2 (February 1992): 72.

Whitelaw, Carolyn A., and Edgardo L. Perez. "Partial Hospitalization Programs: A Current Perspective." *Administration in Mental Health* 15, no. 2 (Winter 1987): 62–72.

Zirul, Doris W., and others. "Respite Care for the Chronically Mentally Ill: Focus for the 1990s." *Community Mental Health Journal* 25, no. 3 (Fall 1989): 171–84.

Endnotes

1. Ridenour, Nina. *Mental Health in the United States: A Fifty-Year History*. Cambridge, Mass.: Harvard University Press, 1961, p. 134.

2. Department of Health and Human Services. *Healthy People 2000: National Health Promotion and Disease Prevention Objectives*. Washington, D.C.: U.S. Government Printing Office, 1991, p. 208.

3. *Ibid*.

4. *Ibid*.

5. Department of Health and Human Services. *Health, United States, 1991*. Washington, D.C.: U.S. Government Printing Office, 1992, p. 241.

6. National Institute of Mental Health. *A National Plan for Schizophrenia Research*. Washington, D.C.: U.S. Government Printing Office, 1989, p. 2.

7. Beers, Clifford W. *A Mind That Found Itself*. New York: Doubleday and Co., Inc., 1906.

8. Ridenour, *Mental Health*, 13–15.

9. Brown, Bertrams. *Trends in Mental Health*. Washington, D.C.: U.S. Government Printing Office, (DHEW) Publication no. (ADM) 76–406 (1976): 2.

10. *Ibid*.

11. Deutsch, Albert. *The Shame of the States*. Salem, New York: Ayer Company, 1948.

12. Department of Health and Human Services, *Healthy People 2000*, 215.

13. Carroll, Charles, and Dean Miller. *Health: The Science of Human Adaptation*, 5th ed. Dubuque, Ia.: Wm. C. Brown, 1991, p. 101.

14. Department of Health and Human Services, *Healthy People 2000*, 214.

15. *Ibid*., 218.

16. Department of Health and Human Services, *Health, United States, 1991*, 241.

17. *Statistical Abstracts of the United States, 1993*. 113th ed. U.S. Department of Commerce. Washington, D.C.: U.S. Government Printing Office, 1993, p. 130.

18. National Institute of Mental Health. *Financing Mental Health Care in the United States*. Washington, D.C.: U.S. Government Printing Office, (DHEW)/Publication no. 73–9117 (1973): 7.

19. Friedman, Emily. "Hospital Psychiatric Services Begin a Changing of the Guard." *Hospitals* 55, no. 9 (May 1, 1981): 53.

20. National Institute of Mental Health. *State and County Hospitals, U.S. 1973–1974*. Washington, D.C.: U.S. Government Printing Office, (DHEW)/Publication no. (ADM) 76–301 (1975): 1.

21. *Statistical Abstracts of the United States, 1993*, 130.

22. *Ibid*.

23. National Institute of Mental Health, *Financing Mental Health Care*, 9.

24. Department of Health and Human Services, *Health, United States, 1991*, 241.

25. Bachrach, Leona L. "The Effects of Deinstitutionalization on General Hospital Psychiatry." *Hospital and Community Psychiatry* 32, no. 11 (November 1981): 786.

26. Tableman, Betty. "Overview of Programs to Prevent Mental Health Problems of Children." *Public Health Reports* 96, no. 1 (January/February 1981): 38.

27. Bloom, B. L. *Community Mental Health: A General Introduction*. Monterey, Calif.: Brooks Cole, 1977.

28. Leaf, Philip J., and others. "Federally Funded CMHS: The Effects of Period of Initial Funding and Hospital Affiliation." *Community Mental Health Journal* 21, no. 3 (Fall 1985): 145.

29. Colton, Sterling I. "Community Residential Treatment Strategies." *Community Mental Health Review* 3, no. 5/6 (September/December 1978): 1, 16–21.

30. Zirul, Doris W., and others. "Respite Care for the Chronically Mentally Ill: Focus for the 1990s." *Community Mental Health Journal* 25, no. 3 (Fall 1989): 171.

31. Nash, Kermit B., and others. "Paraprofessionals and Community Mental Health." *Community Mental Health Review* 3, no. 2 (March/April 1978): 3.

32. American Medical Association. *Archives of General Psychiatry* (February 1993).

33. National Institute of Mental Health. *A National Plan for Schizophrenia Research*. Washington, D.C.: U.S. Government Printing Office, 1989, pp. 14–17.

Whose values, practices, and beliefs are the standards that are taught? At times these standards for health practices may be contrary to family values, beliefs, and morality. How does the school cope with this matter in developing a health curriculum? All too often these difficult questions are not considered when setting goals and establishing learning experiences for the school health program.

In spite of the fact that there are many approaches to health instruction in the schools, the health education curriculum continually needs to be redesigned. Such an effort should focus upon the total entity of health: the *social,* the *emotional,* and the *physical.* Each component must be presented in light of the most current developments and information.

Curriculum Development

The educational curriculum in the United States is determined and controlled locally. According to the Constitution, education is a state responsibility. It is at the community level that decisions are made regarding school funding, curriculum, and other educational matters.

As a result, curriculum development throughout the United States varies significantly from one school district to another. Though there are state education department guidelines and regulations for many subjects in the curriculum, the actual development of what is taught, and how, is usually a local matter.

The process of curriculum design also varies. During the development phase, curriculum specialists, school administrators, teachers, sometimes parents and students, and occasionally others with specific expertise are often consulted. Such an approach to curriculum development leads to a large variance in curriculum organization, topics, methods, and goals.

Health education has seldom been coordinated in a comprehensive K–12 curriculum. All too often school districts do not coordinate the health learning experiences from one grade level to another. The subject matter may be determined by the knowledge and expertise of the teacher or as outlined by the textbook being used. This unplanned scheme of curriculum development often results in overlap, duplication, and repetition. It is not unusual to hear elementary school students complain that the subject being covered this year is the same as that which was studied the previous year. This problem must and can be solved by offering a sequential curriculum. Though other topics can be added, a well-designed school health program should include at least ten major topics.

The National Health Objectives for the year 2000 specifically called for an increase in the number of elementary and secondary school children participating in planned, sequential health education programs.[2] According to the health objectives initiative, several specific topics need emphasis in a comprehensive school health program: injury control, oral health, tobacco use prevention, nutrition, and physical education. Tobacco use prevention should emphasize the short-term and long-term effects of tobacco use, as well as the social factors associated with this problem. Nutrition education is required in twelve states.[3] Physical education must receive a greater emphasis at both the elementary and secondary levels. The skills and activities taught should promote lifetime physical activities, not just sports.

Many people believe that children should receive instruction and help regarding physical and sexual abuse as part of a comprehensive school health education program.[4] Several states now require instruction in these matters and also provide in-service training for teachers. Ohio requires that such instruction be a part of the health education program in grades 1–6. In 1988 New York state passed a law requiring teachers to participate in a training session to help them identify victims of child abuse.

National and State Curriculum Initiatives

At times a national curriculum for certain subject areas has been proposed. However, local control of education in America has forestalled any such development. Despite this opposition, proponents of a national curriculum, particularly for health, continue to argue for its inception.

School Health Education Study

In the mid-1960s, a nationally developed curriculum project known as the School Health Education Study (SHES) was designed and produced. The development of this curricular project was the outgrowth of a nationwide survey that indicated a serious weakness in school instruction of health. In this study, it was found that little coordination of teaching existed between school levels. Students seriously lacked knowledge of basic health. The overall conclusion was that the level and quality of health instruction programs in the schools were poor.[5]

As a consequence of this national study, a curriculum project was initiated. Its goal was to improve health instruction with a nationally recognized curriculum. This project, known as the *SHES Project,* used a conceptual model of curriculum development. It was a well-designed curriculum effort, in which additional concepts were built onto the previous year's conceptual base. Through the latter part of the 1960s and the early 1970s, a number of school districts throughout the country adopted all or parts of this curriculum. However, it never gained widespread use, and the enthusiasm for this curriculum waned by the mid-1970s. One major reason for the lack of interest by many school districts was the cost. In order to use the curriculum on an integrated K–12 basis, the district was forced to spend more money than was usually appropriated for health education.

Health Education Curriculum Models

In more recent years, more than one hundred school health education curriculum models have been developed. These have been received with various degrees of attention and acceptance. Some have been designed specifically as health education curriculums, others as cardiovascular health, fitness, nutritional, dental health, and emotional health programs. Though it is impossible to identify all of the health education curriculum models and resources now available, several are noted in this chapter.[6]

Some of these curriculum models are designed for elementary grades (Health Education Curriculum Guide, Know Your Body, Feelin' Good, Health Skills for Life, Learning for Life), while others are designed for secondary school children (Family and Community Health through Caregiving, Skills for Living—Project Quest, Teenage Health Teaching Modules). Some focus primarily on cardiovascular health (Feelin' Good), others on nutrition (Nutrition Education and Training Program), dental health (School Dental Health Education Curriculum— Tampa), or substance abuse. Most tend to focus on student behavior objectives. They use a variety of values clarification strategies. Discovery activities, decision-making skills, and student-centered materials for self-learning are primary methodologies in most of these programs. Several of the programs involve the home and community, in addition to the school. Such programs usually involve workshops and the involvement of family members in activities along with the students.

These programs rely heavily on audiovisual material. Thus, it is important for teachers to be trained not only in teaching strategies but also in the use of such equipment and materials. For example, before using the Self-Discovery Program, teachers receive five days of training. Training workshops for teachers who use Skills for Living—Project Quest are held regularly.

Some financial support for the development, teacher training, and dissemination of several of these health education curriculum models has originated with various philanthropic foundations. The Kellogg Foundation has provided grants for the Learning for Life Program, the Feelin' Good Curriculum, and the Family and Community Health through Caregiving Program. The Zellerback Family Fund financed the development and piloting in San Francisco of the Growing Healthy

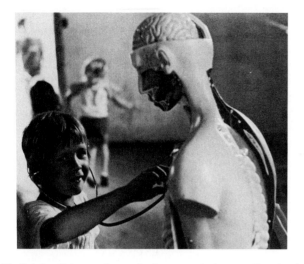

"Feelin' Good" is a cardiovascular fitness curriculum used by school districts in several states. Through education and exercise, health knowledge and values that will last a lifetime are developed.

Curriculum. The Health Education Curriculum Guide was developed with the support of the United Way Health Foundation in Canton, Ohio.

Evaluation studies have been conducted on most of these curriculum models. One three-year comparative study was the School Health Education Evaluation.[7] This study evaluated four projects: the Growing Healthy Curriculum Project, the Health Education Curriculum Guide, Project Prevention of Dalles, Oregon, and the 3Rs and High Blood Pressure Project. More than thirty thousand students in grades 4–7 in one thousand classrooms in twenty states were a part of this study.

In general this study showed that health education instruction in schools is effective. Students in these programs showed improved attitudes toward maintaining a healthy body. Increased knowledge regarding growth and development, human sexuality, and substance abuse was recorded. Also, students in these programs had improved decision-making skills, and less smoking was reported among these students.[8]

The School Health Education Evaluation emphasized the need for administrative support, good teacher training, and the importance of continuity across grade levels.

Growing Healthy Curriculum Project   The curriculum project that has received the greatest national exposure has been the Growing Healthy Curriculum Project. This project, formerly known as the School Health Curriculum and the Primary Grades Curriculum Project, is designed to help students understand how the body functions. Various dimensions that affect the body are studied—both the environment and microorganisms. Students are educated to make appropriate personal health behavioral choices throughout their lives. The goal of this project is to "help the child realize that the body is each person's greatest natural resource in life, that the body is uniquely one's own, that it is exquisitely beautiful and complex in its structure and functions, that it is influenced by one's own choices made throughout life, and that it has the potential to bring experiences in life more exciting than anything imaginable because they will be one's own experiences."[9]

The Growing Healthy Curriculum Project has materials for instruction in grades K–7. The units designed for grades 4–7 focus on the body's systems, while the K–3 material focuses on the senses. Each unit spans a ten-to-twelve-week period, with learning experiences broken down into five phases.

This curriculum employs the problem-solving approach. Investigation, employment of creative learning styles, value clarification, and decision making are the principal means of teaching and learning. The curriculum emphasizes the use of a variety of methods and equipment. Microscopes, books, dramas, experiments, and multiple teaching and learning resources are employed. Multimedia, including films, slides, movies, records, radio, and television, are also incorporated into the program.

Children are encouraged to learn by doing. Learning centers provide a variety of teaching and learning strategies. Classroom teachers must be trained to use this curriculum. The Growing Healthy Curriculum Project is designed for use by regular classroom teachers, not just specialists trained in health education.

Statewide Coalition Networks

Several states have developed and implemented model statewide health curricula. In some instances this has involved revising an already mandated curriculum so as to better meet the needs of school children. In other states it has meant building coalitions to support the introduction and expansion of the health program. The impetus in most instances has come from the state department of education and/or the state health department. Networking coalitions have involved numerous organizations concerned about

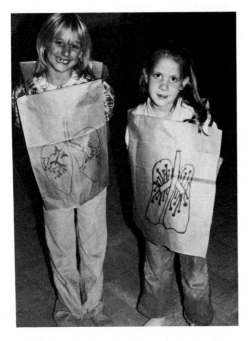

Recently developed curriculum models use a variety of creative activities. Children can learn how their respiratory systems work and what happens during an asthma episode.

the health of schoolage children and adolescents. These coalitions have included the voluntary health agencies, medical associations, and professional and community groups, as well as interested parental groups.

An example of such an initiative is the Michigan Model for Comprehensive School Health Education. Seven state government agencies have worked together with voluntary and professional groups throughout the state to develop and disseminate a basic health and wellness program among the public and private schools of Michigan. The Michigan Model has programs for K–12 health education. In addition a program has been developed for use in preschool programs. Also, the curriculum has been adapted to meet the needs of special education students. There is a strong emphasis on problem-solving, wellness, and abstinence in this curriculum.[10]

An important component of the Michigan Model has been the establishment of several regional sites where classroom teachers can receive training and be provided with orientation to resource materials for implementing a comprehensive health program. Not only are these teachers in-serviced with traditional health topics, but special categorical programs in drug education, AIDS, and other current topics have been part of the training programs.

Some measures being implemented to improve the teaching of health education have focused upon strengthening the professional preparation and health education certification measures in several states. Comprehensive health education teacher training centers have been established in several states. Also, upgrading of college and university health education professional programs and expanding opportunities for health in-service learning have been developments that have taken place in recent years.[11] For example, funding has been made available in Maine to provide a week-long Academy in School Health Education.[12] This program is designed for elementary and secondary teachers to focus on health education content areas and learn effective measures to present material in the classroom setting.

It is believed that health instruction will only become more effective as teachers become more competent in current methodologies and basic health knowledge relating to health behavior and child and adolescent health. Also, in several states measures have been introduced to upgrade the certification requirements for teachers of health.

Contemporary Problems

Often when there are problems in society that affect the schoolage population, school districts are expected to play major educational roles relating to these issues. This has become particularly true during the past decade. Three serious problems face society today; each is a focus of the school health program. These three concerns are teenage pregnancy and human sexuality, substance (drug) abuse, and AIDS.

Curricular development, legislative mandates, program redesign, and teacher training have all emphasized these three problems. Even though the public is aware of the seriousness of each, there is not complete agreement about how the schools should address them. As a matter of fact, many people do not feel the schools can be effective in helping to solve these problems. Despite this opinion, the school health education program must attempt to help children of all ages understand the issues, feelings, and problems associated with human sexuality, drug usage, and AIDS.

Human Sexuality Education

The school health curriculum involves instruction in a number of controversial topics. Possibly the most controversial has been sex education. Many believe that young people, particularly teenagers, must be taught about human sexuality, reproduction, male and female growth and development, family life, and related topics. Attempts to develop a health curriculum that incorporates these topics have met with a great deal of opposition and occasional hostility. This opposition is largely a vocal minority in the community.

Family life education, human reproduction education, sexually transmitted disease education, human growth and development, and even health education are all names for sex education. Unfortunately, many important learning experiences that could benefit children are lost in the emotional response to the single word "sex." It is doubtful that an instructor would discuss sex techniques or emphasize coitus in the curriculum of elementary and secondary school children. Yet, these interpretations are argued by opponents of school sex education programs.

In a speech given in 1986 Surgeon General C. Everett Koop stated that ". . . we need sex education in schools and . . . it must include information on heterosexual and homosexual relationships." The motivation for this strong statement of support for sex education in the school curriculum was the increasing concern about acquired immunodeficiency syndrome (AIDS). It had become increasingly obvious to the medical and political leaders of the United States that the public needed to become more informed about AIDS—its cause, prevention, and treatment.

The Surgeon General suggested that this instruction begin as early as third grade (about eight years of age). It was his contention that school-age children, as well as the adult population, must learn how AIDS is contracted and how it can be prevented.

Such a statement calling for comprehensive school sex education raises problems, questions, and opposition. Is it appropriate to include instruction about AIDS in curriculum material on sexuality? At what age is it appropriate to teach children about human sexuality? Won't such instruction only increase the desire on the part of children to experiment with sex? Is it appropriate for the federal government to provide funding for such a program that includes strong value overtones?

These are just a few of the questions that must be answered if the schools are to respond effectively to the challenge of the Surgeon General.

Human reproduction and sexuality are most often taught as an integrated part of some basic subject in the school curriculum. Usually these learning experiences are a part of health education, biology, or home economics courses. Though some school districts have developed separate school sex education programs, this approach is the most susceptible to opposition.

In the past, attempts have been made to prohibit the teaching of human sexuality either as a separate sex education course or as a part of some other subject. These efforts have been extended to proposed legislative action to ban such courses. However, no state presently has legislation that would prohibit such teaching.[13] In fact, thirty-one states either require, encourage, or permit school districts to include sex education in the curriculum. The remaining states have no legislation or regulations prohibiting sex education.[14]

Sex education has been challenged in the courts on several occasions.[15] Those who introduce such litigation argue that religious freedom, right of privacy, and constitutional rights are infringed upon by exposing children to the subject. The courts have ruled in favor of the schools and found the teaching of sex education to be constitutional and legal.

Opponents also argue that such instruction causes immorality; it has a detrimental effect upon the morals of young people. That such instruction actually leads to sexual activity and experimentation is another view often expressed by those seeking to have sex education removed from the schools. Others simply feel that such instruction will create an unwholesome environment.

A great deal of opposition is based on religious and political positions. Conservative religious groups are usually the most vocal in arguing against school sex education. They feel that such instruction will undermine morals and values.

It is estimated that more than 80 percent of the population supports school sex education.[16] Though sex education is considered legal and its opponents are in the

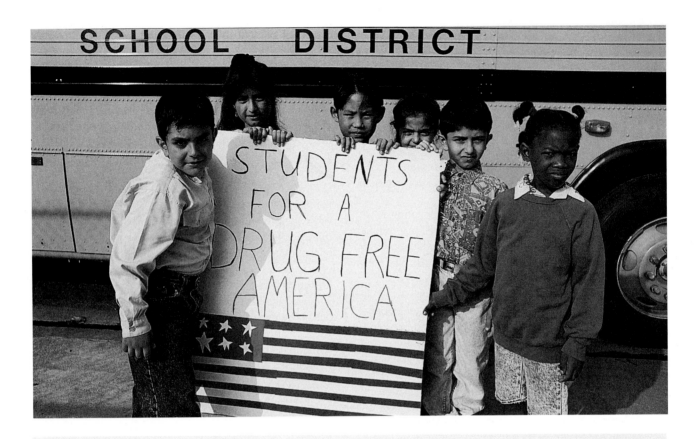

School children need accurate, updated information on drugs. Numerous school drug programs have been developed to educate young people about drug use and abuse, one being the "drug free" schools.

minority, many school administrators are hesitant to incorporate more than basic human anatomy and physiology into the curriculum. Topics such as birth control, abortion, alternative marital life-styles, and other sex-related issues are kept out of the curriculum for fear of controversy.

Considering the problems of teenage pregnancy, teenage sexual activity, and young people's need for information, it is reasonable to suggest that human reproduction and human sexuality should be part of the school curriculum. Sex education programs have been shown to reduce the level of sexual activity by teenagers. Also, sex education programs supplement rather than undermine the influence of parents on matters relating to sexual beliefs and practices.[17] Failure to provide such instruction in the schools may result in continued ignorance and greater problems in sexual adjustment in the future.

Substance Abuse Education

Owing to the increase in drug use, drug education programs have been developed to cope with the problem. It is the perception of much of the general public that the use of drugs by young people is the most serious problem facing the schools today.[18] School-age children need instruction about drugs, their effects, and how to cope with the pressures to use drugs. Drug education initiatives should be developed to achieve a drug-free school environment. This often means that the social, emotional, and physical needs of the students must be considered in such programs.

Comprehensive school drug education programs have been developed in many school districts for all grades, K–12. In the past most substance abuse education initiatives were conducted in the secondary schools. But because drugs such as tobacco and alcohol are being used at earlier ages, it is believed that programs must begin in elementary school. Most states have passed legislation mandating such instruction.[19] The approaches that are taken vary—thousands of school districts include classes, lectures, talks, and assemblies. Law enforcement personnel and reformed drug users, as well as government-funded curriculum, have been used to heighten young people's awareness of the problems associated with drug use. School drug education programs need to be comprehensive, well planned, and have community support.

The development of a useful drug education curriculum must involve a variety of community agencies and experts. It should draw upon a pool of resource people, including those involved in drug intervention and treatment services, the medical profession, law enforcement personnel, parents, and students, as well as teachers.

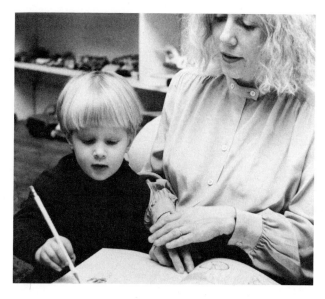

Preschoolers enjoy the antismoking message in the Starting Free program.

Drug-Free Schools

As part of the America 2000 Education Strategy the federal government has set as a goal the establishment of drug-free schools by the year 2000. This federal program is designed to encourage cooperation within communities to work within the framework of the schools to reduce and eliminate the use of drugs of abuse. In particular young people are to be helped and encouraged to avoid use of all drugs, particularly the "gateway drugs," alcohol and tobacco. Recognition of schools that have established drug-free programs has served to encourage the expansion of this federal government initiative.

Seven characteristics have been identified as being necessary for identification as a drug-free school. These seven key characteristics are as follows:[20]

1. Schools must recognize, assess, and monitor the extent and patterns of drug use in their school and the community.

2. Schools must interact and build networks with community groups and agencies who can assist and support student drug use programs.

3. Policies need to be established and then enforced to assist students in refraining from the use of drugs of abuse.

4. Schools should develop their own curriculum, select materials, and then teach prevention of drug use. These curriculum developments are to include all grades, and the information should be integrated into the various academic subjects.

5. Adult school personnel should serve as positive role models for students concerning the use of drugs. This is particularly important concerning the use of alcohol and tobacco.

6. Students should become involved in drug-free activities. They should be able to experience a sense of belonging to an important activity.

7. The involvement of parents in this program is important. Families must realize that substances of abuse can be harmful to the students, and parents need to become motivated to help provide an environment that will support the drug-free school initiative.

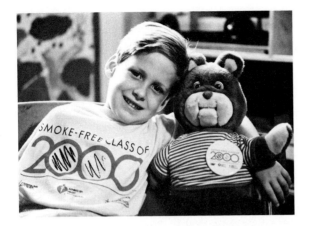

School districts throughout America are supporting educational initiatives designed to encourage preschool and primary school children to not start smoking. The high school graduating class of the year 2000 started first grade in 1988.

More than a hundred schools have developed drug-free programs that have received national notice.[21] Numerous activities and programs have been recognized. Clubs and community groups have been formed to give students leadership roles and to provide an opportunity to associate with peers who are not drug users. Drug-free social activities are planned and conducted to help the students to understand that social life can be active and fun without alcohol, tobacco, and the use of other drugs.

The use of peer counseling has been an effective strategy introduced by some schools. Also, recognizing that the schools do not operate in a vacuum, but are a part of any community, program developers have included a variety of community interactions as part of drug-free programs. For example, members of the community have been involved in working with the students and school personnel in helping to shape goals of a school drug policy and then to develop specific program plans. Many of the activities are designed to help young people develop greater self-esteem and to receive recognition for accomplishments.

AIDS

Acquired immunodeficiency syndrome (AIDS) has had an impact on the nation's schools. This has involved two specific issues. Since there is currently no known cure for this disease, educational initiatives directed toward the U.S. population have been the principal means of prevention. Schools are in a position to play a major educational role for school age children. The second issue, which has been emotionally charged, is whether to permit a student with AIDS to attend school.

It would seem that including AIDS instruction in the school health instruction program would be noncontroversial. However, this has not been the case in many communities. Proper and effective instruction concerning AIDS must present information about human sexuality, for example, that abstinence is the best method of prevention, followed by the use of condoms. Since AIDS has been most prevalent in the United States among the homosexual male population, any instruction will require discussion of homosexuality.

Some parents are opposed to having their children exposed to these topics. Some contend that instruction must emphasize abstinence rather than condoms as a preventive measure. Also, some people feel that information about homosexuality is inappropriate for school age children.

Despite this opposition, most schools today provide instruction about AIDS. In a study conducted by the National School Boards Association in 1990, it was reported that nearly all urban schools and most suburban and rural schools now include such instruction.[22] This report noted that a majority of the school districts permit students to be excused from this instruction at their parent's request.

It is the position of the health objectives for the nation initiative that instruction regarding AIDS should be included as part of the school health education program in grades four through twelve.[23] This has meant development of AIDS curriculum for children in elementary school as well as secondary school. The health objectives for the nation initiative has recommended that such instruction in the school curriculum should include information about how AIDS is and is not transmitted. All students by the time they are in sixth grade should know how to prevent the transmission of the HIV virus and also know something of the risk of this viral infection.[24]

In order to assist school districts in establishing AIDS education programs, the Centers for Disease Control and Prevention has published a set of guidelines.[25] These guidelines include objectives at various grade levels: early and late elementary grades as well as middle school and high school. In addition CDC has been instrumental in supporting many AIDS curriculum development projects throughout the nation.

The question about whether children with AIDS should be permitted to attend school has been controversial. In several instances school officials have excluded children with AIDS from school attendance. In some places parents have boycotted the schools by withdrawing their children from classes when it became known that a child with AIDS was attending. Lawsuits attempting to restrain AIDS children from attending school on the grounds that they are a public health menace were filed in some instances.

Parents who object to school attendance of children with AIDS antibodies point out that states exclude pupils from schools owing to other illnesses. It is their belief that such regulations should also apply to AIDS. Also, in 1986 the Centers for Disease Control announced that no one with AIDS would be permitted immigration into the United States from another country. As a result, parents have pointed out that if the government feels that AIDS is of sufficient danger to prohibit entrance as an immigrant, then the school population should be protected by exclusion of the AIDS patient.

The two principal causes of AIDS in school age children are blood transfusions and birth to a mother with AIDS. Most school-related cases result from the former, but there have been relatively few cases of AIDS among school age children.

There is no evidence that AIDS can be transmitted on a casual basis. It cannot be transmitted by person-to-person contact, such as drinking from a glass, using the same utensil, hugging or touching an AIDS patient, sneezing, or coughing. There is no evidence of sibling transfer of the virus that causes AIDS.

Most state departments of education have developed policies for the local school districts regarding this matter. The states of Connecticut and Massachusetts were the first. In 1985, both states adopted guidelines that advised schools to handle AIDS cases on a case-by-case basis.[26] The National Education Association also recommended that the decision to permit children with AIDS to attend school should be on a case-by-case basis.[27]

In 1985, the Centers for Disease Control issued guidelines for schools that recommended that these children be allowed to remain in school. Each case should be judged separately. The Centers for Disease Control guidelines did recommend that preschool age children not attend school because of their lack of control of body secretions.

Education of the public is vitally important in overcoming this very emotional and controversial issue. Parents must receive accurate information about AIDS. Also, teenagers need information about the causal relationships of AIDS with sexual intercourse and IV transfusion among drug users, since the teen years are a time of experimentation by many with both drugs and sex. Teachers—as well as children with the AIDS virus—and their families—need to be properly educated so as to be able to support the school policy.

Health Services

How comprehensive should health services provided by a school district within the school setting be? Should physicians, dentists, nurses, and other health care providers be employed by the schools? How much money should be spent in developing health facilities at the schools? These and similar questions have been raised when the scope of a school health service program is discussed.

Although health services have been part of the school program since the early years of this century, a broad range of medical care provided within public education facilities has met with only limited acceptance. Most Americans feel that the schools should educate young people, not provide medical care. They do not see a relationship between the provision of health services and the educational process. This has resulted in limited funding of health services in the schools, so rarely do school districts employ dentists, physicians, dental hygienists, or other health care providers (with the exception of nurses) on a full-time basis. It is also unusual for schools to provide a broad scope of health (medical) care in school clinics.

In comparison to other industrial countries in the world, the United States has a relatively underdeveloped system of school health services. In Sweden, 95 percent of the school age children receive dental care through schools. In New Zealand, the rate of service is 98 percent. Dental nurses care for the school children, including such services as cavity preparation and fillings. The school dental services are not always provided in the school buildings, but in district dental health clinics. The program, however, is school managed and school based. The school-based dental health program provides this comprehensive dental care to all children, regardless of economic status, age, or other considerations. In addition, dental health education is integrated with the actual dental care.

By comparison, in the United States there are few school districts that provide dental health care. Instead, most children obtain dental care through private dental practice. Some children do receive dental care at local health departments; however, these visits are rarely coordinated with school programs. At best, dental hygiene is discussed in the school setting.

There are some isolated examples of medical services offered in the context of educational programs. One case involves a miniclinic operated within a high school. Several health care disciplines are united to provide a variety of services. These services include dental care; nutrition counseling and education; and the services of an obstetrician/gynecologist, social worker, drug counselor, public health nurse, and nurse practitioner. The miniclinic is operated as an outreach of a community health center and is funded by a government grant. A number of screening procedures, such as breast examination, Pap smears, and hemoglobin and urinalysis tests, are provided. As a result of this miniclinic, the services of the community health center have been made more accessible to school children.[28]

Other programs involve the use of nonmedical health care providers in school health service activities. The schools involved with these projects have developed relationships with local medical schools and clinics. Usually, the focus of these projects is directed to children from low socioeconomic levels of the community. Of great importance to these medical service programs in schools is the financial support of the federal or state government.

The community agency that is most likely to become involved in the provision of school health services is the local health department, which provides nursing services to the schools and so plays a major role in the health appraisal of school children. The nurses become involved in the screening of vision, hearing, and other functions so that physical and emotional deviations can be identified and referred to medical care for treatment.

In addition, the local health department becomes involved with the school health program by monitoring local and state environmental health and safety regulations.

Immunizations and Physical Examinations

School health services were established at the turn of the century to combat childhood communicable diseases that were a major cause of death and debilitation in school children at that time. In an effort to protect the health of children, schools began to require the immunization of children for certain diseases. Also, children were required to have physical examinations prior to entering school.

Today, immunization is mandated in all states. Though some variance does occur from one state to another, the most commonly required immunizations are for diphtheria, pertussis, tetanus, polio, rubella, rubeola, and mumps. Several states also mandate a tuberculin test for tuberculosis. The tuberculin test does not prevent but provides for detection of tuberculosis. A child cannot attend school unless these immunizations have been received.

Immunization requirements are normally enforced by the school nurse and the local health department. It is the nurse's responsibility to obtain the immunization records of school children, which requires communication with the home and family. When children have not been immunized, the school nurse must work in conjunction with the family, the family physician, or the local health department to see that the regulations are met.

Through the years, many individuals have challenged the legality of school immunization requirements. These people oppose such requirements because of religious beliefs or because they view them as the government's attempt to control private lives. The courts have ruled that state statutes, health department regulations, and school district rules and regulations mandating immunization for school admittance are legal and constitutional, even though state law also requires school attendance.[29] Supporters feel such requirements ensure the protection of the health of the public.

Additionally, periodic physical examinations are also required by the schools. These, too, are monitored by the school nurse. Most school policies stipulate that, in addition to an examination before entering school, children are expected to have other examinations periodically throughout their school years.

One purpose of such examinations is to identify health problems in the growing child. It is also hoped that by encouraging young children to obtain periodic examinations, a lifelong habit will develop. Today, some difference of opinion exists as to whether periodic physical examinations are necessary, and there is little evidence that such behavioral patterns do, in fact, develop in childhood.

For physical examinations obtained during the school years to be most useful, they should be conducted by a family physician. The chances of follow-up when health problems are found is greater than if mass examinations are conducted in a school or public health department. However, when it is not possible to obtain a physical examination from a family physician, for economic or other reasons, the child usually can use the services of a local health department.

Emergency Care

Injuries, accidents, and sickness are common occurrences within the school. It is imperative that school districts take appropriate measures to meet such emergency situations. Policies that specify procedures to be followed during injury or sickness should be developed by the school administration in consultation and cooperation with school health personnel, community medical personnel, legal counsel, and appropriate community agencies. The policies should be available in writing, and all school personnel should be aware of their provisions.

Regardless of the policies developed, it is obvious from legal precedent that school personnel have a responsibility to aid sick or injured children during school hours. Failure to do so has been considered negligent behavior.[30] Concern over the possible legal consequences should never keep a school teacher or other responsible person from caring for a sick or injured student.

The pattern of relying on the school nurse, the physical education teacher, or the school secretary to administer emergency care is not an acceptable policy. All too often, the nurse is not in the building or the physical education teacher is not available. The secretary, though usually available, may not be at the site of injury or may not be properly trained to give the needed care.

Though not commonly required for teacher certification, it seems reasonable that all school personnel should be required to have training in first aid and cardiopulmonary resuscitation (CPR). In addition, appropriate first aid equipment and supplies should be accessible throughout the school. They should not be kept locked in cabinets where they are difficult to secure in emergencies.

Health Assessment Screening

Several health appraisals are usually part of the school program. No health appraisal should be conducted without an effective follow-up. The health assessment should also have an educational value for both the child and the parents, who should be informed of the results and the significance of the testing. Where a potential health problem is identified through the screening process, follow-up medical attention, treatment, and care must be obtained. The responsibility of the school is to assist parents in obtaining this care.

A common, early screening procedure is the weighing and measuring of children. This process, usually performed by the school nurse, the classroom teacher, or the physical education teacher, records the basic growth and development of the child.

Most children are screened for vision and hearing on several occasions during their school years. Both hearing and vision problems can develop gradually and sometimes are not noticed at all. The reduced ability to see or hear can affect learning and, ultimately, success in the classroom. Such conditions may also negatively affect school behavioral patterns. In addition to the formal vision and hearing tests, the classroom teacher can watch for behavioral changes that may indicate a developing problem.

Scoliosis, a lateral curvature of the spine, often becomes noticeable in the upper elementary grades. Early detection of students having scoliosis is important in controlling this health problem, and screening programs conducted by the school nurse, classroom teacher, or physical education instructor have been shown to be effective in identifying early cases.[31] It is important to conduct such screening, which involves little cost or time, before the adolescent growth spurt.

Though the school nurse conducts most health assessment activities, aides and other assistants, along with teachers, can also be trained to screen students. Regardless of who conducts the screening activity, the child's school health record should include the results of each procedure.

Should health clinics designed to provide health care for the students be established in the schools? Should birth control information and contraceptives be made available to teenagers in school-based clinics?

These questions have led to much controversy in a number of localities in recent years. The first school-based clinic was established in 1974 in St. Paul, Minnesota. This clinic provided immunizations, treatments for sexually transmitted diseases, and contraceptive advice and prescriptions. Since then other communities have sought to develop such facilities. Usually, the services at these clinics are provided by a nurse practitioner.

The number of school-based health clinics rose from about a dozen in the early 1980s to more than 327 by the mid-1990s. Most clinics provide a range of primary health care services. For a majority of the students using the school-based health clinic, there is no other source of primary health care. Physical examinations, laboratory tests, diagnosis and treatment of minor injuries, and medication prescription are performed in nearly all clinics, as well as educational and health counseling services.

Despite the many important services provided to children through the clinics, there has been extensive opposition to them. The principal opposition centers on the provision of reproductive health services, even though they account for less than one-fifth of all clinic visits. Pregnancy detection and referral for prenatal care, provision of birth control information, gynecological examinations, and prescriptions for birth control are provided in some clinics. Many people feel that school is not an appropriate place to provide contraceptives and birth control information. Some fear that abortions will eventually be provided.

Do you feel that school-based health clinics would be appropriate in your community? How would your community react if such clinics were established? Is there a need for them in your school district?

The School Nurse

The most visible person in a school health service program is the school nurse. Nursing services in the schools were introduced about the turn of this century as part of childhood disease control efforts.

Today, the services provided by school nurses have increased in number and scope. Most frequently, the school nurse provides direct care to children. The nurse is most often expected to care for a sick or injured child during the hours school is in session. Because such services obviously are not required full-time, the nurse spends much of her time keeping school health records of immunizations, screening results, and other pertinent data. These tasks are secondary, however, to the nurse's responsibilities for the care and supervision of student health.

The school nurse can and should be expected to perform a wider range of tasks than emergency care and record keeping. School nurses can play an important role in conducting immunization programs. Other measures designed to assess the health status of the children should be established and conducted by the nurse. All health assessment efforts should include components to interpret the findings to the parents and, in turn, help them find appropriate follow-up care in the community. The school nurse is in an important position to complete these health counseling tasks.

School nurses have become increasingly involved with special education students since the passage of Public Law 94–142, legislation that opened educational opportunities for handicapped children in the schools. The bill required schools to provide a normal education for all handicapped children within the structure of the regular school program. The nurse is part of the team that assesses the educational needs of the child and develops an individualized educational program (IEP) for each handicapped child.

Many handicapped children need specialized physical care while at school. This may involve the administration of medication or using a special apparatus. Nurses often are expected to provide such services, help the child to become self-sufficient, and assist teachers in overcoming fears and concerns about having handicapped children in their classes.

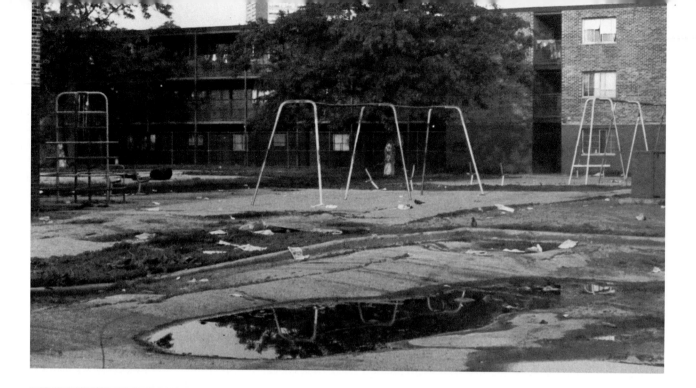

Many school grounds in urban communities are littered with paper, glass, and other debris. This school playground has broken and dangerous play equipment that can cause injury to children at school.

The school nurse is not normally certified to teach health classes. Usually, a health instructor must have a state teacher's certificate and, unless the nurse has taken course work in teacher preparation, it is unlikely that she or he will have earned the necessary credentials.

Nurses do, however, serve as facilitators to the health teachers. In addition to this, they can be helpful resource persons for both the teachers and the students. Because of these functions, any time that a school district is developing a health education curriculum, the school nurse should be included in the planning process.

School nurses usually serve in the schools under one of two administrative patterns: (1) they may be employed by the school district and, as such, work full-time under the control and supervision of the school administration; or (2) public health nurses employed by the local health department may be placed in the schools as part of their work assignments. Usually, public health nurses work in several schools in the community and so are unable to become closely acquainted with the children, faculty, and school administration. Although the

district-employed nurse frequently works in several schools, he or she usually develops a close relationship to the school system, its personnel, children, and overall program.

The School Environment

The school environment can have a direct effect upon student health and well-being. The school is not a vacuum, protected from adverse elements. The environment, physical as well as emotional, must be considered when devising a comprehensive school health program. School buildings need to be clean, properly ventilated, well lighted, and adequately maintained. Conditions within the school building and on the school grounds must be free of hazards that could lead to injuries and fatalities.

Safe School Setting

It is the responsibility of the board of education to provide a safe and healthful environment for students. Often local codes and regulations establish standards for school safety. Then it is the responsibility of the community health department sanitarian to inspect school facilities to make certain the standards are maintained. The food service facility is an example of one part of the school environment that must meet numerous health department regulations. The sanitarian inspects the food preparation facilities, as well as those for serving and eating, on a regular basis. Other state and local regulations assure proper sanitation and a safe water supply. In addition, heating, ventilation, and electrical system regulations, and various fire prevention codes must be met by school districts. These all require periodic inspections by the appropriate community agency.

A major problem in many communities, particularly in large urban settings, is the relatively poor physical condition of school facilities. Schools often are old, poorly maintained, and dirty, with litter covering the school grounds. Monies often are unavailable to repair damaged walls, ceilings, sidewalks, and other parts of the buildings. As school districts find themselves with increasing budget deficits, these adverse environmental conditions will probably worsen.

A report from one school district told of a situation in which a tax referendum for building maintenance and repair was defeated by the taxpayers. This particular district needed funds to repair chipped paint, poor lighting, and a number of other problems. Several days after the referendum defeat, a portion of the ceiling plaster fell on one classroom, injuring several students.

Schools not only have responsibility for children while on school grounds, but also during transport to and from school. Every day, thousands of American school children ride a bus to school. Considering the great number of miles covered each year by school buses, school bus transportation is basically safe; however, over fourteen thousand injuries occur in school bus accidents annually.[32] In one recent year, approximately 110 people were fatally injured in school bus accidents.[33] Of these fatalities, ten were passengers on the buses, twenty-five were pedestrians getting on or off the buses, and the remainder were struck by school buses.

These statistics indicate that measures are needed to assure a safe school bus program. Thus, the selection, training, and supervision of competent school bus drivers is very important. These drivers must maintain control and discipline on the buses to avoid accidents. Children must be taught to follow directions for safety while on the bus and while waiting for the school bus.

Legislation mandating that school buses have seat belts is lacking. After extensive study, the National Research Council reported in 1989 that seat belts on school buses are of minimal value. It stated that raising the minimum height of seat backs and making school bus loading zones safer would be of more value.

The National Transportation Safety Board made a series of recommendations concerning school bus safety in 1989. They strongly urged that all buses constructed before April 1977 be phased out of use. Buses manufactured before that date had unprotected fuel tanks, flammable seat covers, and questionable obstructions at the rear doors. Two major recommendations were that schools conduct bus evacuation drills to instruct students how to safely get off the bus in an emergency and that children receive instruction on how to wait at school bus loading zones.

School responsibility for student safety also extends to field trips, extracurricular events, and other school-related activities. The teacher, coach, or activity sponsor is responsible for the safety and well-being of children while involved in such activities. Not only must school districts establish policy for transportation in these situations, but all school personnel should be covered by liability insurance to protect against possible litigation.

Asbestos in Schools

During the 1950s and 1960s, hundreds of new school buildings were constructed throughout the United States. In most of the buildings a hydrated mineral silicate, asbestos, was used as a soundproofing and fireproofing agent. Asbestos was applied to ceilings, floor tiles, roofing, shingles, cement, and insulation.[34] It was used in the construction of many different types of rooms.

As early as the 1960s, concern began to be expressed about the relationship of asbestos and cancer among workers exposed to high levels of the substance. Studies of individuals in the manufacturing and construction industries who were exposed to asbestos for long periods of time revealed that they were experiencing increased incidences of asbestosis, lung cancer, and cancer of the esophagus, stomach, and colon.[35] These concerns led the Occupational Safety and Health Administration (OSHA)

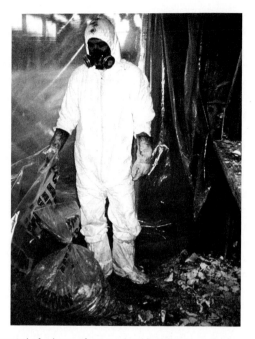

The removal of asbestos from a school building is a rather complex and costly activity. Total removal is the most time-consuming of the three procedures used in coping with the problem of asbestos in schools. The procedure necessitates isolating from the surrounding rooms the area where the asbestos is to be removed. Personnel involved in the removal process must wear protective clothing.

to establish exposure regulations in 1971. In 1973, the Environmental Protection Agency (EPA) banned asbestos for use in fireproofing and insulation.

Concern developed about the effect of asbestos exposure on children in school buildings. This concern was particularly based on the fact that children are in the same buildings over a period of several years throughout their schooling days. Since asbestos fibers are neither chemically nor biologically degradable, the cumulative effect on children might be dangerous.

As a result, school districts have been encouraged to take measures to eliminate this potentially hazardous school environmental factor. Federal legislation passed in 1986, the Asbestos Hazard Emergency Response Act, directed the Environmental Protection Agency to develop rules for assessing and managing asbestos in schools. All school districts are to inspect for friable and nonfriable asbestos in their buildings. Management plans are to be submitted to the state governor.

This legislation did not require removal, but schools must protect human health and the environment.

In 1987 the Environmental Protection Agency issued a plan of proposed rules that specified training and accreditation for five categories of personnel involved in asbestos control in schools. Specific training is indicated for asbestos inspectors, management planners, abatement project designers, contractors and supervisors, and abatement workers.

School administrators must decide whether to totally remove the asbestos or to encapsulate it in some way. Encapsulation may involve spraying the area with a chemical sealant or constructing a permanent partition to enclose the area where the asbestos is present. The procedure of total removal requires much care so that asbestos fibers are not released into the air, contaminating other areas of the schools.

There is no agreement as to which is the best procedure for school districts to take. Total removal is the most expensive. One report indicated that the average cost per school district to remove asbestos was $128,230, compared to $22,703 for encapsulation.[36] Encapsulation, though less expensive, still does not remove the asbestos from the school environment.

Numerous questions have been raised about this problem. In addition to concerns about cost and the most effective risk reduction measures is the basic issue of whether it is necessary. The general public has little interest in asbestos in the schools. There is no evidence that any child has developed cancer or any other ailment as a result of asbestos exposure during school attendance. The evidence linking human health with asbestos centers on individuals who work directly with the substance over a period of years. Nevertheless, it is a community health concern that needs further research and attention.

Violence and Schools

Violence in and around schools has increased dramatically in recent years. Young people, many below high school age, have been reported carrying firearms, knives, clubs, and other lethal objects to school. The federal Center to Prevent Handgun Violence reported in 1993 that there are 100,000 guns brought to school every day.[37] It was reported that gun violence in schools occurred on a weekly basis during the 1992–93 school year.[38] Included were

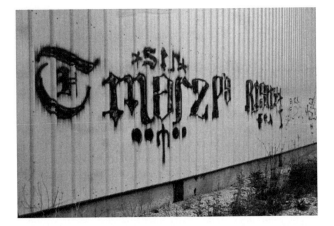

Gang warfare often spills over into the school setting. Graffiti on the walls of urban schools can often be the cause of resulting violence.

killings in the school buildings as well as on the school grounds. Not only were students the victims of shootings, but teachers and principals were also endangered.

Some of the shootings at school occurred while students were playing with guns. Sometimes increased school violence has been for the expressed purpose of harming another student; in other instances it has been for purposes of personal defense while at school or in transit to the school. Romantic disagreements can result in violence. These problems have been noted principally in urban localities. However, it has been reported to be spreading to suburban schools and to smaller towns and communities.

The problem of teenagers carrying weapons has been addressed in the health objectives for the nation initiative. One objective calls for the reduction of the carrying of weapons by teenagers.[39] Many reasons can be cited for the increased possession of lethal weapons by teenagers. In many instances it is the result of increased drug trafficking in the community. The increased presence of gangs is another significant contributing factor.

There always have been gangs, particularly in urban settings. However, in recent years gangs have become more violent because of the use of increasingly more powerful weapons. Gang activities are now being found in communities where gang problems never previously occurred. There are numerous reasons why young people are becoming more involved in gang activities.

Membership in the gang offers status, recognition, acceptance, and often provides identification with the drug trafficking subculture. In many instances violence is demanded for membership in the gang. Warfare between rival gangs often leads to serious problems in the community which spills over onto the school grounds and into the school building.

It is important that schools work with various community and social agencies in attempts to reduce the danger of violence at school. Today, in some cities, students must pass through metal detectors at the building entrances before they can go to their classes. Police presence is far too common in the school hallways of many schools. Random locker searches now are commonplace in many schools. Students in some localities are required to carry their books in mesh bookbags, making it harder to hide a weapon.

Dealing with the problems associated with gangs is no easy task. Defense of turf, a physical territory, is one of the important activities for gangs. It must be understood that schools be neutral territory. Distinctive gang dress, gestures, and jewelry must be banned from schools. School districts need to provide activity at school beyond the normal school hours for gang members. One school district has developed an alternatives to gangs curriculum, designed to capture the interest of teenagers who would otherwise become involved in a gang. The problem of violence at school cannot be solved by the school district acting alone. This is a problem larger than one individual entity. It must be a community effort for there to be any resolution to this increasingly serious school matter.

Emotional Climate of the School

The physical climate within a school and classroom is not the only environmental factor that affects the health and well-being of students. The emotional climate established by the teacher can have direct effects upon children, too. This is particularly important in the elementary schools where the same teacher interacts with the same children throughout most of the school day.

The importance of positive mental health among teachers and other school personnel is essential to the classroom environment. The teacher with mental and emotional problems or with stress-related problems can have a very detrimental effect on the students. The teacher experiencing stress and family or personal problems may contribute directly to the emotional problems of children in the classroom.

Stress is a major problem for many school employees. This tends to produce a number of negative behavior patterns among teachers.[40] Instances have been noted where emotionally disturbed teachers have behaved inappropriately or have exhibited bizarre actions. These actions often take the form of improper discipline and punishment or inappropriate academic demands on children. These inappropriate behaviors may surface in a teacher's conversations with the children, reactions to the students, or attitude toward the class.

One student told of a teacher who placed a telephone on her desk and warned the second-grade students that she could call God on this phone if they misbehaved. The teacher was under severe personal stress and receiving psychiatric care. The trauma, fear, and disruption this caused had a serious effect on the personal and academic growth of the children. It was reported that some children were afraid to attend school.

Schools seldom have plans to assist the emotionally disturbed teacher. School administrators fail to have teachers removed from the classroom when early signs of emotional stress are noted. It is not until a serious episode occurs that such action is taken. By this time, though, the children may be suffering emotionally, too.

In spite of the difficulty in coping with the problem of the emotionally disturbed teacher, school districts need to implement measures for better mental health. Teacher in-service programs on positive mental health and adapting mechanisms would be useful. Also, school districts should grant sick leave for emotional problems, as well as for physical illnesses. Schools must also consider leaves of absence for teachers with mental problems.[41] This would perhaps serve as an incentive for the teacher under stress to seek appropriate care. The teacher's job security and income would not be jeopardized, and so the individual may be more inclined to seek help.

School Nutrition Program

Providing nutritious meals for children at school is one of the most widespread programs in American educational institutions. Each day, nearly twenty-five million school children in about 90,000 schools are served lunch at school. This makes the school lunch program one of the largest "restaurants" in the world. As can be expected, a program this large creates many difficult and controversial issues.

The first school lunch program was developed in New York City in 1853.[42] Children attending a vocational school for the poor were served free meals. Early in the twentieth century, nutrition programs were started in many local communities. This was especially important during the depression of the 1930s, a time when many children received a major portion of the necessary daily nutrients through community school lunch programs.

The National School Lunch Program was authorized by Congress in 1946. Data obtained during World War II suggested that many American men of draft age had nutritional deficiencies. This, plus an available surplus of farm products, resulted in the passage of the legislation. This program was a means both of using surplus farm products and of promoting good nutrition and health in school age children.

In the years since 1946, changes in federal involvement in the school lunch programs have occurred. Federal subsidies have made milk available to school children, too. In the mid-1960s, the program was expanded to provide breakfast at school, particularly for needy children. It was believed that many children arrived at school in the morning without having been given anything to eat, which has a negative impact on learning. The federal government made provision to assist local school districts with food service equipment.

By the early 1970s, large food surpluses were no longer available to give to schools. Thus, the distribution of surplus foods to the schools was replaced by a system of governmental funding to assist local districts in the operation of the school lunch program. As a result, the amount of federal support of school lunch programs rose dramatically during the 1970s.

With the advent of federal budget reductions and reduced involvement in social service programs in the 1980s, the federal government cut subsidies for school lunches. The reductions have had far-reaching effects. Cash assistance for meals was reduced, causing the price charged to students for school lunches to rise. The American School Food Service Association estimated that 10 percent of the school age population dropped out of school lunch programs the first year of program reductions. Many of these children were from low socioeconomic backgrounds, and their parents found it difficult to qualify for free or reduced price meals as a result of tighter school lunch regulations.

The goal of the school lunch program has been to provide at least one-third of a child's daily nutritional requirements as established by the Food and Nutrition Board of the National Research Council. The federal guidelines have required that this lunch, called Type A, include some food from each of the following food groups: milk and milk products, meat and meat substitutes, vegetables and fruits, and bread.

In 1981, the federal government proposed lowering the requirement from one-third of the child's daily nutritional requirements to no more than one-fourth. Because of public and political opposition, this recommendation was not implemented.

The health objectives for the nation initiative has recommended that the Dietary Guidelines for Americans as published by the U.S. Department of Agriculture and the Department of Health and Human Services be used in the planning of school lunch and breakfast programs.[43] These guidelines can serve an important role in planning a healthful menu for school age children.

Despite its good intentions, the school lunch program has generated controversy. There is a great deal of food waste in the program. The United States Department of Agriculture reported that 15 percent of all food served to children in the schools is thrown away, chiefly in the fruits and vegetables groups. Such waste may occur because unpopular foods are served, because food is served in an unappetizing manner, or simply because of the throwaway mentality in the United States today. Government estimates place the dollar value of this waste at over $600 million a year.

In an attempt to reduce this food waste, a method of food service known as "offer versus serve" has been implemented.[44] This system offers five food items, and the child is able to select as few as three of the food items, but not all five. It is assumed that children will not select those foods that they would throw away.

Should schools sell "junk foods" as part of the school lunch program? These foods include soft drinks, candy, and chewing gum. Several state legislatures have attempted to pass laws that would restrict the sale of these items within the school program. Although many people support such actions, most legislative attempts have been unsuccessful. Many feel it is inappropriate; they suggest that local school districts, not federal and state government, should determine whether foods lacking nutritional value are sold at school.

One major reason the banning of such sales is opposed is that the funds earned from selling these foods are often used to support school activities, including athletics, clubs, bands, and other extracurricular activities. Many nutritionists and health professionals believe that it is inappropriate for the schools to make available foods that do not contribute to positive health and well-being.

The school lunch program should extend beyond the mere provision of nutrients for children. School efforts should be designed to educate the students about proper nutrition. Such efforts, it is hoped, will influence eating behavior of school children.

Summary

The schools play an important role in the health status of a community. All of the activities that are focused at the development of healthier individuals constitute the comprehensive school health program.

The school health instruction program introduces the students to health concepts, information, and knowledge. Health instruction is included as part of the total school curriculum at both the elementary and secondary school levels. The school health instruction curriculum should be developed to meet the needs and interests of the children. Even though health instruction is usually not considered a basic subject in the school curriculum, it is required by all state education regulations.

There have been efforts to establish a national curriculum in health education at various times in history. The School Health Education Study Curriculum, or SHES

Project, in the 1960s was one such attempt. In recent years, a variety of health education models have been developed and disseminated throughout various parts of the country. The Growing Healthy Curriculum Project has received the most widespread attention and use. Most of the recently developed curriculum models make use of a broad range of materials and methods, including various audiovisual materials. Teachers must usually attend special in-service training before the curriculum can be used in a school.

Three contemporary problems of those of school age are a particular focus of the school health program: teenage pregnancy and human sexuality, substance (drug) abuse, and AIDS. Education about human sexuality can be found in different formats in the school curriculum. Though supported by a majority of the public, sex education in the schools has been a topic of much controversy.

Increasing concern about substance abuse has put pressure on the schools to develop curriculum initiatives designed to cope with this problem. Such programs have been developed for use in elementary as well as secondary schools. In addition, a variety of activities have been developed to encourage the establishment of drug-free schools.

The growth of incidences of AIDS in the United States has brought about extensive curriculum programming designed to educate school children about this disease. These educational programs have been designed to begin in the elementary grades. Some school districts have had to face the issue of whether to admit an AIDS patient as a student. The Centers for Disease Control and Prevention recommends that these students be permitted to attend school. Most school districts have developed specific policies for coping with the presence of an AIDS patient in their school.

A variety of health services are provided in many school settings. Some health services, such as the enforcement of immunization requirements, are developed to protect against childhood communicable diseases. A number of screening activities designed to assess the health status of children occur at school. Vision and hearing loss and postural deviations are commonly identified by these school screening programs. In addition, the school district must care for all children who become sick or injured while at school. Not only must teachers have the knowledge and skills for emergency care, but the school district should have a written policy that is followed when injury or sickness occurs.

The school nurse is important to the health service program. The nurse can provide a number of services at school, with the families of the children, and in the community. The school nurse is not just a bandage dispenser, provider of first aid, and record keeper. The nurse's skills and training prepare for a broader role as health counselor, facilitator, and educator within the school and community.

The environment within which children spend several hours of each day should be as safe and healthful as possible. The physical environment of the school building and grounds has a profound effect upon the students' well-being. Not only is the physical setting important to the education of the children, but the emotional climate established by the teacher has direct effects that must not be overlooked. Measures need to be taken to help teachers experiencing stress, emotional upset, and family problems.

Violence in communities too often impacts the school. The increase in school violence can be attributed to several factors, particularly the growth of gangs. Schools must take measures to not just protect individuals while in school, but to encourage the development of nonviolent behaviors among school age children.

Many schools have had to cope with the presence of asbestos in their buildings. This substance has been linked with several problems, although none in school settings. Nevertheless, schools have been encouraged to either remove asbestos from the buildings or encapsulate areas where it is present.

The schools have served lunches to school children for years. The school lunch program provides nutrients for many young people, particularly the economically disadvantaged. In spite of the value of the school lunch programs, many questions and issues have arisen relating to the program. These questions concern the quality of food served, the nature of the educational experience, the acceptability of government involvement, and the costs of these programs.

Discussion Questions

1. What is meant by the concept of a comprehensive school health program?

2. Discuss some reasons that school health instructional programs have not affected the behavioral patterns of students.

3. Discuss the relationship of the federal, state, and local governments to the development of health curricula.

4. What is the Growing Healthy Curriculum Project?

5. Identify the main features of several health education curriculum models developed in the past few years.

6. Explain several activities that are part of the Michigan Model for Comprehensive School Health Education.

7. What are some of the topics most commonly found in a sex education curriculum?

8. Describe some of the reasons why people have opposed the teaching of human sexuality in the schools.

9. What topics should be included in an effective substance abuse education program in the schools?

10. Identify the key characteristics of a drug-free school.

11. What are some strategies used by schools in presenting drug-free school initiatives?

12. What should be included in the school health curriculum that pertains to AIDS?

13. Why would people be opposed to teaching about AIDS at school?

14. Discuss the issues involved in the discussion of whether children with AIDS should be permitted to attend school.

15. What position has the Centers for Disease Control and Prevention taken regarding school attendance for children with AIDS?

16. Do you agree with the objective of the national health objectives initiative that relates to teaching about AIDS in the school health program?

17. What immunizations are usually required by the states for admittance to school?

18. Who has the responsibility of caring for an injured child while at school?

19. What items would you include in a school policy for emergency care?

20. Define some screening procedures that are usually part of a school health service program.

21. Identify some of the skills that school nurses use in the school health program.

22. At what point does the school have responsibility for children coming to and going home from school?

23. Discuss the National Research Council recommendations regarding placing seat belts on school buses.

24. Identify some of the uses of asbestos in school construction.

25. Identify the measures that school districts can take to eliminate the potential hazard relating to asbestos.

26. Why has there been an increase in violence in schools in recent years?

27. Discuss measures that a school district can take to reduce the amount of violence in schools.

28. What are some measures that a school district could take to help teachers with emotional problems?

29. Discuss the issue of whether the schools should sell "junk food" as part of the school nutrition program.

30. What are some of the problems that have been noted in the school lunch program?

Suggested Readings

Alan Guttmacher Institute. *Risk and Responsibility: Teaching Sex Education in America's Schools Today.* New York, N.Y.: The Alan Guttmacher Institute, 1989.

Association for the Advancement of Health Education. *Healthy Networks: Models for Success.* The Association (1992): 102 pp.

Brie, James. "Teen Pregnancy: It's Time for the Schools to Tackle the Problem." *Phi Delta Kappan* 68, no. 10 (June 1987): 737.

Connell, David B., and Ralph R. Turner. "The Impact of Instructional Experience and the Effects of Cumulative Instruction." *Journal of School Health* 55, no. 8 (October 1985): 324–31.

Connell, David B., Ralph R. Turner, and Elaine F. Mason. "Summary of Findings of the School Health Education Evaluation: Health Promotion Effectiveness, Implementation, and Costs." *Journal of School Health* 55, no. 8 (October 1985): 316–21.

Education Improvement Center. *Recommendations for School Health Education: A Handbook for State Policymakers.* Report no. 130. Denver, Colo.: Education Commission of the States, 1981.

Farris, Rosanne P., and others. "Nutrient Contribution of the School Lunch Program: Implications for Healthy People 2000." *Journal of School Health* 62, no. 5 (May 1992): 180–84.

Gilbert, Glen G., Roy L. Davis, and Cheryl L. Damberg. "Current Federal Activities in School Health Education." *Public Health Reports* 100, no. 5 (September/October 1985): 499–507.

Griffith, Dan R. "Prenatal Exposure to Cocaine and Other Drugs: Developmental and Educational Prognoses." *Phi Delta Kappan* 74, no. 1 (September 1992): 30–34.

Hawley, Richard A. "Schoolchildren and Drugs: The Fancy That Has Not Passed." *Phi Delta Kappan* 68, no. 9 (May 1987): K1–K8.

Holtzman, Deborah, and others. "HIV Education and Health Education in the United States: A National Survey of Local School District Policies and Practices." *Journal of School Health* 62, no. 9 (November 1992): 421–27.

Horton, Lowell. *Developing Effective Drug Education Programs.* Bloomington, Ind.: Phi Delta Kappa Foundation, 1992, 40 pp.

Jibaja-Rusth, Maria L., and others. "Who Should Teach School Health? Personal and Setting Characteristics." *Health Values* 16, no. 5 (September/October 1992): 46–55.

Kenney, Asta M. "Teen Pregnancy: An Issue for Schools." *Phi Delta Kappan* 68, no. 10 (June 1987): 728–36.

Kenney, Asta M., and Margaret Terry Orr. "Sex Education: An Overview of Current Programs, Policies, and Research." *Phi Delta Kappan* 65, no. 7 (March 1984): 491–96.

Kenney, Asta M., and others. "Sex Education and AIDS Education in the Schools: What States and Large School Districts Are Doing." *Family Planning Perspectives* 21, no. 2 (March/April 1989): 56–64.

Kirp, David L., and Steven Epstein. "AIDS in America's Schoolhouses: Learning the Hard Lessons." *Phi Delta Kappan* 71, no. 8 (April 1989): 585–93.

Lavin, Alison T., and others. "Creating an Agenda for School-Based Health Promotion: A Review of 25 Selected Reports." *Journal of School Health* 62, no. 6 (August 1992): 212–28.

Miller, Dean F. *School Health Programs: Their Basis in Law.* New York: A. S. Barnes, 1971.

Owen, Sandra L., and others. "Selecting and Recruiting Health Programs for the School Health Education Evaluation." *Journal of School Health* 55, no. 8 (October 1985): 305–8.

Pine, Patricia. *Critical Issues Report: Promoting Health Education in Schools—Problems and Solutions.* Arlington, Va.: American Association of School Administrators, 1985.

Price, James H. "AIDS, the Schools, and Policy Issues." *Journal of School Health* 56, no. 4 (April 1986): 137–40.

Reed, Sally. "AIDS in the Schools: A Special Report." *Phi Delta Kappan* 67, no. 7 (March 1986): 494–98.

Rosoff, Jeannie I. "Sex Education in the Schools: Policies and Practice." *Family Planning Perspectives* 21, no. 2 (March/April 1989): 52.

Seidel, John F. "Children with HIV-Related Developmental Difficulties." *Phi Delta Kappan* 74, no. 1 (September 1992): 38–40, 56.

Taggart, Virginia S., and others. "A Process Evaluation of the District of Columbia 'Know Your Body' Project." *Journal of School Health* 60, no. 2 (February 1990): 60–66.

United States Department of Education. *Success Stories from Drug-Free Schools.* Rockville, Md.: National Clearinghouse for Alcohol and Drug Information, 1992, 58 pp.

United States Department of Education. *What Works: Schools without Drugs.* Rockville, Md.: National Clearinghouse for Alcohol and Drug Information, 1989.

Wojtowicz, G. Greg. "A Secondary Analysis of the School Health Education Evaluation Data Base." *Journal of School Health* 60, no. 2 (February 1990): 56–59.

Endnotes

1. Castile, Anne S., and Stephen J. Jerrick. *School Health in America*, 3rd ed. Kent, Ohio: American School Health Association, 1982, p. 9.

2. U.S. Department of Health and Human Services. *Healthy People 2000: National Health Promotion and Disease Prevention Objectives.* Washington, D.C.: U.S. Government Printing Office, 1991, p. 255.

3. *Ibid.*, 123.

4. *Ibid.*, 239.

5. *School Health Education Study: A Summary Report, 1964.* Washington, D.C.: School Health Education Study, 74 pp.

6. A listing of more than one hundred models is available from the Centers for Disease Control and Prevention, Atlanta, Georgia.

7. *School Health Education Study.*

8. Connell, David B., and others. "Summary of Findings of the School Health Education Evaluation: Health Promotion Effectiveness, Implementation, and Costs." *Journal of School Health* 55, no. 8 (October 1985): 316–21.

9. Department of Health and Human Services, Bureau of Health Education. *The School Health Curriculum Project.* Washington, D.C.: U.S. Government Printing Office, 1980, p. 4.

10. Association for the Advancement of Health Education. *Healthy Networks: Models for Success.* The Association (1992): 53–60.

11. *Ibid.*

12. *Ibid.*, 31.

13. "School Sex Ed Required in Three States and D.C., but Most States Allow Local Districts to Decide." *Family Planning Perspectives* 12, no. 6 (November/December 1980): 307.

14. *Ibid.*, 307–10.

15. Miller, Dean F. *School Health Programs: Their Basis in Law.* New York: A. S. Barnes and Co., 1971.

16. Louis Harris and Associates. *Public Attitudes toward Teenage Pregnancy, Sex Education and Birth Control.* New York: Louis Harris and Associates, 1988, p. 24.

17. Forstenberg, Frank F., and others. "Sex Education and Sexual Experience among Adolescents." *American Journal of Public Health* 75, no. 11 (November 1985): 1331–32.

18. Elam, Stanley M., and Alec M. Gallup. "The Twenty-first Annual Gallup Poll of the Public's Attitudes toward the Public Schools." *Phi Delta Kappan* 71, no. 1 (September 1989): 52.

19. U.S. Department of Health and Human Services. *Promoting Health/Preventing Disease: Year 2000 Objectives for the Nation.* Washington, D.C.: U.S. Government Printing Office, September 1989, pp. 4–19.

20. United States Department of Education. *Success Stories from Drug-Free Schools.* Rockville, Md.: National Clearinghouse for Alcohol and Drug Information, 1992, pp. 4–7.

21. *Ibid.*

22. Reported in *USA Today,* February 26, 1990.

23. U.S. Department of Health and Human Services. *Healthy People 2000: National Health Promotion and Disease Prevention Objectives.* Washington, D.C.: U.S. Government Printing Office, 1991, p. 488.

24. *Ibid.*

25. Centers for Disease Control. "Guidelines for Effective School Health Education to Prevent the Spread of AIDS." *Morbidity and Mortality Weekly Report* 37, No. S-2 (January 29, 1988).

26. Reed, Sally. "AIDS in the Schools: A Special Report." *Phi Delta Kappan* 67, no. 7 (March 1986): 494.

27. *Ibid.*

28. Bluford, John W. "Clinic Expands Adolescents' Access to Care." *Hospitals* 53, no. 19 (October 1, 1979): 125.

29. Miller, *School Health Programs,* 104.

30. ———, *School Health Programs,* 67–68.

31. Miller, Dean, and Carol Sue Lever. "Scoliosis Screening: An Approach Used in the School." *Journal of School Health* 52, no. 2 (February 1982): 98–101.

32. National Safety Council. *Accident Facts, 1993.* Chicago: National Safety Council, 1993, p. 74.

33. *Ibid.*, 74.

34. Stavisky, Leonard P. "State Responsibility for the Control of Asbestos in the Schools." *Journal of School Health* 24 (August 1982): 358–64.

35. *Ibid.*, 359.

36. *Asbestos in Schools: Inspection and Abatement.* American Association of School Administrators, Arlington, Va. 22209 (1985).

37. Reported in *USA Today,* June 3, 1993.

38. *Ibid.*

39. Department of Health and Human Services, *Healthy People 2000,* 236.

40. Brodbelt, S. "Teachers' Mental Health: Whose Responsibility?" *Phi Delta Kappan* 53 (1973) 268–69.

41. Miller, Dean F., and Jan Wiltse. "Mental Health and the Teacher." *Journal of School Health* 49 (September 1979): 374–77.

42. Means, Richard K. *Historical Perspectives on School Health.* Thorofare, N.J.: Slack, Inc., 1975.

43. U.S. Department of Health and Human Services. *Healthy People 2000,* 95.

44. National Dairy Council. *Dairy Council Digest* 53, no. 6 (November/December 1982): 33.

CHAPTER **SEVENTEEN**

Health Education/Health Promotion

The Forefront of Preventive Health and Wellness

The basic behavioral patterns of a great many people do not contribute to optimum, positive health and well-being. For example, improper eating habits lead to overweight and the problems associated with it. Despite much evidence linking cigarette smoking to respiratory disease and cancer, many people throughout the world still smoke. Stress is common in the lives of many in our society. Many adults are physically inactive and do not participate in activity that would result in improved levels of fitness. These and numerous other behaviors that have detrimental effects on health are part of the basic life-style of many Americans.

Health Education and Behavioral Change

Traditionally, health services have focused upon curative health care. Most people consult the available health service (the doctor, the hospital, or the clinic) when they are sick with either an acute or chronic problem. Some leave the available health care service with improved (more positive) health and well-being; others do not experience significant improvement. Rarely do people enter health care systems for preventive purposes.

In the past decade increased attention has been given to disease prevention and health promotion. Thus, some changes in the roles and expectations of the health service system have taken place. Greater numbers of people are interested in and now practice preventive measures, and health care providers are expanding health promotion programming.

An important component of this increased emphasis on health promotion is education about health. Community health education initiatives must plan experiences to positively influence health behavioral patterns. Structured health education programs are a necessary element of health promotion. Health education strategies can be designed to meet people's needs, regardless of where they are on the health continuum: from good (positive health and well-being) to bad (negative health, sickness, and debilitation).

The ultimate goal of any health education activity is to change behavioral patterns or to reinforce already positive activity. Influence of health behavior, not just acquisition of additional knowledge, should be the focal point of health education programs. Traditionally, the purpose of education has been to impart specific knowledge about a matter, which would result in the desired behaviors. Many health education instructors still adhere to this practice and impart factual knowledge about a topic to their audience using films, pamphlets, handouts, flip charts, and brochures. There has been little effort to learn if a specific strategy is effective for the population group or the topic under consideration, and behavior often is not influenced by cognitive learning experiences.

Possibly the best example of the ineffectiveness of this approach is the smoking habit. Thousands of people in the United States are very knowledgeable about the potential health hazards associated with smoking cigarettes, yet they continue to smoke. Until *attitudes* can be influenced, certain psychological needs fulfilled, and social influences overcome, the desired behavioral changes may never take place.

Research into human behavior has added to the health educator's available information. Sociological theories of learning behavior and behavioral change can help us understand how changes in health behavior take place. It is important that those conducting a health education program understand how each audience can be persuaded to make certain changes in health behavior. The instructor must be flexible, too; a certain communication strategy that works with a given population is no guarantee that it will be successful with another group. Increasingly, community health educators are creating programs based on behavior dynamics research, not solely upon the techniques of teaching materials and methods used in the past.

Attitudes, cultural beliefs and value systems, teaching and learning strategies, and communication skills all affect the learning process. As a result, each is important to the development of health education programs.

Attitude Formation

An instructor must be aware of the attitudes of the population before planning and conducting a health education program. Every cultural group has established attitudes and values about the topic under consideration, as well as the educational process. Thus, the instructor should ask "What is the general attitude toward the issue under consideration?" and "How will the audience accept me or what I have to say?" Education involving attitude formation and influence can be effective in health modification, but only when the instructor has asked and answered these and other similar questions about the audience and the teacher-student relationship.

Cultural Dimensions

Documented studies have concluded that the cultural mores and background of a group of people must be considered in establishing any successful health education program. However, all too often those who plan and conduct the health education program are unfamiliar with the values, beliefs, language, or life-style of the population. Until the particular cultural group recognizes a need and programming becomes part of their values, it is doubtful that a program will be accepted.

Educational Strategies

An educational strategy or communication skill that has been used to teach health concepts for years is not necessarily the best. Research and experience can tell us much about the most effective ways to present information that will likely result in the desired behavior.

Several different educational learning models have received much attention from health educators and been used for research and program development, including the theory of reasoned action,[1] locus of control,[2] the Health Belief Model,[3] ecological models,[4] and the PRECEDE model.[5] A model of learning theory developed by Brazilian educator Paulo Freire known as *empowerment education* has been useful in adult health education initiatives. Freire's ideas were developed and tested while teaching the poor urban dwellers and peasants of Brazil. First, the community's problems are identified. Then active learning methods including much dialogue take place. Throughout the process the participants determine their own and the community's needs and priorities.

In order for the community health educator to communicate effectively, it is important that the most effective methods and procedures for working with or educating particular groups are used. This necessitates a thorough knowledge of the consumers and their concerns,

Presenting Culturally Appropriate Health Promotion Programming

Many health education initiatives are designed using various social learning theories. These presentations and programs of intervention attempt to bring about certain identified behaviors. In the process of program planning it is important to consider many questions: Just when is the appropriate time for interventions to take place? Whose values and ethical standards should be used in determining the behaviors that are to be the focus of these programs? In a pluralistic society with many different philosophical, religious, racial, ethnic, and social standards, the answers to these questions are very complex.

Development of materials and identification of the most effective interventions depend on an awareness and understanding of the group for which the program is directed. This was taken into account in developing culturally appropriate material relating to AIDS for an Hispanic population group. Some Hispanics did not know the meaning of the Spanish equivalents for anal and oral intercourse. Since this is a very important concept in teaching about AIDS, it was imperative to identify words used and understood by the intended population.

What are some cultural concepts that would be difficult for a health educator in your community to overcome in developing appropriate educational strategies? How can the community health educator cope with the various philosophical and religious beliefs that have an impact on health decision making?

Health promotion programs that will help people change their life-styles toward optimal health must consider physical, emotional, social, spiritual, cultural, and intellectual aspects.

---

interests, background, value systems, and language. Many health education programs are ineffective because they are poorly planned or fail to take into consideration the background and the value system of the prospective population.

For example, attention must be given to the reading level of the material being used in the program. Many pamphlets and brochures used by health educators in community programs are not understood by those for whom they are intended because of a lack of reading comprehension. Some people do not learn from written material as well as they do from oral instruction. For these reasons effective community health promotion programs must include both oral and visual teaching aids and materials designed for the particular population.

Health Promotion

With greater interest in health maintenance and disease prevention, public interest in health education has increased. There are many who feel that through the process of education, health and well-being can be enhanced. But such a development requires a variety of approaches with the same focus: behavioral change. Strategies should consider not only education, but also societal structure and environmental factors.

As a result, a broadened concept of health education known as *health promotion* has been developed and accepted. Health education and health promotion are not synonymous. Health promotion includes education plus related political and economic considerations. Health promotion has been defined as

. . . Any combination of health education and related organizational, economic or political interventions designed to facilitate behavioral and environmental changes conducive to health.[6]

The American Hospital Association has defined health promotion as:

. . . the process of fostering awareness, influencing attitudes, and identifying alternatives so that individuals can make informed choices and change their behavior in order to achieve an optimum level of physical and mental health and improve their physical and social environment.[7]

Health promotion implies that health education has multiple goals. Health education is increasingly turning to the behavioral sciences for a basis for operation. There is increasing focus on behavioral outcomes, with emphasis on how knowledge, attitude, and beliefs contribute to health behavior.

The health educator, more than a dispenser of knowledge, becomes a health advocate to different groups of people, often in the political realm. The health educator might work with community authorities to influence legislation or to establish environmental standards for health protection. Many important health improvements have been thus engineered and have resulted in better sanitation, proper sewage disposal, and a safe water supply. The health advocate also works with disadvantaged people, such as the elderly, the poor, the homeless, or a foreign language-speaking group. Representing the concerns and needs of these people at important decision-making levels in the community is part of health promotion.

The health educator's role has expanded to include program development. This requires skill in setting goals, organizing a project, managing its operation, and then evaluating the effectiveness of the project. Since the funding for such programs often is obtained only through the grant process, the community health educator must also be skilled in grant development and writing.

Health Education/Health Promotion in Operation

Health education and health promotion activities occur in many community settings. They may involve teaching classes in a school, in an industrial setting, or to some neighborhood group. Speaking to different clubs, agencies, or classes may be the means of imparting health concepts. Health education and health promotion activities occur in such locations as hospitals, occupational settings, schools, health fairs, and through the mass media.

The Hospital

Hospitals throughout the United States have become increasingly involved in health promotion programming. Hospitals are providing not only patient educational services but wellness and health promotion activities for residents of the entire community. Nearly 90 percent of hospitals in the United States today offer patient education or community health promotion programs to at least one target population.[8] Hospital-based health promotion programs target inpatients, hospital employees,

outpatients, the general community population, and employees of corporations and industries. These developments expand the hospital's focus from curative treatment for sick and disabled people to health promotion, disease prevention, and improved life-style.

Emphasis on Wellness

Hospital-based community health promotion programs are a recent development. Prior to 1978, few hospitals had such programs.[9] Most hospital-based community education activities that did exist provided first aid instruction and conducted health fairs and occasional seminars. Increasingly, these programs are providing instruction relating to wellness and improved individual life-style.

Today three out of every four hospitals are providing weight reduction and smoking cessation programs.[10] Stress management and fitness classes are other commonly found wellness activities in hospital wellness programs.[11] Even though hospital-based community education programs are conducted for all age groups, most are directed at adults.

The primary purpose of these activities is to promote positive health habits. By conducting health promotion programs, the hospital creates a more positive image in the community. As a result, there is increased community support for the hospital and its activities. Individuals come to accept the hospital as a positive contributor to health and wellness—not just a place to go when injured, sick, or dying. The American Hospital Association has encouraged hospitals to become involved in such community health education efforts:

Hospitals have a responsibility to take a leadership role in helping ensure the good health of their communities.[12]

Hospital-based community wellness programs employ a variety of approaches. One such program screened members of the local unions for hypertension and presented information about positive health behavior. People were encouraged to make life-style adaptations to reduce high blood pressure. Another hospital created health promotion messages for use on cable television. In one city, a wellness center, complete with exercise facilities and classrooms, was established in a shopping center. In yet another location, a school, closed because of reduced enrollment, has been rented by a hospital to house

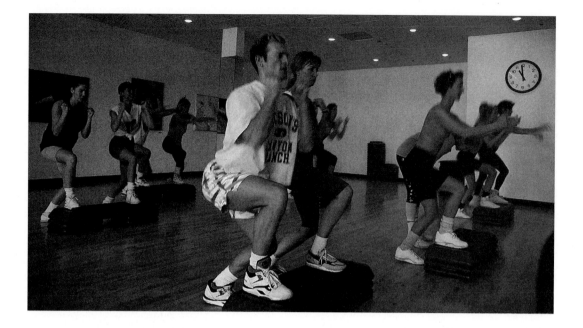

Wellness and health promotion programs include small- and large-group activities.

Hospital-Based Health Promotion Programs

Target Population	Most Common Programs
Inpatients	Diabetes, preoperation education
Hospital employees	CPR, orientation to hospital
Outpatients	Diabetes, nutrition
Community residents	CPR, prenatal
Corporations	CPR, stress management

Source: American Hospital Association. *Hospital-Based Health Promotion Programs: Report and Analysis of the 1984 Survey.* Chicago, Ill.: American Hospital Association, 1984.

community health, nutrition, fitness, and related programs. These approaches are variations of an attempt to convince all sectors of a community to analyze and change their life-styles to promote health.

Patient Education

Hospitals, along with other health care institutions, continue to expand their patient education programs. These programs, available for both the patient and the family, are designed to inform all concerned about specific health problems. It has been recommended that at least 90 percent of all health care institutions should provide patient education programs by the year 2000.[13]

Most patients need more information about their condition than has been traditionally given. Patient education programs provide information about the condition of the patient, the treatment being rendered, and the purposes of medication, and clarify specific directions given the patient. These educational efforts help the patient to cope with the situation and to make any life-style adaptations that might be needed. Patient education sessions may be conducted on a one-to-one basis or in group settings.

Though any disability or health problem can be the focus of a patient education program, two of the more common programs are for diabetic and cardiac patients. Diabetic education programs help the patient understand how to control insulin levels and diet. Cardiac rehabilitation programs assist the heart attack victim in learning how to adjust to a new life-style. The patient is taught to live with heart disease.

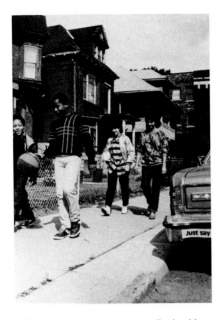

With W. K. Kellogg Foundation support, a pilot health awareness program has been launched in New York's lower Manhattan to prevent young people from adopting negative health behaviors. It is conducted by The Door—A Center of Alternatives, a project of the International Center for Integrative Studies. The program targets inner-city youth who are at high risk for substance abuse, nutritional deficiencies, and other health problems.

One creative diabetic program was a summer camp for young diabetics sponsored by a local hospital. During the one-week session, the children learned about diabetes and how to cope with this condition, and developed skills to enhance their life-styles. Appropriate physical activities and skills were also taught.

Many hospitals and clinics have instructional packages to help the patient and relatives understand operative procedures. Preoperation instructions can be helpful in eliminating some of the misunderstanding and stress associated with surgery. Postoperative education can provide information about how to cope with and assist the recuperation and rehabilitative process.

Patient education programs are often available for both the mother and the father in the clinical setting at the time of and following birth. Matters relating to infant feeding and care, maternal postnatal care, and future birth control are usually of interest to parents at this time.

An important tool in patient education programs is the learning resource center in hospitals or other health care institutions. This center might include a library with a variety of health education materials, as well as audiovisual equipment available for patient use on an individual basis. Learning carrels for independent study and areas for small-group teaching are often available, too. Hospitals have also found the use of closed circuit television and in-house telephone circuits to be effective procedures for conducting patient education programs.

Patient education is likely to continue to expand in the future. Increasingly, educational materials for patients are being provided in smaller clinics, individual physician's offices, and pharmacies. These materials usually include pamphlets that explain in some detail the condition the patient is experiencing, which is useful not only for the patient but also for one's family or care giver.

The cost of patient education programs is currently covered by a few insurance programs. However, until third-party payment provides coverage on a wider basis it is doubtful whether all individuals will be able to obtain useful patient education. Only as more companies extend their benefits will growth in patient education initiatives occur.

Occupational Health

With the rising cost of health insurance coverage for employees, many businesses and industries are establishing health promotion programs. Realizing the cost benefit of preventive health programs, some companies have employed health promotion and health education specialists, constructed facilities for conducting these programs, and taken measures to encourage life-style changes that are conducive to health and wellness.

From the employer's point of view, there are several advantages to health promotion programs: employees involved in such programs perform better on the job and are more productive, and fewer days of work time are lost owing to illness and accident. This, in turn, lowers the cost of medical care coverage.

Health promotion programs also help employees to cope with stress, a major problem for both labor and management. Not only is stress management helpful, but employee morale increases and positively affects the company's output. Where health promotion programs

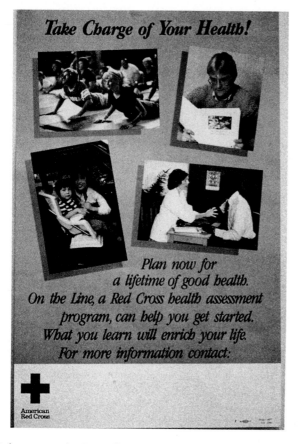

Take Charge of Your Health!

Plan now for a lifetime of good health. On the Line, a Red Cross health assessment program, can help you get started. What you learn will enrich your life. For more information contact:

American Red Cross

Before one can begin an effective health improvement program, it is necessary that some assessment measures be conducted. A number of different health assessment tools are available to help the individual get started in a health promotion program. It is important to understand exactly what kinds of information the particular assessment instrument can provide.

have been established, employees feel that the company is interested in them as persons and not just as "cogs" in the machinery of industry.

The programs that have been developed vary from one locality to another and from one company to the next. Physical fitness programs are one very common component of industrial health programs. Opportunities for the workers to exercise regularly in such facilities as tennis courts, basketball courts, fields for team games, running tracks, and indoor racquetball courts are made available. This availability is an incentive for learning the skills necessary to participate in these fitness activities.

Some occupational health programs focus on reducing the risk of cardiovascular disease. Hypertension screening has revealed numerous individuals who are at risk for heart attacks. Education and risk reduction planning following a screening program can reduce the possibility of a heart attack and help the employee to feel better and so live a more productive life.

Weight reduction programs have been instituted by many companies. Such programs include not only instruction about proper nutrition and nutrition intake surveys but, in some cases, a revamping of the food service facility at the industrial site. In one instance, employees recommended, after several nutrition classes, that the company cafeteria change its menu to include more salads and nonfattening foods.

Safety instruction required by OSHA (Occupational Safety and Health Administration) rules and regulations is an important component of an occupational health promotion program. Instruction in first aid, cardiopulmonary resuscitation (CPR), and accident prevention is often provided.

Regardless of the type of program, the most important component must be health promotion. Industry may create such programs because of economic incentives, but the employees actually benefit by improved health.[14]

The School

Health education has been part of the school curriculum since the 1860s, when Horace Mann, the noted education commissioner in Massachusetts, emphasized in his annual reports the need for effective physiology and hygiene (health) instruction in the schools.[15] Principally as a result of his reviews and urging, Massachusetts became the first state to pass legislation requiring that physiology and hygiene courses be part of the school curriculum. School health programs now include health services in addition to health instruction. The presentation and study of health concepts are a part of the education process from preschool through college. However, coordinated, comprehensive school health education programs are few, and those that do exist lack uniformity.[16]

The curriculum for health education in schools is usually developed at the local level by educators within the school district and is designed to meet the particular needs and interests of students in the community. Though some states require that health education be part of the educational program, the development of comprehensive, statewide school health programs rarely occurs.

Though health education has not been a priority in schools in the United States, it still has the potential, when well organized and well taught, to have lasting positive effects on the health and well-being of school age children. In order for this to happen, support must be gained at the community level from various important decision makers. The importance of school board members, superintendents of schools, principals, curriculum coordinators, and community medical and health leaders must be emphasized in designing school health programs that are effective in the lives of children.

The need for expanded comprehensive school health initiatives in the 1990s has been highlighted by the Year 2000 Health Objectives for the Nation.[17] More than forty-six million children are enrolled in America's schools; the objective states that at least 75 percent of both elementary and secondary schools should provide a planned and sequential health education curriculum by the end of the decade. To achieve this goal, more state and local school districts must develop a K–12 sequential curriculum.

In 1989 the Carnegie Council on Adolescent Development Task Force issued an extensive report giving recommended directions for educational reform of America's middle schools.[18] The task force called for improved school health and fitness programs, noting that if overall academic performance is to be improved, individual health and fitness must be enhanced. The report recommended that every middle-grade school have a health coordinator. In addition, the need for a health-promoting environment was stressed, and schools should play a part in ensuring that all students have access to community health and social services and resources.

To encourage districtwide school health program development, team efforts involving a broad range of personnel working together seem to be the most effective. An approach that has been found to be useful in motivating school districts and getting multidisciplinary teams to begin to work together to set goals has been to bring a team together for a concentrated conference. Here goals and objectives are established and plans initiated. Then the teams return to their communities and begin to work together in coalitions to implement comprehensive school health programs. This approach has been found to be successful in such states as Oregon and Ohio.

Mass Media

The mass media have a tremendous influence on the life-style of the United States citizen. Television, radio, and the printed page reach every home in the country.

The media can have both positive and negative effects on health behavior. From a negative standpoint, mass media, particularly television, often portray unhealthy life-styles. Such portrayal may encourage drunkenness, obesity, drug use, habitual smoking, and violence.

Another media-related contributor to negative health behavior is advertising of products that have detrimental health effects. Though cigarette smoking advertising is banned on television, such advertisements do still appear in print. Advertising is also misleading in its presentation of many health-related products. Health education strategies need to be developed that assist the average citizen in discerning truth in advertising from that which is misleading.

In spite of the negative impact on health behavior made by the mass media, a number of possibilities exist for using television, radio, and periodicals to teach positive health concepts. Simple, one-minute health messages on such topics as accident prevention, immunizations, nutrition, and family planning have been developed and presented. These public service announcements are often presented by local health departments or voluntary health organizations.

Exercise and fitness programs are sometimes offered on television. The viewer is expected to follow the leader in doing a series of exercises in the home. Though interesting to watch and usually well produced, the programs have doubtful value in weight reduction and fitness, and the development of ongoing positive health behavior is doubtful.

With increased public interest in health issues, both television and radio have produced special prime time health programs on topics such as abortion, health care costs, teen suicide, teen pregnancy, and world hunger. Such programs add to the awareness and health knowledge of citizens about these important issues. However, little behavioral effect on individuals is evident from such presentations.

The use of mass media in isolation usually will not bring about positive behavioral change. Such efforts must be reinforced by follow-up activities. One approach to the problem is to relate the message to an appropriate local health agency. The viewers, listeners, or readers are made aware that they can contact the agency for additional information on the topic or for personal counseling and/or services. The mass media message should also encourage listeners and readers to be screened for a health problem when appropriate, particularly diabetes, hypertension, and physical fitness.

The mass media can be used to bring health promotion messages to minority populations.[19] To be effective, these radio and/or television messages must consider the ethnic values, attitudes, and beliefs of the selected population group. To reach non-English-speaking groups, the health messages must be in their primary language. This is particularly important with regard to programs directed at the Spanish-speaking Hispanic population.

The Health Fair

An interesting approach to community health education is the health fair. This exhibition or carnival may be held at an educational institution, a shopping center, as part of a larger county or regional fair, or in any number of other community settings. Many people are exposed to health ideas and concepts in these settings. In this country, nearly two million people visit at least one health fair annually.[20]

Health fairs provide an opportunity to integrate health education activities with multiphasic health-screening activities. Representatives from the community

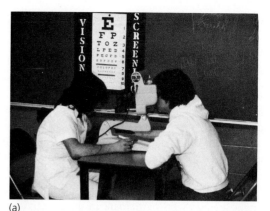

(a)

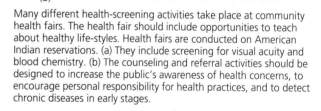

(b)

Many different health-screening activities take place at community health fairs. The health fair should include opportunities to teach about healthy life-styles. Health fairs are conducted on American Indian reservations. (a) They include screening for visual acuity and blood chemistry. (b) The counseling and referral activities should be designed to increase the public's awareness of health concerns, to encourage personal responsibility for health practices, and to detect chronic diseases in early stages.

health agencies, health care providers, and consumers are brought together in these informal settings. This often leads to improved communication within the community.

An important benefit of the health fair is that it often commands media attention. Local newspapers will often present a story or picture from the fair. Also, television finds the health fair an interesting item to show on the local segment of the newscast.

Since learning is best facilitated by doing, health fairs usually provide experiential types of activities. A person may perform a simple exercise to see the effect of the exercise on the pulse rate. A health fair for school age children may have the participants move through a maze of activities, each designed for some learning objective. Audiovisual aids accompany many of these activities.

The health fair stimulates interest in health by providing information and reinforcing already existing positive health behaviors.[21] It is an effective tool that challenges individuals to be informed about community resources.

Though the health fair stimulates a lot of interest and exposes individuals to a great deal of health information, its effect on long-range health behavior has not been documented. In fact, there is some evidence that many people who participate in these activities are already aware of their health status. For example, blood pressure screening is common at health fairs, but those volunteering to be screened are often already aware of their hypertension.[22]

Screening tests are very popular among those attending a health fair. They are most effective when targeted at a specific health risk population. Many kinds of screening procedures can be found. Those tests that have been shown to be reasonably justifiable have included weight measurement, skin fold thickness measurement, blood pressure, serum cholesterol and glucose tests, and stools for occult blood in people over fifty.[23] It is important that people whose screening tests indicate that they are at risk for a particular problem have follow-up treatment. Many times health fair counseling and follow-up are inadequate.

Regardless of problems associated with health fairs, they offer an opportunity to expose people in the community to issues relating to wellness and an improved life-style. The interest and creative approach found in these settings can benefit some individuals who may not be reached in more structured educational settings.

National Health Education/Health Promotion Initiatives

Federal Government

In the early 1970s, an extensive study on health education in the nation was conducted. The study committee, commissioned by President Richard M. Nixon and known as the President's Committee on Health Education, submitted its final report in 1972.[24]

The report noted that federal involvement in health education had been minimal. Only one-half of 1 percent of the total health care expenditures in the United States was for health education.[25] Even worse, about one-fifth of 1 percent of the federal allocation for health was expended on health education.

The study also reported that health education throughout the country was fragmented among many agencies. Even though it is an accepted fact that many major illnesses can be prevented by individual behavioral patterns, health education was a neglected phase of health care.

The committee identified many health needs that could be addressed through health education. Five specific population groups were noted as having unique health education needs: low-income families, mothers, school children and teenagers, middle-aged middle class, and the elderly.

The relationship between low income and poor health, as discussed earlier, was recognized. The poor suffer from malnutrition, have higher rates of infant mortality, and experience a higher incidence of respiratory, emotional, and other disorders than the average population.[26] The ramifications of these health problems are social and political, as well as medical.

Mothers were singled out by the President's Committee as an important audience for health education. Mothers have significant influence on the health and well-being of their young children.[27] Many health behavioral patterns such as nutrition of family members are influenced most by the mother.

Although most young children and teenagers attend school, the commission found health education in the schools extremely poor and ineffective. In the schools, health is often taught as part of another subject, such as biology, home economics, or physical education. There was little evidence that school health education was effective in improving eating habits, reducing teenage smoking, reducing incidence of venereal disease, or stopping the spread of drug usage.[28]

The middle-aged middle class was singled out by the commission because of its low fitness level. Poor nutrition was specifically identified as a negative factor. Obesity, lack of exercise, smoking, and high-cholesterol food intake are common parts of this population's life-style. These conditions lead to a variety of chronic health problems.

Senior citizens have a number of different health needs.[29] The need for attention and health education for this population sector was stressed by this report. Living conditions, as well as health counseling, were noted as being important areas to address in improving the lifestyle of the aged.

The President's Committee made several important recommendations, one of which was for the establishment of a national office for health education. As a result, the Bureau of Health Education was established. The mission of this governmental agency, located within the Centers for Disease Control and Prevention, was to strengthen health programs at the local, state, and national levels.

With the reorganization in 1981 of the Centers for Disease Control, the Bureau of Health Education was combined with two other federal agencies and became known as the Center for Chronic Disease Prevention and Health Promotion. The center supports school health education initiatives along with programming for minorities. Another program responsibility is reproductive health. The center, in conjunction with other agencies, enters into contract arrangements for funding of a variety of health education and health promotion projects.

Congress passed the National Consumer Health Information and Health Promotion Act in 1976, which established an office of health promotion and health information within the Department of Health, Education, and Welfare (HEW). This office is now a part of the Department of Health and Human Services (HHS) and is known as the Office of Disease Prevention and Health Promotion.

The major focus of this federal governmental office is stimulating health promotion and disease prevention through various preventive program activities. Specific program initiatives are directed toward nutrition, school health, worksite health promotion, preventive services, and community/media health promotion.[30] It is the responsibility of this office during the 1990s to coordinate the many initiatives for the Year 2000 Health Objectives for the Nation.

The office's goal of coordinating health promotion efforts throughout the nation is achieved through a series of activities that involve conducting regional forums on various community health promotion issues. The office has provided technical assistance, as well as federal funds, for various community health promotion efforts.

An important project supported by this office is the development of the National Health Information Clearinghouse, a referral system that identifies health information resources. The information provided by these resources is made available upon request to the public, as well as to health professionals. A variety of information on health-related topics is produced and disseminated. The clearinghouse operates a library for the public and maintains a database of health-related groups, agencies, and support groups. Questions concerning rare diseases are answered through the clearinghouse.

Another national program supported by this office has been a national health promotion media campaign. The goal of this project has been to inform the public, with special emphasis on minority groups, of action that would maintain or improve health by reducing health risks. Several mass media approaches have been used—television, radio, newspapers, and magazines, as well as public posters and advertising. Each health message encourages people to write to the National Health Information Clearinghouse for more information on good health. These media health promotion messages have been directed toward the general public, mothers and children, and senior citizens.

A resource center for worksite health promotion has been established within the Office of Disease Prevention and Health Promotion. Various services are made available to employers, employees, labor unions, public policymakers, and others interested in worksite health promotion. One activity has been the development of model programs that are available to small companies not having large numbers of worksite health promotion personnel. Technical assistance is available to start these programs.

Private Sector

Established as a national agency in the private sector to improve health education, the National Center for Health Education has sponsored conferences, workshops, and seminars on a number of topics for many different audiences. It has been prominent in piloting, revising, and updating the Growing Healthy Curriculum Project. The center was also a leading force in the role delineation project, an attempt to identify health educator competencies. During the 1980s the center's activities focused on two areas: (1) school health and (2) health in the workplace.

In addition to the federal funding that has been made available through the Centers for Disease Control and Prevention, operational monies for the National Center for Health Education are made available from a number of sources in the private sector. The Kellogg Foundation and the Ittleson Foundation of New York are the primary backers, although funds have also been received from Aetna Life and Casualty, Bristol Meyers, United States Steel, and the Prudential Life Insurance Foundation. Voluntary agencies, such as the American Cancer Society and the American Heart Association, also contribute to the National Center. Donations from the American Dental Association and the American Hospital Association demonstrate the support of professional health organizations.

Planned Approach to Community Health (PATCH)

The Centers for Disease Control and Prevention has introduced a program designed to support state and local health departments' health promotion programs. This program approach that involves the development of comprehensive community health programs is known as the Planned Approach to Community Health (PATCH). This model is intended to facilitate the development of collaborative, community-based health promotion programs. Strong focus is placed on local empowerment of community health programs.

The program design model involves the inclusion of several specific actions. It begins with the identification of health problems in a particular target population. This assessment is based on the use of local health data. Local support and participation of community people are sought as they become involved in recommending goals, setting objectives, and prioritizing problems where there are multiple problems that have been identified. People within an identified community tend to respond when they recognize the needs and have a strong feeling about

and understanding of the importance of changing the circumstances resulting in the particular problem.

Part of this assessment stage involves the identification of community resources available to bring into play in carrying out the program initiative. This may involve financial as well as personal and agency resources.

Once the needs assessment has been accomplished, specific program planning takes place. During this phase, as well as during the assessment, the population involved in the program focus is included. Implementation of the specific interventions is then carried out.

The final component of the PATCH model involves evaluation. As with any health promotion program, evaluation must consider several factors: the individual outcomes, program component success, as well as attitudes of the community members involved in the specific initiative. The PATCH model has been used for carrying out health promotion programs in public housing communities,[31] among African-Americans in an urban program,[32] and by a state health department.[33]

Health Education Credentialing

Throughout the 1980s several initiatives were designed to upgrade the profession of health education. The primary focus was the development of a professional credentialing system for health educators. Many different professions have been involved in providing health education programming. For some people the medical care provider or nurse comes to mind when health education is mentioned. For others, particularly in school settings, the coach is the person who is thought of. Numerous other related health professionals could be mentioned.

The initiative resulting in health education credentialing had its beginning in 1978 with the establishment of a task force to examine the preparation and practice of health educators. This project, which brought together leaders from several of the professional associations that include health educators, identified a series of competencies that it was felt should be required of any individual considered to be a health educator, regardless of place of employment.

Upon completion of this task, a nonprofit, tax-exempt organization, the National Commission for

Health Education Credentialing, Inc., was created. This commission has become the credentialing association for health educators. Seven basic entry-level competencies that a certified health educator must be able to carry out have been identified. The health educator should have the ability to:

1. *Assess* individual and community needs for health education.
2. *Plan* effective health education programs.
3. *Implement* health education programs.
4. *Evaluate* effectiveness of health education programs.
5. *Coordinate* health education services.
6. Act as a *resource person* in health education.
7. *Communicate* health education needs and concerns.

In 1989 a program of certification for individual health educators was started. Individuals working as health educators voluntarily submit to be certified as certified health education specialists (CHES). The person must meet the entry-level competencies.

It is believed that a credentialing process will be valuable to prospective employers. Employers will be confident that certified health educators meet certain basic skill levels regardless of whether they are employed by a hospital or clinic, a state or local health department, a voluntary health agency, a school system, an industry or business, or any other health-related agency.

This credentialing program should lead to a greater consensus in the health education profession about what basic skills are necessary and thus to less diversity in professional preparation programs. Eventually health education preparation will be improved at both the individual and professional level.

Health Education/Health Promotion Financing

Health promotion activities have received much interest in the past few years. Though many reasons can be cited for this development, the increase in health care costs is primarily responsible. Health promotion is viewed by many as an effective means of reducing the incidence of long-term, expensive health problems.

If health promotion activities are to receive even wider acceptance, insurance coverage for these services must be expanded. Some health education and health promotion activities and services are covered today by health insurance programs. The services most likely to be covered include the following:[34]

1. Educational services delivered to patients as part of the treatment plan for an existing condition
2. Preventive education services delivered to patients to avoid future illness
3. Education services delivered to nonpatients (the "well" community) to promote good health and prevent illness

Most coverage is part of the payment for hospital inpatient and outpatient care. Health education is not separately identified for reimbursement, but it is part of the overall hospital service coverage. In the future, if people are to be oriented to the importance of preventive health, third-party payment must be made more widely available for health education and health promotion services. This is particularly the case where these services are offered apart from the hospital or health care institution.

It is logical that tax incentives should be developed to encourage the purchase and construction of equipment and facilities used in health promotion programs. Maybe the cost of purchasing a stationary bicycle for use in the home could be a tax deduction. The cost of attending sessions on stress management or fitness might also be made tax deductible.

Regardless of the economic incentives, the future role of health education and health promotion in community health seems well established. Focusing upon positive life-style and wellness is much more personally rewarding than centering activities on medical care and curative medicine.

Summary

Health education and health promotion activities are major factors in disease prevention and human wellness. Health education provides learning situations designed to positively affect people's health behavior. A broadened concept of health education now includes the role of political and economic interventions. This focus has been termed health promotion. Health promotion involves program planning, evaluation, and health advocacy in a variety of settings.

Health promotion activities take place in a number of settings, under the sponsorship of different kinds of organizations. Special emphasis should be given to such programming in the occupational setting, in schools and universities, and in the hospital or health care institution. Hospital programs focus upon patient education, as well as community health education activities. Mass media have been used to deliver health messages to the general public. These measures, along with the informal learning environment of the health fair or carnival, reach many people not usually contacted through more structured health programs.

In the past, the United States federal government has shown some interest in health education and health promotion activities. The President's Committee on Health Education noted the relatively low state of health education programming as it existed in the early 1970s. As a result of the recommendations of the study, the Bureau of Health Education was established. Today the Center for Chronic Disease Prevention and Health Promotion in the federal Centers for Disease Control and Prevention supports numerous health education activities. Within the Department of Health and Human Services, the Office of Disease Prevention and Health Promotion has played an important role. In the private sector, the National Center for Health Education has played an important role in the expansion of health education and health promotion programs.

To improve the professional status of health education, a credentialing initiative was designed during the 1980s. A number of entry-level basic skills were identified. The National Commission for Health Education Credentialing, Inc., was established as the certifying agency for health educators regardless of location of employment.

Health care cost containment is the major impetus for the increased interest in health education and health promotion programs. To ensure that interest in this area expands in the future, economic incentives must be established.

Discussion Questions

1. What should be the basic goal of any health education program?

2. Discuss the relationships between knowledge, attitude, and culture in establishing an effective health education program.

3. What are some of the educational learning models that have served as a foundation for development of health education programs in recent years?

4. Explain the significance of being aware of the reading level of material used in a health education activity.

5. What is implied by the various definitions being given to health promotion today?

6. In what ways do health promotion and health education complement each other?

7. How does health promotion relate to disease prevention?

8. Why have hospitals become increasingly active in health promotion programming?

9. Explain some of the components of a patient education program.

10. Identify some of the kinds of activities being carried out by hospital-based health promotion programs.

11. What are some benefits of health promotion programs to industry and business?

12. How would you defend the importance of health promotion activities as part of the school curriculum?

13. What did the Carnegie Council on Adolescent Development indicate in its recommendations concerning the health of adolescents?

14. Identify ways in which the mass media could be used for health promotion.

15. What are the most effective activities carried out at health fairs in terms of individual health behavior?

16. Discuss some of the program activities of the Office of Disease Prevention and Health Promotion.

17. How does the National Center for Health Education differ from the Office of Disease Prevention and Health Promotion and the Center for Chronic Disease Prevention and Health Promotion?

18. Explain the basic underlying concept of the PATCH program.

19. In what ways does the idea of empowerment come into play in the PATCH program?

20. Explain the value of a professional credentialing program for health educators.

21. Should health insurance coverage include the cost of health promotion interventions? If so, why? If not, why not?

Suggested Readings

American Hospital Association. *Hospital-Based Health Promotion Programs: Report and Analysis of the 1984 Survey.* Chicago, Ill.: American Hospital Association, 1984, 110 pp.

Bogan, George, and others. "Organizing an Urban African-American Community for Health Promotion: Lessons from Chicago." *Journal of Health Education* 23, no. 3 (April 1992): 157–59.

Burns, Alvin. "The Expanded Health Belief Model as a Basis for Enlightened Preventive Health Care Practice and Research." *Journal of Health Care Marketing* 12, no. 3 (September 1992): 32–45.

Convissor, Rena B., Robert E. Vollinger, and Phillip Wilbur. "Using National News Events to Stimulate Local Awareness of Public Issues." *Public Health Reports* 105, no. 3 (May/June 1990): 257–60.

Furney, Steven R. "Implementing the Nation's Health Objectives for the 1990s: The Role of the Secondary and Elementary Health Education Specialist." *Health Education* 20, no. 1 (February/March 1989): 22–25.

Higgins, C. Wayne. "The Economics of Health Promotion." *Health Values* 12, no. 5 (September/October 1988): 39–45.

Hutsell, Catherine A. "Creating an Effective Infrastructure within a State Health Department for Community Health Promotion: The Indiana PATCH Experience." *Journal of Health Education* 23, no. 3 (April 1992): 164–66.

Johnson, Elaine M., and Jane L. Delgado. "Reaching Hispanics with Messages to Prevent Alcohol and Other Drug Abuse." *Public Health Reports* 104, no. 6 (November/December 1989): 588–94.

Kelly, Kathryn E. "Building a Successful Health Promotion Program." *Business and Health* 3, no. 4 (March 1986): 44–45.

Kittleson, Mark J., and Vivien C. Carver. "The Status of Health Fairs: Perspectives from the Health Education Profession." *Health Values* 13, no. 4 (July/August 1989): 11–14.

Kreuter, Marshall W. "PATCH: Its Origin, Basic Concepts, and Links to Contemporary Public Health Policy." *Journal of Health Education* 23, no. 3 (April 1992): 135–39.

Miner, Kimberly J., and Susan E. Ward. "Ecological Health Promotion: The Promise of Empowerment Education." *Journal of Health Education* 23, no. 7 (November/December 1992): 429–32.

O'Donnell, Michael P. "Definition of Health Promotion: Part 3: Expanding the Definition." *American Journal of Health Promotion* 3, no. 3 (Winter 1989): 5.

Office of Disease Prevention and Health Promotion. *Screening in Health Fairs: A Critical Review of Benefits, Risks, and Costs.* Washington, D.C.: U.S. Government Printing Office, 1985, 53 pp.

Patterson, Sheila M. "A Historical Perspective of Selected Professional Preparation Conferences that Have Influenced Credentialing for Health Education Specialists." *Journal of Health Education* 23, no. 2 (March 1992): 101–8.

Rivo, Marc L., and others. "Implementing PATCH in Public Housing Communities: The District of Columbia Experience." *Journal of Health Education* 23, no. 3 (April 1992): 148–52.

Robinson, James. "Criteria for the Selection and Use of Health Education Reading Materials." *Health Education* 19, no. 4 (August/September 1988): 31–34.

Rosenstock, Irwin M., Victor J. Strecher, and Marshall H. Becker. "Social Learning Theory and the Health Belief Model." *Health Education Quarterly* 15, no. 2 (Summer 1988): 175–83.

Saunders, Ruth P. "What Is Health Promotion." *Health Education* 19, no. 5 (October/November 1988): 14–18.

Sofalvi, Alan J., and Judy C. Drolet. "Health-Related Content of Selected Sunday Comic Strips." *Journal of School Health* 56, no. 5 (May 1986): 184–86.

Stein, Jane. "Promoting Health by Video." *Business and Health* 2, no. 9 (September 1985): 47–49.

Stewart, Gordon. "With a Little Innovation, Health Promotion Need Not Be Costly." *Occupational Health and Safety* 55, no. 4 (April 1986): 84–87.

Wallerstein, Nina, and Edward Bernstein. "Empowerment Education: Freire's Ideas Adapted to Health Education." *Health Education Quarterly* 15, no. 4 (Winter 1988): 379–94.

Wolle, Joan M, Helen P. Cleary, and Elaine J. Stone. "Initiation of a Voluntary Certification Program for Health Education Specialists." *Public Health Reports* 104, no. 4 (July/August 1989): 396–402.

Endnotes

1. Fishbein, M. "A Theory of Reasoned Action: Some Applications and Implications." In *1979 Nebraska Symposium on Motivation.* Lincoln, Nebr.: University of Nebraska Press, 1980.

2. Wallston, K. A., and B. S. Wallston. "Who Is Responsible for Your Health? The Construct of Health Locus of Control." In *Social Psychology of Health and Illness.* Hillsdale, N.J.: Lawrence Erlbaum, 1982.

3. Rosenstock, Irwin M., Victor J. Strewcher, and Marshall H. Becker. "Social Learning Theory and the Health Belief Model." *Health Education Quarterly* 15, no. 2 (Summer 1988): 175–83.

4. McLeroy, Kenneth R., and others. "An Ecological Perspective on Health Promotion Programs." *Health Education Quarterly* 15, no. 4 (Winter 1988): 351–77.

5. Green, Larry W., and others. *Health Planning: A Diagnostic Approach.* Palo Alto, Calif.: Mayfield Publishing Company, 1980.

6. Green, Lawrence. *Promoting Health: A Source Book.* U.S. Office of Health Information and Health Promotion, Department of Health, Education, and Welfare, 1979, p. 5.

7. American Hospital Association. *Policy and Statement on the Hospital's Responsibilities for Health Promotion.* Chicago, Ill.: American Hospital Association, 1979.

8. American Hospital Association. *Hospital-Based Health Promotion Programs: Report and Analysis of the 1984 Survey.* Chicago, Ill.: American Hospital Association, 1984, 110 pp.

9. Lange, M. E., and A. Wolfe. *Promoting Community Health through Innovative Hospital-Based Programs.* Chicago, Ill.: American Hospital Publishing, Inc., 1984.

10. American Hospital Association. *Ambulatory Care Study.* Chicago, Ill.: American Hospital Association, 1992.

11. *Ibid.*

12. American Hospital Association. *Policy and Statement on the Hospital's Responsibilities for Health Promotion.* Chicago, Ill.: American Hospital Association, 1979.

13. Department of Health and Human Services. *Healthy People 2000: National Health Promotion and Disease Prevention Objectives.* Washington, D.C.: U.S. Government Printing Office, 1991, p. 262.

14. A more in-depth presentation of worksite health promotion is found in chapter 22.

15. Means, Richard K. *Historical Perspectives on School Health.* Thorofare, N.J.: Charles B. Slack, Inc., 1975, p. 87.

16. Issues related to school health are discussed in chapter 16.

17. Department of Health and Human Services. *Healthy People 2000: National Health Promotion and Disease Prevention Objectives.* Washington, D.C.: U.S. Government Printing Office, 1991, p. 254.

18. The Carnegie Commission. *Carnegie Council on Adolescent Development Task Force for Middle Schools.* New York: The Carnegie Commission, 1989.

19. Johnson, Elaine M., and Jane L. Delgado. "Reaching Hispanics with Messages to Prevent Alcohol and Other Drug Abuse." *Public Health Reports* 104, no. 6 (November/December 1989): 588–94.

20. Office of Disease Prevention and Health Promotion. *Screening in Health Fairs: A Critical Review of Benefits, Risks, and Costs.* Washington, D.C.: U.S. Government Printing Office, November, 1985, p. 5.

21. Germer, P., and J. H. Price. "Organization and Evaluation of Health Fairs." *Journal of School Health* 51, no. 2 (February 1981): 87.

22. Wassertheil-Smaller, S., and others. "An Evaluation of the Utility of High Blood Pressure Detection Fairs." *American Journal of Public Health* 68, no. 8 (August 1978): 770.

23. Office of Disease Prevention and Health Promotion. *Screening in Health Fairs: A Critical Review of Benefits, Risks, and Costs.* Washington, D.C.: U.S. Government Printing Office, 1985, 53 pp.

24. *The Report of the President's Committee on Health Education.* New York: The President's Committee on Health Education, 1971.

25. *Ibid.,* 31.

26. Issues related to the health problems of the economically disadvantaged are discussed in chapter 6.

27. Issues related to maternal and child health are discussed in chapter 19.

28. Issues related to school health are discussed in chapter 16.

29. Issues related to health problems of the elderly are discussed in chapter 20.

30. Office of Disease Prevention and Health Promotion. *Fact Sheet.* Washington, D.C.: Office of Disease Prevention and Health Promotion, July 1985.

31. Rivo, Marc L., and others. "Implementing PATCH in Public Housing Communities: The District of Columbia Experience." *Journal of Health Education* 23, no. 3 (April 1992): 148–52.

32. Bogan, George, and others. "Organizing an Urban African-American Community for Health Promotion: Lessons from Chicago." *Journal of Health Education* 23, no. 3 (April 1992): 157–59.

33. Hutsell, Catherine A. "Creating an Effective Infrastructure within a State Health Department for Community Health Promotion: The Indiana PATCH Experience." *Journal of Health Education* 23, no. 3 (April 1992): 164–66.

34. Bureau of Health Education. *Focal Points.* Atlanta, Ga.: Center for Disease Control, June, 1980, p. 1.

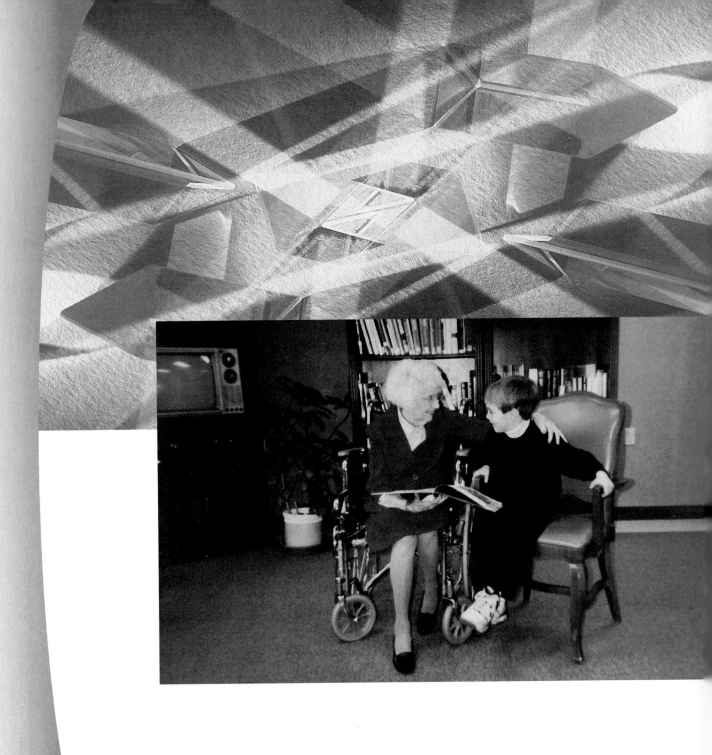

Community Health for Specific Target Groups

CHAPTER EIGHTEEN

Health of Minorities

Socioeconomic Factors Affect Health Status

Blacks, Hispanics, Native Americans, and those of Asian/Pacific Islander heritage have not benefited fully or equitably from the fruits of science or from those systems responsible for translating and using health sciences technology.[1]

Minorities

The United States is a nation of different ethnic groups. As such, many citizens can trace their heritage to several foreign countries. However, there are population groups that can be identified by singular traits and so are known as minorities. Interest in the health status of minorities has increased in recent years, principally because these groups are more likely to be economically disadvantaged. They also tend to have specific value systems and beliefs that affect their use of the health care system. Thus, in providing health care for minorities, it is often necessary to have an understanding of their culture, their beliefs, their language, and their life-style patterns.

The largest minority group in the United States is the African-American population, representing about 12 percent of the national population. The second largest minority is Hispanics, who constitute the most rapidly growing population in the United States, now about 8 percent. Many of these Spanish-speaking people trace their roots to Mexico, although Puerto Ricans, Cubans, and other Spanish-speaking Latin Americans are also classed as Hispanic. A third population group considered an important minority includes Native Americans and Alaskan natives, descendants of the first people to inhabit the North American continent. Many unique health problems are found among this minority population.

The living conditions of many minorities often are not conducive to good health and well-being. These people are more likely to live in overcrowded conditions. Frequently, they are not home owners and, as a result, they encounter many problems caused by renting property owned by absentee landlords. Minorities tend to spend a larger proportion of their income on rent than do other individuals.

Unemployment is much higher among minorities than among the general population. Unemployment breeds discontent, frustration, and lack of self-esteem, and often results in lawless actions. Even more crucial, because unemployment results in less available money, items such as food and health care often are not available.

Additionally, the educational level of minorities is not as high as that of the general population. Literacy is an important tool in adapting to American life, but most minorities cannot read as effectively as can nonminorities.

African-Americans

Generally speaking, the health status of African-Americans in the United States is not as good as that of the white population. A major contributor to this is the lower socioeconomic level of many African-American citizens; many of the problems associated with poverty apply to them.

Cardiovascular heart disease mortality rates are similar in African-American and non-African-American males. Among females the incidence of cardiovascular disease is greater among African-Americans than whites. At as early as nine to ten years of age, racial differences in obesity and blood pressure are being noted.[2] The death rate for cardiovascular disease among African-Americans is more than two to three times greater than for whites under forty-five years of age.

Both hypertension and stroke have been found to occur more often among the African-American population than among whites. The importance of this has been noted in the national health promotion objectives for the nation. African-Americans have been specifically targeted in initiatives to reduce stroke deaths by the year 2000.[3] The death rates of African-Americans are higher for heart disease, cerebrovascular disease, malignancies, diabetes mellitus, and unintentional injuries than those of other ethnic groups.[4] Hypertension is greater among African-American adults than among whites.

Progressive chronic kidney failure, end-state renal disease, is a serious problem closely associated with hypertension and diabetes. African-Americans account for nearly 29 percent of all cases within the United States.[5] The need for dialysis maintenance or kidney transplantation may occur due to the chronic nature of the disease. It is known that this condition may be slowed down in individuals by reducing high blood pressure. The national health objectives initiative has called for reversing the increase in end-stage renal disease by the year 2000.[6]

Studies and reports have indicated that African-Americans are more at risk for conditions associated with heart and cardiovascular diseases. National statistics indicate that a greater percentage of African-American females tend to be overweight.[7] Also, African-American males smoke more cigarettes than do white males. Tobacco is the greatest risk factor for cancer among the African-American population.[8]

The health status of African-American children often reflects serious problems. Many African-American children have not been immunized for the various childhood diseases. African-American children have been reported to be at risk for increased prevalence of blood lead levels, for dental caries, and for growth retardation prior to the age of one.[9] The infant mortality rate for African-Americans is more than twice the projected goal to be achieved by the year 2000.[10]

Diabetes is the seventh leading cause of death in the United States. Its prevalence is 33 percent more common among the African-American population than among whites. Of particular concern when considering diabetes is the relationship of diet, obesity, and diabetes.

Asthma is another debilitating condition that affects the African-American population more than the general population. Death rates from asthma among African-Americans increased significantly during the 1980s.[11]

Lupus is a condition which primarily affects young women. It is three times more common in African-American women than in the general population. Generally the joints, skin, kidneys, lungs, heart, and brain are affected. Something goes wrong with the immune system. Antibodies attack healthy body tissues. As a result redness, pain, and swelling (inflammation) occur. Fever, rash, loss of hair, sensitivity to the sun, and low blood count are other signs noted with this condition. It is not a type of cancer nor is it communicable. Neither is it in any way related to HIV/AIDS. The cause is unknown and there is no cure. However, with medical care most people can lead active fulfilling lives and the symptoms can be relieved.

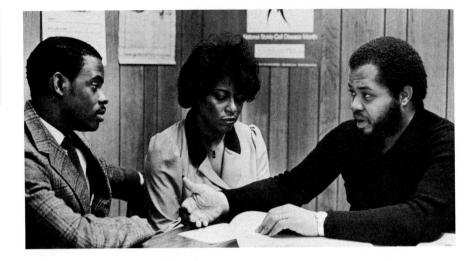

A necessary part of sickle-cell screening is counseling. Couples need to discuss the screening results with a knowledgeable health professional or counselor in order to make life-determining decisions.

Though many reasons can be given for these various chronic conditions, two reasons are especially relevant to community health: (1) cost of the health care, and (2) lack of adequate transportation to obtain the needed health care.

The majority of African-Americans live either in the inner core of urban cities or in rural, isolated communities. Both of these geographical locations have few resources in terms of readily available health personnel and facilities. As a result, it becomes difficult for people to obtain needed medical attention, and individuals do not seek preventive medical care. Not until a major health need arises will a physician usually be consulted. If such a need exists, transportation must be arranged, and this can be costly. The cities offer public transportation, but this is not a viable solution when one is ill and in need of medical care.

Another factor associated with higher incidences of chronic conditions among the African-American population than the non-African-American population is the lesser awareness of preventive health measures. This lack of information is linked to later diagnoses, which in turn reduce the likelihood of curative treatment once a disease is identified. For example, it has been shown that African-Americans have inadequate knowledge about cancer, its diagnosis, detection, and treatment.[12]

Sickle-Cell Anemia

One affliction that is not confined to poverty-stricken African-Americans is sickle-cell trait and sickle-cell anemia. Sickle-cell victims are predominantly African-American; however, other people whose ancestry is Mediterranean, Caribbean, or South American can also be affected. About 8.5 percent of the African-American population in the United States carries the sickle-cell trait. Sickle-cell anemia, the disease itself, is found in approximately 1 percent of the United States African-American population.[13]

Sickle-cell anemia is an inherited disorder of the red blood cells. These cells become sickle shaped and, as a result, can block normal blood flow in the blood vessels. Any part of the body can be affected by this blockage. Sickle-cell disease initially causes pain in the bones, the joints, or other body organs. This pain, called *sickle-cell crisis,* is often precipitated by infection. Death may occur depending on the extent of the blockage and the organs of the body that are affected.

The importance of screening for sickle-cell trait and counseling individuals carrying the trait has led to many sickle-cell community health programs. Programs have been designed to educate people, particularly African-Americans, regarding sickle-cell anemia and sickle-cell trait. These programs also see that as many

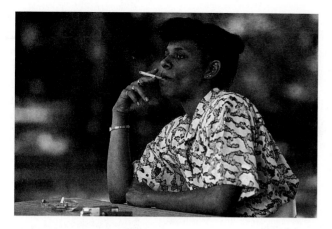

Smoking is the greatest risk factor for cancer among African-Americans.

people as possible are screened and that individuals with sickle-cell trait are made aware of the potential threat to their offspring created by this genetic condition. Information learned through screening procedures can be helpful in counseling couples in various important decisions in their lives regarding childbirth.

Sickle-cell programs also instruct individuals and their families on appropriate action in times of sickle-cell crisis. Because of the importance of maintaining a good level of overall health and well-being, many sickle-cell programs include assistance in good nutrition, dental care, disease prevention, and other general health measures.

Federal funds for sickle-cell conditions have been made available on two fronts. First, research efforts have provided greater understanding of the biological and physiological origins of this problem. Second, programs designed to screen, educate, and assist the African-American population concerning sickle-cell trait or sickle-cell anemia have been put into operation throughout the nation.

Hispanics

Several million Spanish-speaking persons, a majority of them of Mexican descent, live throughout the United States. Others are of Puerto Rican, Cuban, Dominican Republic, and Central and South American heritage. The Hispanic population resides in all fifty states; however, the greatest number live in the southwestern part of the country and in Florida. In several major cities, such as Miami, San Antonio, and Los Angeles, the Spanish-speaking population has major social and political influence.

Many of these individuals, particularly those from Cuba and El Salvador, enter the United States as refugees. Others, particularly those from Mexico, enter the United States as illegal aliens. They cross into the United States in hopes of finding employment and a better way of life. When caught, these illegal aliens are returned to the Mexican-United States border, but many attempt to return another day.

The refugees, as well as the illegal aliens, are often unemployed and lack access to social services that offer health care. Many of the Hispanics who are legal residents are laborers, moving from area to area as the seasons change. Because of poverty, high mobility, and cultural differences, the health of this population is not good. Their nutritional and overall health status is worse than that of the general population.

Hispanics in the United States are a youthful population. Their median age is twenty-three, and nearly 20 percent are children less than ten years of age.[14] Hispanics in the United States have a relatively high fertility rate.

Health Problems

The Hispanic population has been specifically targeted for twenty-seven of the health promotion and disease prevention objectives for the nation.[15] Mention has been given to reducing diabetes among this population, which has a higher incidence of the disease than that found in the general population. Another objective is to decrease the prevalence of overweight persons. Elevated rates of obesity are found to occur in the Mexican-American, Cuban-American, and Puerto Rican female populations. Grain products are dietary staples, while leafy vegetables are not typically a part of their diet. Hispanics in the United States tend to consume few dairy products.[16] Also, reductions in dental caries and gingivitis among Hispanics, who are at particular risk for these oral health problems, was noted.

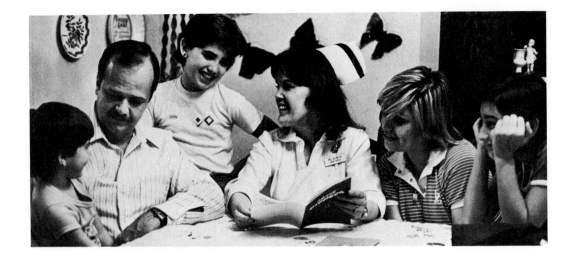

So that health programming for the Hispanic population in the United States is effective, the health worker should be fluent in Spanish. An understanding and acceptance of cultural mores, beliefs, and behavioral patterns are also vital to this programming.

Asthma among children is a significant problem. The highest prevalence of asthma is found among Puerto Rican children in the United States. One reason that has been suggested for this is the exposure to passive smoke from their parents.[17] A greater percentage of Hispanics use tobacco products than does the population as a whole.

The incidence of HIV/AIDS is two and a half times higher in Hispanics than among the non-Hispanic population. It is among this population group that there is the largest proportionate increase of AIDS than of any other racial or ethnic group. The greatest incidence is among Puerto Rican-born Hispanics living in the United States. The lowest rate among Hispanics is found in the Mexican-born population.

Drug use is a major exposure factor among the Puerto Rican-born population.[18] More than 80 percent of Hispanics who get AIDS through heterosexual contact acquire the virus through sexual relations with an intravenous drug abuser.[19] Hispanic children are more greatly affected by AIDS than are other ethnic groups. Usually this is acquired through perinatal transmission related to maternal drug use.

Puerto Ricans living in the United States have infant mortality rates greater than the overall national average. Birth defects are the leading cause of infant mortality among Hispanics. This may be related to the failure of many Hispanic pregnant females to obtain adequate prenatal care and also to poor dietary patterns of many of these individuals.

Cultural Factors

Many Hispanics have a different concept of disease than that of scientific medicine. The germ theory of disease transmission is often misunderstood or unaccepted. Instead, many believe that the body must maintain a balance of the "hot" and "cold" qualities associated with the four humors: blood, phlegm, the yellow bile of anger, and the black bile of depression.[20] A "hot" ailment is treated with "cold" medications, and a "cold" disease is treated with a "hot" medication so that the all-important humoral balance is maintained.

Many migrants rely on traditional folk medicine. These traditional healing measures reflect the influence of custom and religious belief. Folk medicine employs herbs, liniments, diet regulation, massage, and a number of other practices. The dispensers of folk medicine, the *curanderos,* are the most important traditional healers in the Spanish-speaking culture. Integrating these traditional folk medicine practices with modern medical practices is a most difficult problem.

Other cultural problems make programming health services for the Spanish-speaking population extremely difficult. Often they are reluctant to approach a health agency for assistance because of apprehension about governmental agencies and authority in general. Another very important barrier is language. It is difficult to communicate health problems through an interpreter. Many community health agencies do not have Spanish-speaking personnel to communicate with these people. Increasingly, however, health organizations are seeking to employ community health personnel who are bilingual.

Another difficulty is helping the Hispanic people solve their health problems without changing their culture. The family structure of the Spanish-speaking population is complex, with family ties being particularly important. When an individual becomes ill, the health worker must deal not with a single person but with an extended family. This family structure includes the nuclear family and the extended family, plus others selected by the parents who serve as a type of godparent. The elderly members of the family are highly respected, and an illness quite often cannot be treated unless the head of the family is convinced that there is a need and gives approval for medical care.

The need for hospitalization presents the Hispanic with some very difficult decisions. The individual may resist hospitalization because it means leaving the family. For many people, not just the Hispanic, having to go to the hospital is a traumatic experience. Some believe a hospital is the place where a person goes to die. As a result, hospitalization often must include the entire family. Accommodations must be made for other members of the hospitalized individual's family.

The Hispanic culture views childbearing as both a privilege and an obligation. Thus, Hispanic women often resist family planning. During pregnancy, they are very careful to avoid emotional upsets and unpleasant sights, believing this will affect the unborn child. This concern for the welfare of their child does not extend to procurement of adequate prenatal care, however; many complications occur in childbirth, and there is a high rate of miscarriage.

As for all economically disadvantaged people, the cost of health care is a particularly heavy burden for the Spanish-speaking population. Unemployment is high among this group of people, which is one reason why they have the lowest level of health insurance coverage. Because of the inability to pay for health care and a lack of trust and understanding of the health care system, it is not unusual for these people to rely on the traditional medicine and healing procedures of their cultural heritage.

For a health care facility to be used by Spanish-speaking persons, it is important that their individual health needs be well defined. Members from the Hispanic community should be involved in the planning process. This will provide the opportunity for the people to have a voice in the type, organization, and quality of health care that will be provided. It will also give a sense of community involvement to this minority population group.

Female migrants are more likely to visit the health care facility than are the males. Regardless, appropriate treatment is often delayed because of a variety of factors. These include costs, times the clinic is open, fear, working hours, and disbelief in the medical profession.[21]

The necessity of providing bilingual health professionals in those localities with Spanish-speaking residents should not be overlooked. Such a measure is important in communicating not only symptoms of illness, but also feelings, which are often lost when communicating through a translator. Also, use of a translator distances an individual from the health professional. The lack of adequate health care providers who speak Spanish often serves as a barrier for getting needed health care.

The Migrant Worker

It is estimated by the federal Office of Migrant Health that there are more than four million migrant/seasonal farm workers in the United States. Most of these individuals, living in southern Florida, south Texas, and southern California, usually migrate together in families following the agricultural season. They are mobile, following work opportunities in agriculture. All too often the housing, living, and work conditions for migrants are substandard, highly crowded, and conducive to a number of health-related problems.

Many Hispanics, particularly Mexicans, are migrant workers. The migrant worker is likely to experience most of the health problems found in society in general. It has also been found that respiratory diseases, especially tuberculosis, are major health problems for migrant workers. Because of poor sanitary conditions and inadequate water supplies, diarrhea and dysentery plague the migrant. The migrant accident rate is nearly three times the average national rate. Also, the rates of heart disease, diabetes, hepatitis, and cirrhosis of the liver are higher among this population group than for the nation as a whole.

Migrants receive less preventive care than other groups in the United States.[15] Preventive health measures are not practiced by many migrants. They fail to obtain adequate vision care, dental care, and physical examinations.

Many states have established programs to help meet some of the health needs of the migrant. The federal government has provided funds designed to help local communities meet migrant health needs. Some of the projects that have been effective include (1) family clinics where health services can be obtained, (2) services of the public health nurse, (3) health education stressing basic personal health, and (4) sanitation services directed at a more healthful living environment.

The mobility of migrant families creates problems in administering the various local health and social service programs. All too frequently, the moves from one location to another make it impossible for the migrant to qualify for local resident status. As a result, health care may not be available when and where the individual needs it. Medicaid eligibility is also often unobtainable because of the migrant's lack of stability and a permanent address. A federal program has been initiated to promote referrals from one work site to another in an effort to coordinate and continue treatment.

Native Americans

Health care for the Native American and Alaskan native population has been far from adequate. Their health status lags some fifteen to twenty years behind that of the general U.S. population.[22]

Native Americans experience a number of major health problems. The leading cause of death on most Indian reservations is accidents. This is partially the result of the extensive distances over which many must travel. Towns and villages on the reservations are separated by many miles, and connecting roads are often dangerous.

No doubt accidents are also linked to the problem of alcohol consumption. Alcohol-related deaths are more than four times that of the general United States population. Alcoholism is a very serious problem among all age groups of Native Americans. For many, the consumption of alcohol is a means of escape from unemployment, poverty, and frustration. Excessive drinking also leads to malnutrition, infection, mental health problems, and cirrhosis of the liver. Extensive programming at the community level has been established in an attempt to help reduce this heavy alcohol consumption. Such initiatives have included expansion of alcohol treatment centers and aftercare services, as well as alcohol education programs.

The environment in which many Native Americans live contributes to health problems. Crowded substandard housing leads to the spread of disease and illness. Safe water supplies and adequate waste disposal facilities are lacking in many homes on the Indian reservations. The Indian Health Service has established a number of projects to improve sanitation, the water supply, and housing.

The Native American tends to have the various health problems associated with poverty—respiratory illnesses, dental concerns, lack of health education, and malnutrition. Tuberculosis, although a major problem in the past, is not so threatening to the health of Native Americans today. In 1955, there were 55 deaths per 100,000 population from tuberculosis. By the end of the 1980s, that statistic had been reduced to almost 2 per 100,000 population.[23] Though these data show significant progress, the incidence of death from tuberculosis among the Native American population is still four times the overall national figure of 0.05 per 100,000.

Adequate maternal and child health care services among Native Americans have not been available traditionally. Statistics indicate that the birthrate among Native Americans is nearly twice that of the national average.[24] Both maternal and infant mortality are higher than the national average, although the infant mortality rate has been reduced in the past decade. Increased efforts at providing maternal and child health care services in the home and in the community have contributed to this reduction. Among children of preschool age, Native Americans experience three times the rate of injury-related deaths as what occurs among the general American population.

Infant diarrhea is a major problem on many reservations. This is often due to unsanitary water supplies. Many residents of reservations must obtain their

Comparisons of Mortality Rates—Native Americans Compared with Nation as a Whole

Cause of Death	Native Americans	United States
Unintentional Injuries	82.6	34.5
Alcohol-related Motor Vehicle Crashes	52.2	9.8
Cirrhosis of the liver	25.9	9.1
Suicide	15	11.7
Homicide	14.1	8.5

(All data presented on a per 100,000 population basis)
Source: Department of Health and Human Services. *Healthy People 2000: National Health Promotion and Disease Prevention Objectives.* Washington, D.C.: U.S. Government Printing Office, 1991.

water from some distance since they do not have tap water in their homes, and the purity of this imported water is often unacceptable.

Otitis media, an inflammation of the middle ear, has been another major health problem among many Native Americans. In comparison, otitis media is not even considered to be a minor problem for the general United States population. Seventy-five percent of the cases found among Native Americans occur in preschool children.[25] This condition is a special concern because it can result in permanent hearing impairment. The cause of this problem is not known. There is some evidence that poor sanitation in the home environment may be a predisposing factor. Without proper screening for hearing deficiencies and with little knowledge of the problem, many Native Americans develop serious and permanent loss of hearing. Therefore, training in the proper care of the ears is a priority for Native Americans.

Mental health problems are also much greater among Native Americans than the national average. Although hospital stays in mental health facilities have risen in recent years, this is not an indication of an increased incidence of mental illness. Rather, it probably signifies that Native Americans are less resistant to seeking help for mental disorders today than was the case in the past. The most common mental health disorders found among Native Americans are alcoholism, drug abuse, depression, and anxiety.[26]

Homicide and suicide occur with alarming frequency on many reservations. Conflicting values and expectations, as well as changing cultural patterns, produce stress that leads to a diversity of maladaptive behaviors.

Suicide is a special problem among the young Native Americans. It is often associated with alcohol consumption. Suicide epidemics have been reported in some Native American communities.[27]

The Native American population has been specially targeted for thirty-one of the national health promotion and disease prevention objectives for the nation.[28] The reduction of smoking and the use of smokeless tobacco by Indians are two of the objectives. These objectives are significant since it has been shown that the prevalence of smoking is greater among both Native American males and females than among the white population. Also, the health objectives initiative, in recognition of the higher incidences of hepatitis B, bacterial meningitis, diabetes, and end-stage renal disease among the Indian population, set objectives of reducing each of these diseases.

As with other economically disadvantaged population groups, Native Americans tend to have inadequate access to preventive health measures. For example, females are more likely never to have received a breast examination, to have received a mammogram, or to have had a Pap test for cervical cancer than has the general American population.[29] Also, approximately 55 percent of the Native American population has no financial coverage for health care. Those that do are more likely to have lower rates of coverage compared to the national population as a whole.[30]

There have been some efforts made to improve the health status of Native Americans. In 1976, the federal government passed the Indian Health Care Improvement Act. The purpose of this legislation was to authorize funds for the improvement of the health status of Native Americans. As a result, health services on the reservations have expanded, safe drinking water and sanitary disposal facilities have been constructed, and the number of Native Americans trained to serve as health providers has increased. But the future health status of Native Americans is dependent upon even more extensive measures.

The Indian Health Service

Federal health care programs for the nearly two million Native Americans living on reservations are made available through the Indian Health Service. The Indian Health Service, an agency of the Public Health Service, is the only federal program that provides direct health services

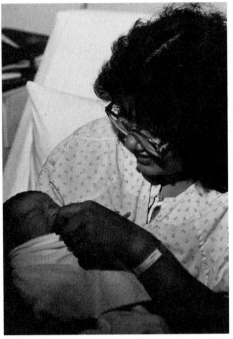

(a)

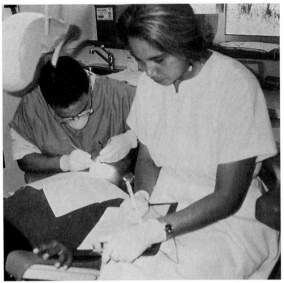

(b)

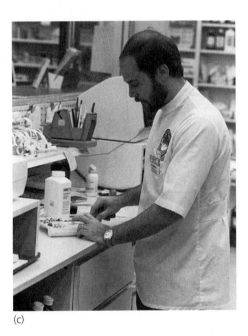

(c)

A variety of health care services are provided to Native Americans in Indian Health Service hospitals. (a) More than 121,000 births occur annually in these facilities. (b) Dental care is available in all hospitals and health centers, with more than two million dental services being provided annually. (c) Pharmacists provide for many hospital and outpatient needs.

to Native Americans. The agency operates hospitals, health stations, village clinics, and health centers throughout the nation; most are in Alaska and the western part of the United States, where the majority of the Native American population lives. In 1990 more than one million Native Americans used the services provided by the Indian Health Service.

For many Native Americans the only available health services are those provided by the Indian Health Service. Access to these health care facilities is often complicated by the isolation of Indian reservations and communities. The difficulty in providing health care to many clients is compounded by the distances that separate homes from medical facilities. It is not unusual to find people living fifty to a hundred miles or more from the nearest health clinic. Many communities, isolated by miles from a clinic or a hospital, may rarely be visited by a physician or a nurse. In these localities serious problems may occur if medical help is needed in an emergency.

Not every facility of the Indian Health Service is located on a reservation. Some of the tribally operated health centers are located in towns and communities near

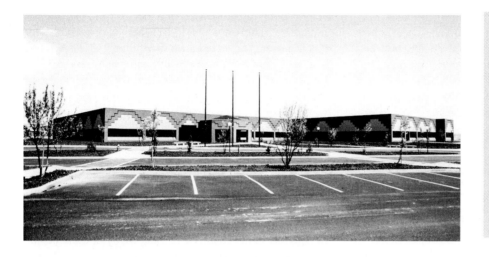

The Public Health Service Indian Hospital, Chinle, Arizona, provides health care services to over 27,000 Navajo people living within 3,600 square miles in Arizona. The hospital provides sixty inpatient beds for medical, surgical, pediatric, obstetrical, and intensive care, as well as renal dialysis, respiratory therapy, physical therapy, dental services, an expanded ambulatory department, and community health service staff. The hospital was designed to provide services in a culturally and aesthetically appropriate environment and contains space for traditional Navajo healing methods.

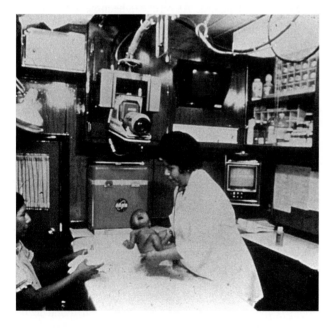

Postnatal medical care is important to the health of newborn infants. For Native Americans living on remote sections of reservations, such care is provided using mobile units.

federal personnel. The tribal health care delivery system is administered by tribes and tribal organizations. In both systems health care services are provided directly by a number of private health care providers.

There are a broad range of comprehensive health care services provided by the Indian Health Service. Both inpatient and outpatient services are available. Health education and prevention services are carried out by health personnel in the communities.

Many maternal and child health care services are provided within the Indian Health Service. Screening and health maintenance services are provided for women. Also midwives and obstetricians are employed to help improve birth outcomes.

Drug and alcohol abuse programs are also a part of the Indian Health Service. Detoxification centers provide assistance to many patients. Daycare and drop-in centers for women and children are provided for individuals receiving treatment and care for alcohol and drug abuse.

Mental health services, emergency medical services, dental services, and medical social work are other programs that are provided within the framework of the Indian Health Service.

Refugees

The United States has always been a nation to which people migrated for a life free of oppression. The founders of this nation came to the new world seeking freedom and independence.

areas with Native American populations. Urban Indian health programs are carried out in several large cities with Indian populations.

The Indian Health Service is composed of two systems: a federal health care delivery system and a tribal delivery system. The federal system is administered by

An alien is any person in the United States who is not a citizen or national of the United States. Most have come to the United States under legal documentation. However, there are others who arrive in the country illegally. An immigrant is an alien who has been issued legal documentation to enter the United States. Refugees are those immigrants who have come to this country to escape persecution, danger, and who are unable or unwilling to return to their native country. There are more than one half million persons a year who are accorded immigrant status in the United States.

Nearly 40 percent of the people who enter the United States each year come from Asia. Since the mid-1970s approximately one million individuals have immigrated as refugees from Southeast Asia. Laotians were the first Asian group to arrive in rather large numbers in the 1970s. Then thousands of Vietnamese immigrated after the war, seeking freedom and protection from the totalitarian government in Vietnam. Most of these people endured extreme physical hardships, including overcrowded boats, hunger and thirst, piracy, and the loss of relatives and friends. A number of these people also experienced total economic loss. During the previous regime, many of these immigrants were merchants, businessmen, government employees, soldiers, and educated professionals. Because of their role in the former society and their affiliations with the United States government in some instances, the new Vietnamese government sought to kill or "retrain" these people. Many lost their positions, their possessions, and even their families.

Following the victory of the Khmer Communist government in Kampuchea (Cambodia) in 1975, thousands of people sought refuge in Thailand. Here these people experienced extreme malnutrition, among other traumas. Some of these Kampucheans have left the Thai refugee camps and been admitted into the United States.

Refugees have come to the United States from other parts of the world. The most recent influx has come from Central America, where civil war has uprooted many people. Many refugees have also come from Cuba and Haiti. In 1980, approximately 125,000 refugees came to Florida from Cuba in what was called the "Freedom Flotilla." However, resettlement of these individuals throughout the country met with numerous problems. Many refugees from Haiti have entered the country illegally, hoping to find a better life, particularly food to eat, land on which to live, and an opportunity for employment. The entrance of these illegal aliens has had a serious impact on many health and social services in a number of communities, especially in the state of Florida.

As refugees come to the United States, they are faced with a variety of adaptation problems. Language presents a significant barrier that must be overcome. Health is another major concern.

Immigrants and refugees coming to the United States must have physical and mental examinations abroad before they can enter the country. These examinations are done by physicians designated by the consulate or embassy in the country of origin. Many of these people come to the United States with a broad range of health problems and concerns. As refugees become a part of our communities, their health has a significant effect on the health of the community in which they reside.

Malnutrition is a common problem faced by refugees. Those who are sponsored for admittance into the United States, however, usually are not malnourished by the time they immigrate. Many do experience food ingestion and diet problems though. Some refugees, particularly Asians, dislike milk and dairy products and often experience diarrhea and stomach cramps if they consume even small amounts of these products.

Refugees often come to the United States with a number of diseases. Tuberculosis, intestinal parasites, skin infections, hepatitis B, and malaria are common. Very few refugee children have obtained the required immunizations for polio, DPT (diphtheria, pertussis, tetanus), and measles before their arrival in the local community.[31]

One disease for which special concern has been noted is tuberculosis. Tuberculosis has been found to be fourteen times more prevalent among foreign-born persons entering the United States than among the national population. Some people enter the United States with active tuberculosis which was missed during the required physical examinations. Others were provided with a waiver because their cases were reported to be inactive. Also, many enter the country having received inadequate drug treatment in their countries of origin. In order to reverse this problem the Centers for Disease Control and

Prevention has recommended that state and local health departments should screen and treat all persons on their arrival. Further, CDC has recommended that tuberculosis screening be mandatory for all foreign-born adults and for children through college age.[32]

Smoking rates are high among Southeast Asian males. Little educational programming has been designed to modify this high-risk behavior among this population. A need exists to develop educational strategies that are culturally and linguistically relevant regarding the dangers associated with smoking.[33] The same findings and recommendations have been noted among the Arab-American population in one large urban locality within the United States.[34]

Many refugees are not familiar with the concepts of modern medicine. For many Southeast Asian refugees it is a cultural belief that it may be inevitable to suffer, hence they will not seek health care when necessary. Also, there are numerous belief systems about disease that impacts their use of health care facilities. For example, some people believe that evil spirits are the cause of disease. Cure for the disease could offend the spirit. Obstruction of a life energy, the *chi*, could cause serious problems if Western healing modalities are used. These beliefs, and many others, result in wide distrust of Western medicine.

Since a visit to a physician or to a clinic is viewed with much uncertainty, mistrust, and fear by many refugees, it is important that someone on the medical staff of the health care facility be present to calm their apprehensions and that a translator is present to interpret the conversation with the patients. It is helpful if the medical staff is sympathetic and familiar with the various cultural beliefs that affect the health practices of the newcomers.

In many instances, reliance upon folk and traditional healing practices is a part of these cultural beliefs. This is particularly the case of the individuals who have come from rural localities. For example, Haitians who believe in voodoo have been difficult to treat in some medical settings.

Some refugee health problems and diseases are difficult to cope with in the United States because most medical providers have had little experience with them. One such disease has been most mysterious. Over a period of about two years in the early 1980s, some twenty-five Laotians died of an unknown condition. These seemingly healthy young males suddenly became ill and died for no recognized reason. The exact cause is still unresolved.

The influx of refugees from Southeast Asia has been supported by the federal Indo-Chinese Migration and Refugee Act. Under provisions of this program, the government provides support for a family to establish itself in a community. This support is discontinued after the English language and marketable skills are learned. After this, the family is expected to become self-supporting. Often this takes a period of months or even years. As a result, many refugees become the recipients of welfare. Medicaid and food stamps are included in the welfare payments. Unfortunately, since refugees are usually better off on welfare than they were in their home countries, some tend to remain on welfare even after they are able to function independently. The unemployment problems in many localities contribute to the difficulty many refugees have in finding work and becoming self-sufficient.

Minority Community Health Initiatives

A number of initiatives have been developed and implemented to rectify the wide disparity in health status between the minority population and the general U.S. population. Community coalitions have brought the resources of many agencies and organizations together to create programs for the prevention of homicide among urban African-American youth. Another coalition, COSSMHO (the National Coalition of Hispanic Health and Human Services Organizations), conducts a variety of programs. One initiative teaches teenage mothers parenting skills designed to prevent child abuse and neglect.[35]

Improving the quality of prenatal care for low-income women has been the emphasis of a number of initiatives, including one designed by the New Jersey Department of Health. In Seattle bilingual Asian women help other Asian refugees with prenatal care and parenting skills.[36]

These many initiatives are designed to inform minorities about the health problems they are experiencing. In addition, model programs of health care delivery have been established in many communities to give lower socioeconomic individuals better access to health care.

This lack of adequate knowledge as well as the failure to practice proper prevention and obtain early care for major chronic diseases has provided an impetus for program development.[37] One initiative has been aimed at lowering the rate of cancer among African-Americans in Chicago.

In 1992 the federal Agency for Health Care Policy and Research announced a major program designed to help prevent, diagnose, treat, and manage illnesses among minorities. Six research centers have been established to focus on a variety of minority health concerns. For example, some programs have been established to encourage mammography screening among Native American females, others to provide treatment of diabetes and asthma among Asian-Americans, and still others to treat substance abuse and depression among Hispanics. Other initiatives have centered on AIDS, tuberculosis, and cardiovascular disease among African-Americans.

The various national institutes of health have established programs directed at improving the health status of minorities. Glaucoma is a leading cause of blindness among African-Americans over the age of forty. It strikes this population group at an earlier age and is often more severe than in other racial populations.[38] There are no early warning signs, the condition often developing undetected until permanent loss of vision occurs. As a result, the National Eye Institute has established a National Eye Health Education Program. This program provides education for high-risk populations, particularly African-Americans over the age of forty. Professional and public education programs to encourage early detection and treatment of glaucoma and diabetic eye disease is a primary focus of this program. Also media campaigns making use of television, radio, and the print media have been designed. An information kit and education program for pharmacists on diabetic eye disease has been made available to help them educate their customers, particularly minorities.

Various community agencies have received funding under the maternal and child health block grant.[39] These funds have been used to provide early infant health care for Native American children, as well as to support programs for Puerto Rican children in certain communities throughout the eastern part of the United States, to improve the nutritional status of Mexican-American children, and to support a program for infants at risk for developmental disabilities among Southeast Asian refugees in California.

Summary

The United States is made up of people of many different nationalities and ethnic groups. Several groups with singular traits, referred to as minorities, tend to experience a number of health-related problems. African-Americans, Hispanic-Americans, Native Americans, and refugees constitute specific groups most often in need of community health programming. Each of these groups tends to have many of the health problems associated with poverty. In addition, each group has unique health concerns.

The health status of a majority of African-Americans in the United States is not what it should be. This is usually because of the lack of health care services in communities where many African-Americans live—the inner-city and rural localities. For many African-Americans, the health provider is not a person with whom they can easily identify.

A specific health problem of major proportion among African-Americans is sickle-cell disease. Screening of blood cells for sickle-cell trait is very important in coping with this problem. Education and counseling are needed so that people understand the results of this screening activity.

The United States is home to a growing Spanish-speaking population. Their health problems are compounded by language and cultural barriers. The mobility of Spanish-speaking migrant laborers also makes ongoing comprehensive health care very difficult.

Several health problems can be found among Native Americans. One of the most serious is alcoholism. Various efforts have been initiated to help the Native American population with this problem. Other health problems that afflict these people include diarrhea and otitis media.

In recent years there has been a large influx of refugees into the United States. They have brought various health problems with them, including respiratory diseases and digestive problems. Treatment of these problems and instruction in preventive measures are hampered by the refugees' unfamiliarity with Western medicine.

Numerous community coalitions have been brought together to improve the health status of minority populations. Examples are initiatives to improve the quality of prenatal care for low-income minority women, to provide educational activities so that the minorities are familiar with measures for improving health, and to support nutritional status programs.

Discussion Questions

1. Discuss some factors that contribute to increased health problems among minorities.

2. How extensive are problems associated with cardiovascular disease among the African-American population?

3. Identify some of the health problems of children of African-Americans.

4. What is lupus?

5. What are the differences between sickle-cell trait and sickle-cell disease?

6. What are some health problems identified in the national health objectives for the nation among the Hispanic population?

7. Why is HIV/AIDS a particular problem among the Hispanic population?

8. What unique dimensions are presented in working in health facilities that serve Hispanics?

9. Discuss some of the specific cultural considerations that influence the concept of medicine among Hispanics.

10. What are the specific problems of providing health care to migrants?

11. Identify several of the more serious health problems of the Native American population.

12. Discuss the problem of alcoholism among Native Americans.

13. What is otitis media, and to what degree is it a problem among Native Americans?

14. Identify some of the problems targeted among the health objectives initiatives as they relate to Native Americans.

15. In what ways do environmental factors affect the health of Native Americans?

16. What kinds of services are provided by the Indian Health Service?

17. What are some considerations that must be taken into account when providing health care to refugees in the United States?

18. What health problems do refugees from Southeast Asia experience?

19. Why does such a large number of immigrants arrive in the United States with tuberculosis?

20. Discuss tuberculosis as a health concern among minorities.

21. Discuss the importance of folk medicine to refugees.

22. Give examples of community coalition programs that have been designed to improve certain health problems of minorities.

23. What are programs operating in your community that are directed at certain minority populations?

24. What are some of the initiatives that are being carried out by various agencies and organizations in attempts to improve the health of minorities in the United States?

Suggested Readings

Beauvais, Fred, and others. "American Indian Youth and Drugs, 1976–1987: A Continuing Problem." *American Journal of Public Health 79,* no. 5 (May 1989): 634–36.

Braithwaite, Ronald L., and Sandra E. Taylor, eds. *Health Issues in the Black Community.* San Francisco, Calif.: Jossey-Bass Publishers, 1992, 410 pp.

Butler, Dennis J., and Lou R. Beltran. "Functions of an Adult Sickle Cell Group: Education, Task Orientation, and Support." *Health and Social Work* 18, no. 1 (February 1993): 49–56.

Carter, Janette, and others. "Tribal Differences in Diabetes: Prevalence among American Indians in New Mexico." *Public Health Reports* 104, no. 6 (November/December 1989): 665–69.

Carter-Pakras, Olivia Denise, and Peter Joseph Gergen. "Reported Asthma among Puerto Rican, Mexican-American, and Cuban Children, 1982 through 1984." *American Journal of Public Health* 83, no. 4 (April 1993): 580–82.

Centers for Disease Control and Prevention. "Health Status of Haitian Migrants." *Morbidity and Mortality Weekly Report* 42, no. 7 (February 26, 1993): 138–40.

Centers for Disease Control and Prevention. "Prevention and Control of Tuberculosis in Migrant Farm Workers." *Morbidity and Mortality Weekly Report* 41, no. RR–10 (June 5, 1992): 15 pp.

Department of Health and Human Services. *Health Status of Minorities and Low Income Groups, Third Edition.* Washington, D.C.: U.S. Government Printing Office, 1991, 376 pp.

Diaz, Theresa, and others. "AIDS Trends among Hispanics in the United States." *American Journal of Public Health* 83, no. 4 (April 1993): 504–9.

Guinn, Bobby. "The Overweight Status of Low-Income Mexican American Children 10 Through 14 Years of Age." *Journal of Health Education* 24, no. 3 (May/June 1993): 132–34.

Heckler, Margaret H., Secretary. *Report of the Secretary's Task Force on Black and Minority Health.* United States Department of Health and Human Services. Washington, D.C.: U.S. Government Printing Office, 1985, 239 pp.

Helsel, Deborah, and others. "Pregnancy among the Hmong: Birthweight, Age, and Parity." *American Journal of Public Health* 82, no. 10 (October 1992): 1361–64.

Hisnanick, John J. "The Prevalence of Alcohol Abuse among American Indians and Alaska Natives." *Health Values* 16, no. 5 (September/October 1992): 32–37.

Hsu, James S. J., and Scott D. Williams. "Injury Prevention Awareness in an Urban Native American Population." *American Journal of Public Health* 81, no. 11 (November 1991): 1466–68.

Lacey, Loretta P., and others. "Social Support in Smoking Cessation Among Black Women in Chicago Public Housing." *Public Health Reports* 108, no. 3 (May/June 1993): 387–94.

Lando, Harry A., and others. "Urban Indians' Smoking Patterns and Interest in Quitting." *Public Health Reports* 107, no. 3 (May/June 1992): 340–44.

Middaugh, John P. "Cardiovascular Deaths among Alaskan Natives, 1980–1986." *American Journal of Public Health* 80, no. 3 (March 1990): 282–85.

Moran, John S., and others. "The Impact of Sexually Transmitted Diseases on Minority Populations." *Public Health Reports* 104, no. 6 (November/December 1989): 560–65.

Munson, Spero M., and others. "Risk Factors for Suicide among Indian Adolescents at a Boarding School." *Public Health Reports* 104, no. 6 (November/December 1989): 609–14.

National Heart, Lung, and Blood Institute Growth and Health Study Research Group. "Obesity and Cardiovascular Disease Risk Factors in Black and White Girls: The NHLBI Growth and Health Study." *American Journal of Public Health* 82, no. 12 (December 1992): 1613–20.

Polednak, Anthony P., and others. "Mammography Use in Hispanic and Anglo Visitors to Community Health Centers." *Health Values* 17, no. 3 (May/June 1993): 42–48.

Public Health Service. *AIDS Knowledge and Attitudes of Black Americans: United States, 1990.* Pub. no. 206 (October 16, 1991): 22 pp.

Public Health Service. *AIDS Knowledge and Attitudes of Hispanic Americans: United States, 1990.* Pub. no. 207 (October 17, 1991): 22 pp.

Public Health Service. *What Black Women Should Know About Lupus.* NIH Pub. no. 91–3219 (July 1991): 7 pp.

Remez, L. "Infant Mortality on an Oregon Indian Reservation Is Almost Three Times Higher Than the Overall U.S. Rate." *Family Planning Perspectives* 24, no. 3 (May/June 1992): 138–39.

Rice, Virginia Hill, and Amahid Kulwicki. "Cigarette Use Among Arab Americans in the Detroit Metropolitan Area." *Public Health Reports* 107, no. 5 (September/October 1992): 589–94.

Samuels, Sarah E., and Mark D. Smith, eds. *Improving the Health of the Poor.* Menlo Park, Calif.: The Henry J. Kaiser Family Foundation, 1992, 185 pp.

Smith, Suzanne M., and others. "Rural American Indian Injury Patterns." *Journal of Environmental Health* 54, no. 6 (May/June 1992): 22–25.

Snider, Dixie E., and others. "Tuberculosis: An Increasing Problem among Minorities in the United States." *Public Health Reports* 104, no. 6 (November/December 1989): 646–53.

Snowden, Lonnie R., and Jane Holschuh. "Ethnic Differences in Emergency Psychiatric Care and Hospitalization in a Program for the Severely Mentally Ill." *Community Mental Health Journal* 28, no. 4 (August 1992): 281–91.

Strogatz, David S. "Use of Medical Care for Chest Pain: Differences between Blacks and Whites." *American Journal of Public Health* 80, no. 3 (March 1990): 290–94.

Sugarman, Jonathan R., and others. "Serum Cholesterol Concentrations among Navajo Indians." *Public Health Reports* 107, no. 1 (1992): 92–99.

Thomas, Stephen F. "Health Status of the Black Community in the 21st Century: A Futuristic Perspective for Health Education." *Journal of Health Education* 23, no. 1 (January/February 1992): 7–13.

Toomey, Kathleen E., and others. "Sexually Transmitted Diseases and Native Americans: Trends in Reported Gonorrhea and Syphilis Morbidity, 1984–1988." *Public Health Reports* 104, no. 6 (November/December 1989): 566–72.

Uba, Laura. "Cultural Barriers to Health Care for Southeast Asia Refugees." *Public Health Reports* 107, no. 5 (September/October 1992): 544–48.

Endnotes

1. *Report of the Secretary's Task Force on Black and Minority Health.* U.S. Department of Health and Human Services: U.S. Government Printing Office, 1985, p. 1.

2. National Heart, Lung, and Blood Institute Growth and Health Study Research Group. "Obesity and Cardiovascular Disease Risk Factors in Black and White Girls: The NHLBI Growth and Health Study." *American Journal of Public Health* 82, no. 12 (December 1992): 1613–20.

3. Department of Health and Human Services. *Healthy People 2000: National Health Promotion and Disease Prevention Objectives.* Washington, D.C.: U.S. Government Printing Office, 1991, p. 398.

4. Comparative data presented in this section is from the Division of Vital Statistics, National Center for Health Statistics, Washington, D.C.

5. National Kidney and Urological Disease Information Clearinghouse, November 1992.

6. Department of Health and Human Services, *Healthy People 2000,* 397.

7. *Ibid.,* 114.

8. *Report of Secretary's Task Force,* 88.

9. Department of Health and Human Services, *Healthy People 2000,* 564–65.

10. *Ibid.,* 565.

11. Centers for Disease Control and Prevention. "Asthma—United States, 1980–1990." *Morbidity and Mortality Weekly Report* 41, no. 39 (October 2, 1992): 733–35.

12. Lacy, Loretta Pratt, and others. "An Urban Community-Based Cancer Prevention Screening and Health Education Intervention in Chicago." *Public Health Reports* 104, no. 6 (November/December 1989): 537.

13. Lin-Fu, Jane S. *Sickle-Cell Anemia: A Medical Review.* Rockville, Md.: Department of HEW, Bureau of Community Health Services, 1978, p. 2.

14. *Report of Secretary's Task Force,* 53.

15. Department of Health and Human Services, *Healthy People 2000,* 599–601.

16. *Report of Secretary's Task Force,* 54.

17. Carter-Pakras, Olivia Denise, and Peter Joseph Gergen. "Reported Asthma among Puerto Rican, Mexican-American, and Cuban Children, 1982 through 1984." *American Journal of Public Health* 83, no. 4 (April 1993): 580–82.

18. Diaz, Theresa, and others. "AIDS Trends among Hispanics in the United States." *American Journal of Public Health* 83, no. 4 (April 1993): 504–9.

19. National Institute on Drug Abuse. *NIDA Capsules.* March 1990.

20. Madsen, William. *The Mexican American of South Texas.* New York: Holt, Rinehart, and Winston, 1964, p. 71.

21. Chi, Peter S. K. "Medical Utilization Patterns of Migrant Farm Workers in Wayne County, New York." *Public Health Reports* 100, no. 5 (September/October 1985): 480–90.

22. Department of Health, Education, and Welfare. *Health, United States, 1979.* Washington, D.C.: U.S. Government Printing Office, 1979, p. 16.

23. Department of Health and Human Services. *Indian Health Service: Trends in Indian Health, 1989.* Washington, D.C.: U.S. Government Printing Office, 1989, p. 54.

24. Department of Health and Human Services. *Indian Health Service: A Comprehensive Health Care Program for American Indians and Alaska Natives.* Washington, D.C.: U.S. Government Printing Office, 1989, p. 17.

25. Goodwin, M. H., J. R. Shaw, and C. M. Feldman. "Distribution of Otitis Media among Four Indian Populations in Arizona." *Public Health Reports* 96, no. 6 (1980): 589–94.

26. Department of Health and Human Services. *Indian Health Service Accomplishments: Fiscal Year 1988.* Washington, D.C.: U.S. Government Printing Office, 1988, p. 12.

27. *Ibid.,* 12.

28. Department of Health and Human Services, *Healthy People 2000,* 602–4.

29. Agency for Health Care Policy and Research. *Personal Health Practices: Findings from the Survey of American Indians and Alaska Natives, Research Findings 10.* Agency for Health Care Policy and Research Publication #91–0034 (1991): 3–4.

30. Agency for Health Care Policy and Research. *Health Care Coverage: Findings from the Survey of American Indians and Alaska Natives, Research Findings 8.* Agency for Health Care Policy and Research Publication #91–0027 (1991): 8.

31. Erickson, R. V., and G. H. Hoang. "Health Problems among Indo-Chinese Refugees." *American Journal of Public Health* 70, no. 9 (1980): 1004.

32. Centers for Disease Control. "Tuberculosis Among Foreign-Born Persons Entering the United States." *Morbidity and Mortality Weekly Report.* 39, no. RR–18 (December 28, 1990).

33. Centers for Disease Control and Prevention. "Cigarette Smoking among Southeast Asian Immigrants—Washington State, 1989." *Morbidity and Mortality Weekly Report* 41, no. 45 (November 13, 1992): 854–55.

34. Rice, Virginia Hill, and Amahid Kulwicki. "Cigarette Use among Arab Americans in the Detroit Metropolitan Area." *Public Health Reports* 107, no. 5 (September/October 1992): 589–94.

35. Office of Minority Health. *Closing the Gap: Homicide, Suicide, Unintentional Injuries, and Minorities,* p. 4.

36. Office of Minority Health, *Closing the Gap: Infant Mortality, Low Birthweight, and Minorities,* p. 4.

37. Lacey, L. P. "An Urban-Based Cancer Prevention Screening and Health Education Intervention in Chicago." *Public Health Reports* 104, no. 6 (November/December 1989): 536.

38. Information provided by the National Eye Health Program, National Institute of Health, Box 20/20, Bethesda, Md. 20892.

39. Hutchins, Vince, and Charlotte Walch. "Meeting with Minority Health Needs through Special MCH Projects." *Public Health Reports* 104, no. 6 (November/December 1989): 621–26.

CHAPTER **NINETEEN**

Child and Maternal Health

A Measure of a Community's Well-Being

The period of time from conception through pregnancy and childbirth and until a child enters school is one of extreme importance to an individual's health and well-being. These years are a time of great growth and development that plays a large role in the future physical and emotional status of a person. Not only do congenital and environmental conditions influence the infant and young child, but the health status of the mother also has a profound effect on the health and well-being of her child.

A variety of maternal factors affects the health of a fetus. For instance, because the fetus is dependent upon the mother for food, water, oxygen, and the disposal of waste products, the physical and emotional state of the mother during this period of time has a direct influence on the fetus. The mother's nutritional status, her age, and the presence of infectious diseases all affect the condition of the fetus. Use of drugs, alcohol, or tobacco by the mother can result in low infant birthweight, a leading cause of infant mortality.

Child health has improved tremendously in the past fifty years. Infant mortality has been reduced significantly, as has maternal mortality. Many of the childhood diseases that caused much suffering and death in the early part of this century have been virtually eliminated by immunization programs. To a great extent, nutrition deficiency diseases have been reduced. Yet in spite of these positive strides in infant and child health, many improvements still require the attention of community health programming and health policy planners. This is particularly the case for children from minority populations and lower socioeconomic environments.

Infant Mortality

Measures of the quality of infants' and mothers' health are an indication of the overall health of a society, a community, or a cultural group. In a community where the infant and maternal mortality rates are high, it is very likely that the inhabitants experience a wide range of health problems. If nutrition and health care are inadequate, communicable diseases cause even more sickness and debilitation. Infant mortality is thus closely allied to poverty.

History has shown that as infant and maternal health improve in a cultural group, so does the overall health of the people. This is evident in the history of the United States. At the turn of this century, the mortality rate within the first year of life exceeded one hundred deaths per one thousand live births. Communicable diseases were the leading cause of these deaths, although many resulted from poor prenatal care.

By 1950 the infant mortality rate had been reduced to about twenty-nine per one thousand live births, and by 1965 it had fallen to below twenty-five per one thousand live births. In the past two decades this statistic has been further reduced by more than one-half; today the infant mortality rate is close to ten (10.1) per one thousand live births.[1]

It is felt that this rate can be reduced even further. There is concern that the lowering of the infant mortality rate seems to be leveling off. The national goal set as part of the Year 2000 Objectives for the Nation is seven per one thousand live births.[2] This goal seems attainable, but major initiatives will need to be directed toward certain high-risk population groups.

In comparison with other nations of the world, the United States ranks twenty-first, despite its great wealth and resources. Japan, with an infant mortality rate of 5.5, ranks first worldwide. A wide discrepancy in infant mortality rates exists among the states, with two states having infant mortality rates of less than eight (Massachusetts and New Hampshire) and four having rates of more than twelve (South Carolina, Georgia, Mississippi, and Alabama).[3]

Even though there has been a measure of success in improving infant mortality rates and the health status of infants and children, not every economic and racial group in the United States has benefited. The infant mortality rate of African-American newborn babies is nearly double the national figure. The same is true among infants born to economically disadvantaged families of all races.

A significant public health problem in our society is teenage pregnancies. Nearly a half million infants are born annually to unwed teenage girls, most of whom are economically poor and culturally disadvantaged. Unmarried African-American teenagers are five times more likely to become pregnant than white teens.[4]

Economically disadvantaged women often receive inadequate prenatal care. Prenatal care should begin as early in the first trimester of pregnancy as possible so that potential risk factors can be minimized. The health status of the pregnant woman can be noted, and appropriate obstetrical and gynecologic care can be planned. As many as 25 percent of all pregnant women in the United States do not receive adequate prenatal care in spite of its extreme importance.[5] The majority of these women are African-American, poor, and less educated.

Infants born to economically disadvantaged women are often not given adequate health care. This is the result of the uneven geographic distribution of health care facilities and providers, particularly the rural areas and in inner-city urban localities. Not only are health services often unavailable, but when available they are usually not used. Mothers may not use the health services for prenatal, postnatal, and early infant primary health care for such reasons as disinterest, lack of money, or poor understanding of the importance of such care. Often there are also racial or language barriers hindering the mothers.

Low Birthweight

Of all infant deaths, two out of three involve babies weighing less than twenty-five hundred grams (5.5 pounds) at birth. Low birthweight has been associated with a number of health problems. Not only is such an infant more likely to die within the first year, but future health can be adversely affected. There is an increased incidence of mental retardation, growth and development problems, birth defects, blindness, cerebral palsy, and various other neurological diseases. Throughout early childhood children who had low infant birthweights tend to have more chronic conditions such as respiratory illnesses and to be hospitalized more often.

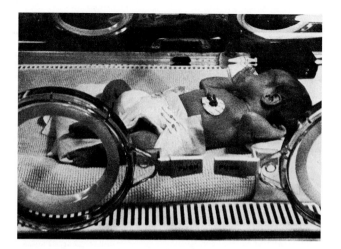

The premature infant begins life with several "strikes" against it, including an increased risk of mental deficiencies, neurological diseases, and possible growth and developmental problems. Fortunately, medical technology has greatly enhanced the future of such infants in recent years.

A number of maternal factors contribute to low birthweight. The chances are three times greater for a pregnant woman to have a low birthweight infant when she has had inadequate prenatal care. This is quite often the case among teenagers and the economically disadvantaged.

Poor maternal nutrition has also been identified as a factor among those who deliver infants of low birthweight. Not only are nutritional habits during pregnancy important, but nutritional status before pregnancy is also relevant. Maternal age is another related risk factor. Greater numbers of premature infants are born to teenage women and to women over the age of thirty-five.

Other factors associated with low birthweight include maternal smoking and use of drugs and alcohol. Pregnant women who smoke have been found to be at higher risk for having a low birthweight baby.

Another concern is fetal alcohol syndrome. This affects infants born to women who drink alcohol during pregnancy. Such infants are often shorter and have low birthweight. Many are mentally retarded, have various body abnormalities, and have such problems as heart defects or eye and ear anomalies. At the present time there is no medical agreement as to what level of alcohol consumption can be considered safe. There is no absolutely safe level of alcohol consumption for the pregnant woman.[6]

The incidences of fetal alcohol syndrome could be reduced by informing women through public education programs about the dangers of ingesting alcoholic beverages during pregnancy. Not only do pregnant women need such information, but men also need to become more aware of the dangers to the fetus associated with drinking. They may be able to encourage their wives and/or other female acquaintances to refrain from the use of alcoholic beverages while pregnant.

The use of illicit drugs during pregnancy has been shown to have major effects on birthweight. Infants born to women who use cocaine and heroin during pregnancy are likely to be premature and to have serious growth impairment. They tend to be malnourished since the drug-using mother often does not have adequate nutrition and prenatal care during the pregnancy. In the case of maternal cocaine or crack use, abnormal behavior is present in the infant within a few days of birth.

Cocaine infants have to endure painful withdrawal symptoms, resulting in lengthy and costly long-term hospital stays. Among babies born to heroin-using mothers, it is estimated that two-thirds are themselves addicted to heroin. Severe birth defects are another commonly noted characteristic of infants born to mothers who use these drugs during pregnancy.

Birth Defects

Second to low birthweight as a cause of infant mortality are birth defects. One out of ten births in the United States results in an infant with a birth defect. Information is continually being documented to add to the store of knowledge already completed on causes of birth defects. Environmental factors, especially, have received considerable attention in these studies.

The fetus is at special risk during the first trimester of pregnancy. During this period there are several recognized dangers associated with exposure to hazardous chemicals and radiation. Women who are exposed to such chemicals as lead, carbon monoxide, polyvinyl chloride, and anesthetic gas during early pregnancy may endanger the well-being of their fetus.

Drugs taken during pregnancy have been linked to birth defects. One of the best-documented cases is the effect of the sedative drug thalidomide on thousands of newborn babies during the 1960s. Thousands of women, principally in Europe, who used this drug during pregnancy gave birth to seriously malformed infants. Most babies were born without arms and/or legs.

Several drugs are known to cause birth defects. For example, use of the tranquilizer chlormazanone by pregnant women has been shown to increase the risk of infant malformation.[7] A hormone, diethylstilbestrol (DES), has been shown to have a relationship to birth defects when pregnant women are exposed to it. The fetus may also be affected by marijuana, and there is much evidence linking heroin use by pregnant women with the occurrence of heroin dependency in newborn infants.

Another high-risk factor related to congenital birth defects is maternal age. Teenage women and women thirty-five years of age and older are more likely to have infants born with birth defects. For example, the risk of having a Down syndrome (a form of mental retardation) child increases when the mother is thirty-five years of age or older.

Several medical advances have helped to reduce the number of birth-related injuries and birth defects. One such medical development is electronic monitoring of the fetal heart rate, which can detect fetal distress during early labor. Such indications provide the physician with information that is helpful in delivering the baby. Potentially injurious complications can often be avoided.

Electronic fetal monitoring is not without its detractors. Some feel it leads to unnecessary cesarean operations. Others suggest that maternal infections are more prevalent when such procedures are used.

Amniocentesis has helped to identify the risk of birth defects in infants. By removing a small amount of amniotic fluid from the amniotic sac, certain birth defects can be identified early in pregnancy. Through genetic and medical counseling, decisions can be made about whether to continue a pregnancy or to terminate it.

Sudden Infant Death Syndrome

Nearly seven thousand infant deaths occur annually from sudden infant death syndrome (SIDS), usually during a child's first six months. The infant is put to bed in apparently good health and is later found dead in the crib, having stopped breathing for no apparent reason. This syndrome has been referred to as "crib death."

There are presently no known causes of sudden infant death syndrome, though several theories and relational observations have been noted.[8] Some feel that SIDS might be the result of a minor viral infection in the airway. Others have noted that SIDS occurs quite often among premature infants and in infants with central nervous system abnormalities. Abnormalities of autonomic regulation of respiratory and cardiovascular functions have been noted. Whether this is due to genetic or environmental factors is unknown.[9] There also seems to be a relationship with low socioeconomic status. African-Americans and Native Americans have a two to three times greater risk of SIDS than whites.[10] SIDS cannot be predicted nor prevented by physicians. It is not contagious nor does it cause suffering to the child.

Some reports suggest that SIDS may be associated with certain other risk factors. One associated risk factor is maternal age—being less than twenty at the first pregnancy. Other risk factors that have been identified are sex (more males die of SIDS than females), maternal smoking, and certain prenatal problems. Many SIDS victims have had hypoxia (a condition where there is a reduced supply of oxygen) during this period. There are also increased incidences of sudden infant death syndrome during the winter months.

In addition to the trauma of losing an infant, most SIDS parents carry heavy guilt over the loss. They often wonder if in some way their seemingly normal child may have died as the result of their negligence. It is common for prolonged depression to follow the initial shock of a SIDS death. Physical as well as psychological indications may present themselves for some time after the death of the child. There is little that parents can be taught to prevent SIDS owing to the lack of information regarding its etiology.

Parents and Birth Crisis

Parents experiencing a birth-related crisis, such as the death of an infant, a stillbirth, or the birth of a baby with a defect, need support and comfort. Such an experience is emotionally difficult. Parents of a retarded child or of an infant needing long-term hospital care are usually not prepared to cope with the situation. Therefore, it is important for communities to establish support programs for parents. Some hospitals have provided meaningful assistance activities. Volunteer groups in many localities come to the aid of grieving and distressed couples. Such aid must be extended over a period of weeks, months, or even years, until the mother and father have learned to cope with the crisis.

Genetic counseling, which is the interpretation of medical information about genetically induced defects, can help couples cope with the birth of an infant having a birth defect. It is possible to help couples understand the various factors relating to birth defects. In situations of a family history of genetic-linked abnormalities, counseling can help the couple make important family planning decisions.

Carriers of potentially harmful genetic traits can be identified using a variety of diagnostic tests, including simple blood tests that can identify carriers for the traits of sickle-cell anemia and Tay-Sachs disease. If either individual is a carrier for a given trait, genetic counseling can help the couple make decisions about whether or not they should have a child.

With appropriate and effective genetic counseling, many couples will decide not to have children, thus avoiding the anger, sorrow, and disappointment of having a child with a birth defect. The counseling process can also help couples deal with situations in which they choose to proceed with a pregnancy that results in the birth of an infant with a defect.

Immunization

For many years communicable diseases were the leading cause of death among children. But increased public health efforts at immunizing children of preschool age have resulted in a significant reduction in fatalities due to communicable diseases. There has also been a reduction in incidences of such diseases as diphtheria, pertussis, tetanus, measles, mumps, rubella, and polio.

Today all states require children to have certain immunizations prior to enrolling in school for the first time. However, there are various degrees of enforcement. In spite of school attempts, health department informational programs, and public media announcements, it has been estimated that as many as one-third of American children between the ages of one and four have not been fully immunized against one or more of the childhood diseases.[11]

The state health department in each state is responsible for establishing the standards for immunization. To assist the states, the Centers for Disease Control and Prevention has published a recommended immunization schedule for the states to follow.

Through the 1980s immunization levels for mumps, rubella, and measles increased. Mumps, though usually the least serious of the three diseases, has been known to cause serious complications. Central nervous system problems and deafness have occasionally resulted from mumps. In adults, mumps may cause sterility if the reproductive organs are affected.

Rubella is of great concern to pregnant women. The fetus may be affected if the woman has rubella early in her pregnancy. Immunization of young women should only occur when there is no chance of pregnancy.

Measles is considered the most serious of the childhood communicable diseases. The most dangerous measles complication is encephalitis, an inflammation of the brain that can cause permanent brain damage and retardation. In the mid-1980s an increase in the number of cases of measles was observed.[12] The increase was observed in all age groups, with most occurring among preschool children and teenagers. The outbreaks in preschool children occur among those who have not been properly immunized. The incidences reported among the teenage school population were predominantly among students who had been immunized prior to one year of age. The Centers for Disease Control and Prevention today recommends that children not be immunized until about fifteen months of age. There is evidence indicating that the vaccine does not provide lasting protection if administered prior to this. However, in localities where a measles epidemic occurs, it is recommended that the measles vaccine be given between the ages of six and twelve months, instead of waiting until fifteen months.

Today there are still many children of school age who are not adequately immunized for measles, and serious attention must be given to measles preventive measures for preschool children over fifteen months of age.[13]

There are two additional childhood diseases for which vaccines have been developed: the Haemophilus influenzae type b (Hib) and hepatitis B. The Hib vaccine provides protection for a child from such diseases as meningitis and epiglottitis—a throat infection that can cause choking, pneumonia, and infections of several organs of the body. Hepatitis B virus can cause infection of the liver. Presently vaccination for Hib and hepatitis B is not required for school admittance in any state.

Some public health concern has arisen over the decrease in immunizations for diphtheria, pertussis, tetanus, and polio over the last several years. The incidences of all four of these diseases have been reduced to very low levels.[14] But possibly because of these low incidence levels, parental concern for having children properly immunized has decreased. Greater public health and school health service efforts are needed to keep immunization levels at a safe and effective level.

As with many health problems, the preschool age children who are not immunized are most likely the poor and those residing in the inner city. Immunization of these children is often made available through the programs of local health departments and community health centers. The parents need to be informed and educated as to when each immunization should be given. The combined efforts, then, of the public health agency and school officials can effectively increase immunization levels and decrease the number of communicable disease cases.

Teenage Pregnancy

One of the major public health problems in the United States today is teenage pregnancy. Over a million girls under the age of nineteen become pregnant each year. This averages to at least one in ten teenage girls becoming pregnant.[15] Four out of five teens who become pregnant are unmarried. Twenty-five percent of all teenage females in the United States have had at least one pregnancy, and many of these have had multiple pregnancies before reaching the age of twenty. Among teenage mothers, more than 25 percent become pregnant again within the first year after their first delivery.[16] Teenage pregnancy is a problem of increasing intensity with little indication of abatement in the future.

The large number of teenage pregnancies can be attributed to several factors, but increased sexual experience by young adolescents is a major reason. At least twelve million adolescents between the ages of thirteen and nineteen are sexually active. Fifty percent of teenage girls in the United States have had premarital sexual intercourse. The average age at which teenagers begin to experience intercourse is about 16.1 for males and 16.9 for females.[17]

Another reason for the increase in teenage pregnancies is that the most effective medical methods of contraception—the pill and the intrauterine device (IUD)—are not commonly used by teenagers. Instead, less effective contraceptive measures—the diaphragm, withdrawal, and rhythm—are being employed.[18] The reduction in the use of the pill and the IUD can be attributed to several factors, but primarily to the publicity given to the health risks of each. Nearly two-thirds of unwed teenagers do not practice contraception at all, or they are inconsistent in their use of a particular method. This ineffective use of contraceptives is demonstrated by the fact that nearly one-half of all teenage pregnancies occur in the first six months after beginning sexual intercourse.

Most teenage pregnancies are not wanted. In fact, more than four out of every five (84 percent) are unwanted.[19] Such a dramatic figure points out the severe social problems caused by teenage pregnancy. Because of these consequences and because adolescents are not using effective contraceptives, it seems important to educate them on birth control measures.

However, providing contraceptive information to young adolescents is a controversial issue. Most teenagers have little accurate information about birth control measures. Ideally information regarding human sexuality with emphasis on contraception should be obtained from one's parents. Unfortunately many adolescents have never carried out such discussions with their mothers and/or fathers. What they do know has usually been obtained from friends, the movies, or other nonstructured sources. Thus, any public health activity directed at preventing adolescent pregnancy should include sex education and information about contraceptives and their effective use.

The school would seem the likely place for sex education classes that include instruction about contraception. However, many school districts fail to provide such instruction. In many school districts where sex education is part of the school curriculum, birth control information is expressly prohibited.

Since the schools have been ineffective in providing appropriate contraceptive information to teenagers and because parents fail to inform their children about this matter, it becomes evident that community health agencies must fill this void. This has been one of the important services provided by various family planning agencies. Other agencies with programming for young adolescents help the sexually active teenager make responsible decisions about birth control. Not only should educational and counseling services be available for females, but the adolescent male also needs information regarding contraception, pregnancy, and sexuality in order to make decisions on responsible sexual behavior.

Health Effects

There are many health problems associated with teenage pregnancy. Childbearing during the teen years is a high-risk experience. Infant and maternal mortality rates are much greater in teenage births than in other maternal age groups. Infant mortality is twice as high in teenage births as in other age groups, while maternal mortality is nearly two and a half times as great.

Low birthweight infants are a serious problem. A teen mother is twice as likely to have a low birthweight baby as is a mother between the ages of twenty and thirty-five. Infants born weighing less than twenty-five hundred grams (5.5 pounds) are more than twenty times as likely to die before the age of one year.[20] The number of premature infants born to teenagers has increased since 1980, with the majority being born to economically disadvantaged racial minorities.[21]

There are a number of factors that result in low birthweight babies being born to teenage mothers. Lack of prenatal care and the expectant mother's poor nutrition are often the source of the problem. As many as 50 percent of all pregnant teenagers fail to receive prenatal care during the first trimester. Also, the use of tobacco, alcohol, and drugs has been associated with premature deliveries.

In order to protect against low birthweight, the expectant mother needs improved prenatal health care and improved nutrition. Early prenatal medical care is very important. Such care should include pregnancy testing and then appropriate checkups during the pregnancy. Once the infant is born, both baby and mother should receive postnatal medical attention. Although for many young mothers the only medical services available are those of the local health department or of a community family planning agency, even these would improve the well-being of both mother and child.

Social Services

Many social problems are associated with teenage pregnancy and motherhood. Today it is uncommon for an unmarried teenage mother to give up her baby for adoption or for care by friends or relatives. Ninety-six percent of unmarried teenage mothers keep their infants.[22] Various health and social services for both mother and infant and daycare services for the infant are needed in many communities as a result.

In all likelihood the child will be raised in a single-parent family. Because of a lack of education and job skills, the teenage mother is usually unable to support her family financially. As a result, many teenage mothers and their infants live in economic poverty and encounter related social problems.

Social services must include counseling, financial support, daycare services, and legal services. It is also important for the mother to have the opportunity to further her education, which has more often than not been interrupted because of the pregnancy.

Family Planning Services

Another important community service that assists not only pregnant teenagers but also individuals of all ages and social groups is family planning. Family planning services have come a long way since the early twentieth century when Margaret Sanger opened the first birth control clinic in 1916 in Brooklyn, New York. Operation of this clinic was illegal according to the laws of that time. On several occasions it was raided by the New York vice squad, and Sanger was frequently arrested and put in jail. In time, however, Margaret Sanger organized a group

Norplant Contraceptive Implants Provided at School

The Norplant subdermal implant contraceptive has been used effectively in a number of European countries for several years. This contraceptive provides protection against pregnancy over a relatively long period of time and does not interfere with the woman's future fertility. Implants have been used that were in place for as long as five years and have been shown to provide 99 percent effectiveness in preventing pregnancy.

The Norplant contraceptive is a small six-capsule contraceptive which is placed under the skin of the woman's upper arm by a physician or physician's assistant. Low doses of progestin are released from the capsules into the circulatory system, thus preventing conception. After five years the capsules can be removed and fertility resumed.

A school-based health clinic in Baltimore has introduced a program of giving the Norplant contraceptive to sexually active teenagers, to already pregnant girls, and to new teenage mothers. This program is designed to help reduce the likelihood of teenagers who have already had a pregnancy from becoming pregnant again as well as reducing the numbers of pregnancies among all teenage girls in the community.

Many questions can be asked about this practice. Who is to determine what students in the school should be encouraged to receive the Norplant contraceptive? Since the implants are relatively expensive, between $500 to $750, who is going to provide the money, particularly for those teens most at risk, the economically disadvantaged?

Another important factor is the possibility that these young women having the Norplant implants will no longer be requesting that their partners use condoms. Without condom use it is feared by many that sexually transmitted diseases and HIV/AIDS will be transmitted.

Even though the Norplant contraceptive has been approved for use by the Food and Drug Administration, there are many questions needing discussion regarding its distribution among sexually active teenagers through school-based health clinics:

1. Are the schools an appropriate place for providing the implants?
2. What types of counseling will be necessary for teenagers who receive the implants?
3. What should be done to help protect these young people from being at greater risk for sexually transmitted diseases?

---

called the Birth Control League. This organization was the forerunner of the present Planned Parenthood Association, which provides family planning services to the nation's communities.

Many women become pregnant and bear children who are neither planned nor wanted. Although the exact number of such pregnancies is unknown, accumulated data leave little doubt that most of the nearly one million teenage pregnancies are not planned. Many other couples wish to plan their families and have some time between children. For these parents contraceptive information and family planning services are very important. But others have not conceived for a variety of reasons. Information on conception is as important to those individuals as contraception is to others. All of these circumstances show why comprehensive family planning has become an important community health activity.

Ideally, all pregnancies should be wanted pregnancies. Therefore, family planning services must include information about how to space a family and how to care for infants, as well as information about contraception. The services provided for family planning should be viewed as a part of primary and preventive health care.

Family planning services are provided in many different settings. For many couples a personal physician, a general practitioner, or an obstetrician may be the source of information, counseling, and service concerning these matters. The physician can help the couple to better understand contraception, family planning, child spacing, and infant care, and can provide needed services to the couple.

For other individuals and couples there may not be a physician to whom they can turn. As a result, family planning services have been established in different

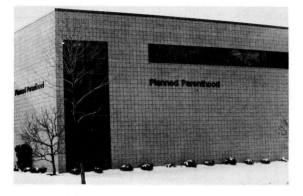

The services of Planned Parenthood include a broad range of family planning services. An individual can receive prenatal care, birth control information and contraceptives, educational services, and counseling, as well as preventive emphasis relating to family planning, at Planned Parenthood Centers throughout the nation.

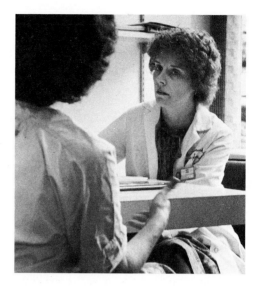

Family planning agencies have provided birth control information and contraceptives to young people. Without the opportunity to obtain this reliable birth control counseling, the number of teenage pregnancies would be even greater.

community health agencies and programs. Local health departments and community neighborhood health centers usually provide these services. Hospitals or specific agencies such as Planned Parenthood affiliates offer family planning services. Most family planning clinics tend to serve primarily low-income individuals.

Family planning agencies provide a number of services, but education is the most important component of their family planning program. Educational activities include information about reproductive anatomy and physiology as well as about various contraceptive methods. Studies have shown that many young people, particularly teenagers, have little accurate information about human reproduction. This is due in part to the failure of parents and the schools to provide this information to young people.

Counseling is another important aspect of family planning. Counseling must be designed to help an individual or couple make intelligent decisions concerning contraception, medical procedures needed during pregnancy, and other pertinent matters.

Many family planning centers perform pregnancy screening, a relatively simple procedure. This screening, however, should be accompanied by counseling. If a woman is pregnant, it is important that prenatal care is discussed. Appointments for periodic follow-up should be established. If the woman is not pregnant, counseling, particularly about contraception, is still useful.

Many teenagers will not consult with a family planning service out of fear of parental reactions. Either they do not want their parents to know of their sexual activity or the relationship of the two sexual partners is unstable.

The question of teenagers being given counseling and the services of a family planning center involves several complex issues. Many family planning clinics do not require parental consent or notification prior to providing such service to a teenager. The United States Supreme Court has ruled it unconstitutional to legally require parental consent before contraceptives can be given to teenagers. However, the federal government attempted to impose a regulation that would have required any federally subsidized health clinic to notify the parents of any teenager under eighteen years of age who applied for contraception. This regulation, referred to by many as the "squeal rule," has been opposed by many family planning specialists, educators, social workers, and young people. The assumption is that many teenagers needing contraceptives would not seek them because they do not wish their parents to be aware of their sexual activity. These people contend that such a regulation would lead to more unwanted pregnancies and have no impact on the level of sexual activity among teenagers. The position of the federal government in requesting such a regulation was that it would help restore parental authority in the lives of teenagers and would thereby reduce sexual activity. This hotly contested governmental regulation has been overruled by the courts.

Several medical services can be found in family planning centers. A pregnant woman may undergo a comprehensive physical examination that includes a complete health history, along with blood and urine laboratory analysis, so that as much as possible is learned about the health status of the woman. Other tests available through family planning centers include Pap smears, gonorrheal cultures, serologic tests for syphilis, and tests for other sexually transmitted diseases.

Increasingly, comprehensive prenatal care services are being provided by some family planning clinics. Many of these are located in Planned Parenthood affiliates.[23] This expanded service was supported financially by Congress when it broadened the eligibility requirements for Medicaid coverage for prenatal care in 1988. Increased funding through maternal and child health block grants has also provided financial support.

Both male and female sterilization have become increasingly common in the past decade. This procedure is now the most commonly used form of contraception in the United States among married couples.[24] These procedures are often performed in family planning centers. As with any major medical procedure, it is important that the individual be properly informed about the permanent nature of this action.

All too often family planning services are directed only toward the female. A need exists to provide services to the male. The issue of male responsibility in adolescent pregnancy is often not dealt with by many family planning counselors and program planners. When one realizes that most sexual activity is initiated by the male, it becomes obvious that no major resolutions to problems of teenage pregnancy will occur without focusing on the male, as well as the female. Increasingly, the need to focus contraceptive and family planning educational programs on the key role the male plays is being considered by many family planning organizations and agencies.[25]

Not all family planning services involve pregnancy or contraception. Many couples are unable to have children. Because of this, it is often necessary for both the male and the female to undergo infertility testing and to receive appropriate instruction and counseling. Though not as common, these services are available in some community family planning centers.

Abortion

Possibly the most controversial and emotional issue in public health today is abortion. Prior to the 1960s, it was illegal to obtain an abortion in the United States unless certain medical reasons made the procedure necessary. When an illegal abortion was performed, it usually resulted in complications, diseases, and sometimes death.

Throughout the 1960s there were several unsuccessful attempts to legalize abortion. But not until 1967, when the state of Colorado passed a liberalized abortion law, did states begin to change their laws and permit abortion. By January 1973, when the United States Supreme Court declared existing state laws prohibiting abortion unconstitutional, sixteen other states had passed liberalized abortion laws. The Supreme Court announced its decision in the cases of *Roe v. Wade* and *Doe v. Bolton*.

In these landmark legal decisions it was concluded that the unborn is not a person and therefore has no rights under the law. The woman's right to have an abortion was supported by the Supreme Court; the state could not interfere with this right. This legal ruling left the decision to have an abortion to the pregnant woman and her physician, but only during the first twelve weeks of pregnancy. After the first trimester, the state could permit abortion only in cases that would preserve and protect the health of the mother. Abortion during the third trimester was prohibited unless the measure was necessary to preserve the life of the pregnant woman.

Since the Supreme Court decisions, the number of abortions performed each year has increased dramatically. One-fourth of all pregnancies end in abortion. There are about 1.5 million abortions in the United States each year. One in three is obtained by a teenager.[26] Most of these procedures take place in nonhospital abortion facilities such as abortion clinics, outpatient surgical centers, and private physicians' offices.

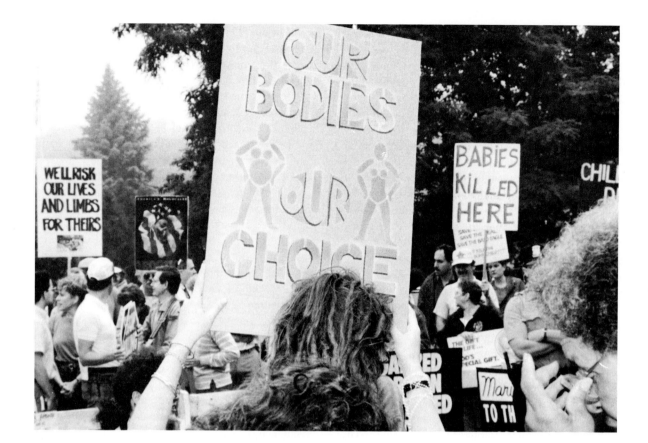

Both pro- and antiabortion activists demonstrate outside the Dobbs Ferry Woman's Medical Pavillion, Dobbs Ferry, N.Y.

The availability of abortion services and facilities has met with increasing opposition, which has taken on political and religious dimensions. It has resulted in a clash between two groups with different value systems and viewpoints. Each is asking government to impose their viewpoint on the other.

The major opposition, or "pro-life" groups, voice theological or religious arguments. These opponents contend that abortion is an act of murder or the direct taking of life, since they believe that life begins at conception. An embryo has human characteristics and therefore is a person. Any action that destroys this fertilized egg is tantamount to murder and should be ruled unconstitutional.

The pro-abortionists, or "pro-choice" group, argue the scientific and medical feasibility of the procedure and the issue of "the right of the mother." This group does not believe that a fertilized egg is a person, particularly during the first three months of pregnancy. Their concern is more toward an emphasis on individual rights than on reproduction. They believe that a woman's freedom rests in having control over her reproductive process. The woman has a right to make decisions regarding her bodily functions. It is their position that reproductive choice protects women from the dangers of illegal abortion and enhances the health of children as well as women.

During the congressional and the national presidential campaigns of the 1980s and in 1992 the question of abortion attracted much attention. In most political conflict there is a common ground where a compromise can be worked out. However, it appears there is no such area of compromise when the conflict concerns abortion.

In the legal realm there have been several important decisions rendered that have affected the abortion issue. In 1976 the United States Congress approved the Hyde Amendment. This legislation forbade the use of federal monies for funding abortions except when the woman's life was threatened. This action halted Medicaid reimbursement for abortions. As a result, many women, particularly indigent women, could not obtain legal abortions. In 1980 the Supreme Court upheld the constitutionality of the Hyde Amendment.

The Supreme Court has been asked to rule on several important abortion cases. In 1989 the Supreme Court ruled that individual states could implement restrictions on the provision of abortions.[27] In this case a law in Missouri placed certain limitations on the obtaining of an abortion. This law required viability tests before an abortion could be performed after twenty weeks of pregnancy.

Ruling for the state in this case, the Supreme Court suggested that abortion is no longer to be considered a fundamental right guaranteed to all women. The states now have greater responsibility in determining what is legal regarding abortion.

In another decision given in 1992,[28] the Supreme Court supported several state-imposed restrictions on obtaining abortions as long as they do not pose an "undue burden." In this case a Pennsylvania law was ruled to be constitutional which required that women be given information about abortion and childbirth before having an abortion. The Court said that the informational materials must be truthful and not be misleading. In addition the Supreme Court supported the idea of "informed consent." This was a regulation that required the physician to inform a woman of the nature of the abortion procedure, of the health risks of abortion and of childbirth, and of the gestational age of the fetus at least twenty-four hours prior to performing the procedure.

In the case the Supreme Court also supported the Pennsylvania mandate that minors must receive parental consent before getting an abortion. Also records must be kept. In the case of publicly funded clinics, records are to be made public. The one provision that the Supreme Court did not support was the mandate that husbands must be notified before an abortion can be carried out.

As the result of the appointment of several new Supreme Court justices in the 1980s, the position of the court is now considered to be more supportive of the antiabortion stance. Opponents of abortion are optimistic that the Supreme Court will overrule *Roe v. Wade* in the 1990s and declare abortion unconstitutional.

Upon assuming the presidency in 1993 President Bill Clinton issued governmental directives which eliminated several previously imposed federal government restrictions on abortion. This presidential declaration has resulted in much anger and opposition on behalf of those opposed to abortion.

One of the directives ended a five-year ban on fetal tissue research. Many biomedical scientists had been frustrated by the restrictions placed on such research. There is considerable belief that biomedical research using fetal tissue may have important benefits for individuals with Parkinson's disease, Alzheimer's disease, and other serious health problems.

Also, the presidential directive now allows abortions to be performed at United States military hospitals located overseas. Payment for these abortions must be made with private, nongovernment funds. The directive also overturned governmental restrictions on abortion counseling at federally funded family planning clinics. Also, an order issued in 1984 that prohibited the United States from giving foreign aid to international agencies that perform or promote abortion was overturned by the 1993 directive.

The presidential directive also revoked prohibitions on the importation of the French "abortion pill," RU 486. However, approval for its use in the United States rests with the Food and Drug Administration.

Political action is now occurring in many states; antiabortion proponents are putting pressure on state and local governments to pass laws and ordinances that would restrict the availability of abortions. For example, some states have passed laws prohibiting the use of public funds for abortion as well as for abortion counseling. Abortions cannot be performed in publicly funded clinics in some localities. Other states have passed laws that require parental notification before a teenager can obtain an abortion. It remains to be seen what additional changes and challenges to abortion will come about in the 1990s, both judicially and legislatively. As states entertain a variety of laws on abortion in the coming years, much confusion will reign at every state level on this issue.

New advances in medical technology have compounded this issue. Physicians are able to save the lives of premature babies at earlier stages of the pregnancy. Today twenty-four-to-twenty-six-week-old fetuses can survive with major life-sustaining efforts. With the use of sonograms the medical profession can now view in much detail the developing fetus. Such technology has led many health care providers to have reservations about conducting abortions late in the first trimester and during the second trimester of pregnancy. In spite of the fact that most abortions occur during the first trimester, at times, owing to improper timing, the abortion is performed during the midtrimester. One is left with the question as to whether these fetuses are "viable."

An unfortunate recent development in this conflict is the use of violent tactics against abortion clinics by the opponents of abortion. Demonstrations of harassment against those coming to abortion clinics have occurred. Picketing of abortion clinics, threats to doctors and nurses working in the clinics, and bombings of these facilities have taken place. Some clinics have difficulty getting physicians to perform abortions owing to fear for personal safety. There have been a number of instances in which abortion clinics have been damaged or destroyed by fire bombs.

When the positions are so extreme and tenaciously held, consensus is obviously unattainable and will not be reached in the near future. In many respects, it is unfortunate that a medical and health issue has turned into a political one. It can only be hoped that other measures of contraception will become so widely accepted that the need for abortion will be reduced. In theory this sounds good; in practice it is not likely to happen. The result? Continued bitter animosity.

Cesarean Delivery

An operative procedure whereby the fetus is removed directly through the abdomen is known as cesarean section. This procedure is a relatively safe operation. It is necessary under certain circumstances, such as when there is a small pelvic opening in relation to the baby's head size, when there is malpresentation of the fetus for delivery, or when other obstacles are present, interfering with a normal delivery.

The number of cesarean deliveries increased fivefold between 1965 and the early 1990s. Of all births, one in four occurs through cesarean delivery. There are several concerns resulting from this development. Cesarean delivery is a more expensive procedure than normal delivery. It requires a longer hospital stay—twice the time experienced by women having a normal vaginal delivery. Since cesarean deliveries are more costly than vaginal births, women of lower socioeconomic status and those without health insurance are less likely to have them.

There is a greater risk of injury or death to the mother from a cesarean delivery. Delivery complications are more common. There is increased risk of respiratory distress in infants born by cesarean section. The cesarean delivery must be considered a major operative procedure and as such the various potential problems associated with surgery accompany the birth process.

The important question being raised by this increase in cesarean deliveries is whether there is legitimate reason for such deliveries. Since for many women the operative procedure is covered by insurance, the reason for cesarean delivery may be economic. Hospitals with intensive care units for newborns and more sophisticated technology are more likely to perform cesarean deliveries. The possession of such equipment by many hospitals, some say, makes it necessary to encourage its use from an economic point of view.[29]

To encourage the reduction of the numbers of cesarean deliveries, the American College of Obstetricians and Gynecologists recommended in 1988 that repeat cesareans no longer need be routine; vaginal deliveries could be considered for women who had previously had cesarean deliveries.[30] Previously, most women assumed, or were told, by their physicians that once they had delivered by cesarean it was necessary that all subsequent births be in the same manner. The federal government in the health promotion and disease prevention health objectives initiative has taken note of this matter. It has been recommended that there be a reduction of cesarean deliveries by nearly 40 percent by the year 2000.[31]

Maternal and Child Health and the Government

The overall health of infants, children, and mothers has improved steadily throughout the twentieth century. Numerous reasons can be given for such improvement: increased medical technology, development of immunizations, improved nutritional status, and overall advanced knowledge relating to health. Some would suggest that improvement has been due in part to the increased involvement of government spending and programming in activities designed specifically to improve health.

The federal government has supported child health programs for many years. Several programs have made some positive contributions to the improved health of mothers and children. Though it would not be possible to review all public health accomplishments through the years, highlights should be noted.

As early as 1935, under provisions of the Social Security Act, maternal and child health programs were funded. In the years since, several federal assistance programs have included child health.

During the 1960s a number of public programs not specifically designed for health included maternal and child health components. The Vaccination Assistance Act of 1962 made funds available to help local health departments immunize all preschool children. The Model Cities Programs established neighborhood health centers where preschool children could be given health services. Often these centers were the only source of health care for the poor and disadvantaged children.

The Head Start Program provides services to preschool children of low-income families. The program includes educational activities, medical provisions, social services, and nutritional services. Over 80 percent of the children enrolled in the Head Start Program receive medical screening. Most children who have had problems identified through these screenings have also received appropriate follow-up measures. Dental care and immunizations are also provided.

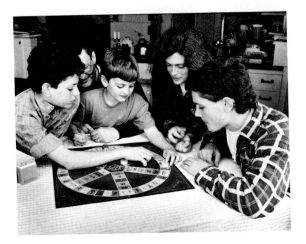

Every child deserves as healthy a home environment as is possible. This sometimes necessitates the support and assistance of various community health and social services agencies.

Early and Periodic Screening, Diagnosis, and Treatment (EPSDT) for all young people under age twenty-one who are eligible for Medicaid was legislated in 1967. This program is a multiphase program of preventive health for children of low-income families. The purpose of EPSDT is to detect health problems and take corrective action to improve the health status of children. EPSDT provides the following services: taking a health history, physical assessment, check on immunization status, various screening tests such as blood tests for lead poisoning and sickle cell, urine tests for albumin and sugar, tuberculosis tests, and hearing and vision screening. The purpose is to identify problems, not to diagnose disease.

In several states materials in both English and Spanish have been developed for use with media campaigns promoting prenatal care.

The effectiveness of EPSDT as an intervention in providing good health has been noted in a number of studies. It has been concluded that this program is cost-effective and beneficial to child health.[32] Its value is evidenced by the periodic screening, which shows a decrease in the incidences of health problems requiring extended care.[33]

Healthy Mothers, Healthy Babies Coalition

Since 1982 a coalition of some eighty national voluntary health and official governmental organizations have come together to improve maternal and infant health. The primary focus was education. The activities of this coalition are directed toward:

1. Providing information that encourages positive health habits for pregnant women
2. Motivating pregnant women to seek regular prenatal care and good nutrition
3. Informing women of health risks related to childbearing
4. Developing understanding among men of the supportive role they play in pregnancy and infant care

State coalitions have been developed in over forty states. A broad range of programs bringing together private and public governmental agencies has been involved. Activities have been as widespread as conducting statewide television and radio media campaigns, providing crisis phone service and pregnancy hotlines for expectant women, working as lobbyists for increased funding for maternal-child health programs at the state legislative level, and establishing similar coalition programs in various cities.

Source: Arkin, Elaine Bratic. "The Healthy Mothers, Healthy Babies Coalition: Four Years of Progress." *Public Health Reports* 101, no. 2 (March/April 1986): 147–56.

Several other federal programs have also had as a major goal the improvement of maternal and child health. The Supplemental Feeding Program for Women, Infants, and Children (WIC) has been administered by the United States Department of Agriculture. Realizing that maternal nutrition is a vital factor in infant health, the WIC program has provided supplemental foods and nutrition education to women who are at risk nutritionally. Similar federal programs include the Family Planning Program and the Maternal and Child Health Program.

The major source of public funding for prenatal and postnatal care and for delivery for low socioeconomic women is Medicaid. Over a half million deliveries are paid for each year by this federal health insurance program for the poor. The major component of these payments is for hospitalization.

During the latter part of the 1980s Congress expanded the eligibility of young children for Medicaid. Even if parents have left the welfare roles owing to increased earnings, their children are entitled to Medicaid coverage for one year. As of the early 1990s, all states must provide coverage to all pregnant women and infants (up to one year of age) when the family income is below the federal poverty level.

As with many health and social service programs, federal budget reductions during the 1980s led to reductions in federal maternal and child health program support. The Omnibus Budget Reconciliation Act of 1981 created the health block grants.[34] One of these was the maternal and child health care block. This block-grant program brought together several former categorical programs: maternal and child health care programming, genetic disease research, adolescent pregnancy services, sudden infant death syndrome research, hemophilia research, crippled children research, and lead-based paint poisoning research. Under provision of the maternal-child health block-grant program, individual states must match spending (three dollars state share for every four dollars of federal money received). The states now have greater control over maternal-child health programming. This places a great responsibility for programs relating to child health and maternal health on state and local health departments.

These developments shifted the emphasis from federal mandate, support, and control to specific state programming. Families on Medicaid with small children are more likely to use public health centers or health department clinics than physicians' offices. Because the local health department is often the prime provider of health care for many poor mothers and children, greater emphasis has been placed on providing comprehensive primary services and family planning services in these settings.

Many infant and child health services are most useful when available in the home. For this reason, local health departments must provide adequate personnel, particularly public health nurses, to enter the homes and provide these important maternal and child health services.

Summary

The health and well-being of infants, preschool children, and mothers is an important factor in any culture. In the United States, maternal and child health has improved significantly in this century.

However, there are still many health problems related to maternal and child health. Infant mortality has been reduced to below eleven per one thousand live births. Yet this ratio is nearly double for the economically disadvantaged. The principal causes of infant mortality are low infant birthweight and congenital disorders.

Not only are babies born with a low birthweight more likely to die in infancy, but their future health status is often adversely affected. A number of maternal factors have been identified as contributing to low birthweight.

Birth defects are second only to low birthweight as a cause of infant mortality. Maternal health and environmental factors have been shown to result in certain birth defects.

Once a major cause of death among children, communicable diseases have been greatly reduced throughout the past several decades. This is due in large measure to the development of effective vaccines for several different communicable diseases. Today seven once fatal childhood diseases are of minor consequence owing to immunization: (1) diphtheria, (2) pertussis, (3) tetanus, (4) polio, (5) measles, (6) rubella, and (7) mumps. In spite of these major improvements, parents must still be aware of the need to update all immunizations for their children.

One of the more rapidly expanding health problems in the United States today is teenage pregnancy. The increase in teenage pregnancy is due to many factors: increased sexual experience among adolescents, poor information regarding contraceptives, and a permissive society. Most teenage pregnancies are not wanted and as a result many social problems occur. Teenage pregnancies often involve low infant birthweight, poor maternal nutrition, and inadequate prenatal care.

Family planning services are available in communities throughout the nation. Educational services are important to improve family planning. Educational efforts include family planning counseling and other medical services.

One of the most controversial issues in public health is abortion. Since 1973, when the United States Supreme Court ruled abortion legal, thousands of abortions have been performed. However, many people are opposed to abortion. They view abortion as murder, suggesting that the fetus is a human life. This has lead to extensive political and religious debate as well as legal decisions concerning the procedure. This issue will not be easily resolved in the near future.

Within the past decade a significant increase in cesarean deliveries has taken place. This major operative procedure produces greater risks to both the mother and the infant and is much more costly in terms of economics and use of medical resources.

The federal government has for many years supported and provided maternal and child health programs to various populations. Many public health observers suggest that this federal involvement has resulted in the improved status of maternal and child health care in the nation. But a change in government philosophy in the early 1980s placed increased responsibility for maternal and child health programming on the local and state governments. Regardless of the source of the services, the vigilance, resources, and efforts in coping with health problems of infants and children and of mothers should not be reduced.

Discussion Questions

1. Discuss what can be learned about the health status of a society by reviewing its infant and maternal mortality rates.

2. What are some of the dynamics that have resulted in a reduction in the infant mortality rate in the United States in the past fifty years?

3. What goals have been established regarding infant mortality rates in the Year 2000 Health Objectives for the Nation?

4. What is meant by the term "low birthweight"?

5. Discuss some of the maternal factors that have been identified as contributing to low infant birthweights.

6. Explain the relationship between fetal alcohol syndrome and infant mortality and debilitation.

7. In what ways are infants affected by the maternal use of cocaine?

8. What is electronic fetal monitoring?

9. What are some of the possible causes of sudden infant death syndrome?

10. Explain some of the purposes and values of genetic counseling.

11. Discuss the effect immunization of preschool children has had on childhood communicable diseases.

12. Discuss some of the causes of increased teenage pregnancy.

13. Do you feel that sex education in the school curriculum could reduce the teenage pregnancy rate? Why or why not?

14. Why should family planning services be made available to males as well as females?

15. What are some social services available to pregnant teenagers in your community?

16. What are some of the services provided by family planning agencies?

17. Should nonmarried teenagers be given contraceptives without their parents' consent? Why or why not?

18. Explain the position rendered by the Supreme Court regarding abortion in 1973.

19. What changes did the Supreme Court initiate with its 1989 decision regarding abortion?

20. How has the 1989 Webster abortion decision affected states' actions regarding abortion law?

21. What are four regulations concerning abortion that the Supreme Court supported in the 1992 Pennsylvania case?

22. Discuss some of the laws and ordinances that restrict the availability of abortions that have become law in various states and localities.

23. Discuss the arguments heard during a debate concerning abortion.

24. In what ways have new advances in medical technology compounded the issues relating to abortion?

25. What is the significance of the terms "pro-choice" and "pro-life"?

26. Discuss reasons why there has been an increase in the number of cesarean deliveries during the past several years.

27. Discuss the need for government involvement in maternal and child health programming.

28. Identify ways in which federal support for maternal and child health programming has changed since 1980.

29. What are the maternal and child health block grants?

Suggested Readings

Alan Guttmacher Institute. *Teenage Pregnancy in the United States: The Scope of the Problem and State Responses.* New York: The Alan Guttmacher Institute, 1989.

American College of Obstetricians and Gynecologists (ACOG). "Guidelines for Vaginal Delivery after a Previous Cesarean Birth." *ACOG Committee Opinion No. 64.* Washington, D.C.: American College of Obstetricians and Gynecologists, 1988.

Apte, Dipali V. "A Plan to Prevent Adolescent Pregnancy and Reduce Infant Mortality." *Public Health Reports* 102, no. 1 (January/February 1987): 80–86.

Arkin, Elaine Bratic. "The Healthy Mothers, Healthy Babies Coalition: Four Years of Progress." *Public Health Reports* 101, no. 2 (March/April 1986): 147–56.

Brown, Sarah S. "Can Low Birth Weight Be Prevented?" *Family Planning Perspectives* 17, no. 3 (May/June 1985): 112–18.

"Court Reaffirms Roe but Upholds Restrictions." *Family Planning Perspectives* 24, no. 4 (July/August 1992): 174–77, 184–85.

Donovan, Patricia. "Providing Prenatal Care Services at Family Planning Clinics: Problems and Opportunities." *Family Planning Perspectives* 21, no. 3 (June 1989): 127–30.

Dryfoos, Jay. "School-Based Health Clinics: A New Approach to Preventing Adolescent Pregnancy?" *Family Planning Perspectives* 17, no. 2 (March/April 1985): 70–75.

Flick, Louise H. "Paths to Adolescence Parenthood: Implications for Prevention." *Public Health Reports* 101, no. 7 (March/April 1986): 132–47.

Haglund, Bengt, and Sven Cnattingius. "Cigarette Smoking as a Risk Factor for Sudden Infant Death Syndrome: A Population-Based Study." *American Journal of Public Health* 80, no. 1 (January 1990): 29–32.

Harris, Stanley. "Services and Educational Approaches to Adolescent Pregnancy." *Journal of Community Health* 11, no. 1 (Spring 1986): 31–34.

Lesser, Arthur J. "The Origin and Development of Maternal and Child Health Programs in the United States." *American Journal of Public Health* 75, no. 6 (June 1985): 590–98.

Maddox, Mary, and Eugene Edgar. "Implementing EPSDT Screening in the Public Schools: Resolving Some Issues." *Journal of School Health* 53, no. 9 (November 1983): 536–40.

Makinson, Carolyn. "The Health Consequences of Teenage Fertility." *Family Planning Perspectives* 17, no. 3 (May/June 1985): 132–39.

Malloy, Michael A., and others. "Sudden Infant Death Syndrome and Maternal Smoking." *American Journal of Public Health* 82, no. 10 (October 1992): 1380–82.

Mariner, Wendy K. "The Supreme Court, Abortion, and the Jurisprudence of Class." *American Journal of Public Health* 82, no. 11 (November 1992): 1556–62.

Marsiglio, William, and Frank L. Mott. "The Impact of Sex Education on Sexual Activity, Contraceptive Use, and Premarital Pregnancy among American Teenagers." *Family Planning Perspectives* 18, no. 4 (July/August 1986): 151–62.

Metropolitan Life and Affiliated Companies. "Cesarean Section in America: Dramatic Trends, 1970 to 1987." *Statistical Bulletin* 70, no. 4 (October/December 1989): 2–11.

Overpeck, M. D., and others. "A Comparison of the Childhood Health Status of Normal Birth Weight and Low Birth Weight Infants." *Public Health Reports* 104 (1989): 58.

Philliber, Susan Gustavus, and others. "Age Variation in Use of a Contraceptive Service by Adolescents." *Public Health Reports* 100, no. 1 (January/February 1985): 34–40.

Pitt, Edward. "Targeting the Adolescent Male." *Journal of Community Health* 11, no. 1 (Spring 1986): 31–34.

Polit, Denise F., and Janet R. Kahn. "Early Subsequent Pregnancy among Economically Disadvantaged Teenage Mothers." *American Journal of Public Health* 76, no. 2 (February 1986): 167–71.

Randolph, Linda, and Melita Gesche. "Black Adolescent Pregnancy: Prevention and Management." *Journal of Community Health* 11, no. 1 (Spring 1986): 10–18.

Rosenfield, Allan. "Mifepristone (RU 486) in the United States: What Does the Future Hold?" *New England Journal of Medicine* 328, no. 21 (May 27, 1993): 1560–61.

"Sexual Behavior Among High School Students—United States, 1990." *Morbidity and Mortality Weekly Report* 40, no. 51–52 (January 3, 1992): 885–88.

Torres, Aida, and Jacqueline Darroch Forrest. "Family Planning Clinic Services in the United States, 1983." *Family Planning Perspectives* 17, no. 1 (January/February 1985): 30–35.

Zelnik, Melvin, and John F. Kantner. "Sexual Activity, Contraceptive Use and Pregnancy among Metropolitan-Area Teenagers: 1971–1979." *Family Planning Perspectives* 12, no. 5 (September/October 1980): 230–37.

Endnotes

1. United States Bureau of the Census. *Statistical Abstracts of the United States, 1993, 113th ed.* Washington, D.C.: U.S. Government Printing Office, 1993, p. 89.

2. Department of Health and Human Services, *Healthy People 2000: National Health Promotion and Disease Prevention Objectives.* Washington, D.C.: U.S. Government Printing Office, 1991, p. 368.

3. *Child Health, USA 1989.* HRS-M-CH8915 (1989): 22.

4. Randolph, Linda, and Melita Gesche. "Black Adolescent Pregnancy: Prevention and Management." *Journal of Community Health* 11, no. 1 (Spring 1986): p. 11.

5. Ryan, George. "Review and Assessment of the Current Status of Knowledge, Services, and Deficiencies," in the *Surgeon General's Workshop on Maternal and Child Health—Report* (1981), p. 27.

6. Kruse, Jerry. "Alcohol Use During Pregnancy." *American Family Physician* 29, no. 4 (April 1984): 199.

7. Heinonen, O. P., D. Stone, and S. Shapiro. *Birth Defects and Drugs in Pregnancy.* Littleton, Mass.: Publishing Sciences Group, 1977, p. 516.

8. *Fact Sheet: What is SIDS?.* McLean, Va.: National SIDS Clearinghouse, 1989.

9. "Premature Mortality Due to Sudden Infant Death Syndrome." *Morbidity and Mortality Weekly Report* 35, no. 14 (March 21, 1986): 169–70.

10. *Ibid.*

11. *Child Health, USA 1989,* 35.

12. "Measles—United States, First 26 Weeks, 1986." *Morbidity and Mortality Weekly Report* 35, no. 33 (August 27, 1986): 525–33.

13. *Ibid.,* 533.

14. *The Status of Children, Youth, and Families.* Washington, D.C.: U.S. Government Printing Office 1979: 25.

15. Alan Guttmacher Institute Report, *Teenage Pregnancy: The Problem That Hasn't Gone Away.* New York: The Alan Guttmacher Institute, 1981.

16. Surgeon General's Report on Health Promotion and Disease Prevention. *Healthy People.* Washington, D.C.: U.S. Government Printing Office, 1979, p. 48.

17. "Selected Behaviors that Increase Risk for HIV Infection among High School Students—United States, 1990." *Morbidity and Mortality Weekly Report* 41, no. 14 (April 10, 1992): 231–40.

18. Zelnik, Melvin, and John F. Kantner. "Sexual Activity, Contraceptive Use and Pregnancy among Metropolitan-Area Teenagers: 1971–1979." *Family Planning Perspectives* 12, no. 5 (September/October 1980): 231.

19. Department of Health and Human Services, *Healthy People 2000,* 189.

20. Surgeon General's Report on Health Promotion and Disease Prevention, *Healthy People,* 24.

21. Friedman, Emily. "The Health Lifeline: Out of the Reach of Women and Children?" *Hospitals* (October 20, 1986): 46–51.

22. Alan Guttmacher Institute Report, *Teenage Pregnancy,* 27.

23. Donovan, Patricia. "Providing Prenatal Care Services at Family Planning Clinics: Problems and Opportunities." *Family Planning Perspectives* 21, no. 3 (June 1989): 127–30.

24. Bachrach, Christine A., and William D. Mosher. "Use of Contraceptives in the United States, 1982." *Advance Data* (U.S. Department of Health and Human Services) no. 102, December 4, 1984, p. 1.

25. Harris, Stanley. "Services and Educational Approaches to Adolescent Pregnancy." *Journal of Community Health* 11, no. 1 (Spring 1986): 31–34; Edward Pitt. "Targeting the Adolescent Male." *Journal of Community Health* 11, no. 1 (Spring 1986): 45–48.

26. Henshaw, Stanley, and others. "Abortion in the United States, 1978–1979." *Family Planning Perspectives* 13, no. 1 (January/February 1981): 15.

27. *Webster v. Missouri Reproductive Services,* 1989.

28. *Planned Parenthood of Southeastern Pennsylvania v. Casey,* 1992.

29. "Who Receives Cesearans: Patient and Hospital Characteristics." NCHSR Publications, Information Branch, National Institutes of Health, Rockville, Md. (1985).

30. American College of Obstetricians and Gynecologists (ACOG). "Guidelines for Vaginal Delivery after a Previous Cesarean Birth." ACOG Committee Opinion No. 64. Washington, D.C.: American College of Obstetricians and Gynecologists, 1988.

31. Department of Health and Human Services, *Healthy People 2000,* 378.

32. Currier, Richard. "Is Early and Periodic Screening, Diagnosis, and Treatment (EPSDT) Worthwhile?" *Public Health Reports* 92, no. 6 (November/December 1977): 536.

33. Irwin, P. H., and Rosemary Conroy-Hughes. "EPSDT Impact on Health Status." *Health Care Financing Review* 2, no. 4 (Spring 1981): 39.

34. Block-grant programs are discussed in detail in chapter 2.

CHAPTER **TWENTY**

Senior Citizens

Needs, Services, and Hope for Life's Later Years

Medical advances have enabled many people to live longer lives than past generations. Not only are people living longer, but for many the quality of the extended life is greatly improved compared to that experienced by their forebearers. Senior citizens today are able to travel throughout the world; they provide hundreds of thousands of hours of volunteer time to civic and religious organizations, and many continue to be productive within their community and family structure.

Many communities have established senior citizen centers for this ever increasing population of elderly citizens (usually those who are at least sixty-five years of age). People who frequent these centers can meet for social events, educational experiences, recreational opportunities, and a variety of other services. The later years of life should be a time of positive activity that encourages a feeling of contribution and meaning.

In spite of the great potential that the elderly possess, a variety of factors, including increased mobility and separation of families, have resulted in numerous problems. This is particularly true when these individuals are faced with illness and disability that require some type of care. The situation has created a number of social responsibilities for communities, hence involving the field of community health for direction and action.

Old Age

When does old age begin? At what point is an individual considered elderly—a senior citizen? There is no magical day or year at which the status is attained. As with other factors in human development and life-style, all individuals vary.

In the United States, age sixty-five has been designated by the 1935 Social Security legislation as the time in life when an employee can retire and receive Social Security benefits. Because of this, many people consider sixty-five as that point in life when elderly status is achieved. And once this status is reached, our society assumes that life-style changes will occur.

But nothing magical occurs physiologically, emotionally, or socially at sixty-five that is different from earlier ages. Many individuals in their late sixties, seventies, and beyond can still be productive. History was made by leaders who achieved greatness and world renown after reaching the age of sixty-five. For example, Winston Churchill was sixty-five before he became the Prime Minister of Great Britain and led his nation during World War II. Some of the great works of art were created by artists who were in their seventies. Michelangelo was over seventy when he completed his work in the Pauline Chapel in Rome. When Picasso died in 1973, at the age of ninety-one, he was still active in his artistic endeavors. The Chinese philosopher Confucius was teaching until his death at the age of seventy-two.

With today's increased life expectancy, it is important that people not be required to retire from productive, regular employment at the age of sixty-five. From an analysis of other cultures, it is obvious that the elderly can be very productive far beyond the traditional retirement age of sixty-five. In fact, in many nations the elderly are highly respected and often consulted for the wisdom they have earned with age. They remain a very integral part of the family unit and lead very fulfilled lives.

This is usually not the state of affairs in the United States; the opposite is often true. Early retirement is a goal for many working people. However, upon retirement retirees often find it difficult to find meaning and satisfaction in their lives. Their ideas are considered "old-fashioned" by the younger generation, and they are not sought out for their experiences and knowledge. Rather, they are encouraged to retire as soon as retirement age is reached.

The current status of the elderly in the United States indicates that they must be encouraged to lead a more productive life-style, and they must be provided with opportunities to do so. Such developments will necessitate a reorientation of our concept of aging and the redesigning of many social structures. This challenge requires creative thinking but also offers great opportunity for the future of millions of Americans.

Demographics of the Elderly

Today one person in eight in the United States is over sixty-five years of age—nearly thirty million people. The number of people reaching sixty-five years of age is increasing daily, and projections indicate that the percentage of senior citizens will double by the year 2020. The fastest growing segment of the American population is over seventy-five years of age.[1]

There are many reasons for projected increases in the over sixty-five population. Primarily, though, improved health status and health care have resulted in longer life expectancy.

With increased numbers of people expected to live beyond sixty-five in the years ahead, many social issues need to be addressed. Will there be resources to meet the demands that this population group will create? Economic problems will plague many elderly citizens in the future. Inflation, which reduces the buying power of the dollar, will inhibit the elderly citizens' efforts to purchase food or obtain health care and other services.

Social Security, established in 1935, is a social insurance program for the elderly. It provides old age insurance for retired workers and their dependents. Also eligible are the survivors of deceased or disabled workers and their dependents. For a number of people, Social Security has been a very helpful program. Even though many retired individuals have other retirement programs, some rely totally upon Social Security for financial support.

There are serious problems concerning the future of Social Security as it has existed for more than fifty years. Inflation, high interest rates, increasing Medicare

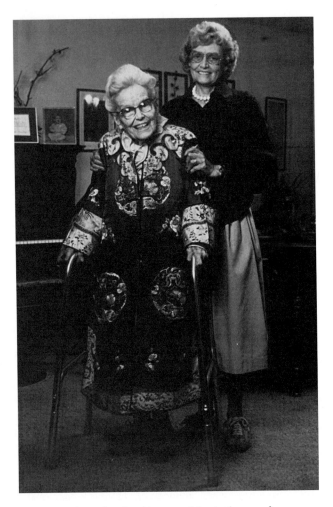

Greater numbers of senior citizens are living to the age of one hundred. These individuals can make very useful contributions to their communities, their families, and their friends.

the benefits available to the recipient. Others suggest raising the costs to employers and employees and requiring groups not now paying into Social Security to do so. Also, there is a suggestion receiving much consideration that the age of eligibility to be able to receive Social Security benefits should be raised two or three years to the ages of 67 or 68. These options would increase the amount of funds in the system. However, the elderly American public has not been very accepting of such proposals. As a matter of fact, major opposition has been raised by senior citizen groups to any proposed changes in the Social Security System.

Although the elderly make up only 12 percent of the U.S. population, they account for over one-third of the nation's health care costs, use twice as many prescription drugs, make an average of eight visits to physicians each year, and account for 42 percent of all days in short-stay hospitals.[2] The demise of the Social Security System would have a dramatic effect on the ability of senior citizens to pay for their health care needs and services.

Elderly Health Concerns

The improvement in the general level of health in America has led to greater longevity. Life expectancy at birth today is 72.1 years for males and 79 years for females. At age 65 life expectancy is 15 years for men and 19.5 for women.[3] It has been reported that the elderly tend to have better personal health habits than the nonelderly.[4] Individuals over sixty-five are less likely to smoke, drink, and be overweight. Despite overall improved health status, widespread provisions of health care, and advanced health technology, certain health problems continue to plague the elderly.

Chronic Diseases

Chronic and degenerative diseases are the major health problems of the elderly. Arthritic conditions (particularly rheumatoid arthritis and osteoarthritis), hypertensive disease, heart disease, hearing impairment, and orthopedic impairment are the most prevalent chronic conditions experienced by senior citizens.[5] Some of these chronic conditions are eventually fatal. The leading causes of death among the elderly are heart disease, malignant neoplasms, cerebrovascular disease, influenza and pneumonia, and chronic obstructive pulmonary disease.[6]

costs, governmental spending, and, of course, the surge in the number of recipients have brought the Social Security System to the edge of bankruptcy. Some economic and political experts predict that the Social Security System will be broke in the near future, possibly before the year 2000. Political discussions and debates and legislative attempts have been undertaken to keep the program solvent, but no easy solution to the problem has surfaced.

Chaos would result if Social Security funds were not available for those who have paid into the system and planned to rely upon these retirement monies. In an effort to "save" Social Security, some have suggested reducing

As people age, hearing and vision problems frequently develop. Since these problems often develop gradually, the individual is unaware of the loss until a serious problem occurs. An accident may result because the individual is unable to hear a warning sound.

Limited vision and blindness can have emotional as well as physiological effects on the elderly. Cataracts, once a leading cause of vision loss in many senior citizens, are not as threatening anymore. Fortunately, surgical procedures to remove cataracts have improved and have helped many elderly to see and function productively in their later years.

Senior citizens are at particular risk for glaucoma, the second leading cause of blindness in America. The eyes should be checked regularly after the age of sixty so that this problem can be identified at an early stage. Individuals at risk for glaucoma—those with a family history of the problem and diabetics—should be especially aware of the importance of regular screening.

Chronic diseases create adjustment problems for the elderly. Whereas most younger people are able to receive health care, medicine, and therapy to cure an illness or sickness, chronic diseases are longer lasting. Many are debilitating, with ongoing pain and discomfort. The long-term nature of chronic diseases is both costly and depressing to individuals.

Chronic illnesses result in an increase in the number of pharmaceutical drugs taken on a routine basis. The elderly consume a major portion of all prescription medications used annually in the United States. There is increasing evidence that as one grows older certain physiological changes affect the action of drugs on the individual. For example, there is often reduced efficiency of the kidneys, the primary mode of excretion of drugs.

There is no cure for most chronic conditions experienced by the elderly. Unfortunately, the exact cause of these conditions is often unknown (as in the case of cancer, arthritis, and heart disease). In spite of the fact that certain risk factors can be identified for these conditions, it is impossible to prescribe a pill, perform an operation, or provide therapy to cure the problem. The individual must adapt to the pain, debilitation, and other problems caused by the chronic conditions. Many elderly people resign themselves to the problem because they view it as "a sign of getting old" or "something with which I must learn to live."

Most chronic diseases are now known to originate in early life. The life-style of earlier years has a very definite effect on the development of chronic conditions later in life. Diet, the use of alcohol and tobacco, and activity patterns are just a few of the life patterns that relate to chronic diseases.

Nutrition

The nutritional status of the elderly is a major public health concern because many senior citizens are malnourished. The healthy senior citizen needs about the same amount of essential nutrients as do younger people. However, they usually require fewer calories to maintain satisfactory weight levels. In an attempt to reduce calorie intake, the elderly often do not eat nutritionally balanced meals. In addition, there is evidence that as one grows older certain nutritional needs change.

Economics are a major factor in elderly malnutrition. The rising cost of food makes it necessary for many senior citizens on fixed incomes to purchase less nutritious foods. Thus, the high food costs have a definite negative effect on the health and well-being of the economically disadvantaged elderly.

Other factors, isolation and loneliness, also lead to poor eating patterns. The individual living alone is not likely to prepare nutritious, well-balanced meals. It seems unimportant or a waste of time to prepare a nutritious meal when there is no one with whom to share it. Because of this reasoning, the elderly are more likely to snack on less nutritious, inexpensive food that does not contain needed vitamins and other nutrients.

For this reason, many communities have social centers where the elderly can meet and eat with others for a relatively low cost. These services are provided in schools, churches, public housing, union halls, and community centers. This opportunity to socialize leads to improved intake of nutritious food. Elderly individuals who are unable to go to such a community nutrition center may be able to have meals delivered to their homes. These programs are referred to as "meals on wheels."

The United States Department of Agriculture and the Department of Health and Human Services through the Food Distribution Program and the Elderly Feeding Program provide the states with funds as well as donated food. States then have the responsibility of providing meals to senior citizen groups. Food assistance programs also benefit community soup kitchens and nursing homes.

Reduced mobility is another major factor that affects shopping and cooking habits of the elderly. Many people with arthritic handicaps are fearful of cooking for fear of spilling hot food on themselves. Others do not have the energy or capacity to stand in the kitchen to prepare a full meal.

Chronic diseases also affect the nutritional status of the elderly. These conditions impede physiological processes such as digestion and absorption. Drugs, too, will sometimes undermine the nutritional status of an individual. For example, prolonged use of laxatives can alter the absorption of vitamins or result in diarrhea, weight loss, and fatigue.[7]

As individuals grow older, certain taste buds do not function as efficiently. Foods often taste more sour and bitter than they did before. For this reason, foods are not as appealing, and as a result many senior citizens lose their appetites. Though it is possible to adjust to this problem, many elderly refuse to eat certain nutritious foods that now do not taste as they did in earlier years.

Dental problems also prevent the elderly from having a well-balanced diet. Dental caries, gingivitis, and periodontal disease, important health problems for the elderly, are major causes of tooth loss among senior citizens.[8] Dentures, the only alternative when teeth are lost, make it difficult to eat certain foods. Those elderly who cannot afford dentures are forced to eat only liquids and soft foods. Not only do they fail to eat well-balanced meals, but certain nutrients are not as readily available.

Since tooth loss among the elderly is primarily the result of untreated dental caries and periodontal disease, it is recommended that through education and regular dental care beginning in childhood such loss can be minimized. There has been a steady decline in total loss of teeth among senior citizens the past several decades. This reduction in tooth loss has not been noted as much among people of lower socioeconomic status. With this understanding the federal government has established an objective to be achieved by the year 2000 of reducing the proportion of people over sixty-five years of age who have lost all of their natural teeth. Special emphasis for achieving this objective should be placed upon individuals with an annual income of below $15,000.[9]

Osteoporosis

Another physiological development that affects the elderly, particularly older women, is a thinning of the bones. Beginning in the midthirties, slight bone loss begins and continues throughout life. This gradual bone loss, which occurs over a period of years, usually goes unrecognized until a bone is broken, resulting in pain and disability. Healing of the fracture often is very time-consuming. This condition is known as *osteoporosis*.

Osteoporosis, a serious debilitation for many, requires prolonged medical and therapeutic care. Thin, small-framed females are more at risk for osteoporosis than larger females. Because of denser bone structure, males are less likely to get this condition. Early indication of having osteoporosis is loss of body height. The vertebrae become compressed with age owing to a weakening of the spinal bones. A curvature of the spine is often noted in elderly females.

The cause of osteoporosis is not known. Several factors may play a role in its development.[10] These include decrease in hormonal levels—it is principally found in postmenopausal females—inadequate calcium in the diet, inadequate exposure to sunlight, and inactivity.

Treatment of individuals with osteoporosis involves taking measures to prevent further bone loss. Diet is an important preventive factor. People should eat foods that are high in calcium. In addition, vitamin D will often be added to the diet, as it helps in calcium absorption. Calcium and vitamin D may slow the rate of bone loss, but they will not cause new bone to form. Excess protein should be avoided, as it can lead to bone loss.

Estrogen slows the process of bone loss in postmenopausal women. For this reason some physicians prescribe estrogen replacement therapy for females at risk for osteoporosis. However, there are some concerns about the possible risks associated with estrogen use. Therefore, it is necessary for research to continue that will provide indication as to whether estrogen can be used widely as a preventive for osteoporosis. It is known that estrogen replacement will not reverse established osteoporosis. It is also unclear as to whether it is effective beyond the first decade after menopause.[11]

Regular exercise can be helpful in prevention of osteoporosis and in the treatment of the patient. Exercise may stimulate formation of new bone and helps maintain strength of the skeletal system.

Unintentional Injuries

Nearly a third of all fatalities resulting from unintentional injury occur to individuals over sixty-five years of age. Motor vehicle collisions cause the most fatalities through the age of seventy-nine. Beginning with the age of eighty, falls cause the most fatalities.[12] In addition, fatalities among the elderly result from drowning, suffocation, and fires. In addition to fatalities, many accidents among the elderly result in serious injury, hospitalization, lengthy disability, and the need for long-term and expensive rehabilitation.

Most falls, both fatal and nonfatal, occur in the home. Falls among the elderly have been attributed to a number of factors. As one ages there is loss of muscle strength and endurance which can precipitate an injury situation. With reduced vision and hearing acuity an individual is at greater risk for an injury-resulting fall.

The older individual also is not able to adapt as easily to darkness. This results in many falls and injuries occurring where there is inadequate lighting. Reaction time tends to slow down as one ages. This is a major contributor to causing one to lose balance and fall.

For many senior citizens a fall often results in hip fracture. This community health problem was highlighted in the Year 2000 Objectives for the Nation; one of the objectives calls for a reduction in hip fractures among people over the age of sixty-five.[13] Hip fractures occur more often in women than in men. Because of the nature of the injury, long-term hospitalization accompanied by nursing home care is often necessary. It has been estimated that annual costs associated with this problem may run as high as $10 billion in the United States.

As a person grows older the ability to drive an automobile is often impaired. Slower reaction time, reduced adaptation to darkness, and a lessening of depth perception all contribute to poorer driving skills. Senior citizens must recognize these changes and be willing to change driving patterns. The elderly individual may need to drive more slowly, reduce night driving, drive fewer miles at one time, and adapt to winter driving conditions.

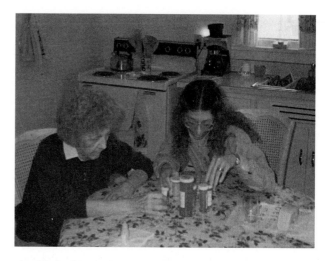

The elderly often need the assistance of public health nurses to understand the proper use of medications.

Medication Use and Misuse

The elderly use twice as many prescription drugs as the nonelderly. Because of the nature of chronic diseases, senior citizens often take various medications. The concern that many older people are seriously overusing prescription medications is growing.

A variety of reasons for this problem have been identified. Overuse of medications occurs among the elderly living in nursing homes, those receiving home health care, those in adult foster care, and those living alone. In some nursing homes drugs have been used to calm patients or to induce sleep, or even as chemical restraints.

Without proper supervision, older people may take drugs in the belief that they need them, when in fact these drugs are not necessary. In addition, there is a tendency for the elderly to go to several different physicians. If the physicians do not carefully manage medication use, it is not unlikely that the individual will be given several different prescriptions by the different health care providers. This can lead to taking drugs that interact in a negative way and to medication errors, as well as to confusion on behalf of the patient.

Both the physicians and the patients themselves need to know more about the effects of drugs on the elderly. Many physicians do not realize that as people age, they become more sensitive to certain medications. This may lead to prescribing too high a dosage and to certain drug interactions. Better education of health care providers in the effects of medications on the elderly is needed.

The Surgeon General's Workshop on Aging in 1988 made several strong recommendations regarding this problem. It called for medication management to reduce adverse reactions. It urged that the role of pharmacists be expanded to include geriatric medication management and that drugs for senior citizens be limited whenever possible. It was emphasized that the pharmacists, as well as other health care providers and care givers, should provide information to the elderly regarding medication management.

Mental Health

The emotional health of the elderly is a concern of community mental health services. An estimated 15 percent of the elderly population in the United States have some mental disorder.[14] Many experiences in the later years of life have such a profound effect upon mental and emotional health that individuals need help in order to cope with their reactions.

Mental illnesses among the elderly may be functional, organic, or a combination. Functional disorders are problems related to psychological stressors. For example, the loss of one's spouse of many years often causes emotional problems. As people grow older they tend to become more fearful of being robbed, of being injured, or of sickness. Personality disorders, such as suspicion, and development of nonsocial behavioral patterns are other examples of functional disorders which are observed in many senior citizens.

Organic disorders result from physiological impairments. Some organic disorders may result from infection, drug reaction, poor nutrition, cerebral arteriosclerosis, or a variety of other physical problems. Major concerns related to organic disorders are those physical impairments that affect the functioning of the brain.

Depression

A common cause of functional mental illness is depression. During the later years, the death of a spouse or close friend has an emotional effect with which the elderly often find it difficult to cope. The nature of chronic illnesses and the uncertainty of cure can also depress people. The trauma of retirement can lead to depression and psychological problems since many people no longer feel wanted or productive after retirement. Economic pressures during the senior citizen years have contributed to the emotional instability of many. Some individuals are uncertain about how they can pay for the necessities of life, such as food, housing, and medicine. Because of these problems, depression and schizophrenia are the most common causes of psychiatric admissions among the elderly.[15]

Depression often goes untreated because people will not go for care. There is no one specific test that is used to diagnose depression. People often do not tell their physician that they are feeling depressed. For many individuals depression is considered a sign of personal weakness. However, it is important that elderly people who are experiencing depression receive medical care. There are very effective antidepressant drugs available which can provide significant help to the patient.

In days gone by, the elderly were often placed in state mental health institutions if they had emotional and psychological problems. This often occurred when the family physician was unable to provide the needed medical care for a patient. Once placed in such institutions, they were often forgotten, received poor or inadequate care, and seldom received the psychological rehabilitation that would permit them to return to their communities.

The development of community and mental health centers has been a positive step in upgrading care for the elderly.[16] Much of the needed care is available on an outpatient basis so the individual is able to live at home with relatives or friends; it is unnecessary for the person to be institutionalized for long periods of time.

In spite of the potential for improved psychiatric care for the elderly, many community mental health centers have not been successful in meeting the inpatient needs of many elderly.[17] Psychiatric treatment is often long-term and can have detrimental effects on the patients. The treatment of depression often uses drugs that, in turn, may result in the loss of appetite, insomnia, or even personal withdrawal. As a result, clinical care for the elderly mental health patient sometimes compounds the individual's health problems.

Organic Disorders

Some organic disorders may be acute in nature. This means that they may be short-term, lasting as long as the person is experiencing the particular physical problem. Usually, through medical treatment this disorder is reversible if the individual receives appropriate care. However, greater concern must be expressed for chronic organic disorders. These disorders result in loss of memory and inability to function normally because of physiological disruptions of the brain.

It is not uncommon for an elderly individual to experience memory loss to some degree. In some instances, this may be simply the inability to remember a person's name. For others it may be a more complex and serious problem involving forgetfulness, confusion, and/or changes in personality and behavior. Although it is often assumed that senility affects all the elderly, the vast majority of senior citizens are actually not affected.

The two most common forms of organic mental impairment experienced by the elderly are: (1) dementia and (2) Alzheimer's disease.

Dementia

The term *dementia* refers to a group of symptoms related to a decline in intellectual functioning. It has been estimated that approximately 5 percent of all people over sixty-five are affected by dementia.[18]

Dementia is caused by the degeneration of brain cells. It may be caused by a variety of different occurrences. There is evidence that use of alcohol over years can cause degeneration of the cells. In many cases the condition is the result of a series of minor strokes caused by a narrowing of the blood vessels that supply the brain with oxygen. This impediment to the oxygen supply disrupts brain functioning and results in the death of brain tissue. Some problems referred to as dementia can be treated and cured, whereas others can only be treated. Lost brain function may be restored, but the dead brain tissue cannot.

Alzheimer's Disease

A disorder common to many senior citizens that produces memory loss and disorientation is Alzheimer's disease. It has been estimated that this impairment is present in some 2.5 million adults in the United States.[19]

A German pathologist, Alois Alzheimer, first described this disease in 1907. No particular population is at risk; it affects all races, geographical groups, and cultural populations. The cause is not known, but those afflicted by Alzheimer's disease have neurofibrillary tangles (clumping and distortion of fibers in the nerve cells) and clusters of degenerating nerve endings of the cerebral cortex. These areas of degeneration are called plaques. They disrupt the passage of electrochemical signals between the cells. The greater the number of tangles and plaques, the more serious is the disturbance of intellectual function and memory in the individual.

An early indication of Alzheimer's disease is forgetfulness, particularly of more current events. As the disease progresses memory loss increases, often accompanied by confusion, restlessness, and various personality and behavioral changes. In the most severe stages the patient becomes incapable of self-care.

Research supported by the National Institute on Aging has been studying three potential factors in the development of Alzheimer's disease.[20] These are (1) traces of aluminum in the brain, (2) viral infections of the central nervous system, and (3) genetic defects. The brains of people with advanced cases of Alzheimer's disease have been found to contain high amounts of aluminum.

So far the most consistent finding is that the activity of certain chemicals in the brain changes. These chemicals are part of the *cholinergic system,* which is involved in memory and learning. The change that is most commonly found in Alzheimer's disease occurs in the proteins of the nerve cells of the cerebral cortex.[21] Changes in these proteins lead to an accumulation of neurofibrillary tangles, which are associated with memory loss and disorientation. Some studies suggest that drugs

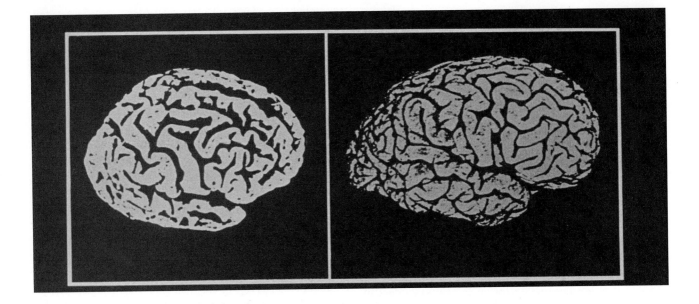

Comparison of Alzheimer and normal brain.

can be used to block the breakdown of the cholinergic activity in the brain and so improve the memory and learning in Alzheimer's patients.[22]

Other research conducted on brain cells grown in culture has shown that a protein, beta amyloid, found in plaque deposits in the brains of Alzheimer's patients produced degeneration of brain cells in the test tube. Alzheimer's patients have excessive amounts of beta amyloid. Verification of these findings in humans needs to take place.

There is no single effective diagnostic test for Alzheimer's. Usually diagnosis is made only after various physiological, psychiatric, and neurological evaluations are carried out. The only way to confirm a diagnosis of Alzheimer's disease is to examine the brain tissue with a microscope.

No treatment or cure is currently available to stop or reverse the onset or progression of this disease. The basic care given an Alzheimer's patient is management of the various symptoms with different medications.

Major research initiatives are currently being carried out to find a cure for Alzheimer's disease. Much of what is known was discovered through autopsies of the brains of deceased Alzheimer's patients. Distinctive changes in the brain have been identified. Researchers have also investigated the theory that Alzheimer's disease is caused by a slow-acting virus. So far there is a lack of evidence to support this theory. Some genetic studies suggest that the form of Alzheimer's often developed prior to fifty years of age is inherited.

Until the cause of Alzheimer's can be determined, it will be impossible to find a cure for this disease. Unfortunately, the burden of caring for an Alzheimer's patient often falls on the family. As the condition becomes progressively worse, continual care is necessary. This places tremendous pressure on the care givers.

Obtaining outside help for the care of the Alzheimer's patient becomes very expensive. Estimates place the annual cost at between twenty thousand and twenty-five thousand dollars.[23] Health insurance, both private and Medicare, provides no help. Before Medicaid can be sought for financial assistance it is necessary to qualify. All too often, families end up spending their own resources until they are depleted. Only then do they qualify for coverage under Medicaid.

Quality of Life as Opposed to Life Enhancement

It is possible to keep a terminally ill individual alive with medical technology for years. However, all too often the quality of life has been negated by such factors as damage to the brain, severe debilitating conditions, continuous pain, as well as physical and mental handicaps of many types.

There is much debate as to how far medical science should go in maintaining one's life. Where do we draw the line? The question often is raised—Who should play God?—in determining whether a patient should be permitted to live or die. Legislation tends to be passed that keeps people alive regardless of the condition of the patient.

Why do we get upset when a chronically ill individual wants to die? For example, the piano artist with severe, painful, crippling arthritis may have no desire to continue to live. Or what should be the responsibility of the family and/or caretaker of the totally incapacitated patient suffering from Alzheimer's disease or stroke with no hope of recovery and being kept alive by medical technology?

The issue of "assisted suicide" has gained much attention in recent years. Do physicians have the right to help a patient with a long-term, chronic condition die, if they so desire? The state of Michigan in 1993 passed legislation that forbade physicians to provide assistance to such patients. This legislation was in response to the actions of a physician in that state who had assisted more than a dozen suicides to terminally ill patients.

These are not easy questions to answer. On one hand it does seem illogical to keep an individual alive on a respirator, or some other type of medical equipment, when there is no hope of recovery. However, the issue becomes very personal where it is a close relative or friend who is involved. There is always the thought that maybe a different medication, treatment modality, or time might result in a change of condition resulting in recovery. These issues must be addressed from the perspective of ethical and value beliefs. It does seem inappropriate for government to legislate what can and cannot be carried out in such circumstances.

Suicide

The loss of a spouse, separation from family or loved ones, and feelings of hopelessness and uselessness are common among the elderly. These factors, along with many others, result in depression, and all too often, in suicide among many senior citizens. Twenty-five percent of reported suicides are committed by the elderly (more than ten thousand per year).[24]

Most suicides among the elderly tend to be well-planned acts. Use of a firearm is the most common method of committing suicide among both male and female senior citizens. However, overdosing on drugs, hanging, and inhalation of carbon monoxide are other procedures that are used.

There are a number of risk factors that are identified as being principle causes of suicide among the elderly. Lack of economic assets is a primary cause. Also lack of social support, depression, use of alcohol, and chronic illness tend to cause many suicides.

Coping with this problem is no easy matter. Programs and activities designed to prevent suicides among the elderly are needed. Most crisis services for suicide prevention have been designed to prevent adolescent suicide, not suicide among the elderly. For the elderly there is a need to prevent social isolation and economic stressors, and to provide opportunity for establishing relationships with others. Supportive services, day care, and senior citizen centers can help to increase the social support and decrease the felt isolation. Activities should include not only community counseling agencies, but also therapeutic services.

Health-Related Social Problems

Many problems faced by the elderly are not primarily health concerns. However, these problems do have an impact on the ability to obtain health care, on the emotional health of the individual, and on the quality of life experienced. Two such health-related social problems are transportation and housing.

Transportation

Mobility is a problem for many senior citizens. As long as a person is able to drive and can afford to operate an automobile, that person is usually able to care for personal needs. However, advanced age frequently forces an individual to rely on others for transportation to appointments, to obtain the essentials of life, and to recreate outside the home. Independence is lost.

Inadequate transportation, in addition to the loss of independence, affects the health of the elderly. They need transportation in order to grocery shop and to travel to medical facilities. But in many communities there is no comprehensive transportation system, so it becomes extremely difficult to go to the physician's office when care is needed.

Reliance upon others for transportation has a negative effect upon the emotional health of the elderly. Psychologically, it tends to produce an attitude of dependence. Not only is the person dependent upon others for transportation, but this characteristic often carries over into other areas of living as well.

Some community social service agencies provide transportation for the elderly. However, this usually is limited to travel to and from a specific agency. Within some communities there are several agencies providing transportation, but unfortunately, this, too, is usually limited in destination and route. Measures need to be designed that would provide unrestricted mobility within the community for the elderly.

Mass transportation in urban communities is often the only means of travel for the senior citizen. In many communities, public transportation offers reduced fares to this age group. In spite of this, many people are hesitant to use public transportation because they fear crime, because of inappropriate time schedules, or because of unacceptable routes.

Housing

In spite of the belief that most elderly live in an institutional setting, the vast majority of senior citizens, in fact, live in a house, an apartment, a condominium, or some type of public housing within the community. Only 5 percent of those over sixty-five years of age are institutionalized.

Often the elderly reside in older houses that have structural deficiencies. The United States Senate Special Committee on Aging reported that at least 30 percent of the elderly population live in substandard, deteriorating housing.[25] This is particularly the case in urban communities among the economically disadvantaged. As a home becomes older, major repairs are often needed to maintain the structure. But the costs of construction, building repair, and maintenance make it very difficult for the poor to maintain a home. These rising construction and maintenance costs, along with the rising expenditures needed to heat a home and the potential for crime, pose serious problems for many elderly citizens.

Rent and property taxes have increased dramatically in recent years. For the elderly living on fixed incomes, this increase has forced them to sell their homes and move to less desirable locations. But rental property is often not maintained at an acceptable level, thus exposing the elderly to a number of the same health problems encountered in their own homes.

Housing quality has a direct relationship to the health and well-being of people. Not only is this related to physical well-being but in the case of the elderly also to emotional health. Emotional health often deteriorates when an individual is forced to move from an area where he or she has lived for many years.

In order to help provide good living conditions for all citizens, including the elderly, many local health departments have units that conduct housing inspections. These activities ensure that housing meets local building codes. These health department employees also inspect facilities where the residents have complaints about conditions. Such inspections usually result when the landlord fails to make repairs requested by tenants.

Long-Term Care Facilities

The very nature of illness experienced by the elderly frequently results in long-term care and treatment. This medical care often must continue even after leaving the hospital. As a result, long-term health care facilities are very important in meeting these needs.

The present long-term institutional concepts originated in the late 1800s and the early part of the twentieth century. Before the depression of the 1930s, the major form of government-supported institutional care for the elderly was the county poorhouse. These facilities were known as "almshouses" or "county farms." They were financed by local government. The poorhouses were often known for their poor living conditions. Most disappeared following passage of the Social Security legislation of 1935. This legislation provided income maintenance for the elderly and the disabled and specifically denied payment to "inmates of public institutions" to prevent the program from supporting residents of county poorhouses.[26]

Since the passage of the Medicare and Medicaid legislation in 1965, the number of beds in nursing homes and the number of elderly living in long-term institutional settings has increased. However, it is important to note that the vast majority of senior citizens will never live in a long-term care facility. Only about 5 percent of the United States population over sixty-five years of age resides in long-term care institutions.[27]

There are several types of long-term facilities, including nursing homes, extended care facilities, home care services, and community-based services. These facilities provide medical and rehabilitative care, and various social services, for those individuals who either cannot obtain the needed care in the home or who are in situations where there are not adequate support systems for them.

Even though most senior citizens are able to receive the care they need while living in a noninstitutional setting, conditions may arise that require long-range, around-the-clock nursing and medical care. Also, many elderly do not have family or friends who can provide the necessary support.

Nursing Homes

The principal health care facility providing long-term care is the nursing home. Most nursing home residents are white, widowed females older than seventy-five years of age. A majority need assistance in such personal care as dressing, bathing, and use of the toilet. Most have difficulty controlling the bowels and/or bladder. Nursing homes are licensed to care for individuals who must have nursing care on a daily basis.

About half of all nursing home patients are admitted following hospital inpatient care. The Medicare prospective payment program, which requires limitations on hospital stays, has resulted in more individuals with terminally ill and chronic conditions being placed in nursing homes. These individuals often have several chronic conditions but are admitted for a particular functional disorder. In the past nursing care was primarily provided in nursing homes; today more medical care is necessary. For example, 40 percent of nursing home admissions are related to cardiovascular diseases.[28]

Placing an individual in a nursing home can be very expensive. The average cost of nursing home care usually exceeds two thousand dollars per month. This is the cost of board, room, and general care; medical services are extra. The long-term nature of nursing home care compounds the cost factor for many families.

Medicare covers medical expenses for those in nursing homes up to a certain limit. However, it does not cover the cost of custodial services. Medicaid will pay for nursing home care, but only after the person qualifies for this coverage. This means that individuals must divest themselves of their financial resources so that they qualify as being economically disadvantaged under the rules of Medicaid within the state in which they reside. Today Medicaid covers the cost of almost half of nursing home expenditures.[29] Most of the rest is paid by the patients' families from their personal resources.

Most nursing homes are not reimbursed in ways that provide incentives for them to provide high-quality care. The individual states usually set flat daily reimbursement rates that are equal for all Medicaid recipients, regardless of the costs of the particular individual. As a result, nursing homes tend to admit the healthiest of the sick elderly. Those individuals who are in need of the most expensive care are less likely to be admitted. Also, expensive therapy is not provided in many nursing homes because of the failure of Medicaid to reimburse for such services. As a result there is no incentive for a nursing home to provide care that would improve the health status of the patient.

Until 1987 each nursing home was classified as either a skilled nursing facility or an intermediate care facility. These categories were eliminated by federal legislation in 1987. A system involving several variables is now used to classify nursing homes. These variables include the extent of patient care, types of programs available for the residents, and the type and amount of professional staff available.

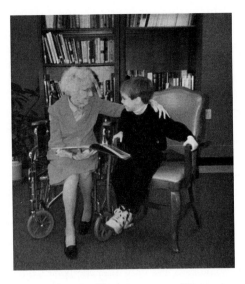

Positive interaction between the young man and his great-grandmother at the nursing home helps both to have basic human needs met. The boy better understands his great-grandmother is an individual who can help him to learn to read. The elderly resident can feel she is playing a useful role in the young boy's life.

It is expected that nursing services and rehabilitative care are available on a twenty-four-hour-a-day basis. Patients who cannot function without medical supervision or those undergoing long-term medical convalescence are often placed in nursing home facilities. Individuals needing a special diet may receive special assistance in such facilities. In addition, residents often require and receive assistance in dressing, bathing, mobility, and elimination.

When placement in a long-term care facility is necessary, a major life change for an individual usually occurs. For this reason, placement in an institution must involve very careful decision making. Several factors are important in this process:[30]

1. The physical and emotional care needs of the individual

2. The degree of support received from family, friends, and neighbors

3. The attitude of the patient regarding institutional placement

The needs of the elderly are a primary factor in determining the type of care and services required. Assessment of these needs must include a medical evaluation, a functional ability evaluation, a psychological evaluation, and a social evaluation.[31]

Placement in a long-term care facility should be a decision reached only after all alternatives have been discussed. It should not result simply as a matter of convenience for the health care providers or the person's family. This action must be taken only out of concern for the well-being of the patient involved.

Even though elderly persons are placed in long-term care facilities for a variety of reasons, two types of problems in particular result in the most admissions.[32] These are (1) the need for rehabilitative care following an acute illness and (2) the need for care owing to chronic disabling disease. These conditions require the services of personnel who cannot work effectively in the home setting.

Some nursing homes are exclusively for people who are mentally retarded. These facilities, however, are licensed as residential nursing homes.

Until the 1960s, most mentally impaired elderly were placed in state or local mental hospitals for care and treatment. However, nursing home services for the mentally impaired senior citizen have replaced the hospital as the psychiatric care center. The two principal reasons for this change are economic and humanitarian. Patients receive better nursing services and rehabilitative care in nursing homes than they do in large public mental health hospitals.

Under federal legislation passed in 1987, nursing homes are required to screen and to treat individuals with mental illness. Nursing homes must screen all applicants for admission for mental disorders. Also, all individuals who have been residents in nursing homes must be screened. Those in need of treatment must be identified through this mandated screening process. Measures must be implemented to provide treatment for those in need of psychological care while in the nursing home. If this is impossible, the patient is to be discharged to an appropriate psychiatric treatment facility.[33]

Many Americans regard long-term institutionalization as a last resort and usually approach it with various degrees of "apprehension, guilt and revulsion." [34] These negative feelings may pertain to the physical characteristics of the nursing home. They may also be due to the nature of the staff. Numerous problems inherent in nursing home care also contribute to such feelings. Common problems include infrequent and brief physician visits, usually by someone untrained in geriatric medicine; understaffed nursing services; and a lack of social workers, psychologists, and/or mental health workers with experience and knowledge in geriatric patient care.

Institutionalization is frequently used to relieve the burden on families due to the lack of any alternatives. The need for alternatives to long-term institutional care for the elderly stems not only from a physical and emotional level but also from financial constraints.

Alternatives to Long-Term Care

Respite Care

In order to relieve the family of the necessity for institutionalization of the elderly and also of the need for twenty-four-hour care, there are several alternatives available. One area that provides planned, short-term care is referred to as *respite care*. This type of care provides periodic relief to the family and makes available expanded health support services such as food preparation and shopping as well as supervision of the older person as needed. Unfortunately these services are not reimbursed by Medicare and most private insurance.

One type of respite care is the adult daycare center. There are more than fourteen hundred adult daycare centers in the United States. Daycare services for the elderly began in England in the late 1950s and have been available there and in other European countries for some time. This facility provides an alternative to the isolation of home and to institutionalization in a nursing home.

Adult daycare facilities may be rehabilitative, or they may focus on a specific type of health problem. Three models of adult daycare centers exist. The day hospital has a strong health care orientation, and physical rehabilitation is the primary goal.[35] Most day hospitals are closely associated with health care institutions, the patients having been released from inpatient status.

The second model of adult daycare centers focuses on social services, nutrition, and social activities. Participants in these settings have fewer diagnosed medical problems and are less dependent.

The elderly person is brought to the center and left for all or part of the day. He or she is picked up after a designated time and returns home. Daycare emphasizes health maintenance, health promotion, health restoration, and rehabilitation for physical problems. Some provide dental care and dietary guidance, as well as emotional counseling. Physicians, occupational therapists, social workers, physical therapists, and nursing personnel provide their services. The senior citizen can participate in a social environment during the day. Usually these individuals do not need constant care, yet they cannot, or should not, stay at home alone. Most patients in adult daycare facilities are stroke and arthritis patients, diabetics, and amputees. An important goal for these individuals is the prevention of problems that require hospitalization. Adult daycare also relieves the family of the continual care of the elderly person.

A problem associated with adult daycare is that the medical costs are not covered by Medicare and only a few states cover such costs in their Medicaid programs.

Another form of adult daycare emphasizes socialization and activity rather than physical health care and rehabilitation. The senior citizen center offers the opportunity for the elderly to socialize, learn new roles, maintain and develop involvement in the community, and gain a sense of usefulness and dignity. The elderly come to the center, where they may have contact with other community agencies providing health screenings.

Adult Foster Homes

The adult foster home is a private residence licensed to care for a few disabled adults. There is a live-in manager who provides personal care and housekeeping services to the residents. Meals are served family style. The residents are encouraged to socialize and to help with the various housekeeping chores and with the cooking.

These homes provide a place to live for individuals in need of health care provided by home health agencies. They tend to serve low-income persons with mental illness or developmental disabilities who are in need of a supportive environment.

Most adult foster homes are located in privately owned homes. It is important that strong regulations be established so as to protect those who are living in these foster care settings.

Home Health Care

Perhaps the most popular alternative to long-term institutional nursing home care for the elderly is the home health care program, where medical care and related services are provided in the home of the patient. A sick or partially disabled senior citizen should not always assume that they must enter a residential nursing home following illness and hospitalization. There is increasing interest in home health care for the elderly in this country.

Services that can be provided in the home include basic nursing care, rehabilitative therapy, nutritional assistance, home health aide services, and counseling. The health care specialists come to the home on a regular basis to provide these services. The physician is responsible for prescribing the medical treatment that the individual will need at home. Treatment may include medication, skilled nursing care, and physical, occupational, speech, and/or hearing therapy. The nurse is responsible for determining the type of nursing care needed to carry out the plan established by the physician.

There is evidence that patients respond to therapy more quickly in their own homes than in residential nursing homes. Studies have also shown that health improves more with patients involved in home-based care programs than with those in nursing homes.[36] The patient is more relaxed at home around familiar and comfortable surroundings. As a result, there is greater motivation to follow instructions. The psychological benefit to the individual also contributes to rehabilitation.

Home health care is provided by public health departments, hospitals, and some private agencies. Regardless of which type of home health agency a person chooses, the initial step in developing a home care plan rests with the physician.

Home health care is of interest to the government and private health insurance agencies as one approach to controlling hospital costs. Home health care is less expensive than extended hospitalization. However, before the concept of home health care is widely accepted, it will be necessary for hospitalization insurance, both private and Medicare and Medicaid, to extend coverage for the services.

For many of the seven million elderly who need long-term assistance at home, care is provided by family members. Often the care givers are their spouses, children,

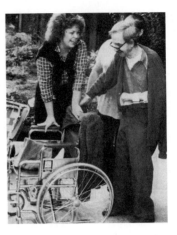

Many community health projects support the preparation of geriatric nurse practitioners to improve nursing within the long-term care field. These projects also support the coordination of services offered by community health agencies to improve home care for the elderly.

other relatives, or friends. But spouses are usually elderly and frail, and children, who are often in middle age, may be experiencing chronic health problems themselves.

Medicare does not reimburse the costs of personal services such as general household services and assistance with dressing, bathing, meal preparation, and shopping. Medicare rarely provides for long-term care for chronic conditions in the home. It provides only for care when one is confined at home owing to injury or illness. To be eligible for home health care services reimbursed by Medicare, one must have been hospitalized for three consecutive days for the same illness, have documented evidence that one is considered homebound, and need skilled nursing services, physical therapy, speech therapy, or other types of therapy. A plan of treatment must be established by the physician and recertified every sixty days.[37]

Aging—The Future

The demand for services for the elderly will increase in the future. This is due partially to the fact that the number of elderly will grow in the years ahead. The elderly in the early part of the twenty-first century will have greater expectations of services than has been the case in the past. Most of today's younger generation have had educational

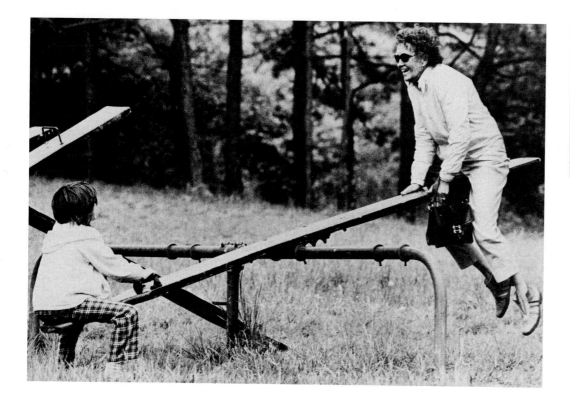

opportunities, health services, and other services that many in the present elderly population did not have. This younger generation also has had greater financial freedom than previous generations. As this population group grows older and begins to experience the problems of chronic illnesses and the need for certain health and social services, expectations will rise as well. These expectations will be complicated by the escalating costs of such services. Increased medical care costs, hospital expenses, and finances needed for institutional care negatively affect both the present and future senior citizen.

The elderly population in the early twenty-first century will be more highly educated and politically aware than previous generations. As a result, the problems and needs of the elderly will receive greater interest, attention, and concern in the years ahead. The elderly population will be a force that cannot be shunned by politicians, economists, and society. "Gray power" is a force that will definitely be heard in the future.

More is being understood about health promotion for all ages, including senior citizens. This was

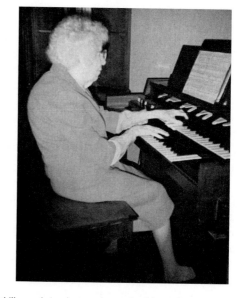

Music skills can bring hours of meaningful satisfaction to the elderly.

particularly highlighted in 1988 with the numerous recommendations that came out of the Surgeon General's Workshop on Health Promotion and Aging. The importance of leading an active life-style throughout the senior years was strongly emphasized. Research needs to identify the types and levels of activity that will most benefit the health status of the elderly, and community resources need to be available to provide opportunities for more active life-styles.

The American society must accept the role of the elderly. It is important that we realize that the elderly person need not be isolated from society in the institutional setting but instead must be included as a vital figure in the life of the family as well as the community. The elderly should be encouraged to remain useful in their later years. This can be accomplished in numerous ways: as foster grandparents and by helping in child day-care centers and other similar programs. Senior citizens might even be encouraged to continue in their professions at reduced levels of involvement as they grow older.

Summary

A number of medical advances in the past century have lengthened the life span of many people in the United States. This, accompanied by other factors, has contributed to a growth in the number of people living past the age of sixty-five. Today over 12 percent of the U.S. population is over sixty-five, and it is projected that this figure will surpass 20 percent in the next forty years.

There is no one point at which a person automatically becomes elderly. The Social Security legislation passed in 1935, retirement policies, and American culture have all influenced the establishment of the age of sixty-five as the point at which people are classified as elderly. However, for many people, both in the past and in the present, life has been productive beyond sixty-five.

In spite of the general improvement in the health of Americans, health problems continue to plague the senior citizen. Chronic and degenerative diseases are a major health care problem for most of the elderly. The various chronic diseases, such as arthritis, cancer, and cardiovascular diseases, are usually long-term and have no known cures.

Other elderly health problems include inadequate nutrition and a variety of physiological changes that occur in old age. Bone structure changes, metabolic performance is affected, and dietary patterns change. Alzheimer's disease is a disorder that produces memory loss and disorientation, and there is no treatment or cure. Extensive research initiatives are currently being carried out to find a means of reducing its impact on thousands of individuals and their families.

A variety of social problems affect the health status of the elderly. Independence is greatly reduced. Transportation modes are limited, so the individual is forced to rely on others for mobility. Adequate, safe, and affordable housing is another concern for many senior citizens.

The very nature of elderly illnesses results in long-term care. About 5 percent of the elderly reside in long-term health care facilities. The principal long-term care facility is the nursing home. In the nursing home, the patient can receive medical care on a twenty-four-hour-a-day basis.

There are several alternatives to long-term institutional care for the elderly. Respite care provides a place where certain services can be made available to the elderly on a daily outpatient basis. The individual can live with family and friends, yet receive needed care.

Another alternative to the long-term care institution is health care provided in the home. In these situations, the provider comes to the home and gives medical care, therapy, or rehabilitative assistance in the familiar setting of the patient's home. This approach has been the object of great attention. In order for alternative elderly care programs to become more widely accepted and used, it is important that costs for these services be covered by third-party insurers, such as private health insurance companies, Medicare, and Medicaid.

Discussion Questions

1. What factors have contributed to the increased longevity of people in the past century?
2. In your opinion, when does old age begin?
3. Discuss the various issues that must be considered by a person thinking about retiring.
4. Discuss the effect of economics on the health and well-being of the elderly.
5. In what ways do chronic illnesses affect the quality of elderly life?
6. Why are senior citizens often malnourished?
7. What are the risk factors associated with osteoporosis?
8. Physiologically, what happens in the human body that results in osteoporosis?
9. Why are the elderly more likely to suffer hip fractures than younger people?
10. Identify some of the factors associated with unintentional injury among the elderly.
11. Discuss some of the issues concerning medication misuse among the elderly.
12. What role might a pharmacist play in controlling the prescription use of senior citizens?
13. Explain the differences between functional and organic mental illnesses.
14. Why is depression rather common among the elderly?
15. Explain the cause, the signs, and the symptoms of Alzheimer's disease.
16. What has been learned from research in the past few years about Alzheimer's disease?
17. Are there preventive measures that can be taken to reduce the possibility of getting Alzheimer's disease?
18. Why is suicide a concern among the elderly?
19. What measures can be taken to reduce the risk of suicide among senior citizens?
20. Explain why transportation must be considered as a problem for many senior citizens.
21. What are some factors related to housing that impact the well-being of elderly persons?
22. What are the different kinds of long-term health care facilities?
23. Discuss the economic pressures on the elderly and their families resulting from long-term institutional care.
24. Identify some alternatives to long-term institutionalization of the elderly.
25. What does federal law now require nursing homes to do relating to mental illness of patients?
26. What is an adult foster home?
27. What is provided for in a home health care program?
28. Identify some of the services available in your community to make for a more positive life-style among the elderly.

Suggested Readings

Aging America: Trends and Projections. An information paper to the Special Committee on Aging. United States Senate, Serial no. 101–J. Washington, D.C.: U.S. Government Printing Office, February, 1990.

"All about Alzheimer's." *Newsweek* (December 18, 1989): 54–63.

Beers, Mark H., and others. "Screening Recommendations for the Elderly." *American Journal of Public Health* 81, no. 9 (September 1991): 1131–40.

Branch, Laurence G. "Health Practices and Incident Disability among the Elderly." *American Journal of Public Health* 75, no. 12 (December 1985): 1436–39.

Burns, Barbara J., and others. "Mental Health Service Use by the Elderly in Nursing Homes." *American Journal of Public Health* 83, no. 3 (March 1993): 331–37.

Cohen, Gene D., and others. "Workshop: Alzheimer's Disease and Other Dementias." *Public Health Reports* 103, no. 5 (September/October 1988): 543–45.

Corolli, Connie H. "Osteoporosis: Significance, Risk Factors and Treatment." *The Nurse Practitioner* 11, no. 9 (September 1986): 16–35.

Cowart, Marie E. "Policy Issues: Financial Reimbursement for Home Care." *Family and Community Health* 8, no. 2 (August 1985): 1–10.

Douglas, Kaaren, C., and Michael C. Hosokowa. "Better Health for Elderly Patients." *Medical Times* 114, no. 10 (October 1986): 52–60.

Fox, Patrick. "From Senility to Alzheimer's Disease: The Rise of the Alzheimer's Disease Movement." *The Milbank Quarterly* 67, no. 1 (1989): 58–102.

Greenfield, Carol A. "Improving Elderly Access to Health Care Information." *Business and Health* 3, no. 7 (June 1986): 26–30.

Gurwitz, Jerry H., and others. "Treatment for Glaucoma: Adherence by the Elderly." *American Journal of Public Health* 83, no. 5 (May 1993): 711–16.

Hemmink, Elina, and others. "Clustering and Consistency of Use of Medicines among Mid-Aged Women." *Medical Care* 27, no. 9 (September 1989): 859–68.

Kahl, Anne, and others. "Geriatric Education Centers Address Medication Issues Affecting Older Adults." *Public Health Reports* 107, no. 1 (1992): 37–47.

Kane, Rosalie, and others. "Adult Foster Care for the Elderly in Oregon: A Mainstream Alternative to Nursing Homes?" *American Journal of Public Health* 81, no. 9 (September 1991): 1113–20.

Kutner, Nancy G., and others. "Measuring the Quality of Life of the Elderly in Health Promotion Intervention Clinical Trials." *Public Health Reports* 107, no. 5 (September/October 1992): 530–39.

Latta, Viola B., and Roger E. Keene. "Use and Cost of Skilled Nursing Facilities under Medicare, 1987." *Health Care Financing Review* 11, no. 1 (Fall 1989): 105–06.

Libow, Leslie, S., and Perry Starer. "Care of the Nursing Home Patient." *The New England Journal of Medicine* 321, no. 2 (July 13, 1989): 93–96.

Meehan, Patrick J., and others. "Suicides among Older United States Residents: Epidemiologic Characteristics and Trends." *American Journal of Public Health* 81, no. 9 (September 1991): 1198–1200.

Melin, Anna-Lisa, and others. "The Cost-Effectiveness of Rehabilitation in the Home: A Study of Swedish Elderly." *American Journal of Public Health* 83, no. 3 (March 1993): 356–62.

Morford, Thomas G. "Nursing Home Regulation: History and Expectations." *Health Care Financing Review, 1988 Supplement,* pp. 129–39.

Peterson, Steven, A., and Robert Maidon. "Older Americans' Use of Nutrition Programs." *Journal of Nutrition for the Elderly* 11, no. 1/2 (1991): 49–67.

Piano, Lois A. "Adult Day Care: A New Ambulatory Care Alternative." *Nursing* 16, no. 8 (August 1986): 60–62.

Scanlon, Wm. J. "A Perspective on Long-Term Care for the Elderly." *Health Care Financing Review* (1988—Suppl.): 7–15.

Sorenson, Susan B. "Suicide among the Elderly: Issues Facing Public Health." *American Journal of Public Health* 81, no. 9 (September 1991): 1109–10.

Task Force on Older Women's Health. "Older Women's Health." *Journal of the American Geriatrics Society* 41, no. 6 (June 1993): 680–83.

Tolstoi, Linda G., and Robert M. Levin. "Osteoporosis—The Treatment Controversy." *Nutrition Today* 27, no. 4 (July/August 1992): 6–12.

Waxman, Howard M. "Community Mental Health Care for the Elderly—a Look at the Obstacles." *Public Health Reports* 101, no. 3 (May/June 1986): 294–300.

Weinberger, Morris, and others. "Expenditures in Caring for Patients with Dementia Who Live at Home." *American Journal of Public Health* 83, no. 3 (March 1993): 338–41.

"Who Can Afford Nursing Homes?" *Consumer Reports* 53, no. 5 (May 1988): 300–309.

Endnotes

1. *Aging America: Trends and Projections*. An information paper to the Speical Committee on Aging. United States Senate. Serial no. 101–J, Washington, D.C.: U.S. Government Printing Office, February, 1990.

2. *Ibid.*

3. *Ibid.,* 16.

4. *Ibid.,* 79.

5. *Ibid.,* 81.

6. *Ibid.,* 90.

7. Posner, Barbara M. *Nutrition and the Elderly*. Lexington, Ky.: D.C. Heath and Co., 1979.

8. Wolf, Colleen A. "Oral Health Care of the Elderly." *Ohio's Health* 34, no. 1 (1982): 11.

9. Department of Health and Human Services. *Healthy People 2000: National Health Promotion and Disease Prevention Objectives*. Washington, D.C.: U.S. Government Printing Office, 1991, p. 354.

10. Department of Health and Human Services, Public Health Service, National Institute on Aging. *Age Pages* (November 1985): 66.

11. Department of Health and Human Services, *Healthy People 2000*, 467.

12. National Safety Council, *Accident Facts, 1993 Edition*. Chicago, Ill.: National Safety Council, 1993, p. 4.

13. Department of Health and Human Services, *Healthy People 2000*, 279.

14. Department of Health and Human Services, Public Health Service. *Changes . . . Research on Aging and the Aged*. NIH Publication no. 81–85 (October 1980).

15. Surgeon General's Report on Health Promotion and Disease Prevention. *Healthy People*. Washington, D.C.: U.S. Government Printing Office, 1976, p. 375.

16. The subject of community mental health centers is discussed at length in chapter 15.

17. Gaitz, Charles M., and Roy V. Varner. "Principles of Mental Health for Elderly Patients." *Hospital and Community Psychiatry* 33, no. 2 (February 1982): 132.

18. Department of Health and Human Services. *Promoting Health/Preventing Disease: Year 2000 Objectives for the Nation*, pp. 7–16.

19. Department of Health and Human Services, Public Health Service, National Institutes on Aging. *Alzheimer's Disease: Fact Sheet*. GPO #92–3431 (1992).

20. *Aging America: Trends and Projections*. An information paper to the Special Committee on Aging, United States Senate, p. 92.

21. Department of Health and Human Services. *Special Report on Aging*, 1980.

22. Emr, Marian. "Senility: The Outlook Is Bright." *World Health* (February/March 1982): 14.

23. "All About Alzheimer's." *Newsweek* (December 18, 1989): 62.

24. Department of Health and Human Services, *Healthy People 2000*, 210–11.

25. United States Senate Special Committee on Aging. *Developments in Aging, 1976*. Washington, D.C.: U.S. Government Printing Office, 1976.

26. U.S. Senate Committee on Finance. *The Social Security Act and Related Laws*. Washington, D.C.: U.S. Government Printing Office, December 1978.

27. Department of Health and Human Services, *Healthy People 2000*, 448.

28. U.S. Bipartisan Commission of Comprehensive Health Care, 1990.

29. *Aging America: Trends and Projections*. An information paper to the Special Committee on Aging United States, p. 105.

30. Freece, Debbie. "Issues Relating to Long-Term Care Placement." *Ohio's Health* 34, no. 2 (February 1982): 5.

31. Ham, R. "Alternatives to Institutionalization." *American Family Physician* 21, no. 7 (July 1980): 95–100.

32. Freece, "Long-Term Care," 5.

33. U.S. Congress. The Omnibus Budget Reconciliation Act of 1987.

34. Krause, D. "Institutional Living for the Elderly in Denmark: A Model for the United States." *Aging* (September/October 1981): 29–38.

35. Burris, K. C. "Recommending Adult Day Care Centers." *Nursing and Health Care* 2, no. 8 (October 1981): 437–41.

36. Mitchell, J. B. "Patient Outcomes in Alternative Long-Term Care Settings." *Medical Care* 16, no. 6 (1978): 439–52.

37. DePaoli, T., and P. Zenk-Jones. "Medicare Reimbursement in Home Care." *The American Journal of Occupational Therapy* 38, no. 11 (November 1984): 739–42.

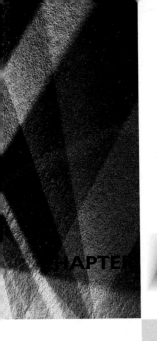

CHAPTER **TWENTY-ONE**

Substances of Abuse

Drugs, Alcohol, and Tobacco

The people of the United States use drugs extensively. In many instances, there is a definite purpose and value for such use; drugs have numerous medicinal purposes. Medications may be either prescribed drugs or nonprescription medications. Over 1.4 billion prescriptions are filled each year by pharmacists in the United States. Several billion dollars are spent each year on nonprescription medications. Thus, it is obvious why the United States is often termed a drug-taking society.

All too often, however, drugs are used to satisfy underlying psychological needs. There are substances that cause alterations in the mood and psyche of an individual. With habitual use of these substances, the person can become dependent either physiologically or psychologically. The individual may feel it is impossible to meet the responsibilities of a day without the use of a drug.

It is this unnecessary use of alcohol, tobacco, and other drugs of abuse that causes problems in society. As such, this drug overuse has become important in community health programming. The extent of the problem is highlighted by the economic costs, the number of deaths caused by use of these mood-modifying substances, and the upheaval or disturbance of family and personal social structures, as well as society as a whole.

Whereas in the past substance abuse was considered to be a medical and community health issue, during the decade of the 1980s it became a concern of our whole society. Government at many different levels has become involved in measures designed to control illegal drug use. The matter has international ramifications, with illegal drugs being brought from other countries of the world to the United States. Policy decisions have been influenced by the problems associated with substance abuse.

It is doubtful that a totally drug abstinent society is possible, or even desirable. A more realistic goal is for controlled, responsible use of chemicals. The behavioral patterns of drug abuse must be curtailed and eventually eliminated. Drug use, as it negatively affects the health and well-being of others, must be abolished. This is an important challenge for community health in the years ahead.

Drugs of Abuse

Drug use and abuse are community health issues that the medical community cannot deal with in isolation. Though there certainly are medical and health considerations associated with drug abuse, many community agencies and services are also extensively involved in comprehensive community drug abuse programs. In addition to medical personnel, the behavioral scientist, the educational expert, and social and vocational rehabilitators are important in planning activities to help the drug abuser. Today local, state, and federal law enforcement agencies and governmental legislative bodies, plus numerous other federal agencies, are involved in programming and funding designed to win the "War on Drugs."

Illicit use of drugs has always been a part of society. However, most communities have viewed it as a serious problem only in recent years. Prior to that, drug abuse was usually perceived to be a problem for social outcasts who were living in poor, slum conditions and who were not considered part of the mainstream of community life.

As drug use and abuse have increased, their growth has extended beyond the boundaries of race, geography, and socioeconomics. Though it is very difficult to ascertain the cost of drug abuse, estimates indicate that it exceeds $76 billion a year, and there is speculation that this figure is too low.[1] This estimate includes expenditures for drug control, prevention, treatment, and enforcement as well as lost and damaged resources resulting from the drug use. These costs will continue to significantly affect the nation's economy in the years ahead.

Though drug abuse is found at all ages, significant use of drugs for nonmedical purposes decreases with age. Most drug abuse is found among adolescents and young adults, those in the eighteen-to-twenty-five-year-old age group. Unfortunately, a greater percentage of substance abuse is found among minority populations and the economically disadvantaged.

Why People Abuse Drugs

Why do people abuse drugs? What has accounted for the serious increase of drug abuse in the United States? A number of social factors are associated with the misuse of drugs in society. Drug misuse often begins during adolescence, at a time when peer pressure is most significant. Young people tend to adopt the behavioral patterns of their peers. Peer pressure, because of its inherent power, is one of the major influences leading to drug use.

Taking drugs has become a part of normal living in many households. Alcohol consumption is considered a natural activity in the lives of many people, and people in the United States consume hundreds of thousands of over-the-counter and prescription drugs each year. These drug consumption models have an effect on young people. As young people see adults taking a drink or "popping pills" to alleviate such problems as headaches or inability to sleep or to help them relax, it seems only natural to seek drugs as a solution to their problems as well. Thus adults must realize the relationship between their drug and alcohol use and their children's behavior.

Young people use drugs, particularly marijuana, as a display of their alienation from authority. They see their parents and other authority figures using alcohol and other drugs to "get through the day." For the young person marijuana is the drug of choice to relax or to release stress and pressure. They see no reason why marijuana use is not acceptable behavior for them if alcohol use is the "norm" for adults. As a matter of fact, they often resent adult opposition to their drug use behavior and consider parental and authority figures' opposition to their drug use patterns hypocritical.

Drug use is often a way to satisfy certain sociological and psychological problems. It may be the means for gaining support, respect, and meaning from a social group or an individual. When a person is unable to find meaning in life or personal identity in socially approved activities, the alternative is often drug use.

Such behavior is often accompanied by apathy and decline in school or work performance. This is referred to as the "amotivational syndrome." The person cannot find success or interest in sports, clubs, or academic achievement, so becomes involved in drug abuse. It is still not known, however, whether drug use causes the syndrome or whether the syndrome is a forerunner of drug use.

The extent of fatalities resulting from drug abuse cannot be precisely measured because such fatalities are often categorized as "unknown," or "accidental," or are listed as an "overdose." It is known that in approximately

War on Drugs

Much has been said and written about a "War on Drugs." Politicians have spoken out concerning actions that need to be taken to reduce the drug problem. The mass media has presented various options directed toward improving this problem.

The abuse of illicit drugs cost the United States economy $76 billion in a single year.[*] This includes expenditures for law enforcement, lost resources, and drug control, prevention, and treatment. It does not consider the additional costs of behaviors exhibited while under the influence of drugs and alcohol, such as violence, homicide, robbery, and child abuse.

Toward whom should this "war on drugs" be directed—the user? the seller? the importer of the drugs? the peasant in a Third World nation growing the coca leaves that become cocaine? What procedures should be taken? How is such a "war" going to be financed? Such questions have increasingly brought the issue of drug abuse into the political spectrum.

Law enforcement has been the principle measure in the past to control drug use. Local and state law enforcement agencies along with the U.S. Drug Enforcement Administra-tion have carried out drug busts, made arrests, and attempted to stop the flow of drugs into our communities.

Some believe that increased public drug education programs can be an effective activity in this "war." However, it must be pointed out that there is little evidence that school drug education programs have been effective in halting the increase in drug usage. Whether mass media appeals to not use drugs by popular personalities are effective is open to question.

Military operations have been used. In 1986 the United States military conducted operations in Bolivia designed to destroy cocaine laboratories, confiscate equipment used in drug manufacturing, and damage jungle airstrips used by drug manufacturers. In Bolivia 80,000 acres of coca are grown. The leaves of these plants are chewed and brewed as tea by Indian tribes living in the Andes. Doubt exists as to how effective military might is in winning a "war on drugs."

What priorities need to be established in countering the increasing use of drugs in American society? How would you relegate resources—financial, personnel, media, and the like—to be most effective in this campaign?

[*]University of Southern California study reported in *The Nation's Health* (September 1992): 2.

50 percent of all traffic-related fatalities alcohol is the contributing cause. The increase in the use of crack cocaine has resulted in the death of thousands, either directly or indirectly. The violent crime associated with cocaine use has led to a serious escalation in the number of homicides and other violent crimes.

Commonly Abused Drugs

Several drugs are considered drugs of abuse. The most commonly abused drugs are alcohol, hallucinogenic drugs, marijuana, nicotine, opiates, sedatives, and stimulants.

Alcohol

Alcohol consumption is a multibillion-dollar-a-year business in the United States. Approximately 70 percent of the American population drinks alcoholic beverages.

Drinking in America is a social phenomenon. Alcoholic beverages are advertised extensively on television, on the radio, and in print. This advertising portrays drinking as being normal, socially acceptable, and healthy. Many people feel it is inappropriate to have a party or gathering without serving alcoholic beverages. Mention a New Year's Eve party or a wedding reception, and most people picture an affair where various alcoholic drinks will be served. A significant amount of business is also transacted over cocktails, so many businesses and corporations budget large amounts of money for entertaining and social functions that usually involve alcohol consumption.

Most people drink socially and are able to control their level of liquor consumption. But the problem of alcohol misuse among those who do not know their "limit" has become a major social problem and as such is an important public health problem.

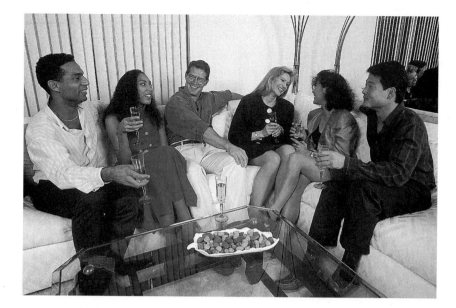

Millions of Americans consider alcohol consumption an important part of socialization. Alcoholic beverages are served at such social functions as parties, receptions, and business luncheons.

There are a number of problems related to alcohol use. Of increasing concern are alcohol-related birth defects, the most common of which is fetal alcohol syndrome. There is a definite association between the alcohol consumption of pregnant women and birth defects in newborn infants. How much alcohol must be consumed before the syndrome develops is not known, but it is known that a variety of physiological abnormalities and mental retardation occur when the pregnant woman is a moderate-to-heavy drinker.[2]

Heavy drinking is associated with increased risks of cancer of several parts of the body: the tongue, mouth, larynx, and liver. Alcohol consumption has also been associated with deterioration of the heart muscle, diminished cardiac output, and decreased ability of the heart muscle to contract. In fact, alcohol consumption is considered one of the major factors of cardiovascular disease.

Malnutrition is also linked to alcohol consumption. Alcohol is high in "empty" calories. The individual who drinks moderately to heavily often is deficient in vitamins and other essential nutrients needed for bodily functions.

One of the main organs affected by alcohol is the liver. An inflammation of the liver is known as *cirrhosis,* and is almost always associated with alcohol consumption.

Nicotine

Nicotine is a central nervous system stimulant that is present in the tobacco leaf and so is inhaled into the body when a person smokes cigarettes. Though nicotine is partially destroyed by the burning cigarette, as much as one-third passes into the body unchanged in the inhaled smoke.[3] Nicotine increases respiratory and heart rates as well as the blood pressure of cigarette smokers. The stimulant has also been know to increase peristalsis of the intestines.[4]

The Surgeon General has said that smoking is the most important public health issue of our time. Tobacco use is the single most important preventable cause of death and disease among the American population.[5]

Many health problems are associated with cigarette smoking, including cardiovascular disease, chronic bronchitis, emphysema, and cancer. Respiratory infections and stomach ulcers are also linked to cigarette smoking. Nearly a third of all cancer deaths in the United States are related to smoking; it is the major cause of lung cancer and contributes to cancer of the bladder, kidney, and pancreas.[6]

Marijuana

After alcohol and cigarettes, marijuana is the third most frequently used drug in the United States. This drug has been used in various cultures for centuries in religious ceremonies and in important social celebrations. Today, though, marijuana is an illegal drug in most parts of the world.

Marijuana use has been a part of various cultures in the United States for decades. In the early part of the twentieth century many professional musicians were known to use this drug. However, the use of marijuana among the general mainstream population first became a problem in the United States during the 1960s when it was heavily used by the counterculture population. In the past two decades, the use of marijuana has increased and expanded to people of all social, economic, and cultural groups, not just the young. Though marijuana can be chewed, it is usually smoked in the form of marijuana cigarettes. The cigarettes contain a low potency level of the drug.

Despite this diffusion of marijuana use, it is still found principally among adolescents and young adults. The highest usage rates are found in the eighteen- to twenty-five-year age group. Marijuana use is increasing in a younger age group—among teenagers. As many as one-third of the high school seniors who use marijuana admitted that they began using the drug in ninth grade or earlier.[7] Marijuana use, however, declines with age.

Marijuana is derived from the Indian hemp plant *Cannabis sativa*. The flowering tops and leaves of this plant are dried, crushed, and then rolled into cigarettes. Marijuana cigarettes, known as "joints" or "reefers," are smoked by inhaling deeply into the lungs. The deep inhalation increases the absorption of the active ingredient that causes the euphoric effects. This psychoactive ingredient in marijuana is *tetrahydrocannabinol* (THC).

The psychoactive effect on an individual depends on the depth of the smoke inhalation, the strength (concentration) of THC, and the extent to which an individual has used the drug. Reactions to marijuana often include feelings of anxiety, depression, fatigue, nausea, and dizziness. Other noted physiological effects include an increase in pulse rate and blood pressure, dryness of the throat and mouth, and reddening of the whites of the eyes. Further intoxication can affect motor skills, reflexes, behavior, vision, and memory. In addition, sensitivity to pain has been noted among marijuana users.

Marijuana use has a depressant effect upon motor skills. As a result, motor vehicle operation and complex psychomotor performance are impaired, as they are when an individual is under the influence of alcohol. Habitual marijuana users tend to have more accidents than nonusers. This problem is compounded by the fact that marijuana is commonly used in conjunction with alcohol. The combined effect results in greater impairment than that which would result from the use of either alone.[8] There is sufficient evidence to recommend that marijuana users not drive while under the influence of the drug, just as they should not drive while intoxicated with alcohol.

Though the evidence is inconclusive, there seems to be a relationship between biological health and marijuana use. There have been reported instances of impairment of the body's natural defense system against disease among marijuana smokers. However, other reports contradict this.[9]

Another relationship involves the effect of marijuana use on reproduction. The drug decreases the number and mobility of sperm among males who use marijuana on a regular basis. Also, abnormal chromosomes have been noted among marijuana users. Both of these concerns, however, are subject to difference of opinion since much of the evidence has been gathered in animal research studies.

Marijuana affects short-term memory, leading to impairment of intellectual performance.[10] Though this impairment varies according to the dose of the drug, the individual's level of motivation, and other variables, it does have definite implications for young people of school age.

Marijuana use has been an extremely controversial issue. Some contend that the drug is no more dangerous than alcohol. Thus, they argue, it should be legalized so its use is free from the stigma of drug abuse. Others believe that marijuana must be banned from society and its users punished. Between these two poles are a spectrum of opinions as to how society should cope with the problem of marijuana use.

It is interesting to note that marijuana has been used in medical treatment. It has been effective in the treatment of glaucoma, and there have been instances where it has been used to help control nausea and vomiting in cancer chemotherapy patients. Marijuana dilates the bronchial tubes, so some medical personnel working with asthma patients have suggested that it might be helpful in treating this respiratory condition.

Hallucinogenic Drugs

Several drugs create illusions in the mind of the user. These drugs alter perception, thought, and mood when taken in even very small amounts. The user may see objects change color, shape, and appearance. In addition, different sights and sounds may be seen and heard. *Synesthesia,* crossing of sense responses—hearing colors and seeing sounds—may occur.[11] Hallucinogenic drugs also produce a variety of physiological and psychological effects.

The best-known hallucinogenic drugs are lysergic acid diethylamide (LSD) and mescaline (peyote). Other drugs that produce hallucinations, disorientation, and other mind-altering patterns are psilocybin, DMT (dimethyltryptamine), and PCP (phencyclidine).

LSD has received the most attention of the hallucinogenic drugs, probably because it causes many serious physiological and psychological problems. It has been shown that LSD use impairs intellectual processes. The effects of LSD are unpredictable depending on several factors: the amount taken, the mood of the individual, expectations, and the environment in which the drug is being used.[12] Prolonged psychosis and neurosis have also resulted from the use of this drug.

Much of the concern over LSD is generated by the effect it has on chromosomes. Studies have shown chromosome breakdown in human white blood cells and in the fetus when exposed to LSD.[13] Extensive research in this area continues in an effort to find more definite relationships.

Mescaline is an alkaloid found in the peyote cactus. Peyote is especially interesting because Native Americans have the legal sanction to use its derivative, mescaline, in religious ceremonies. The Native Americans believe that the visual hallucinations that occur with its use are a way of communicating with the spirits.[14]

Opiates

The opiates are drugs derived from opium. These drugs, the opium alkaloids, are narcotics. Opium derivatives include codeine (a prescription drug), morphine (a prescription drug), and heroin (an illegal drug). Narcotics have a depressant effect on the central nervous system so are used for pain relief by producing drowsiness and sleep. Codeine is often prescribed as a cough suppressant, morphine as a pain reliever. When used in moderation, there are few side effects of codeine and little risk of addiction.[15]

Morphine, used as a pain killer and as an anesthetic, is more addictive. When used over a long period of time with increasing dosage, a person becomes psychologically and physically dependent upon the drug. An individual develops a tolerance to the drug, and consequently, larger doses are required to achieve the desired effect. This leads to physical dependency.

Heroin is considered to be the most seriously abused drug. Because of its adverse effect on users, it is illegal in the United States. The use of heroin causes a euphoric or pleasurable sensation for most users.

Heroin can be used in several forms. It is most frequently mixed with a liquid and injected directly into the vein, a practice called *mainlining.* This intravenous injection results in the most rapid and most euphoric sensation. Heroin may also be taken orally or inhaled. In both of these procedures, the euphoric effect is often not as strong and is more delayed than when injected.

The danger of overdose resulting in death or physical disability is always present. Often the drug user is unaware of the exact strength or dose of the heroin and so uses too much. Unless emergency help is available to assist the abuser through the overdose crisis, serious consequences may occur.

Heroin use can indirectly cause disease, especially hepatitis. Hepatitis develops when contaminated drug paraphernalia is used to inject the heroin into the bloodstream.

Addiction to heroin can result if there is continued use of the drug. An addicted individual finds it extremely difficult to break this reliance on heroin. The process of detoxification, described later in this chapter, can be both painful and difficult.

Heroin is very costly in terms of both physiological and social problems. For example, malnutrition is often found among heroin users. All too often the individual using heroin is unemployed so resorts to crime in order to support the habit. Any incoming money is applied directly to heroin purchase, not to the purchase of nutritious food.

Since the use, possession, and sale of heroin are illegal in this country, a user can only obtain the drug through illegal and black market sellers. This practice creates many serious social problems. The quality of the purchased heroin often is questionable, in terms of both strength and purity. Purchasing "bad" heroin may result in overdose, disease, or other problems.

Sedatives

Drugs that cause depressant effects on the central nervous system and upon the various physiological processes of the body are known as sedatives. Sedatives are prescribed for a variety of medical purposes. Certain sedatives are used in treatment of the psychotic mental patient. The antipsychotic drugs alleviate pain, fear, delusions, and tensions in the psychotic patient.

Thousands of sedatives are used daily to help people to relax, to encourage sleep, and to relieve nervous conditions. More prescriptions are written for tranquilizers than for any other drug in the United States.[16] This reliance upon tranquilizers to "make it through the day" provokes a variety of problems. For example, young people who see their parents using tranquilizers use this behavior as justification for their own use of drugs for pleasure. Physiologically, the use of tranquilizers to induce sleep can have a detrimental effect on the normal sleep pattern. The induced sleep is not as sound or complete as when these drugs are not used.

Sedative abuse refers to (1) the increasing reliance upon the drug or (2) overdose, either accidental or intentional. Overdose reduces the body's physiological functioning and can cause death. If the respiratory functioning becomes depressed to the point where breathing stops, the individual is likely to suffer long-term impairment or death. Sedatives are the major prescription drugs used by people in the United States in attempts to commit suicide.[17] When combined with alcohol, serious depressing effects occur.

Stimulants

Central nervous system stimulants are also heavily used in the United States. Stimulants are used by dieters to lose weight, students at exam time, and long-distance truck drivers to keep awake. Because of their extensive use and despite their medicinal benefits, stimulants are frequently abused.

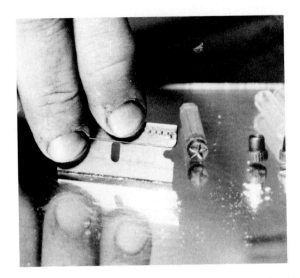

A razor blade is being used to divide the contents of a vial of crack in a crack house in N.Y. South Bronx.

The abuse of stimulants begins innocently enough. Often the individual begins to take amphetamines (stimulants) for a specific medical purpose. The euphoric feeling produced becomes increasingly desirable. As a result, the user increases the dosage in order to obtain even greater effects from the drug. Physical dependence does not occur, but the psychological dependence necessitates progressively greater doses of the drug. The mental depression that follows a high is avoided by taking another round of the given drug.

Cocaine Possibly the most serious substance abuse problem in America today is the use of cocaine. It is particularly dangerous because occasional use can easily lead to heavy involvement with this drug. It is considered to be the drug of choice for millions of adults and adolescents. In the past, cocaine use was found most prevalently among entertainers, professional athletes, and wealthy businessmen. However, today it is widely used by middle- and working-class people. Because of the low cost of crack, a form of cocaine, it has become widely used by the economically disadvantaged of America's inner cities.

Cocaine is an alkaloid extracted from the leaves of the coca plant found in parts of South America. In the late 1800s cocaine was thought to be a miracle drug having medicinal values.

Cocaine is usually taken by snorting—sniffing or inhaling through the nostrils—and free-basing (smoking).

In either case, the effect of the drug on the central nervous system is immediate. Smoking, or freebasing, of cocaine results in a quicker, more intense, euphoric, and addictive effect. It is usually smoked in a glass water pipe using a lighter as a heat source. Cocaine is also smoked in cigarettes.

Upon inhalation of the smoke, cocaine is absorbed in the lungs directly into the circulatory system. It is transmitted to the brain in as quickly as ten seconds. Hence instantaneous euphoria is attained. This is followed by a rebound dysphoria (crash), with intense craving for another euphoric state.

Cocaine increases the respiratory rate, the heart rate, and the blood pressure. It can interrupt the normal electrical impulse control of the heart, resulting in a sudden onset of seizures and cardiac arrest. In addition, it causes an acceleration of many other of the body's physiological functions. This produces restlessness, euphoria, excitement, and an inability to relax. Serious overdose reactions often occur. These include such respiratory problems as chest congestion, chronic cough, wheezing, and the development of black phlegm. Following the "highs" produced by the drug, depression, anxiety, and other psychological problems occur.

It has been known for some time that cocaine is psychologically addicting. Irritability, violent behavior, hallucinations, and short temper have been associated with its use. The individual using cocaine must cope with depression as well as sleep and appetite disturbances. Though not considered physically addictive in the past, recent clinical data indicates that cocaine use leads to physical dependence.

The cocaine user is often in need of the support of a substance abuse treatment program. Initial hospitalization is often needed to disrupt compulsive use. Total abstinence is difficult to achieve, often requiring extensive rehabilitative care including counseling.

A smokable form of cocaine that has received much attention since the 1980s is crack cocaine. Crack is extracted in a simple procedure using sodium bicarbonate (baking soda), heat, and water. It is easily manufactured and extremely addictive. This form of cocaine is called "crack" because of the "crackling" sound that is produced when it is being heated. It is sold as tiny "rocks" for under twenty dollars. It is cheap, readily available, and desired by the users because of its highly addictive feature. For the drug dealer "crack" provides extremely high profits and is very easy to handle. The addictive feature assures continuing need by the users.

Crack can be smoked alone or in mixture with other substances, such as marijuana. It is absorbed into the bloodstream and reaches the brain in a very short time. As a result, the feeling of euphoria is experienced very quickly. It is very addictive, causing the user to desire additional crack experiences.

The addictive nature of crack cocaine has led to a serious escalation of crime in America. Various acts of violent crime are carried out by individuals using crack because they need money to pay for additional amounts of the drug. Prolonged use of the drug can result in violent behavior.

Caffeine   The most widely ingested central nervous system stimulant in America is caffeine. Caffeine is found in a number of substances consumed by the American public: cola drinks, tea, over-the-counter preparations, and most specifically, coffee. Caffeine stimulates the cortex of the brain where breathing, the thought processes, and other vital activities of the body are controlled. Greater sensitivity to stimuli, wakefulness, and better physical functioning result from use of this drug.

The widespread use of caffeine has raised concern for various population groups. At particular risk are young people, cardiac patients, the elderly, and pregnant women. It may cross the placenta in expectant women, and caffeine has been detected in the milk of breast-feeding mothers. Although most research has been conducted on animals, warnings have been issued about the possible relationship between caffeine intake and birth defects. Educational programs must be developed to inform the public of the potential dangers of too much caffeine and to encourage its reduction in the diet.

Treatment and Rehabilitation

Treatment of drug abusers was not a public health concern until the early part of the twentieth century. At that time, treatment was a medical procedure conducted by private physicians. Since drug addiction was considered a physical disease that could be cured by gradual withdrawal, there was little concern for the psychological and sociological aspects of drug use. For this reason, care was provided in a quiet manner by the individual's private physician with as little public attention as possible.

With passage of the Harrison Narcotic Act in 1914, the availability of certain drugs, the opiates and cocaine, became restricted to medical professionals. Physicians and dentists had access to these drugs only for use in their professional practice. This legal restriction led to the development of an illegal drug market. As with many other social issues, illegal markets compound problems, usually by introducing crime and skyrocketing costs. Since drug abuse was considered a felony, the prisons became populated with drug addicts.

In response to these problems, the federal government established two drug abuse treatment hospitals in the 1930s—in Lexington, Kentucky, and in Fort Worth, Texas. Here drug addicts underwent withdrawal. This was accompanied by vocational rehabilitation, counseling, and various social services. Unfortunately, all too often the withdrawal was only temporary. A large number of patients in these facilities reverted to drug abuse after their release.

Until the early 1950s, these two facilities were the only major drug abuse treatment facilities in the United States. But as drug abuse increased during the 1950s and 1960s, several drug treatment programs were developed. At the present time, treatment for drug dependency is effective only for opiate and alcohol addiction. There is no chemotherapy for treating the abuse of amphetamines, barbiturates, and hallucinogens.

Therapeutic Communities

Residential programs, called *therapeutic communities,* have become important in drug abuse treatment. These programs attempt to effect behavioral change, leading to a reduction in drug use.

The first therapeutic community program for drug addicts, Synanon, was founded in 1958. The residential therapy concept instituted there involves a group of individuals living and working together while striving to solve their drug abuse problems. The psychological dimension of drug abuse is emphasized using group therapy, group interaction, and mutual support activities. The principles of behavior modification are the foundation of the program of the therapeutic community. Because this frequently demands small-group participation, residential

therapeutic programs are only somewhat successful. The number of individuals that can be treated is limited.

The value of residential treatment centers is that the individual can receive social support during the rehabilitative process. Social and medical professionals help the patient to gradually work his or her way back into the community setting. The patient is still able to "lean" on the support of the residential center during this time.

Therapeutic community programs require individuals to remain in the program for different periods of time. In some instances, this may be for months, and it is not unusual to find an individual involved in such a program for several years. It is for this reason that the operation of a therapeutic community can become a very expensive form of treatment. Many drug users do not have the financial resources to continue the treatment until their drug usage is in remission.

Methadone Maintenance Treatment Programs

The primary method of treating heroin use is through the methadone maintenance treatment programs. These programs were developed in the 1960s by Doctors Dole and Nyswander of Rockefeller University. These researchers noted that methadone, a synthetic narcotic drug, could serve as a substitute, or a blocking agent, for heroin and morphine to ease the pain of withdrawal.

Methadone maintenance treatment programs are found in many communities throughout the country. In this drug therapy, the drug user is stabilized with daily doses of methadone, taken orally. Methadone is a synthetic opiate which reduces the craving for heroin and permits the patient to become more acclimated to a pattern of living that does not include drugs.

These programs can be conducted on an outpatient basis and so are much less costly than other treatment programs that require inpatient care. Even though the patient does not have to be hospitalized, it is necessary to return to the treatment center daily for methadone maintenance. As long as the individual takes the methadone on a daily basis, the craving for heroin does not occur. Methadone creates a "blocking effect" to the euphoria created by the opiate drug. The dependence is then shifted from heroin and morphine to methadone. For this reason some critics of methadone maintenance believe that this program is simply substituting one drug for another. Those who support the program point out that methadone is a far less serious drug than heroin.

Because the long-term cure rate is not good, addicts must be kept on methadone maintenance for years. The ultimate goal of methadone maintenance treatment programs should be complete detoxification, a drug-free state. Unfortunately, these programs have not been successful in total detoxification.

Federal regulations require methadone maintenance programs to provide services other than administering methadone. Group therapy, vocational training, and social services must be a part of the treatment program, too. Thus, the needs of the total person are met. The individual's craving for heroin is relieved by the methadone, and the psychological and sociological needs are met through involvement in the additional services.

Drug-Free Outpatient Services

Another approach to drug treatment offers drug-free services on an outpatient basis. In this approach, group or individual psychotherapy is usually provided, as are counseling, health services, and vocational and educational training. Some detoxification measures are taken, but the program centers more on group support for a drug-free life-style. This approach, though somewhat successful for the young drug experimenter, is of less value to the addict. The outpatient nature of this program places the drug addict back into the community with no support mechanisms to withstand the social and personal pressures that forced the drug use originally.

Detoxification

The process whereby a person who is physically dependent upon a drug is gradually withdrawn from the drug is known as *detoxification*. The goal of detoxification is to provide a safe withdrawal by administering decreasing doses of the drug. Detoxification is necessary in order to prevent pain, discomfort, and other related problems created by abrupt termination of drug use.

In a drug detoxification program (which should be joined voluntarily) the patient receives enough of the substitute drug to suppress severe withdrawal symptoms. Usually a long-acting drug is substituted for the short-acting drug of addiction. For example, methadone is substituted for heroin, phenobarbital for short-acting barbiturates, and Valium and Librium for alcohol.[18]

Detoxification must be part of an integrated long-term treatment program, because besides removal from drug dependency, the treatment must attempt to resolve the underlying social and psychological factors that led to the drug abuse. This social and psychological rehabilitation requires effective counseling, positive education, and the support of the community.

Hospitalization

Considered to be the least effective form of treatment, hospitalization is also the most expensive, as the patient is usually treated over a long period of time. When hospitals have been used for drug treatment, the relapse rate after release has been very high.

Hospital emergency room services are used when an individual is experiencing a drug crisis. But after the crisis passes, the patient is released and often does not receive the rehabilitative treatment needed. If there are associated health needs in addition to the drug dependency, it is likely that hospital inpatient care will be necessary. However, this inpatient care often does not include treatment for the drug abuse problem itself.

Multimodality Approach

There is no single treatment that is effective for all drug users. For this reason, most treatment and rehabilitation programs for drug abusers have used a multimodality approach. The need for prevention, treatment, education, and rehabilitation must be met in one drug treatment program that integrates these services. For example, a treatment program may include the use of methadone maintenance, detoxification, inpatient drug-free treatment, outpatient services, and a therapeutic community. The patient may be transferred from one type of program to another as the need arises. Some suggest that the multimodality approach may be the most effective method of treating abuse within the local community.

Alcoholism

For many people the term alcoholism evokes thoughts of poorly clothed, dirty, unemployed, transient men found on the skid rows of large urban communities. The stereotyped picture is often a homeless, lonely person who has spent years moving about, drowning loneliness in drink.

With the growing alcohol consumption in American society, alcoholism has taken on larger dimensions. Alcoholics are people who cannot control their intake of liquor, yet who are still employed and able to lead an outwardly reasonable life-style. When confronted with the accusation of being alcoholics, they will almost always deny having a drinking problem.

Owing to society's negative attitude toward the alcoholic, family members and close associates of an alcoholic often will not take measures to assist the individual until the condition has become obvious. These support people often do not understand the problem and therefore refuse to talk about it.

The Disease

Is alcoholism a disease or is it the result of a weakened personality? For many years the alcoholic was considered a deviate who simply could not, or would not, control the amount of alcohol consumed. This alcohol intake often led to intoxication or to non-social behavior. For many people, this problem had moral dimensions. The drunk was often put in jail; the alcoholic was hidden from society by family and friends; and certain groups taught that the problem was the result of evil or sin. There was relatively little success in the few attempts to rehabilitate the alcoholic.

Since the 1950s, the American Medical Association has considered alcoholism a disease, a deviation from normal health and well-being. Today most rehabilitation programs are based on the disease theory of alcoholism rather than on the personality deviation theory.

Exactly what causes alcoholism is not known. No chemical in alcoholic beverages, nor any metabolic, physiological, or genetic defects in individuals have been identified that cause alcoholism. Research has examined hormone deficiencies, allergic reactions, and body metabolism as possible causes of alcoholism. In spite of such extensive efforts to find a cause, "The nature of the addictive process, the developmental sequence of events and the central nervous system alterations which define the condition of alcohol addiction are unknown. . . . The development of approaches to these very basic questions constitutes perhaps the major challenge to the biological scientist concerned with addiction."[19]

Today, most professionals treat alcoholism as a chronic disease. The alcoholic can never be cured, but can be treated and the disease arrested. With appropriate care and treatment, the alcoholic can resume a happy, healthy, and productive lifestyle. This is not an easy task, however. The person must completely refrain from the use of any alcoholic beverage. Failure to do so only precipitates a renewed problem with alcohol.

Alcoholism is a progressive disease in that the person's condition deteriorates without appropriate care. Physiological processes are affected, mental health is impaired, and social relationships deteriorate. Without proper care, alcoholism can eventually result in death.

A serious problem with alcoholism is that the alcoholic often is not aware of the problem. This may be the failure to admit to the condition, but it is more likely the result of the physiological effects of alcohol on the body. Alcohol depresses the neurological system, and often an alcoholic does not remember anything related to the drinking episode. Since the problem usually is not recognized in the early stages by those who could treat it, the diagnosis of alcoholism occurs at an advanced stage. The patient is then unable to control personal drinking, organic damage has begun, and social relationships are endangered.

Treatment

Unfortunately, in the case of alcoholism, the individual is in need of medical treatment but fails to obtain the care voluntarily. This often leads to forced medical care, a process known as *intervention*. Intervention is a method of obtaining help for the alcoholic before it is physiologically too late to reverse the problem or before death occurs. People who care about the alcoholic seek treatment for the person. If necessary, the alcoholic is forced to enter a treatment program. Once in the program, it is hoped that the individual will recognize the problem and then take action to solve the problem. Intervention is usually only effective if more than one person is willing to help.

Treatment of alcoholism is a complex process involving time, patience, professional competence, and the understanding of friends and relatives. Physical, psychological, and social factors are measures included in alcohol treatment programs.

The process begins with detoxification. Through medical supervision, the alcoholic is taken off alcohol and other mood-modifying chemicals, a procedure that is best accomplished in a general hospital. Withdrawal is often very difficult for the patient. Dietary measures to improve the nutrition of the individual are usually a part of the treatment. Emotional support, as well as physical modalities, is an important need at this time. Psychotherapy, involving talking between the patient and a counselor, is used to help the individual modify attitudes and personal behaviors that resulted in the reliance upon alcohol.

In the past, general hospitals did not offer long-term inpatient care for alcoholism. Most inpatient alcoholism treatment was conducted in state mental hospitals. If such care was available in the general hospital, it was usually quite costly. This denied treatment to those who could not afford it. As a result, the alcoholic was treated in the emergency department for related injuries, then discharged to other agencies, such as the jail or mental hospital, in order to sober up.

Even though state mental hospitals and community mental health centers still provide extensive alcoholic care, the American Medical Association and the American Hospital Association recommend that alcoholic patients be treated in the general hospital. Hospitals now have developed treatment programs for the alcoholic. The number of hospital inpatient addiction treatment programs more than doubled in the past decade.

The services provided include activities for the family and associates. Another part of the treatment process involves educational measures to inform the alcoholic, family, and friends about the disease. These efforts provide information about how alcoholic beverages affect the body. Group therapy allows the patient to interact with others who have faced the same problems. Therapy sessions help the patient to understand and accept the disease, as well as to prepare for reentry into the community when the inpatient part of the treatment is completed. The patient must be prepared for problems that will occur when he or she returns home, to his or her job and to social settings. Usually an alcoholic patient faces personal, family, and financial problems created by the drinking problem, all of which need therapeutic attention before release from the treatment center.

When hospital treatment ends, recovery from alcoholism becomes a lifetime process. The recovering alcoholic must from that time on take measures to stay well. This extremely difficult task usually requires the understanding, concern, and support of family, friends, and associates. The education, counseling, and therapy assistance family members receive during the treatment phase help them assist the patient in abstaining from drink.

Most communities have several organizations that help the recovering alcoholic. These agencies, usually staffed by nonmedical personnel, aid the patient in adjusting to the new life-style of a recovering alcoholic. Possibly the best-known agency is Alcoholics Anonymous.

Alcoholics Anonymous (AA) is a voluntary fellowship of recovering alcoholics who come together to help each other stay away from alcohol. Before becoming involved in AA, a person must recognize a lack of control over alcohol and desire assistance from a therapeutic group.

Another organization modeled after Alcoholics Anonymous is Al-Anon. This organization is for relatives of alcoholic patients. The spouse or other relative is able to learn how to cope with the situation from the experience of others. Alateen is a similar organization for the teenage children of alcoholics.

In addition to these organizations, community professionals are available to counsel the alcoholic and his or her family. Clergy are often called upon for counseling. Public health nurses, vocational rehabilitation counselors, and parole officers have also received special training to assist the alcoholic. The key to successful alcoholic rehabilitation is recognition and use of these available resources in the community.

A number of governmental agencies have alcohol treatment programs. The Veterans Administration hospital system conducts the largest alcohol treatment program in the country. Veterans receive this care free of charge. Other programs are sponsored by various state and local government authorities.

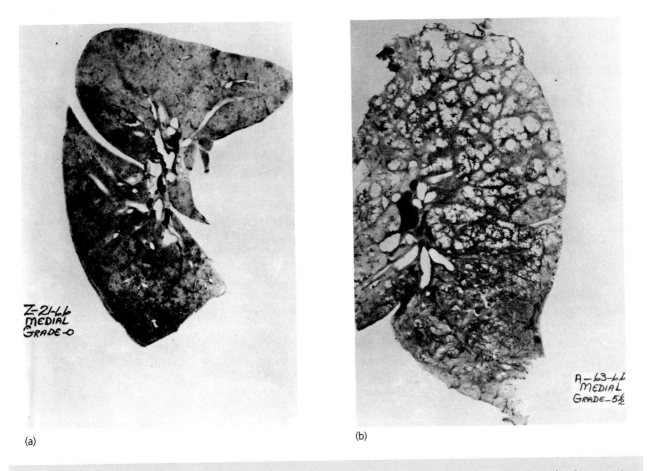

(a)

(b)

An examination of lung tissue leaves little doubt about the harmful effects of cigarette smoking. (a) In normal lung tissue the air sacs are too fine to be visible. (b) The lung tissue of a heavy smoker shows an abundance of greatly enlarged air sacs.

Industry has shown increasing interest in the establishment of alcohol treatment programs. The first industrial alcohol treatment programs were established in the 1940s. Since then, hundreds of companies have developed similar programs. These industrial alcoholic rehabilitation programs are designed for early recovery from alcohol misuse. Usually such efforts are quite effective.

Tobacco Use

Smoking and Health

For many years, there was no clear association between smoking and disease. It was not until 1964, with the publication of the first *Surgeon General's Report on Smoking and Health,* that clear associations between smoking and specific diseases were noted. The report by the Surgeon General's Advisory Committee identified an association of lung cancer, emphysema, coronary artery disease, and chronic bronchitis with cigarette smoking.

A second *Surgeon General's Report on Smoking and Health* was released in 1979. This report updated the data on smoking in the United States and provided a foundation for the establishment of an antismoking campaign established by the Department of Health, Education, and Welfare (HEW). Cigarette smoking was designated "Public Health Enemy Number One" by the federal government. Since that time, additional reports have been issued, more than one a year, each focusing upon some aspect of the hazards related to cigarette smoking. The various publications have reported links between cigarette smoking and cancer, particularly lung cancer; the close relationship between smoking and cardiovascular disease; the relationship between smoking and chronic obstructive lung disease; plus a variety of other matters.

Since the publication of the first report, many people have quit smoking and the proportion of adult smokers has declined from about 42 percent in 1965 to under 26 percent today.[20] Though cigarette smoking has declined, there are still an estimated 390,000 deaths each year related to smoking.[21] Smoking rates for males have declined more rapidly than for females, and the gap between male and female smoking is narrowing.[22] The fact that the percentage of smokers in all groups has declined does not eliminate smoking as a major community health concern.

Smoking is a particular problem among African-Americans, blue-collar workers, and those with less education than the overall population. The Surgeon General noted that educational attainment appears to be a significant predictor of smoking. High school dropouts, the unemployed, and minorities are more likely to smoke.[23]

Women of childbearing age should seriously consider the hazards of cigarette smoking. Women who smoke and use oral birth control pills have a greater risk of having a heart attack or other cardiovascular diseases than those who do not smoke. There is also evidence that maternal smoking can have an effect on the fetus and on childbirth. Frequently, children of smoking women are born prematurely or with birth defects. The risk of spontaneous abortion, fetal death, and infant death is also greater among smoking mothers.[24]

Not only should concern be expressed for the person who smokes, but there is evidence that those who live and/or work around smokers may be at danger for certain problems. For example, it has been noted that children of smoking parents have more respiratory diseases such as bronchitis and pneumonia. There is a possibility that lung cancer may be caused by passive inhalation of smoke by nonsmokers. Women who are nonsmokers but whose husbands are smokers have shown an increased incidence of lung cancer. The matter of passive effects of smoking, or *secondhand smoke,* as many refer to it, is receiving an increasing amount of concern and research. The federal government has called for a reduction by the year 2000 in exposure to passive, secondhand smoke at home for children six years of age and younger.[25]

Smoking among Young People

By law it is illegal to sell cigarettes to minors under the age of eighteen in 45 states and the District of Columbia. Yet three million young people under eighteen smoke cigarettes or use smokeless tobacco in the United States. More than half of these individuals begin use of tobacco in the early teens, many as early as thirteen and fourteen years of age. It is also pointed out that more than one billion packs of cigarettes are sold to minors annually at a cost of $1.25 billion.

It seems that laws banning the sale of tobacco products to minors are of minimal effect. There are a number of reasons that can be given as to why this is the case. One reason is that cigarettes can be easily obtained from relatives and friends who are of legal purchasing age. Also many retail stores, drug stores, grocery stores, and convenience stores sell to minors with little demand to be shown evidence of age. Another source of cigarettes for minors is purchasing them from vending machines.

Many recommendations have been made for reducing the sale of tobacco products to minors. Among the many suggestions would be outlawing of cigarette vending machines. Even though there may be signs on vending machines saying that it is illegal for minors to purchase cigarettes, there is no means of control. Another recommendation is to place all tobacco products behind counters in stores where they are sold. It has also been recommended that raising the legal age of tobacco purchase to twenty-one would be effective in reducing sales to minors. A point raised by those who support this action is that most high school students have friends who are eighteen years old who can obtain cigarettes for them. They are not as likely to have friends who are twenty-one.

It has been suggested that more effective enforcement of the laws and institution of penalties should be placed upon those retailers who sell tobacco products to minors. Possibly licensure of all merchants selling tobacco products would help. The federal government has recommended that free distribution of cigarettes and smokeless tobacco should be outlawed. All too often these free samples get into the hands of minors.

A great amount of discussion has gone on about advertising of tobacco products that seem to be directed toward adolescents. Though the tobacco industry will argue that their advertising is not focused on this population group, many question this contention. The one issue that has received much attention is the use of cartoon characters in cigarette advertising. RJR Nabisco has used such a cartoon character, Joe the Camel, in its advertising. This character delivers the message that it is smooth and appropriate to use this corporation's tobacco products. It is doubtful that this character was designed with adults and senior citizens in mind. The success of this cartoon character has led other tobacco corporations to explore the development of such an advertising message.

Another initiative that has become increasingly a part of school district policies is prohibiting the use of tobacco products in school, on school grounds, and at school sponsored events. These regulations have been focused not just upon the students, but also upon adults when in the school environment.

In an attempt to assist individual states in developing legislation to restrict tobacco use among minors, the Department of Health and Human Services has proposed a "Model Sale of Tobacco Products to Minors Control Act." This proposed act would:

1. Set nineteen years of age as the minimum age for purchasing tobacco products.
2. Create a tobacco sales licensing system.
3. Establish a graduated schedule of penalties for illegal sales of tobacco products to minors.
4. Place primary responsibility for enforcement with a designated state agency.
5. Assess fines using civil penalties.
6. Ban all cigarette sales vending machines.

National Health Objectives for the Year 2000

Tobacco Use among Minors

1. Establish tobacco-free environments in all schools.
2. Include tobacco use prevention programs in the school curriculum.
3. Enact and enforce state laws prohibiting the sale and distribution of tobacco products to young people under nineteen.
4. Develop plans at the state level to reduce tobacco use among youth.
5. Eliminate or restrict all forms of tobacco product advertising and promotion to which minors under eighteen are likely to be exposed.

Source: Department of Health and Human Services. *Healthy People 2000: National Health Promotion and Disease Prevention Objectives.* Washington, D.C.: U.S. Government Printing Office, 1991, pp. 147–53.

Smoking Cessation Programs

Different programs have been developed to help people stop smoking. Most smoking cessation programs are either self-help strategies or assisted strategies. Self-help smoking cessation strategies include stopping the smoking behavioral pattern "cold turkey." A number of materials, books, and manuals have been developed to assist people wishing to stop smoking on their own. Self-help strategies tend to be more successful in the long-term than are the assisted strategy initiatives.

The assisted strategies include attendance at clinics, use of hypnosis, the application of acupuncture, and the substitution of nicotine gum or the nicotine patch. Smoking cessation clinics are more likely to attract the heavier smoker. In many instances physician counseling intervention has been shown to be helpful in helping smokers to quit. The clinic approaches tend to have limited long-term effect.

Several educational programs make use of the mass media. These programs include public interest statements that focus upon high-risk groups, including pregnant women, teenagers, and workers in potentially dangerous environments.

The American Cancer Society and the American Lung Association have smoking cessation programs. The American Lung Association introduced a program in

1981 entitled *Freedom from Smoking*. This program is based on extensive research, development, and evaluation, and encourages ongoing support activities for the individual. It is designed to free cigarette smokers of the habit in as short a period as twenty days, primarily through behavior modification. It incorporates ways to improve eating habits, to reduce stress, and to assert feelings. The material employed is very attractive and seems positive in its approach and appearance.

The American Cancer Society smoking program is entitled *Fresh Start*. The program actively involves smokers in initiatives leading to a positive smoke-free life-style. The program is designed to assist smokers to stop within two weeks.

In 1991 the National Cancer Institute began a science-based smoking intervention project. This project, the American Stop Smoking Intervention Study for Cancer Prevention (ASSIST), is a demonstration project being carried out in seventeen states. The primary objective of this project is to reduce smoking to 15 percent of the population or less by the year 2000. It is estimated that this project can result in 4.5 million adults quitting smoking and prevention of 1.2 million smoking related deaths.[26]

Most people who quit smoking seem to have some motivation to do so. Four factors have been identified as being of major importance in smoking cessation: (1) a concern about some health problem, (2) a desire to set an example for others, (3) a desire for self-control, and (4) aesthetic reasons.[27] The highest proportion of smokers who are successful at quitting are males among the white population, individuals with college degrees, and older smokers.

Smokeless Tobacco

The increasing concern related to smoking and its effects on health has led many individuals to turn to the use of smokeless tobacco. Smokeless tobacco has been promoted by the tobacco industry as a safe alternative to smoking. An estimated twenty-two million people in the United States use smokeless tobacco.[28] Sales of smokeless tobacco have increased more than 10 percent each year in the past decade, with annual sales now being nearly one billion dollars.[29]

Smokeless tobacco has been used throughout the history of this country. However, the major concern in recent years is its increasing use by young adults, women, and school age children. It has not been uncommon to find children in elementary and junior high schools "chewing" tobacco.

Smokeless tobacco is available in two basic forms—as snuff (powdered tobacco) and as chewing tobacco. Snuff is powdered tobacco made from finely cut tobacco leaves. In the United States there are three main types of chewing tobacco: (1) loose leaf, (2) plug, and (3) twist.

"Dipping and chewing tobacco have . . . become a social activity. In some areas, schools set aside student lounge areas for smokeless tobacco use with names like 'cowboy corner,' and chewing clubs for young men have sprung up with mottos such as 'don't spit on me.' Companies . . . are . . . producing copycat products—bubble gum, for example—packaged to look, taste, and spit like smokeless tobacco."

Source: Koop, C. Everett, Surgeon General. "The Campaign against Smokeless Tobacco." *The New England Journal of Medicine* 314, no. 16 (April 17, 1986): 1042.

With this increase in use of smokeless tobacco have come increasing concerns about its effect on health. An increase in the incidence of oral cancer, particularly cancers of the cheek and gums, has been noted among users. Oral cancers usually appear at the site most in contact with the tobacco. Snuff users have been shown to be 4.2 times more likely to develop oral cancer, and their risk for gum cancer is fifty times that of nonusers.[30] Increased dental problems are found among users of smokeless tobacco, with greater gum recession and advanced periodontal destruction of the tissue of the mouth. Smokeless tobacco users are two to three times more likely to lose their teeth.

Smokeless tobacco may be more addictive than cigarette smoking. Nicotine is absorbed more slowly than is the case in cigarettes. As a result, the nicotine levels are higher than among smokers.[31]

Recognition of the health hazards of use of smokeless tobacco has led to legislation directed toward reducing its use, particularly among younger children and teenagers. In 1985, Massachusetts became the first state to enact legislation requiring that warning labels be placed on all smokeless tobacco products. In 1986, the United States Congress passed legislation that barred television and radio advertising of smokeless tobacco products.[32]

This legislation required that, as of 1987, health warnings be placed on smokeless tobacco cans. The warnings indicate that use of the product may cause oral cancer, gum disease, and tooth loss. The consumer is also warned that smokeless tobacco is not a safe alternative to cigarette smoking.

Public Policy

Legal Control of Drug Abuse

Legal action involves preventing or minimizing the use of drugs that impair health and well-being. If a substance results in abnormal behavior that affects the individual and society, legal action is appropriate.

Since the early years of this century, there have been several federal laws designed to control narcotic drugs. The Narcotic Drug Import and Export Act prohibited the import of narcotic drugs except for use in certain medical and scientific environments. The Harrison Narcotic Act established regulations for the control of narcotic drugs within the country.

In 1970 Congress passed the Comprehensive Drug Abuse Prevention and Control Act, better known as the Controlled Substances Act. It repealed and superseded other federal drug laws, particularly the Harrison Narcotic Act. This federal law was designed to control the distribution of all stimulants, depressants, and other abused drugs.

The Controlled Substances Act established five different classifications, or schedules, of drugs. Every drug is classified from I to V depending on its potential for abuse, its acceptability for medical use, and its potential for causing physical or psychological dependency.

Drugs with high abuse potential and for which there is no current medical use are classified in Schedule I. Heroin and marijuana are two drugs in this classification. All drugs in Schedule I are illegal, and penalties for sale, use, and possession have been established.

Drugs classified in Schedule II have a high potential for abuse, but they are also acceptable for certain medical purposes. Morphine and codeine are examples of drugs in this classification. A characteristic of these drugs is that, when abused, they can result in severe physical or psychological dependence. A prescription for a drug in this schedule can only be written by typewriter or with indelible ink and must be signed by the physician. The law forbids refill of a prescription of a Schedule II drug.

Schedule III drugs have less abuse potential than those in Schedules I and II. Use of these drugs leads to high psychological dependence or low physical dependence. Drugs in this classification have medical use and may be obtained with either a written or an oral prescription. They may not be refilled more than five times per each prescription.

Drugs with a low abuse potential and recognized as having an accepted medical use are classified in Schedule IV. Use of these drugs may lead to limited physical or psychological dependence. These drugs, most often tranquilizers, may be prescribed either in writing or orally and are limited to no more than five refills. They may not be refilled more than six months after the date of the original prescription.

Drugs that can be sold without a prescription are described in Schedule V. They have a low potential for both physical and psychological abuse. The drugs in this classification are often referred to as "over-the-counter" drugs.

The Controlled Substances Act sets specific penalties for illegal possession, manufacture, distribution, and use of the drugs. The penalties include both fines and imprisonment; penalties for selling drugs to minors are greater than those for distribution of drugs to persons over the age of eighteen.

Additional legislation and regulatory action have occurred at the state and local levels in attempts to further reduce the incidence of drug abuse. In particular, states and local communities have passed laws and ordinances

Comprehensive Drug Abuse Prevention and Control Act (Controlled Substances Act)

Class		
I	High abuse potential No medical use	Heroin, marijuana
II	High abuse potential Some medical uses	Morphine, codeine
III	Less abuse potential Medical use with written or oral prescription	Prescription cannot be refilled more than five times
IV	Low abuse potential Accepted medical use	Prescriptions may not be refilled more than six months after date of original
V	Low abuse potential	Over-the-counter drugs

designed to control the paraphernalia used by the drug abuser. For example, the possession of hypodermic needles that can be used to inject a drug are illegal in some localities. An individual having such a needle can be arrested and fined or sentenced to a jail term. Pipes and other gadgets that are used to smoke drugs are controlled by such laws, too. There is a significant difference from one locality to another in what is legal, as well as in what is considered a felony or a misdemeanor.

Several states have passed legislation decriminalizing marijuana. These legal regulations reduce the penalty for possession and use of small amounts of the drug. In the past conviction was usually a misdemeanor, which carried an accompanying criminal record. With decriminalization, the charge is reduced to a lesser offense and the criminal factor eliminated. On the other hand, laws relating to the sale of marijuana have continued to be severe.

The control of drug use has put a great deal of responsibility on several federal law enforcement agencies. The Federal Drug Enforcement Administration investigates major narcotics violators who operate at international or interstate levels, and enforces narcotics laws and regulations. The Federal Bureau of Investigation (FBI) gathers information relating to trafficking in drugs. The Narcotics and Dangerous Drugs Section of the United States Department of Justice carries out prosecution and conviction of drug traffickers. Major responsibility for stopping the illegal flow of drugs into the country belongs to the Customs Service. Illegal drugs are regularly seized by personnel of this agency.

Alcohol

There is no clear resolution to the problem of alcohol abuse. In the past, many laws were passed to eliminate the excessive use of alcoholic beverages. Early in American history, in 1619, a law was passed in the Virginia Colony decreeing that ". . . any person found drunk for the first time was to be reproved privately by the minister; the second time publicly; the third time to 'lye in halter' for twelve hours and pay a fine."[33]

In the early 1800s, the temperance movement was started and gained momentum in the United States. Originally the goal of this movement was to encourage moderation in drinking, but through the years the meaning of temperance shifted from moderation to total abstinence. At the beginning of the twentieth century, increased public demand led to total prohibition of alcoholic beverages.

In 1919 the United States tried to solve the problems of alcohol use with passage of the Eighteenth Amendment to the Constitution. This amendment made it illegal to manufacture or sell alcoholic beverages. This period of national prohibition extended from 1920 to 1933, when the Eighteenth Amendment was repealed.

Many problems arose during Prohibition. By most standards, the effort was not successful. No other measures have been successful in reducing the problems of alcohol consumption since the Eighteenth Amendment was rescinded.

Nevertheless, efforts need to be taken to reduce the many emotional, social, and economic problems resulting from drinking. This includes the drinking of the vast majority of Americans, not just alcoholics. One report suggested several measures that, if made public policy, would reduce some of the problems associated with the use of alcohol:[34]

1. Place higher taxes on alcoholic beverages. This would raise the cost of drinking and hopefully reduce liquor consumption in the nation.

2. Develop effective communitywide educational programs. Such programs would be designed for people of all ages.

3. Disallow tax deductions on alcoholic beverages bought as part of business-related meals. Extensive alcohol consumption frequently occurs in connection with business affairs.

4. Enforce drunken driving laws more strictly, and raise the legal age for drinking in many states.

Specific national health objectives to be achieved by the year 2000 have been identified for both alcohol and drug abuse.[35] Three of the objectives relate to reducing fatalities in alcohol-related motor vehicle crashes, deaths from cirrhosis, and fatalities associated with the use of drugs of abuse. Several of the objectives focus upon reduction of the use of alcohol and other drugs among adolescents and young adults.

Tobacco

For many years, little consideration was given to the nonsmokers who had to endure cigarette or cigar smoke in rooms, restaurants, airplanes, and other public locations. Often, the smoke was more than just a nuisance. For some people, this passive smoking was not only discomforting but even a hazard to health. Yet not until the 1970s were any major efforts made to protect nonsmokers.

Nonsmoker rights have become an important public policy issue because it has been shown that measurable levels of nicotine enter the bloodstream of nonsmokers exposed to tobacco smoke. Breathing air polluted by tobacco smoke on a regular basis can result in unsafe levels of carbon monoxide. Asthma, respiratory infections, and certain allergic conditions may be agitated.

Three movements—the consumer movement, the environmental pollution movement, and the individual rights movement—have led to legislation and regulatory measures for the prohibition of smoking in certain localities. The state of Arizona was the first state to prohibit smoking in public places with legislation passed in 1973.

In 1974 the state of Connecticut became the first state to pass a law restricting smoking in restaurants. A Clean Indoor Air Act legislated in 1975 in Minnesota prohibited smoking everywhere except where specifically permitted. What this legislation did was make nonsmoking the norm. Since the mid-1970s most states, as well as city and local governments, have enacted laws restricting smoking. These laws vary, but they usually prohibit smoking in general office space, lobbies, restrooms, elevators, libraries, conference rooms, and classrooms. Generally, the smoker can still smoke in his or her private office, however some businesses and corporations are placing restrictions on this practice. The federal government has recommended that all states pass clean indoor air legislation that would prohibit smoking in all enclosed public facilities, such as schools, hospitals, workplaces, and public transportation.[36]

Federal regulation has banned smoking on all domestic airline flights originating and ending in the United States. In 1986, the United States Army established a regulation that prohibits smoking in enclosed public spaces, such as auditoriums, conference rooms, dining halls, and military vehicles. One base commander went so far as to prohibit smoking for all basic recruits.

The restriction of smoking in the workplace has increased. Regulations vary from state to state and between industrial sites. In some cases smoking is limited to certain locations within the building. In others smoking is prohibited in areas where it can have an effect on others, such as in open office space, counsel rooms, and other meeting rooms. Generally, worksite smoking policies have been implemented by the larger companies.

It is the objective of the Year 2000 Health Objectives for the Nation initiative that every state have smoking restriction laws designed to provide clean indoor air and that at least 75 percent of worksites have some type of smoking policy prohibiting or restricting smoking in the workplace.[37] This would mean that the number of industries and companies with policies would need to double during the 1990s.

In 1984 Congress passed legislation that required cigarette manufacturers to place warning labels on every pack of cigarettes. These warnings must be precise and disease specific. Four labels have been determined that appear on a rotating basis. The warning labels include the following:

Smoking causes lung cancer, heart disease, emphysema, and may complicate pregnancy.

Quitting smoking greatly reduces serious health risks.

Smoking by pregnant women may result in fetal injury, premature births, and low birth weight.

Cigarette smoke contains carbon monoxide.

This same legislation required that cigarette companies must disclose to the Department of Health and Human Services a list of all chemicals and other ingredients added to cigarettes during the manufacturing process.

"We're moving toward a smoke-free society by the year 2000"—U.S. Surgeon General C. Everett Koop, 1986.

National Health Objectives for the Year 2000

Tobacco Use

1. Reduce cigarette smoking among all adults by about 50 percent.
2. Reduce the start of smoking among young adults.
3. Increase smoking cessation initiatives among women smokers during pregnancy.
4. Reduce smokeless tobacco use by males.

Source: Department of Health and Human Services. *Healthy People 2000: National Health Promotion and Disease Prevention Objectives.* Washington, D.C.: U.S. Government Printing Office, 1991.

Economics of Substance Abuse

Substance abuse is a multibillion-dollar-a-year enterprise. Hundreds of thousands of people rely on money made from the manufacture, sale, and marketing of drugs, alcohol, and tobacco: the subteen on the streets of a large American city who sells drugs for money to friends, a peasant farmer in rural Colombia or Peru who raises coca plants that end up as crack cocaine in the United States, an employee of a tobacco-manufacturing plant in North Carolina, or a beer salesman for a major brewing company. Others have invested in the stocks of tobacco companies.

In some nations, such as Colombia, the economy and political stability have been greatly affected by the actions and power of major drug kingpins who have made billions of dollars in recent years. The need for money to maintain drug habits has led many into crime and violence.

In spite of strong evidence linking cigarette smoking to various diseases, there still exists a strong opposition to antismoking programs and strategies. Tobacco is a multimillion dollar agricultural business in several southeastern states, and efforts to reduce the level of tobacco use have posed a serious economic threat to people living in these localities.

In recent years the tobacco-manufacturing companies have diversified their businesses by purchasing or buying major financial interests in a broad range of other companies and corporations. For example, the Philip Morris Company purchased the General Foods Corporation for $5.75 billion. This meant that the Post Cereal line of Grape Nuts, Honeycomb, Alpha Bits, Sugar Crisp, and

Fruit and Fiber is now owned by a tobacco company. Other products of the General Foods Corporation included Maxwell House Coffee, Kool-Aid, Oscar Mayer meats, Minute Rice, Tang, Log Cabin syrups, and a variety of other products. Philip Morris had already purchased the Miller High Life Beer, Lowenbrau, 7-up, and Meister Brau lines.

In the latter part of the 1980s the United States government threatened several Third World countries, notably Asian nations, with trade sanctions if they forbade the advertising and sale of United States-manufactured cigarettes in their countries. This action was based on the 1974 Trade Act. With the decline of cigarette consumption in the United States and America's trade deficit, the tobacco industry has lobbied heavily for government support in this matter.

In the late 1980s markets in Japan, Taiwan, and South Korea were opened to American tobacco products, and heavy advertising campaigns and vigorous marketing practices were begun by the tobacco companies. As a result, smoking has increased in these nations in recent years.

Use of the threat of trade sanctions has led to controversy. For example, is it ethical for the United States to force Thailand to permit the advertising and sale of U.S. cigarettes to maintain trade relations? At the present time this nation prohibits any cigarette advertising and does not allow importation of foreign cigarettes.

The Tobacco Institute takes the position that as a legally manufactured product, tobacco should receive the same trade protection as other products do. On the other hand, opponents question whether it is ethical to place general trade sanctions on a nation that refuses to permit

American tobacco company advertising, that has quotas on importing cigarettes, or that has high tariff rates on imported cigarettes. It seems hypocritical for the United States government to export a product that causes disease and death while at the same time passing legislation to ban cigarette use in the United States.

Price-Support Program

The federal government supports the tobacco-growing industry with the tobacco price-support program. This program, like other agricultural price-support programs, guarantees the farmer a certain price for a product. In the case of the tobacco farmer, if the tobacco fails to bring a certain determined price guaranteed by the federal government, federal subsidies will be paid to assure a given income.

Public health officials and some legislators believe that federal price support of tobacco should be terminated. In their view it is paradoxical and inconsistent to fund a product (tobacco) through price supports while developing and funding programs that deal with the detrimental effects of smoking. It seems reasonable then, from a health perspective, that governmental price-support programs for the tobacco industry be eliminated. However, because of the economic importance of tobacco farming in several southeastern states and because of the tax revenues obtained from the sales of cigarettes and other tobacco products throughout the nation, legislation that would eliminate tobacco price-supports has not yet been approved.

Advertising

Not only has the tobacco industry lobbied political bodies to stop antismoking programs and to open foreign markets for sales of cigarettes, but major advertising campaigns have been designed to show the pleasures of smoking. In 1970, cigarette advertising was banned from television and radio. The tobacco industry could no longer advertise its products over the airwaves. Despite this, cigarettes are one of the most heavily advertised commercial products in the United States today.

It is estimated that tobacco industries spend more than $3.5 billion a year on cigarette advertising.[38] Much of this money is used to sponsor sporting and public

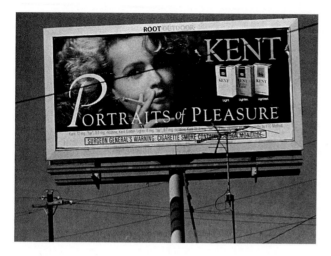

Cigarette advertising on outdoor billboards can be seen by everyone, including minors for which the purchasing of cigarettes is illegal in most states. Cigarette smoking is portrayed as glamorous, cool, and an appropriate activity for all.

entertainment events, such as golf and tennis tournaments and automobile racing.

Next to automobiles, cigarettes are the second most heavily advertised product in the mass media, including the newspapers and magazines. Other advertising can be found on outdoor billboards, where anyone can read the messages. In these advertisements smoking is depicted as pleasurable, masculine, and appropriate for adolescents. It never suggests the danger to health. Many question the ethics, as well as the legality, of such advertising.

Many suggestions have been put forth to counter cigarette advertising. Some have suggested that government should mount an antismoking campaign. Others feel that ordinances and regulations should be passed prohibiting cigarette advertising on outdoor billboards. It has also been strongly suggested that tobacco advertising directed toward adolescents, the minority population, and women be banned. This would include advertising of cigarettes in magazines that are principally directed toward these groups.

The constitutionality of banning all tobacco advertising must be considered. It is the position of the tobacco industry that they have every legal right to advertise their product, just as does any other manufacturing industry. There is little doubt that this issue will continue to be discussed in the decade of the 1990s.

Mass media advertising of alcoholic beverages is big business. It accounts for over $700 million of income for the mass media each year. Many have questioned the appropriateness of advertising alcoholic beverages and at the same time having legislation which prohibits advertising of tobacco products. It has been suggested that short of a total ban on alcoholic beverage advertising, legislation should be passed that would require that broadcast time with messages about the health effects and the risks of alcohol use match the time allotted for alcohol advertising.[39] When one realizes the tremendous effect of mass media advertising and the dangers of alcohol use and driving, such measures would seem to be reasonable considerations.

Concerted efforts to reduce alcohol consumption, bring about more positive behavior in the social use of alcohol, and reduce the advertising of the alcohol industry have not occurred in the United States. These measures must be addressed in our society, either individually or as a part of public policy, if the problems associated with alcohol abuse are to be reduced. Failure to do so will only result in increased problems in the community health field.

Summary

A number of drugs are widely abused in America. Drugs of abuse include alcohol, hallucinogenic drugs, marijuana, nicotine, opiates, sedatives, and stimulants. Cocaine has increasingly become the drug of choice of a large segment of the American population. The extent of abuse differs, depending on age, race, economic status, and geographical location. For all substances, federal, state, and local agencies have taken measures attempting to control abuse and related problems.

Various treatment and rehabilitation programs for drug abusers are found throughout the country. Residential therapeutic communities, methadone maintenance treatment programs, hospitals, drug-free services provided on an outpatient basis, and multimodality programs are the most common drug rehabilitation programs. There are benefits, as well as deficiencies, in all drug treatment and rehabilitation programs. Unfortunately, the percentage of totally rehabilitated drug abusers is relatively low.

Alcohol consumption is a common behavioral pattern for a majority of Americans. Responsible drinking is a socially acceptable activity in much of modern civilization. The majority of people in the United States drink socially and can control their level of consumption. Nevertheless, there are a variety of problems associated with alcohol use, including economics, physiological matters causing certain diseases and health problems, accidents, and alcoholism.

Alcoholism is a disease requiring special attention, care, and treatment. The alcoholic is often unaware of the condition that has progressively affected him or her. Treatment of alcoholism includes, in addition to medical attention, group and individual therapy. The family and friends of the alcoholic must also be involved in any effective rehabilitative effort.

Tobacco use is another major concern in the United States. Habitual use of tobacco can result in a number of health problems. A relationship exists between cigarette smoking and cancer, chronic bronchitis, and emphysema. With increasing concern about cigarette smoking, many people are turning to the use of smokeless tobacco. The relationship between smokeless tobacco and oral cancer and dental problems is causing many to warn about the dangers of tobacco use in any form. Concern about the negative health effects of cigarette smoking has led to the development of smoking cessation programs conducted by voluntary agencies and industry, as well as public health departments.

Legal regulatory controls and law enforcement have played important roles in the control of and the use and sale of illegal drugs. In 1970, federal legislation was passed that provides a framework for classifying drugs as illegal or legal for restricted medical purposes. In addition, this legislation set penalties for illegal use, possession, and sale of illegal drugs.

Throughout the country many jurisdictions have passed laws and ordinances prohibiting smoking in public facilities. Current initiatives are under way to limit the sale of cigarettes to minors. In an attempt to reduce the incidence of cigarette smoking, federal legislation expanded the number and types of warnings to be placed on cigarette packages.

Billions of dollars are spent each year on drugs, alcohol, and tobacco. The tobacco and alcohol industries have been very effective in political lobbying, marketing, and advertising programs to encourage the purchase of their products.

Discussion Questions

1. Why have the problems associated with substance abuse become a concern of our whole society rather than just a concern of community health?

2. What are some social and psychological reasons found for involvement in substance abuse?

3. Explain how hallucinogenic drugs affect one's behavior.

4. What are some of the physiological effects of nicotine?

5. Explain some of the long-term effects of marijuana on the chronic user.

6. What is cocaine, and how is it taken by the drug user?

7. Explain some of the reasons why use of crack cocaine has become a serious problem in the United States.

8. What are therapeutic drug treatment programs?

9. Discuss some of the issues involving methadone maintenance.

10. What is the basic concept underlying detoxification for drug abuse?

11. Is alcoholism a disease? Give reasons for your answer.

12. What is intervention as it relates to alcoholism?

13. Explain the difference between Alcoholics Anonymous and Al-Anon.

14. Do you agree that smoking is the "single most important preventable cause of death and disease?" Why or why not?

15. What are some measures that you feel should be taken to reduce cigarette smoking in our nation?

16. Discuss issues concerning the use of tobacco products by minors.

17. Do you feel that the "Model Sale of Tobacco Products to Minors Control Act" is a useful piece of legislation? Explain your answer.

18. Discuss the different approaches to smoking cessation programs.

19. What have been some of the factors contributing to an increase in the use of smokeless tobacco since the 1980s?

20. Explain some of the negative ways in which the use of smokeless tobacco can affect one's health.

21. Explain the various provisions of the Comprehensive Drug Abuse Prevention and Control Act of 1970.

22. What is meant by decriminalization of marijuana?

23. Should there be legislation outlawing the use of alcohol? Defend your answer.

24. Should taxes be increased on alcoholic beverages and cigarettes? Why or why not?

25. What are some local ordinances that have been passed that limit smoking in your community?

26. Discuss the issue of eliminating the sales of cigarettes from vending machines.

27. Explain your position on the issue of placing trade sanctions on nations that prohibit the advertising and sale of American cigarettes in their countries.

28. Why has diversification by the tobacco companies occurred in recent years?

29. Should the advertising of tobacco and alcohol products be banned from public billboards?

30. Do you support the elimination of price-support subsidies for tobacco? Why or why not?

31. Do you believe that requiring warning labels on cigarette packages is effective in reducing smoking? Explain your answer.

32. What are some measures that you would recommend to counter cigarette advertising?

Suggested Readings

Allen, John P., and others. "Screening for Alcoholism: Techniques and Issues." *Public Health Reports* 103, no. 6 (November/December 1988): 586–92.

Caan, Bette J., and Marilyn K. Goldhaber. "Caffeinated Beverages and Low Birthweight: A Case-Control Study." *American Journal of Public Health* 79, no. 9 (September 1989): 1299–1300.

Carroll, Charles R. *Drugs in Modern Society.* Dubuque, Ia.: William C. Brown Publishers, 1989.

Centers for Disease Control and Prevention. "Minors' Access to Tobacco—Missouri, 1992 and Texas, 1993." *Morbidity and Mortality Weekly Report* 42, no. 7 (February 26, 1993): 125–28.

Centers for Disease Control and Prevention. "Public Health Focus: Effectiveness of Smoking-Control Strategies—United States." *Morbidity and Mortality Weekly Report* 41, no. 35 (September 4, 1992): 645.

Centers for Disease Control and Prevention. "State Tobacco Prevention and Control Activities: Final Report." *Morbidity and Mortality Weekly Report* 40, no. RR-11 (August 16, 1991): 40 pp.

Chen, Ted T. L., and Alvin E. Winder. "The Opium Wars Revisited as U.S. Forces Tobacco Exports in Asia." *American Journal of Public Health* 80, no. 6 (June 1990): 659–61.

Conolly, Gregory N., and others. "The Reemergence of Smokeless Tobacco." *New England Journal of Medicine* 314 (April 17, 1986): 1020–27.

Cullen, Joseph W., and others. "Health Consequences of Using Smokeless Tobacco: Summary of the Advisory Committee's Report to the Surgeon General." *Public Health Reports* 101, no. 4 (July/August 1986): 355–73.

Fiore, M. C., and others. "Methods Used to Quit Smoking in the United States: Do Cessation Programs Help?" *Journal of the American Medical Association* 263 (1990): 2760–65.

Goodwin, Frederick K. "Alcoholism Research: Delivering on the Promise." *Public Health Reports* 103, no. 6 (November/December 1988): 569–74.

Hinds, M. Ward. "Impact of a Local Ordinance Banning Tobacco Sales to Minors." *Public Health Reports* 107, no. 3 (May/June 1992): 355–58.

Hodgson, T. A. "Cigarette Smoking and Lifetime Medical Expenditures." *Milbank Quarterly* 70 (1992): 81–125.

Koop, C. Everett, Surgeon General. "The Campaign against Smokeless Tobacco." *The New England Journal of Medicine* 314, no. 16 (April 17, 1986): 1042.

Lando, Harry A., and others. "Comparative Evaluation of ACS and ALA Smoking Cessation Clinics." *American Journal of Public Health* 80, no. 5 (May 1990): 554–59.

Petitti, Diane B., and Charlotte Coleman. "Cocaine and the Risk of Low Birth Weight." *American Journal of Public Health* 80, no. 1 (January 1990): 25–28.

Public Health Service. *Strategies to Control Tobacco Use in the United States: A Blueprint for Public Health Action in the 1990s.* NIH Publication No. 92–3316 (October 1991): 307 pp.

Wallen, Jacqueline. "Alcoholism Treatment Service Systems: A Health Services Research Perspective." *Public Health Reports* 103, no. 6 (November/December 1988): 605–11.

Endnotes

1. University of Southern California study reported in *The Nation's Health* (September 1992): 2.

2. These relationships were discussed in chapter 18.

3. Liska, Ken. *Drugs and the Human Body.* New York: Macmillan Publishing Co., 1981, p. 145.

4. Ibid., 146.

5. Office on Smoking and Health. *Reducing the Health Consequences of Smoking: 25 Years of Progress. A Report of the Surgeon General.* DHHS Pub. No. 89–8411. Washington, D.C.: U.S. Government Printing Office (1989).

6. Department of Health and Human Services. *The Health Consequences of Smoking, the Changing Cigarette: A Report of the Surgeon General.* Washington, D.C.: U.S. Government Printing Office (1981).

7. National Institute on Drug Abuse. *Marijuana Research Findings: 1980.* Series no. 31. Research Monograph, 1980.

8. Ibid., 37.

9. Ibid., 23–25.

10. *NIDA Capsules, Marijuana Update.* Press release, National Institute on Drug Abuse, 1989.

11. Carroll, Charles, and Dean Miller. *Health: The Science of Human Adaptation,* 5th ed., Dubuque, Ia.: Wm. C. Brown Publishers, 1991, p. 198.

12. Ibid., 199.

13. Girdano, Dorothy Dusek, and Daniel A. Girdano. *Drugs—A Factual Account.* Menlo Park, Calif.: Addison-Wesley Publishing Company, 1976, p. 88.

14. Ibid., 93.

15. Tanner, Ogden. *The Prudent Use of Medicines.* Alexandria, Va.: Time-Life Books, 1981, p. 55.

16. Girdano and Girdano, *Drugs—A Factual Account,* 137.

17. Ibid., 140.

18. National Institute on Alcohol Abuse and Alcoholism. *Facts About Alcohol and Alcoholism.* 1976, p. 20.

19. Ibid., 24.

20. Centers for Disease Control and Prevention news release, April 1993.

21. Department of Health and Human Services. *Healthy People 2000: National Health Promotion and Disease Prevention Objectives.* Washington, D.C.: U.S. Government Printing Office, 1991, p. 136.

22. Centers for Disease Control. *Smoking and Health: A National Status Report.* Rockville, Md.: Public Health Service. DHHS Publication no. (CDC) 87–8396 (1986).

23. U.S. Department of Health and Human Services. *Reducing the Health Consequences of Smoking, 25 Years of Progress: A Report of the Surgeon General.* 1989, p. 11.

24. Centers for Disease Control, *Smoking and Health: A National Status Report,* p. 123.

25. Department of Health and Human Services, *Healthy People 2000,* 146.

26. Public Health Service. *Strategies to Control Tobacco Use in the United States: A Blueprint for Public Health Action in the 1990s.* NIH Publication #92–3316 (1991): pp. IX–XII.

27. Public Law 91–513, passed in 1970.

28. Council on Scientific Affairs. "Health Effects of Smokeless Tobacco." *Journal of the American Medical Association* 255, no. 8 (February 28, 1986): 1038–44.

29. National Institute of Health Consensus Development Conference on Smokeless Tobacco. "Health Implications of Smokeless Tobacco Use." *Public Health Reports* 101, no. 4 (July/August 1986): 349.

30. Winn, D. M., W. J. Blot, C. M. Shy, and others. "Snuff Dipping and Oral Cancer among Women in the Southern U.S." *New England Journal of Medicine* 304 (March 26, 1981): 745–49.

31. Ibid., 172.

32. Comprehensive Smokeless Tobacco and Health Education Act, 1986, Public Law 99–257, 1986.

33. Moore, Mark H., and Dean R. Gerstein. *Alcohol and Public Policy: Beyond the Shadow of Prohibition.* Washington, D.C.: National Research Council, National Academy Press, 1981.

34. Department of Health and Human Services. *Promoting Health/Preventing Diseases: Objectives for the Nation.* Washington, D.C.: U.S. Government Printing Office, 1980, pp. 67–72.

35. Department of Health and Human Services, *Healthy People 2000,* 164–78.

36. *Ibid.*

37. *Ibid.,* 148–49.

38. American Public Health Association. *The Nation's Health* (November 1992): 20.

39. American Public Health Association. *The Nation's Health* (September 1985): 15.

CHAPTER **TWENTY-TWO**

Occupational Safety and Health

Protection and Prevention at the Worksite

More than one hundred million Americans spend a portion of each day at work. The working conditions often have profound effects upon the health and well-being of these Americans. Some working conditions are much more dangerous than others: mining, construction, transportation, agriculture, and heavy industrial settings are far more dangerous than offices, schools, and retail stores. Nevertheless, there is the potential for injury, exposure to health hazards, and stress-producing situations in every occupational setting.

Innumerable efforts have been made to improve working conditions, some instituted by industry and management, others as the result of union demands agreed to in the bargaining process. Often, however, it has been necessary for the government to pass legislation and to establish regulations to improve the health and safety of the workplace.

In spite of the far-reaching improvements in working conditions, accidents, exposure to harmful and toxic industrial agents, and disease-causing conditions still occur and exist too frequently in industrial settings. It has been estimated that the total cost to society of occupational injuries is more than $115 billion annually.[1] These costs are measured in terms of lost wages, increased insurance premiums, medical care, fire and destruction in the workplace, and administrative overhead.

Job-related accidents account for more than eight thousand fatalities annually.[2] More than three million workers a year suffer some disabling injuries, the result of "on the job" accidents. An estimated seventy-five million work days are lost each year from work-related injuries.[3]

Health and the Workplace

Not only is it costly to industry and business, but occupation-related diseases negatively affect the work force. Governmental statistics indicate that an estimated 125,000 occupation-related diseases occur each year. This data amplifies the importance of improving the health and safety conditions of employees in the workplace.

Occupational health programs date back many years. An example of an early employee health program can be traced to 1894. In Dayton, Ohio, the National Cash Register Company introduced a program of morning and afternoon exercise breaks for the employees. This same company installed a gymnasium on the fourth floor for employee use in 1904, and in 1911 opened a 325-acre park for employees.[4]

Unfortunately, not all businesses and industries have been as progressive in employee health care as has National Cash Register. As a matter of fact, the working conditions of many have remained deplorable. For example, hundreds of coal miners still suffer serious respiratory diseases at a very early age owing to inhalation of coal dust. Many times industry does not establish appropriate safety standards nor provide employee health care coverage until either mandated by legislation or negotiated with the union as part of the benefit package.

Several industrial developments have been designed through the years to protect the health and safety of employees. These developments include the addition of health and safety medical personnel to the payroll. Medical services in a clinic are found in some industrial settings, usually among large companies with hundreds of employees. Smaller companies have to rely upon the services of a nurse for emergency care and leave the associated medical care to individual workers' private physicians.

A comprehensive occupational safety and health program includes environmental monitoring and safety review. Other occupational health activities include such health promotion and education activities as corporate fitness programs, employee stress management, nutrition and weight control education, smoking cessation programs, health counseling, and alcoholism and drug abuse rehabilitation.

Occupational health and safety programs should extend beyond the needs of the employees since the health of the employees, their families, job fulfillment, industrial production, and the community as a whole are all interrelated. Without question, this programming is a far-reaching community health program affecting many people.

The American Medical Association has suggested that the scope of occupational health programs include the following.[5]

1. Protect employees against health and safety hazards at work

2. Protect the general environment

3. Place workers in job capacities without endangering their health and safety or that of others

4. Assure adequate medical care and rehabilitation of the ill and injured

5. Encourage and assist in measures designed for personal health maintenance

Comprehensive Health Service Programs

Health problems are among the main causes for absenteeism from work. These problems may include physical and mental illnesses, or they may be the result of accidents. A variety of personal behaviors, such as drinking, drug usage, stress, and other preventable problems, also result in absence from work.

In the past, some businesses and industries required a preemployment health examination. Such examinations provided the company with baseline health information that could be useful for reference in later years of employment. However, in 1990 the federal government passed the Americans with Disabilities Act. This legislation requires employers to make reasonable accommodations for employees or applicants with disabilities. Employers cannot discriminate against qualified workers with potentially costly disabilities. This includes elderly individuals, people returning to work after an injury, as well as disabled persons.

Young people with disabilities who have been educated must now be included in the work force instead of being placed in sheltered employment situations. Also people who have been excluded from promotion in the past due to disability now must be given equal consideration with other nondisabled individuals.

Under provisions of the Americans with Disabilities Act companies cannot conduct a medical examination before offering a job to a person. Neither can a prospective employee be asked about a disability. The employer can require a medical examination only after an offer of employment is made, and the offer cannot be withdrawn because of illness or disability found in the examination.[6]

Many companies pay for a routine annual health examination. These examinations may be conducted by the industrial medical staff, in some instances by a group prepaid medical staff contracted by the industry, or by private, personal, or family physicians where the company provides payment.

The Occupational Safety and Health Administration (OSHA) has mandated that employees exposed in the workplace to certain toxic substances such as asbestos, benzene, and ethylene oxide be provided with a medical screening program by their employers. It is mandated that the employee have a preplacement examination, a yearly medical examination, and a termination examination.[7] Though this provides for medical examinations for certain employees working with toxic agents, it does not mandate them for all workers.

From a humanitarian point of view, business and industry should provide health and safety programs for their employees. Unfortunately, it is often necessary to

Scenario of Health in the Workplace by the Year 2010

1. Health promotion and wellness programs will no longer be viewed as "luxury" benefits by business.
2. Health promotion research and development will increasingly focus on the role of mental health in enhancing physical health.
3. Hospitals, clinics, nursing homes, and other health institutions will lose influence, yielding to job sites as settings for the pursuit of health.

Source: Bezold, Clement, Rick J. Carlson, and Jonathan C. Peck. *The Future of Work and Health.* Auburn House Publishing Company, 1985, 191 pp.

argue the cost benefits rather than the humanitarian reasons in support of such programs. If it can be shown that a specific health or safety activity has cost benefits, then there is greater likelihood that the activities will be implemented.

Clinical Services

Some companies and industries provide health care services for their employees. This may simply be an arrangement with local physicians to provide emergency care when accidents and injuries occur. In these circumstances, any required health care, services, or examinations are the responsibility of the individual employee's physician. But in other instances, larger companies will provide in-plant health clinics of various sizes. Some industries operate comprehensive health maintenance organizations for employees, relatives, and, in a few cases, for community residents.

The clinical services include preplacement as well as periodic medical examinations. Laboratory services are also found in some occupational clinics. Most commonly, though, emergency care is provided. On occasion industries will have well-trained emergency medical personnel available, but in most instances only the occupational nurse and a few first aid supplies are provided.

Not all Americans work in factories and offices that have well-staffed occupational health clinics. In fact, 70 percent of the labor force work in settings with fewer than five hundred employees, where such facilities are often too costly. These smaller companies usually have to refer injuries and health problems to the private sector.

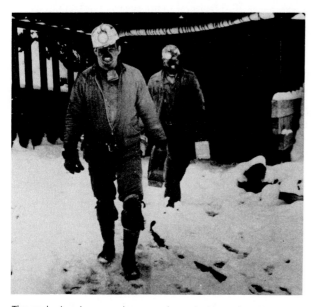

The coal miner is exposed to many hazards. Not only is the underground environment dangerous, but black lung disease, *pneumoconiosis,* has debilitated thousands of miners.

Occupational Health and Safety Personnel

Larger companies usually have a program, administered by a medical director, that employs occupational health and safety professionals. The four professionals most commonly found in occupational health and safety are (1) occupational physicians, (2) occupational health nurses, (3) industrial hygienists, and (4) safety engineers.

Occupational Physicians The occupational physician is a medical doctor who services the medical needs of the worker in the occupational setting. The physician is familiar with the occupation-related diseases, both their causes and treatment. This individual usually serves as the medical director for the health program of a company, industry, or business.

Only the largest corporations employ physicians having knowledge, training, and experience in occupational medicine on a full-time basis. This knowledge and skill is usually obtained through experience on the job, since very few medical schools provide instruction in occupational medicine.[8] Most companies unable to afford a full-time medical director employ a physician on a part-time, on-call, or consultative basis.

Occupational Health Nurses The occupational health nurse is a specialist having specific knowledge and skills that are different from the clinical nurse. This individual sees a fairly stable group of well people rather than the sick and disabled.

The occupational health nurse provides primary nursing care in the workplace for injuries and illnesses, both work-related and nonoccupational. In addition, this nurse plans and administers nursing services for all company employees. This involves assisting with physical examinations, recording health histories, and collecting other data. The position may also involve providing immunizations, screening for health defects, or evaluating activities relating to the health status of the workers.[9]

Often when a health problem is noted, the occupational health nurse makes the appropriate referral to health care facilities in the community. This role as counselor also includes working with employees on health behavior and personal life-styles. Increasingly, the occupational nurse is involved in health promotion and disease prevention.

The occupational nurse must be knowledgeable about the harmful substances and working procedures to which the employees are exposed in the industrial environmental setting. He or she not only works to reduce such hazards but also is expected to educate employees about the hazards.

An example of the importance of educating employees about the unique health conditions that can develop in specific work settings relates to Raynaud's phenomenon.[10] A certain metal manufacturing process in which vibrating hand tools are used was causing this syndrome. This condition of pain, numbness, and tingling in the hands, accompanied by a paleness of the fingertips, is reversible if caught in the early stages. It is estimated that approximately 1.2 million United States workers are at risk for Raynaud's phenomenon. The National Institute of Occupational Safety and Health has issued a recommendation that jobs be redesigned to minimize the use of vibrating hand tools. It is easy to see the importance of education relating to this condition and how workers can learn to prevent it.

With the growing interest in health promotion and cost containment of medical expenditures by industries, there may be an increase of nurses employed in industrial settings. They will provide a broad range of educational services, including counseling and others that are beyond the traditional nursing role. In fact, the occupational nurse is often the only source of health information available to the employees and their families.

Industrial Hygienists The industrial hygienist deals with the environmental factors that may cause sickness and injury or otherwise impair health. This individual is trained to survey and analyze the various chemical, physical, and biological agents that can affect the health of workers. Not only does the industrial hygienist assess hazardous agents, but this individual is also responsible for control of these hazards in the workplace.

These tasks are complicated by the thousands of potentially hazardous agents. The *Registry of Toxic Effects of Chemical Substances,* published by the National Institute of Occupational Safety and Health, lists over twenty-five thousand chemicals that are found in industrial use. Every year some five hundred to one thousand new chemical compounds are produced in the United States to which the worker is exposed during the manufacturing, processing, and packaging processes.[11] Some of the more common compounds are pesticides, plastics, and hydrocarbons.

Many of these toxic agents cause industry-related diseases. These diseases result from dusts such as silica, asbestos, coal, and cotton. Other toxic agents include gases, fumes, and vapors. The industrial hygienist must also be familiar with the biological agents that cause disease such as bacteria, viruses, metazoa, fungi, and rickettsiae.

The industrial hygienist must make sure that federal exposure limits are not exceeded. Should the levels exceed the federal standards, it is necessary to remove the hazard, to substitute a less hazardous material into the manufacturing process, or to require the use of protective devices.

Safety Engineers The safety engineer is concerned with hazards in the workplace that can cause injury to workers. This person's responsibilities include the identification of potential hazards and the development of ways to control or eliminate them.

Implementation of regulations resulting from the Americans with Disabilities Act will require numerous adaptations in the workplace. Safety engineers have major responsibilities to modify the workplace settings to accommodate the disabled. This necessitates changes in machinery, in the basic structure of the worksite to permit mobility of the disabled employee, as well as adaptations in safety measures.

Accident and safety education programs are designed by this specialist. The focus of activities in the industrial setting is upon both accident prevention and the creation of a safer working environment. In recent years, since the passage of the Occupational Safety and Health Act, it has become a very difficult task to monitor all industrial safety regulations established by the federal government. But despite the difficulty, this remains the primary task of the safety engineer in the industrial setting.

Occupation-Related Diseases

Occupation-related diseases account for approximately one hundred thousand deaths annually, with nearly four hundred thousand new cases developing every year.[12] Many work-related diseases develop only after long and continuous exposure to an environmental substance in the work setting. Sometimes these diseases develop as the result of a combined effect: exposure and smoking, drinking, or life-style.

Occupational disease surveillance has not been particularly effective. A congressional subcommittee concluded that occupational disease surveillance ". . . is . . . 70 years behind (surveillance of) communicable disease."[13] There are numerous reasons why such surveillance is lacking. With workers being exposed to hundreds of different chemical, biological, and physical agents, it is extremely difficult to pinpoint specific disease-related causes. The Occupational Safety and Health Administration has established regulatory standards for only about five hundred agents of more than eight thousand potential exposure agents.[14] One can see the tremendous difficulty of being aware of all potential disease-producing agents in the workplace.

Skin diseases account for the largest single group of occupational illnesses.[15] These result from exposure to corrosive and irritating agents that cause dermatitis. For example, creosote is the oldest and most common form of oil-based preservative. It is used as a wood preservative and as a waterproofing agent. When the skin is exposed to creosote, it can cause burning, itching, and reddening. Occupational exposure standards have been published for this chemical.

Skin diseases may also result from an accident in which a toxic substance comes in contact with the skin and causes irritation, burning, or other damage. Dirt, too, causes skin problems for many. Skin disorders are found to be a very extensive problem among agricultural workers. Most skin diseases associated with the workplace can be prevented with protective clothing. Workers should be given gloves, shirts, and other clothing that will protect against the specific irritant. Proper emergency care should be followed when toxic agents are accidentally spilled on the skin. Workers should also be educated to clean their skin after exposure to dirt and other substances.

Programs have been designed to increase employee awareness of the toxicity of substances used in the workplace and to improve protective clothing for workers. Not only has the National Institute of Occupational Safety and Health (NIOSH) been working to develop better protective clothing, but educational efforts to motivate employees to use such clothing have been developed and conducted.

A number of respiratory diseases are caused by exposure to substances in the workplace. Yet, proof that the work environment, not other factors, causes the problem is difficult to find. For example, asbestosis is found in a significant number of construction and shipyard workers who have been exposed to asbestos. Asbestosis has a latent period of between ten and twenty years. Hence, its symptoms may not appear for years after the individual has been exposed. Asbestos exposure causes extensive scarring of the lungs that gets worse even after the direct exposure ends.

Silicosis is prevalent among workers exposed to silica. This condition is found among workers in mines and foundries and among those individuals involved in glass, stone, and clay manufacturing. Another respiratory disease, known as byssinosis or "brown lung," is noted among textile workers, particularly those in the cotton industry and in yarn manufacturing.

Pneumoconiosis, or "black lung disease," results from exposure to various dusts. This is most frequently found among coal miners who inhale coal dust. Black lung disease may be responsible for as many as four thousand deaths a year.[16]

Pneumoconiosis is not a curable condition. Like most of the other occupational respiratory diseases, measures can only be taken to help the person to adapt to the condition. The victim must learn to live with the lung impairment and make life-style adaptations to counter its debilitating effects.

Work-related back injuries create significant costs to industry. Back injuries are considered the number-one source of absenteeism, accounting for approximately twenty-five million lost work days each year.[17] Most back problems are not the result of a single incident but of improper use of the anatomical structure over a long period of time. Quite often these problems are the result of poor posture, inadequate exercise and activity, or change in body weight. If employees know about proper lifting and body carriage, the incidence of low back pain can be reduced.

Industrial health programs must not only inform employees about how to prevent low back pain, but measures must also be available to provide emergency care when a back injury occurs on the job. The occupational health personnel, particularly the nurse, need to work with the employee in rehabilitation efforts after a back injury.

Musculoskeletal injuries that cause damage due to wear of the musculoskeletal system at a rate faster than the body can be repaired are known as cumulative trauma disorders. Tendinitis, shoulder injuries, and carpal tunnel syndrome are examples of these disorders. They result from a number of different causes such as poor work habits, poor posture and fitness, as well as repetitive movement over extensive periods of time.

Concern over cumulative trauma disorders has been noted in the health objectives for the nation. One objective calls for the reduction in cumulative trauma disorders by the year 2000.[18] Among the various strategies that can be instituted to overcome these traumas are job rotation, improvement in the design of work equipment, ergonomic improvements, and providing opportunity for the employee to perform stretching exercises during the work day to permit a relaxation in continuous tension on the musculoskeletal system.

An example of cumulative trauma disorder is carpal tunnel syndrome. This is a condition caused by irritation of the median nerve passing through the carpal tunnel in the wrist. It leads to pain and/or numbness of the hand and occurs among many workers who perform repetitive tasks that stress the hand and wrist. Left untreated, hand disability results. Occupational work involving the use of vibrating hand tools or the use of the hands in repetitive movements or awkward positions places individuals at risk for this condition. It has been associated with assembly line workers such as those in the automotive industry and manual laborers. Also, secretaries working on computer and typewriter keyboards for lengthy periods of time have developed this condition. Women tend to be at greater risk for carpal tunnel syndrome than men.

Loud noise in the workplace has the potential for causing hearing loss among workers. Loud noise produces irreversible damage to the auditory system. The hair cells of the organ of Corti in the cochlea are destroyed by continued exposure to loud noises over a long period of time. Hearing loss is initially limited to the high frequencies, but over time the hearing loss can affect all levels of hearing.

Noise-induced hearing loss occurs so gradually that it is likely a person will not be aware of the loss until permanent damage is done. For this reason, employees should undergo periodic hearing screening. Workers should be informed of the dangers associated with continual exposure to loud sounds, and they should be required to wear such noise resistant devices as plugs or muffs.

The protection of workers' hearing has been important for centuries. As early as 600 B.C., a law was passed in ancient Greece barring metalwork hammering in populated areas because of the excessive noise.[19] In recent years, because of the Occupational Safety and Health Act, standards for noise exposure in the workplace have been specified. Currently, no worker should be exposed to a noise level above ninety decibels. Any time that workers are exposed to noise limits over eighty-five decibels, protective equipment must be worn and workers must submit to periodic hearing testing.

In addition to requiring workers to wear hearing protection devices, industry must also seek ways to limit the noise generation at the source. This may involve modifying the machine or instrument causing the noise.

According to the National Institute for Occupational Safety and Health, some 850 chemicals have been identified as being toxic to the human nervous system. Eight million employees in the United States are regularly exposed to these chemicals.

Various signs and symptoms resulting from chemical exposure present themselves. Many are simply minor influenzalike symptoms, sleep disturbances, and lethargy in the early exposure stages. However, with increased exposure more serious difficulties occur. Mental disorders, sexual disorders, and even death can result. For example, a condition known as peripheral neuropathy has been reported. Body tremors, feelings of numbness, and tingling in the feet or hands are early indications of this problem. These symptoms are followed by muscle weakness and eventual problems with vision and perception.

Indoor air pollution has become an increasing problem in many occupational settings. This is particularly a factor in recently built office and service buildings that are air conditioned and mechanically ventilated. Since the 1970s many buildings have been constructed so as to be energy efficient. This has resulted in buildings being constructed that are airtight, having an inadequate exchange of outside air because of increased use of insulation and reduction of any small pockets around windows where exchange of air might occur. Energy conservation has been an important factor in building construction. This development has become known as the "sick building syndrome."

The problem comes to the attention of employers when employees working in newly constructed or remodeled buildings begin to report respiratory irritation, particularly of the eye, nose, and throat. Headache, dizziness, fatigue, and nausea are other symptoms that develop. Various odors are reported by occupants of these buildings. The symptoms may be mild and only present a nuisance to basic comfort. However, in many cases people are unable to work on a regular basis because of the associated symptoms, and there have been a number of reports of individuals having to be hospitalized.

Identifying the cause of these problems is often a very difficult task. There have been cases where a newly constructed and occupied building has had to be evacuated and left unoccupied for several weeks until the source of the problem can be identified and corrected.

Four general sources of these problems have been identified: the presence of household chemicals, formaldehyde, asbestos, and radon.[20] Several different household chemical agents used for cleaning are known or suspected of contributing to these problems. For example, methylene chloride used in aerosol paints has been one contributing factor. Formaldehyde found in several building materials and in room furnishings, such as draperies and carpets, is another related cause. Paints

Ten Leading Work-Related Diseases and Injuries, United States

1. Occupational lung diseases
2. Musculoskeletal injuries
3. Occupational cancers (other than lung)
4. Amputations, fractures, eye loss, lacerations, traumatic deaths
5. Cardiovascular diseases
6. Diseases of reproduction
7. Neurotoxic disorders
8. Noise-induced hearing loss
9. Dermatological conditions
10. Psychological disorders

Source: National Institute of Occupational Safety and Health as reported in CDC, *Morbidity and Mortality Weekly Report* 32, no. 14 (April 15, 1983): 190.

National Health Objectives for the Year 2000

Occupation-Related Conditions

1. The incidence of occupational skin disorders and diseases should be reduced.
2. Four occupational diseases—asbestosis, byssinosis, silicosis, and pneumoconiosis—should be prevented.
3. The prevalence of occupational noise-induced hearing loss should be reduced.
4. There should be a reduction of Hepatitis B among occupational exposed workers.

Source: Department of Health and Human Services. *Healthy People 2000: National Health Promotion and Disease Prevention Objectives.* Washington, D.C.: U.S. Government Printing Office (1991).

and stains, organic compounds in the carpeting, and cleaning compounds have been found to cause problems. Resolution to this problem awaits further research and developments.

The working environment is an excellent place to encourage preventive measures for the two major causes of death in the United States—heart disease and cancer. It has been estimated that United States industries lose more than 140 million work days owing to heart disease each year. The cost to industry in terms of lost work days, disability payments, medical expenses, and substitute personnel is approximately $50 billion per year.[21] Educational programs, screening procedures, and facilities to encourage an active life-style are measures that the industrial and business world can take to help reduce the incidence of cardiovascular disease.

One person in four will get cancer. It is uncertain how much cancer is the result of occupation-related factors—estimates range from as low as 5 percent to as high as 40 percent.[22] It is very difficult to determine a direct cause-and-effect relationship. For many cancers various cofactors, such as smoking, alcohol consumption, and the environment, as well as certain conditions in the work setting, may be the causative agents.

However, there are several agents found in the workplace that have been closely linked to an increase in cancer incidence among workers. Benzene, a highly flammable liquid that is used as a gasoline additive and in the manufacture of dyes, linoleum, and varnishes, has been linked to blood disorders, particularly leukemia. Nickel, which is used in the manufacture of steel and in petroleum refining, batteries, ceramics, and coins, has been linked to cancer of the nasal cavity, the lung, and the larynx. Benzidine, used in textile and silk dyes, has been linked with an increased incidence of cancer of the bladder.

Several occupations have been closely linked with the occurrence of cancer.[23] For example, coal miners and rubber workers are prone to stomach cancer. Increase in lung cancer has been noted in heavily industrialized locations. Cancer of the mouth and pharynx is prevalent among textile workers and newspaper printing press operators.[24] More research and regulatory measures are important so that the worksite is no longer a contributing factor in the development of cancers.

The occupational setting is an ideal place to inform adults about cancer. Occupational health programs should include cancer education and screening. For women employees, regular self-examinations for breast cancer and Pap tests for uterine cancer should be encouraged. For males, a proctoscopic examination for cancer of the colon and rectum should be performed annually after the age of forty. Any indication of respiratory congestion should be noted for the possibility of lung cancer. Surveillance of the worksite must be increased in the years ahead to identify specific relationships between the work environment and cancer, and measures must be expanded to inform employees of the dangers, signs and symptoms, and prevention of cancer.

A number of studies, as well as the Surgeon General's Report on Health in 1986, have documented that nonsmoking individuals can be at risk for various respiratory illnesses as the result of exposure to the "sidestream" smoke of others. This has raised a number of questions about whether nonsmokers should be placed at risk for respiratory illnesses, lung cancer, and other debilitating conditions in the worksite.

Increasing numbers of state and local regulations and ordinances have been passed that restrict smoking in the workplace. Some corporations have levied a surcharge on employees who smoke. Those who smoke must pay an increased amount on their health insurance premiums.

The economic consequences of smoking have been a concern and consideration of many companies.[25]

1. Business loses $26 billion in productivity each year owing to smoking.
2. Smokers are 50 percent more likely to take sick leave than nonsmokers.
3. Job-related accident rates are twice as high for smokers as nonsmokers.
4. Employers spend an average of three hundred dollars more in insurance claims each year for smokers than for nonsmokers.

Numerous issues arise relating to the employee and smoking.

1. Do you feel that smoking at work should be restricted?
2. Does the company have an obligation to provide a place for the smoking employees to smoke?
3. If a company charges employees who smoke a surcharge for health insurance, does the company have a moral obligation to provide some type of smoking cessation program at the worksite?

Safety and the Workplace

In spite of the importance of occupational health measures, most emphasis in industrial health and safety has focused upon safety. This is partly because of the simplicity of identifying a cause-and-effect relationship in accidents. When an accident in the workplace occurs, it is obvious who is injured and what caused the incident. But if a disease is related to the workplace, it is often quite difficult to ascertain the specific disease-causing agent.

Fatalities in the workplace occur all too often. It is difficult to accept any accidental death; however, when a person goes to one's place of employment, it is expected that the surrounding circumstances will not be life-threatening. In spite of such expectations, it is estimated that approximately 8,500 lives are lost annually in work-related accidents.[26] Even though most fatalities occur on a one-by-one basis, multiple fatality tragedies do occur. In 1991 a fire at a chicken processing plant in a small North Carolina community resulted in twenty-five deaths, fifty-six injuries. In this situation fire broke out in a facility where the exit doors were locked or bolted shut and the employees could not escape through the emergency exits.

More than 3.3 million disabling injuries occur annually in the workplace.[27] In addition to fatalities and disabling injuries, lost work time results from injury-producing occurrences while on the job. It is estimated that over 105 million work days are lost each year due to workplace accidents.[28] This places very heavy economic burdens on businesses and industries to pay for lost wages, medical expenses, insurance costs, as well as capital losses, as in the case of fires.

Industrial safety programs are the responsibility of both management and employees. Management is interested in maintaining a safe working environment so that productivity is not hindered or reduced. An accident may lead to the shutdown of the production line. It may mean that the time, money, and effort put into training a skilled worker is lost if the person is injured while on the job. All too often, however, even though management is interested in safety, it fails to pay for measures to improve the safety of the workplace unless forced to do so by law and worker demand.

Employees, particularly through the collective bargaining process, have been able to effect changes in the work setting. Safer working environments have

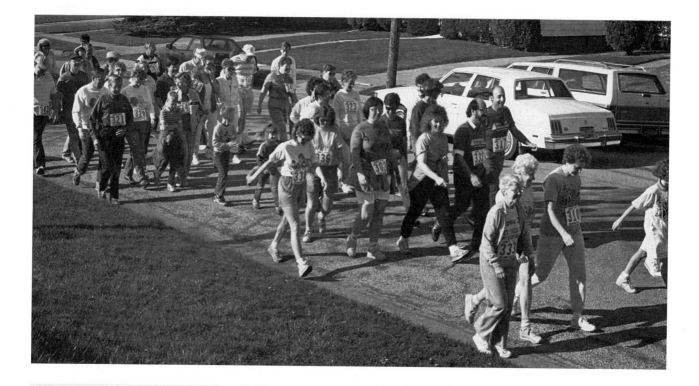

Several companies, including the Kimberly-Clark Corporation, sponsor health promotion activities. In the "Walkers Club" employees receive rewards (gym bags, etc.) after logging a certain number of miles. The employees are encouraged to participate in community walk-a-thons.

resulted from negotiation, strikes, and legislation. Nevertheless, accidents are still too frequent in such industries as mining, construction, and agriculture. Continuing surveillance and effort by both management and labor are needed to improve the safety of such workplaces.

Health Promotion Programs in the Workplace

In addition to providing medical care facilities and surveillance of the work environment, industry and business have become more interested in health promotion. An increasing number of occupational health promotion programs have been established in recent years. These initiatives are seen as part of human resource management programming by the corporations.

The continuing escalation of health care costs in the United States and the subsequent costs for business and industry of providing health insurance have become a major influence on worksite health promotion programming. Companies are recognizing the relationship between physical and mental health and increased efficiency among their employees. Employee productivity is improved, as is morale. Absenteeism has been shown to be reduced.[29] Health promotion is now considered a part of the employee compensation package in many instances.

Industry has realized a number of benefits from providing these programs, including reduced absenteeism, illness, injuries, and disabilities and less use of sick leave. Such reductions result in higher employee morale, more productive work, and greater output. Employee benefits include improved health, a greater feeling of well-being, and a more positive attitude. These benefits, in turn, affect the company, because the employees are motivated to do quality work and productivity increases.

Through health promotion activities, business and industry can encourage its employees and their families to become more responsible for their health. The establishment of such activities and provision of corporate facilities assist employees in becoming more productive persons, both on and off the job. A physically fit person is most likely to be a mentally and socially well-adjusted individual.

A number of health promotion activities are provided in the industrial health setting: fitness programs, alcohol and other substance abuse rehabilitation programs, hypertension and cardiovascular screening, stress management, weight control, smoking cessation, and health education.

Fitness

Many companies are developing physical fitness programs for their employees for a variety of reasons. With the cost of health care escalating rapidly, many businesses and industries are recognizing the potential cost benefits of health promotion measures. It is hoped that with the provision of health programs, the need for curative health services will be reduced. Because of this, more than four hundred major corporations now have exercise facilities.[30] Mobil Oil, Exxon, Adolph Coors, Boeing, Ford Motor Company, Xerox, Kimberly-Clark, and Rockwell International are examples of corporations that employ physical fitness directors. A professional organization known as the American Association of Fitness Directors in Business and Industry has been formed.[31]

Physical fitness programs range from highly structured workouts using fully equipped company facilities to low-profile walking and jogging programs using in-house facilities or grounds. Where companies do not have their own facilities, local health clubs, YMCAs, school gymnasiums, and other community resources have been used.

Such programs are important and often help improve the employee attitude about the management of the company. As employees participate in a variety of fitness activities, they generally become better acquainted. The impersonal relationships so often present in industry are then replaced by more personal relationships.

One industrial fitness program is the *Health Management Program* for salaried employees developed

"... most employees who take their fitness program seriously are happier people. They adjust well. They are enthusiastic and positive about their jobs; and they seem to enjoy hard work, mental or physical."

Source: Darwin E. Smith, Chairman of the Board and Chief Executive Officer, Kimberly-Clark Corporation, Neenah, Wisconsin (Press release dated September 21, 1981).

by the Kimberly-Clark Corporation in Neenah, Wisconsin.[32] This program, which emphasizes wellness, consists of a computer-analyzed medical history and health risk profile, multiphasic screening, physical examination, exercise testing and treadmill, and health review. The company has an exercise facility where a variety of aerobic exercise programs are conducted. The goal of this program is to help employees maintain or improve their health. Employees not only are made aware of health risks and how to control them but are encouraged to make positive changes in their life-style.

The Kimberly-Clark program is conducted in a company-owned facility. However, other industrial physical fitness programs for employees may be designed and conducted by community agencies. Urban YMCAs often schedule a fitness program for area business people during the lunch hour or before and after working hours. Some businesses send their employees to these fitness programs as an alternative to staffing and maintaining in-house programs.

Other fitness activities provided by industries include tennis lessons, bowling and golf leagues, and access to outdoor jogging paths on employer-owned land. For several years the Adolph Coors Company has conducted a cardiac rehabilitation program.[33] It has been estimated that nearly $1.5 million has been saved over a six year period of time.

To encourage fitness program participation, some firms offer incentives to motivate employees. The Hospital Corporation of America in Nashville pays exercisers by the mile. Runners and walkers receive sixteen cents for each mile; bicyclers, four cents per mile; and swimmers, fifteen cents a mile.[34]

In addition to on-site activities, some companies offer corporate discount rates on memberships in health clubs. Others provide a subsidy for participation in exercise programs and in health club membership.

A rather unique program was introduced in 1987 by Union Pacific Railroad in Omaha, Nebraska.[35] In order to provide service for work crews on their various railroad lines, a railcar was outfitted as a mini-health center. Exercise equipment, videotapes, and literature were available in the cars, which traveled to remote locations along their lines where employees were working.

Alcohol, Chemical Abuse Treatment, and Smoking Cessation Programs

A growing number of industries and businesses offer alcohol and chemical abuse and alcoholism programs. As employee performance and output have been affected by the use of these substances, business has recognized a need to do something about the situation.

Alcoholism on the job causes a range of problems: lost time from work and additional medical expenses and workers' compensation, as well as many safety and social problems. Thus, alcoholism affects both the employee and management.

The first employee alcoholism treatment programs were established in the early 1940s by the E. I. Dupont Company of Wilmington, Delaware, and the Eastman Kodak Company of Rochester, New York. Since then, a number of programs have been established that include not just the employees but also family members.

With increasing use and abuse of drugs, it has been necessary to develop chemical abuse programs in addition to those dealing with alcoholism. Industry's alcohol and drug rehabilitation programs have proved to be successful. General Motors reported a savings of $9,878 in disability insurance benefits and 10,850 work hours that would have been lost from twenty-five alcoholic employees. In another General Motors drug and alcohol rehabilitation project that cost the company $11,114, a 49 percent decrease in lost employee hours, a 29 percent decrease in disability insurance benefits, and a 56 percent decrease in leaves of absence among 117 hourly workers were reported.[36] These returns justify such rehabilitation efforts.

Supervisors at the worksite and the occupational nurse learn to identify early indicators of alcohol and drug abuse. The first signs of such abuse include tardiness, sick time, long lunch hours, irritability, and declining quality of work.[37]

The major benefit to employers of treatment programs for problem drinkers is improved work attendance. Other benefits include reduced labor turnover, fewer job accidents, improved worker morale, and lower medical care costs.[38]

Approximately 15 percent of United States businesses have programs designed to help employees quit smoking.[39] It is estimated that smoking costs approximately $3 billion annually in lost wages.[40] Smoking contributes to a number of chronic diseases including lung cancer, emphysema, and chronic bronchitis.

Smoking cessation programs in industry and business are usually developed in cooperation with community agencies involved in similar programs. The American Lung Association, the American Cancer Society, and various other voluntary and private organizations have programs that are used by various companies.

Some companies have used economic incentives to encourage employees to stop smoking.[41] The employees are awarded cash bonuses for not smoking over a given period of time. Other incentives include a weekly bonus for not smoking while on the job. This uses group support and encouragement to help people stop smoking and also reduces nonsmoker exposure to the smoke. These bonuses are considered worth the cost in terms of a more healthy and productive employee, the decreased group health insurance rates, and the reduced risk of debilitating respiratory illness, which could result in long-term physical disability payments by management. On the other hand, it is important to question the ethical nature of corporations using economic incentives for health promotion. An important issue that must be considered is whether the use of such incentives is in some ways coercive in nature. Also, is such practice discriminatory? In reality nonsmokers are excluded from the opportunity to receive economic benefits simply because they do not have the negative health habit.

The most successful smoking cessation programs make use of group smoking withdrawal clinics and counseling on an individual basis.[42] These sessions make use of various behavioral modification strategies and permit the participant to draw on the experiences of others.

Hypertension Screening

A health problem that affects employees in all businesses and industries is high blood pressure (hypertension). As many as fifteen million working Americans have high blood pressure. This condition results in more than fifty-two million lost workdays a year.[43]

Many industries have incorporated blood pressure screening into their health promotion programs. The screening procedure often reveals employees with potential high blood pressure problems who may never have suspected there was a problem. In addition to the hypertension screening, information about high blood pressure, referral, and follow-up are necessary components of these programs. At-risk individuals should be informed that hypertension can be treated through stress reduction, exercise, sodium restriction, weight reduction, and careful life-style monitoring. The employee may be referred to a private physician, a medical resource in the community, or an in-house program designed to reduce the hypertension.

Nutrition and Weight Control

The diet of millions of Americans results in a weight problem. Such eating patterns have a serious effect upon the well-being of employees and their productivity. Thus, industry has begun to develop nutritional awareness programs for employees.

Nutritional awareness can be encouraged in company cafeterias and dining facilities. Information about foods and diet can be displayed and food offerings modified to provide a nutritious diet.

Instruction about proper nutrition is an important part of the program. There is a significant amount of ignorance about the subject and about how to evaluate the many commercial diets on the market. Instructional programs and company publications can combat some of the ignorance about diet and nutrition.

Weight reduction and control programs in industry are usually components of a larger exercise and fitness program. Because of this, the emphasis of industrial nutrition programs should be on general dietary guidelines. Specific diets should be prescribed in cooperation with the individual's physician. After the employer's physician has examined the individual, a registered dietitian or nutritionist can work with the person to provide an appropriate diet.

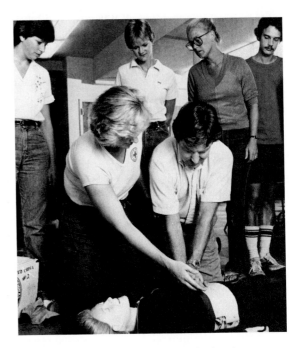

Instruction in cardiopulmonary resuscitation is given in many industrial health promotion programs. This provides the workers with skills that can be useful not just at the worksite, but also at home.

Stress Management

Stress is the cause of many work-related problems. Often the pressures of the job lead to emotional and physical problems. Symptoms of stress include emotional upset, cardiovascular problems, increased use of medication, abuse of alcohol and other drugs, and other chronic ailments.

Stress is a problem for employees in industry at both the management and the labor levels. Since stress reduces the effectiveness of work capabilities, it has become increasingly important that industry and business develop programs in stress management. These programs are designed to help individuals cope with the pressures of work, home, and their personal lives. Such programs include measures to help understand the need for relaxation as well as how to relax. Oftentimes this is accomplished with the use of counseling and biofeedback.

Health Education

If conducted through the workplace, health education can be a very effective means of promoting health and understanding about all the previously mentioned health problems and concerns. Health education activities in the industrial setting include health counseling in connection with health examinations, safety and first aid training classes, distribution of printed materials in employee newspapers, pamphlets, and posters, and the use of films.

The effectiveness of any health education activity depends on a number of variables. The efforts should be directed toward the employee, as well as the employee's family, and must be designed to incorporate effective theories of adult learning. Industrial management wants assurance that the health education strategies will result in improved health behaviors that, in turn, will affect the productivity of the worker and, as a result, the productivity of the company. Experience has shown that health education is most effective when the employer demonstrates a sincere and continuing interest in the health of the employees and when employees are encouraged to participate in the planning and conducting of health education activities.[44]

Worksite Health Promotion Effectiveness and Future Directions

Extensive studies of health promotion initiatives carried out by companies have revealed their many economic benefits. A savings in health expenses of 37 percent was attributed to employee fitness programs in a survey of some fifteen hundred companies.[45] In addition, improved employee morale and better employee job satisfaction were reported.

The General Mills Company has developed a program called Tri-Healthalon. Not only have they reported significant reduction in job absenteeism but also a three to four dollar payback for each dollar spent on this health promotion program.[46]

A grain merchandising company in Nebraska has estimated that it saved one million dollars in 1990 on health care costs as a result of their health and fitness programs. General Electric Aircraft in Cincinnati estimates it saves a half million dollars a year in medical costs and has reduced hospitalization of employees by 760 hospital days a year as a result of their health promotion program.

Other studies have noted that employee fitness programs tend to enhance the company's ability to recruit new workers. Also, there are improved attitudes and greater loyalty on the part of employees. Increasing

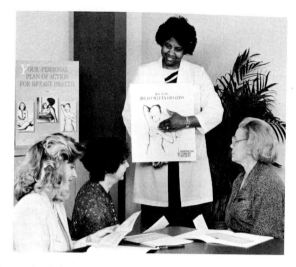

Instruction in breast self-examination is given as part of many corporate health promotion programs.

interest in the well-being of the employees' families has been noted by many corporations.[47]

IBM provides exercise, safety, and first aid courses for spouses of company employees and their children between the ages of fifteen and twenty-two. Company retirees and their spouses may also participate in this program.

A prenatal care program is provided by the Whitman Corporation of Chicago. Female employees and their spouses are required to contact a counselor within thirty days of learning they are pregnant. Counselors monitor the pregnancy to be sure that the individual is getting proper prenatal care. The company pays 90 percent of the cost of the pregnancy if the woman follows through with this program.[48]

In the future worksite health promotion must be directed toward smaller businesses. The major initiatives have been carried out by the larger corporations. Often the smaller company, employing fewer than ten to fifteen employees, has no program for their workers. It seems logical to suggest that community agencies cooperate with these companies to provide the same programs that the big companies provide.

Worksite health promotion programs should increasingly focus on the specific problems of minorities and of women. Minorities are more likely to smoke, to not use seatbelts, and to not exercise regularly. Often members of this population employed in the industrial setting

Issue—Case Study

Drug Abuse, Drug Testing, and the Workplace

Today a number of concerns confront the corporate world regarding drug abuse among employees. It has been estimated that business and industry lose $60 billion a year due to substance abuse. These losses are the result of lost productivity, increased absence from work, accidents occurring due to alcohol and drug use, thefts, and medical costs. For example General Motors estimates that they spend one billion dollars a year due to drug abuse. Many other companies have reported that as much as 40 percent of their health care costs are attributable to substance abuse.

Not only do drug and alcohol abusers put themselves at risk, but their coworkers also are endangered, particularly for injuries resulting from accidents. As a result they are more likely to file worker's compensation claims, thus raising the costs to the companies.

These factors have led many to suggest that companies should consider mandatory drug testing for their employees. Failure to pass the drug tests could either result in required placement in alcohol and drug rehabilitation programs or in the individual being removed from employment.

Mandatory drug and alcohol testing for employees is a very controversial matter. Many suggest that it is an infringement on one's personal freedoms and individual rights. They argue that if a person meets the job requirements the company has no right to take action against an individual because of alcohol and/or drug use patterns. Opponents also question the accuracy of testing procedures.

On the other hand, proponents suggest that it is a necessary safeguard to assure quality in the work production and safety among the work force. Also, supporters feel that mandatory drug testing for employment is necessary to help in some way to lower health care costs.

Should employees be required to undergo drug/alcohol testing prior to being employed by a company?

Is there a circumstance upon employment that should require mandatory drug testing?

If an employee fails to pass a drug/alcohol test, what is the responsibility of the corporation for this individual?

If there is workplace drug/alcohol testing of all employees, who should pay for this program—government, the corporation, the individual, the union, or other agencies?

---

have not completed a high school education. There is a need to ascertain the specific problems of employed minorities and women and then initiate activities for them.

Employee Assistance Programs

Many corporations and companies have Employee Assistance Programs (EAPs) as part of their human resource management activities. These programs are designed to help employees define personal problems in their lives and to motivate them to act, thus bringing about effective and productive change. EAP counselors and community resources are brought together to assist the individual employee.

EAPs were originally developed to help those individuals with problems related to alcohol abuse. The recognition that alcohol abuse and alcoholism can have a serious detrimental effect on work productivity led to the establishment of EAPs. In more recent years the program focus has expanded to include help and support for employees with substance abuse problems, emotional problems,

burnout, family discord and personal relationship problems, job stress, eating disorders, and other factors affecting work performance.

Employee Assistance Programs help industry to save money and also promote the welfare of the employee. Because of their common program goals, EAPs and health promotion and wellness programs need to be brought together. A well-developed comprehensive employee health program should include services of an EAP.

Occupational Safety and Health Act

The data collected on job-related accidents resulting in fatalities, work-related disabilities, and the extent of occupation-related diseases led to the congressional passage of the Occupational Safety and Health Act (OSHA) in 1970. This federal legislation had as its goal a safe and healthful working environment for all employed men and women.

This goal was to be achieved through several programs. The act created a National Institute for Occupational Safety and Health (NIOSH). NIOSH conducts health hazard evaluations when requested by either industry or by individual workers. These evaluations involve a number of health-related problems and safety issues.

NIOSH, administered by the Department of Health and Human Services, the Centers for Disease Control and Prevention, is responsible for conducting research that leads to the establishment of occupational safety and health standards. After conducting the appropriate health hazard evaluation, NIOSH issues a report, including recommendations that must be followed. Since its inception in the early 1970s, the institute has issued some 130 criteria documents with over six hundred recommended exposure limits. Some criteria documents take several years to complete before they are made public. It would be impossible to identify all the health hazard evaluations conducted by NIOSH, but the following examples should indicate the types of requests made for such evaluations.

Employees working at a public roadway were tested for exposure to carbon monoxide, lead, sulfuric acid, particulate matter, benzene, and noise.[49] Hospital employees were tested for exposure to elementary mercury. Employees in a battery manufacturing plant were tested for exposure to lead, arsenic, sulfuric acid, benzene, and several lesser-known chemicals.

In one request by several workers, a survey found overexposure to inorganic lead. Recommendations were presented on personal hygiene and for the installation of an exhaust system.

Study of pneumoconiosis among coal miners has been an important program of NIOSH. The institute also investigates the effects of work-related traumas such as crushing injuries and injuries resulting in amputations.

Guidelines have been established designed to avoid trauma of the back in work-related circumstances. NIOSH has also conducted research on various cumulative trauma disorders. These include such conditions as shoulder problems, tendinitis, and carpal tunnel syndrome.

Often requests are made for health hazard evaluations where employees are experiencing certain signs and symptoms of illness. Such symptoms have included respiratory and gastrointestinal problems, headaches, nausea, and eye and throat irritation.

Research programs have been designed, conducted, and financed with respect to the numerous agents that are potentially hazardous. An outgrowth of such research was the establishment of specific exposure criteria for toxic materials and harmful physical agents in the workplace. The most obvious benefit of this research has been the determination of harmful levels of exposure by a specific agent and the measures needed to control the hazard. Agents such as asbestos, beryllium, carbon monoxide, noise, lead, mercury, benzene, and arsenic have been identified by the National Institute for Occupational Safety and Health for study and recommendation.

In 1987 the recommended exposure level for benzene was lowered. Standards were identified for short-term exposure, that is, a fifteen-minute period, and for long-term exposure, that is, an eight-hour period. Evidence that overexposure to this substance can result in blood diseases, particularly leukemia, led to concern about safe levels.

Employees have the right to file a complaint with the Occupational Safety and Health Administration (OSHA) and request an inspection if they feel that working conditions are unsafe or unhealthful. The act protects employees who make such requests from discharge or discrimination by the employer. OSHA will not release names of employees who submit a complaint about working conditions.

The Occupational Safety and Health Administration conducts worksite inspections of hazardous conditions and substances. These inspections identify safety hazards and evaluate the level of conformity to specified standards. OSHA inspections are conducted by compliance officers who have been specifically trained in the regulations developed as a result of the act.

It is impossible for OSHA compliance officers to inspect all worksites on an annual basis. In reality, it is possible to inspect only about 3 percent of American businesses each year.[50] As a result, OSHA has established a system of inspection priorities. A number-one priority is assigned to situations where there is imminent danger to the life or physical well-being of employees. A second priority is the inspection of a worksite where an accident resulted in death or the hospitalization of five or more employees. It is required by the law that whenever either of these situations occurs, OSHA must be informed within forty-eight hours. Employee complaints rank third in priority, and the fourth priority is random inspections.

OSHA inspections have created controversy. Many people oppose the inspections because OSHA compliance officers are often poorly prepared to understand the specific manufacturing process of a given industry. The penalty for failure to meet regulations has tended to be "soft." For example, inspectors cannot give penalties for first-offense, non-serious violations unless they are able to cite ten or more specific violations.

Congress passed legislation in 1991 designed to stiffen the OSHA inspection penalty system. The maximum allowable penalty for willful or repeated violations was increased from $10,000 to $70,000. Maximum penalties for each serious or other than serious violation was increased to $7,000 from $1,000. It is hoped that these increased monetary penalties will be more effective in having companies comply with OSHA regulations.

Legal opposition to the inspections has been raised, also. The issue involves the legality of OSHA compliance officers' inspecting a business or industrial establishment without a search warrant. Even police authorities must have a warrant before they can search a private home or business establishment. This concern was taken as far as the Supreme Court in 1978. In the Barlow case, which originated in Idaho, the owner of a plumbing and electrical supply store refused to permit a compliance officer to enter his place of business. The Supreme Court supported the store owner's right to refuse admission of a warrantless OSHA inspector to private premises. As a result of this decision, warrantless inspections cannot be carried out. However, once an authorized search warrant is issued, the OSHA inspectors may proceed.

Many other questions have been raised regarding whether the Occupational Safety and Health Act has achieved a significant impact on employee health and safety. It is very difficult to learn from a review of statistics how effective this legislation has been. There has been a slight reduction in the number of fatalities in worksite accidents since the passage of the act. However, the incidences of disabling injuries have remained about the same. Even though standards have been established for a number of toxic and potentially dangerous agents, there are still many other hazardous agents in the work environment.

Smaller businesses are not inspected by OSHA unless there is an accident. Employees of smaller businesses are less likely to complain of potential dangers in the workplace owing to the fear of losing their jobs. Smaller companies tend to be nonunionized and have fewer technical personnel to deal with possible dangerous substances in the workplace. Exposure to metals, chemicals, noise, and many safety deficiencies are often found in these settings. Lack of proper air ventilation can contribute to respiratory problems.

For example, individuals employed in dry cleaning establishments are often exposed to various cleaning solvents that can cause dermatitis. Most automobile body repair and paint shops employ a small number of employees, and the use of dust respirators is not always enforced in these shops. In addition, proper storage of flammable objects is not always practiced.

OSHA opponents feel that many of the regulations are arbitrary and often have little effect on the well-being of the employees. Without question, the act has resulted in additional administrative paperwork for businesses and industry. This, combined with the necessity to comply with measures mandated by the act, has increased costs. The increased costs have been passed on to the consumer and have contributed to inflation.

Supporters of OSHA point out that the private industrial sector has never been particularly effective in policing its own safety and health standards. Labor has been supportive of the Occupational Safety and Health Act and has opposed political efforts to eliminate the regulations or to radically change the act. Organized labor feels that the act ensures the rights of the working person and has built-in safeguards for better health and safety in the workplace.

Current political thinking is unclear regarding the authority of OSHA. Some believe it is inappropriate for the federal government to police private industry. Possibly, the federal government should suggest useful health and safety research, but the monitoring and establishing of regulations should be accomplished by state and local government, not by the federal government. Business and management have been particularly supportive of these changes.

With opposition to federal regulatory programs and tightened federal budgets for occupational safety and health programs, it is possible that the shape and emphasis of OSHA and NIOSH will change in the future. However, it is the position of others that the OSHA regulatory process must be accelerated and that stricter regulatory enforcement, including increased fines and better safety reporting, is needed. The form that occupational safety and health legislation will take in the remainder of the twentieth century is uncertain.

Summary

People are exposed to a variety of disease-causing agents and conditions, as well as accident situations, while at work. Though management and labor have attempted to reduce these problems, injury, death, and economic loss are still serious concerns in the American industrial and business world.

Occupation-related diseases often develop only after exposure to a substance over an extended period of time. Respiratory diseases, such as pneumoconiosis and asbestosis, cause the debilitation of thousands of workers. Work-related back injuries result in significant cost to industry. Skin diseases and damage to hearing due to continual exposure to loud noise over a long period of time are other health-related problems in the workplace.

Many individuals experience cumulative trauma disorders. These are musculoskeletal system injuries which result from repetitive movement over extensive periods of time. Several different conditions have been noted, particularly carpal tunnel syndrome.

Indoor air pollution has caused an increasing amount of sickness among people working in newer office and service buildings. A variety of physical conditions have been reported. Often finding the cause of these problems is difficult. The underlying cause tends to be inadequate exchange of clean air.

A number of health and safety services have been provided in an effort to improve employee well-being. Some companies provide clinical health services for their workers. Through these services, employees are provided preemployment and periodic medical examinations; or they may receive emergency care or rehabilitative services.

Four categories of occupational health and safety personnel are found in the workplace. The occupational physician usually serves as medical director of the company's health program. Some physicians are employed by industry on a full-time basis and others on a part-time or consultant basis. Occupational health nurses provide primary nursing care at the industrial worksite. Other occupational health and safety personnel include the industrial hygienist and the safety engineer.

Industry and business have become increasingly involved in developing health promotion programs. The emphasis in these efforts is to improve the health and well-being of the employees. Such developments should result in greater employee productivity, better morale, and economic benefits for the company. Corporate health promotion initiatives include programs of physical fitness, smoking cessation, alcoholism, drug and substance abuse, hypertension screening, nutrition and weight control, stress management, and health education.

Fatalities and unintentional injuries are all too common at the worksite. Accidents cause death, disability, and economic loss. Safety programs are varied and widespread throughout the industrial world.

In 1970 the United States Congress passed the Occupational Safety and Health Act. This legislation was established to provide for a safe and healthful working environment for all employed Americans. The act created a mechanism whereby numerous health and safety regulations were established. The Occupational Safety and Health Administration (OSHA) was established to monitor, inspect, and enforce federal health and safety regulations. In addition, the National Institute of Occupational Safety and Health (NIOSH) was established to conduct extensive research programs in occupational safety and health matters.

Discussion Questions

1. What should constitute the scope of an occupational health and safety program?
2. Discuss several of the occupational safety and health objectives for the nation to be achieved by the year 2000.
3. Explain the significance of the Americans with Disabilities Act for business and industry.
4. Identify some of the clinical services that are provided as part of an occupational health program.
5. Discuss some of the responsibilities that the occupational health nurse fulfills.
6. What are the roles of occupational physicians?
7. What is an industrial hygienist?
8. Explain the difference between a safety engineer and an industrial hygienist.
9. Why are skin diseases a particular concern in the occupational setting?
10. What are cumulative trauma disorders?
11. Explain the signs and symptoms associated with carpal tunnel syndrome.
12. What are some of the signs and symptoms noted in the condition referred to as "sick building syndrome"?
13. In what ways does the work-related environment cause different types of cancers?
14. Describe what might be included in a well-designed and executed industrial fitness program.
15. Why is alcoholism a problem in industry and business?
16. Should employees who smoke cigarettes be permitted to smoke at the worksite? Discuss the reasons you have for your answer.
17. What kinds of stress management activities do local industries in your community conduct for employees?
18. What relationships should be encouraged between an industry's food service department and a program of nutrition and weight control?
19. Discuss the effectiveness of worksite health promotion programs as reported in various studies.
20. Explain the scope of focus of Employee Assistance Programs.
21. In what ways should EAPs and worksite health promotion programs be working together?
22. What are some of the provisions of the Occupational Safety and Health Act?
23. Describe some of the responsibilities of the OSHA compliance officer.
24. Describe the significant outcome of the Barlow Decision made by the United States Supreme Court.
25. Explain changes in the OSHA penalty system implemented in 1991.
26. Do you believe that the Occupational Safety and Health Act should be strengthened or eliminated? Explain your answer.

Suggested Readings

Abramson, Leonard. "Boost to the Bottom Line." *Personnel Administrator* 33, no. 7 (July 1988): 36–39.

Banning, Margaret N. "The Occupational Health Nursing Puzzle." *Ohio Monitor* 59, no. 4 (April 1986): 4–7.

Bezold, Clement, Rick J. Carlson, and Jonathan C. Peck. *The Future of Work and Health*. Auburn House Publishing Company, 1985.

Blair, Brenda R. "EAPS: Essential Elements and Approaches." *Health Values* 13, no. 1 (January/February 1989): 28–31.

Brody, Bruce E. "Employee Assistance Programs: An Historical and Literature Review." *American Journal of Health Promotion* 2, no. 3 (Winter 1988): 13–19.

Connors, Nancy. "Wellness Promotes Healthier Employees." *Business and Health* 10, no. 3 (1992): 66–71.

Coughlin, Kenneth M. "Expanding Employee Assistance Programs Is Paying Dividends." *Business and Health* 10, no. 9 (1992): 45–49.

Dedmon, R. E., and others. "Employees as Health Educators: A Reality at Kimberly-Clark." *Occupational Health and Safety* 49, no. 4 (April 1980): 18–24.

Falkenberg, Loren E. "Employee Fitness Programs: Their Impact on the Employee and the Organization." *Academy of Management Review* 12, no. 3 (July 1987): 511–22.

Feldman, Robert H. L. "Worksite Health Promotion, Labor Unions, and Social Support." *Health Education* 20, no. 6 (October/November 1989): 55–56.

Fielding, Jonathan E. "Banning Worksite Smoking." *American Journal of Public Health* 76, no. 8 (August 1986): 957–59.

Friedman, James M., and Todd S. Davis. "Controlling Pollution of Indoor Office Air." *Occupational Health and Safety* 61, no. 9 (September 1992): 16–22.

Grzelka, Constance. "Smoking at Work: No Ifs, Ands, or Butts." *Health Link* 2, no. 1 (March 1986): 39–41.

Ham, Faith Lyman. "How Companies Are Making Wellness a Family Affair." *Business and Health* 7, no. 9 (September 1989): 27–32.

Hebert, Lauren A. "Body at Work." *Occupational Health and Safety* 61, no. 10 (November/December 1992): 48–58.

Henritze, Joanne, and H. L. Brammell. "Phase II Cardiac Wellness at the Adolph Coors Company." *American Journal of Health Promotion* 4, no. 1 (September/October 1989): 25–31.

Lawton, Bryan. "EAPs in the 1990s: Challenges and Opportunities." *Health Values* 13, no. 1 (January/February 1989): 43–45.

Massachusetts Medical Society. "Leading Work-Related Diseases and Injuries—United States." *Morbidity and Mortality Weekly Report* 35, no. 12 (March 28, 1986): 185–87.

Millar, Donald. "NIOSH Director Millar Speaks Out on Trends in the Health and Safety Industry." *Occupational Health and Safety* 61, no. 10 (October 1992): 26–27.

Myerson, William A., and Joel Farb. "EAPs: Essential Elements and Approaches." *Health Values* 13, no. 1 (January/February 1989): 28–31.

"Occupational Disease Surveillance: Carpal Tunnel Syndrome." *Morbidity and Mortality Weekly Report* 38, no. 28 (July 21, 1989): 485–89.

Ostwald, Sharon K. "Changing Employees' Dietary and Exercise Practices: An Experimental Study in a Small Company." *Journal of Occupational Medicine* 31, no. 2 (February 1989): 90–97.

Parkinson, Rebecca S., and others. *Managing Health Promotion in the Workplace.* Palo Alto, Calif.: Mayfield Publishing Company, 1982.

Pender, Nola J. "Health Promotion in the Workplace: Suggested Directions for Research." *American Journal of Health Promotion* 3, no. 3 (Winter 1989): 38–43.

Penner, Maurice. "Economic Incentives to Reduce Employee Smoking: A Health Insurance Surcharge for Tobacco Using State of Kansas Employees." *American Journal of Health Promotion* 4, no. 1 (September/October 1989): 5–11.

Polakoff, Philip L. "Ergonomics: Diagnosis and Treatment for Ailing Workplace Performance." *Occupational Health and Safety* 61, no. 10 (October 1992): 64–66.

Rekus, John F. "Lead Poisoning." *Occupational Safety and Health* 61, no. 8 (August 1992): 14–26.

Schilling, Robert F., and others. "Smoking in the Workplace: Review of Critical Issues." *Public Health Reports* 100, no. 5 (September/October 1985): 473–79.

Smith, R. Blake. "OSHA Reform." *Occupational Health and Safety* 61, no. 8 (August 1992): 30–34.

Sundin, David S., and others. "Occupational Hazard and Health Surveillance." *American Journal of Public Health* 76, no. 9 (September 1986): 1083–84.

Tichy, Anna Mae. "Wellness, the Worker and the Nurse." *Occupational Health Nursing* 29, no. 2 (February 1981): 21–23.

Tuskes, Paul M., and Marcus M. Key. "Potential Hazards in Small Business—A Gap in OSHA Protection." *Applied Industrial Hygiene* 3, no. 2 (February 1988): 55–57.

United States House of Representatives, Committee on Government Operations. *Occupational Illness Data Collection: Fragmented, Unreliable, and Seventy Years Behind Communicable Disease Surveillance.* Washington, D.C.: U.S. Government Printing Office, 1984.

Wagener, Diane K., and Deborah W. Winn. "Injuries in Working Populations: Black-White Differences." *American Journal of Public Health* 81, no. 11 (November 1991): 1408–14.

White, Peggy. "Does Employee Fitness Decrease Employee Absenteeism and Medical Cost?" *Health Matrix: The Quarterly Journal of Health Services* 5, no. 4 (Winter 1987–88): 10–15.

Wood, E. Andrew, and others. "An Evaluation of Lifestyle Risk Factors and Absenteeism after Two Years in a Worksite Health Promotion Program." *American Journal of Health Promotion* 4, no. 2 (November/December 1989): 128–33.

Endnotes

1. Data is from National Safety Council, *Accident Facts, 1993.* Chicago, Ill.: National Safety Council, 1993, p. 35.

2. *Ibid.,* 34.

3. *Ibid.,* 34.

4. Martin, Jack. "The Business Boom—Employee Fitness." *Nation's Business* (February, 1978): 68–73.

5. American Medical Association. "Scope, Objectives, and Functions of Occupational Health Programs." Chicago: American Medical Association, 1971.

6. Americans with Disabilities Act of 1990, sec. 102 (c).

7. *Federal Register.* June 20, 1986, 22612–790.

8. Department of Health, Education, and Welfare. *Healthy People: The Surgeon General's Report on Health Promotion and Disease Prevention.* Washington, D.C.: U.S. Government Printing Office, 1979, p. 397.

9. Lee, Jane. *The New Nurse in Industry.* Washington, D.C.: U.S. Government Printing Office, 1978.

10. Banning, Margaret N. "The Occupational Health Nursing Puzzle." *Ohio Monitor* 59, no. 4 (April 1986): 4–7.

11. Department of HEW, *Healthy People,* 390.

12. Department of Health and Human Services. *Promoting Health/Preventing Disease: Objectives for the Nation, Fall, 1980.* Washington, D.C.: U.S. Government Printing Office, 1980, p. 39.

13. U.S. House of Representatives, Committee on Government Operations. *Occupational Illness Data Collection: Fragmented, Unreliable, and Seventy Years Behind Communicable Disease Surveillance.* Washington, D.C.: U.S. Government Printing Office, 1984.

14. Sundin, David S., and others. "Occupational Hazard and Health Surveillance." *American Journal of Public Health* 76, no.1 (September 1986): 1083–84.

15. Department of Health and Human Services, *Promoting Health/Preventing Disease,* 39.

16. *Ibid.*

17. Goldberg, Henry M. "Diagnosis and Management of Low Back Pain." *Occupational Health and Safety* 49, no. 6 (June 1980): 14.

18. Department of Health and Human Services. *Healthy People 2000: National Health Promotion and Disease Prevention Objectives.* Washington, D.C.: U.S. Government Printing Office, 1991, p. 300.

19. Woodford, Charles M. "Noise-Induced Hearing Loss." *Occupational Health and Safety Physician* 50, no. 3 (March 1981): 62.

20. Friedman, James M., and Todd S. Davis. "Controlling Pollution of Indoor Office Air." *Occupational Health and Safety* 61, no. 9 (September 1992): 18.

21. Chenoweth, David. "Risk-Reduction Strategies Improve Industrial Completions." *Occupational Health and Safety Physician* 50, no. 4 (April 1981): 22.

22. Payne, Mike. "Cancer: How Many Lives Lost?" *Ohio Monitor* 62, no. 10 (October 1989): 8.

23. Department of HEW, *Healthy People,* 390–91.

24. *Ibid.,* 390–91.

25. Grzelka, Constance. "Smoking at Work: No Ifs, Ands, or Butts." *Health Link* 2, no. 1 (March 1986): 39–41.

26. National Safety Council, *Accident Facts, 1993,* 34.

27. *Ibid.,* 34.

28. *Ibid.,* 35.

29. "Health Promotion Initiatives." *Business and Health* 10, no. 10 (1992): 18.

30. Hitchings, Bradley. "The Healthy Trend Toward Corporate Exercise Programs." *Business Week* (April 3, 1978): 91.

31. American Association of Fitness Directors in Business and Industry, 700 Anderson Hill Road, Purchase, New York.

32. "Kimberly-Clark Health Management Program Aimed at Prevention." *Occupational Health and Safety* 46, no. 6 (November/December 1977): 25–27.

33. Henritze, Joanne, and H. L. Brammell. "Phase II Cardiac Wellness at the Adolph Coors Company." *American Journal of Health Promotion* 4, no. 1 (September/October 1989): 25–31.

34. "As Companies Jump on Fitness Bandwagon." *U.S. News and World Report* (January 28, 1980): 36–39.

35. Nancy Connors. "Wellness Promotes Healthier Employees." *Business and Health* 10, no. 3 (1992): 66–71.

36. Chamber of Commerce of the United States. *How Business Can Protect Good Health for Employers and Their Families.* Washington, D.C.: National Chamber Foundation, 1978, p. 13.

37. "Solving the Problem of the Drinking Worker." *Occupational Health and Safety* 48, no. 1 (January/February 1970): 43.

38. Schramm, Carl J. "Measuring the Return on Program Costs: Evaluation of Multi-Employer Alcoholism Treatment Program." *American Journal of Public Health* 67, no. 1 (January 1977): 51.

39. Reported in *Occupational Safety and Health* (May 1970): 31.

40. Bennett, Diane, and Barry S. Levy. "Smoking Policies and Smoking Cessation Programs of Large Employers in Massachusetts." *American Journal of Public Health* 70, no. 6 (June 1980): 630.

41. *Ibid.,* 630.

42. Thompson, E. L. "Smoking Education Programs, 1960–1976." *Public Health* 68 (1978): 250–57.

43. Penn, Ann C. "Finding the Silent Killer: High Blood Pressure." *Job Safety and Health* 4, no. 10 (October 1976): 16–22.

44. Henry Forbush Howe. "Organization and Operation of Occupational Health Program." *Journal of Occupational Medicine* 17, no. 6 (June 1975): 367.

45. Wagstaff, B. "Executive Health Update." *Dunn's Business Month* 128, no. 1 (1986): 50–54.

46. Wood, E. Andrew, and others. "An Evaluation of Lifestyle Risk Factors and Absenteeism after Two Years in a Worksite Health Promotion Program." *American Journal of Health Promotion* 4, no. 2 (November/December 1989): 133.

47. Ham, Faith Lyman. "How Companies Are Making Wellness a Family Affair." *Business and Health* 7, no. 9 (September 1989): 27–32.

48. *Ibid.,* 30.

49. Examples presented in this section are taken from *Health Hazard Evaluation Summaries, May 1981,* publication of the National Institute of Occupational Safety and Health, Cincinnati, Ohio.

50. Bingham, Eula. "What OSHA Expects of Physicians Serving in the Industrial Community." *Journal of Occupational Medicine* 20, no. 12 (December 1978): 818–19.

CHAPTER **TWENTY-THREE**

Violence

Interpersonal Actions Needing Community Health Services

Throughout the history of humankind, violence has had a major impact on people's lives. Death and debilitation resulting from natural phenomenon, warfare, and interpersonal violence have affected millions of individuals. Violence not only results in debilitation and death, but it often leads to upheaval in the personal lives of those affected. Violence results in more than physical injury. It may produce psychological problems with which individuals must cope for the remainder of their lives. Numerous social problems necessitating community action are created by violence. Violence is closely related to poverty, lack of employment, fear, misuse of alcohol and drugs, as well as the loss of personal material possessions.

Interpersonal violence results from those actions between people on a personal basis. It is this type of violence that is more commonly seen by community health personnel in the United States. Interpersonal violence may occur in a number of different settings, involving strangers as well as family members and close acquaintances.

Interpersonal Violence and Community Health

No one agency or organization has total responsibility for solving problems related to interpersonal violence in our society. Current services for victims of abuse are fragmented and often inadequate. A number of different kinds of professionals become involved in working with the victims of violence as well as those responsible for violent actions. One agency may treat the physical injuries of the abused while another may provide legal advice; another may provide shelter and council; yet others may provide financial help.

Often law enforcement personnel are the principal individuals to deal with acts of violence. The judicial system comes into play as charges are brought against the person who commits the act. Personnel in the various social service fields must provide help, assistance, and counsel to both the abused and the abuser. Therefore, the need exists for a multidisciplinary approach in coping with the problems of interpersonal violence.

Violence is an increasing concern within the field of community health. Health care personnel and other workers in the various fields of community health must learn how to prevent or deal with the many different kinds of abuse and violence. Health care providers often are required to respond to the physical wounds left by violence. Emergency room personnel in hospitals need to know how to help the victims of violence. They must be able to treat all forms of injuries associated with violence. Health care providers must know how to recognize the indicators of violent behavior. It is important that they learn how to diagnose potential abuse victims and help the victims deal with the psychological, emotional, and social stigma attached to the abusive situation.

In order for health care providers to be more effective in providing services to the victims of violence it has become necessary to develop professional in-service programs. The American Hospital Association, the American Medical Association, and the Educational Development Center of Massachusetts have combined to establish a series of activities designed to help health care providers better identify and treat victims of abuse. An increasing number of health care institutions are joining forces to provide help and services to those who are abused. Also, the American Medical Association has published diagnostic and treatment guidelines on domestic abuse. Among the several different emphases of these guidelines is help for the interviewing process, a skill often lacking in the training of health care providers. The Nursing Network on Violence Against Women has been conducting national multidisciplinary conferences on prevention and treatment strategies for several years.

Although the epidemiological model has been used in identifying the etiological factors of abuse, a need exists for more reliable and valid data. Unfortunately, accurate data are unavailable since most interpersonal violence is greatly underreported. Health care personnel need to know what types of questions to ask, what physical and emotional signs to look for, and how to help the victim recover from both the physical and the emotional wounds.

The importance of including acts of violence in health promotion and disease prevention programming

National Health Objectives for the Year 2000

Violence

1. The death rate from homicide should be reduced. Special note is given to homicides among African-American and Hispanic males between the ages of fifteen and thirty-four.
2. Suicides should be reduced, with special note of teenagers, males between the ages of twenty and thirty-four, elderly males, and Native Americans.
3. Fatalities resulting from the use of firearms should be reduced.
4. Injuries and deaths to children inflicted by abusing parents should be reduced.
5. Incidences of rape should be reduced, with special note given to women between the ages of twelve and thirty-four.

Source: Department of Health and Human Services. *Healthy People 2000: National Health Promotion and Disease Prevention Objectives.* Washington, D.C.: U.S. Government Printing Office, 1991, pp. 228–34.

and planning was noted in the Year 2000 Objectives for the Nation. Specific objectives relating to homicide, child abuse, suicide, rape, personal assault, and firearms injury were included.[1]

The family is often perceived as an environment that is a safe haven for most individuals. Ideally, the home should be a place where love, understanding, and support can be found. However, violence within the domestic setting has become an increasing problem to society. In the past, familial problems usually were kept isolated from the public. With increased openness about such problems, child abuse, spouse abuse, and elder abuse have become major health and social concerns.

Child Abuse

One of the most rapidly expanding social and community health problems in America today is child abuse. Some cases of child abuse are easily recognized: the small child with multiple bruises on the face or the infant with doughnut-shaped burns on the buttocks. On the other hand, there are numerous other more subtle forms of abuse that rarely come to the attention of authorities. This form of abuse may include verbal abuse, overly strict discipline, or poor supervision and negligence. All are factors that need the attention of personnel working in the fields of education, community health, and social work today.

Although the exact extent of child abuse is impossible to determine, government data indicates that somewhere between one and four million children suffer some type of child abuse each year. Many of these children experience long-term physical and emotional scarring or even die. It is estimated that two thousand to five thousand children die each year from child abuse.

Children who are abused are always negatively affected by these experiences. Not only do they often come to accept the abusive actions as being normal behavior, but they often carry such behavior into other relationships. Abused children are likely to strike, hit, or exhibit other abusive behavioral patterns in their relationships with schoolmates, brothers and sisters, and other acquaintances. All too often they become abusive parents when they grow up.

Forms of Abuse

The forms of abuse vary. The most prominent and identifiable is *physical abuse.* This type of abuse is manifested by the presence of bruises, lacerations, fractures, burns on various parts of the body, and in a variety of other ways. *Child neglect* is a more difficult problem to identify. Generally, neglect refers to failure by parents or guardians to provide the child with minimum needs such as food, health care, shelter, clothing, and other necessities. The third form of abuse is *sexual abuse;* another form is *emotional abuse.*

Physical Abuse

Younger children are more likely than older children to be physically abused. They may be beaten, kicked, thrown about, or handled in such a way that physical injury and disability occur. Bruises, wounds, burns, lacerations, and abrasions, dental damage, and skeletal and head injuries are often indicators of physical abuse. Such mistreatment can lead to brain damage, mental retardation, or a variety of other psychological and emotional problems.

However, not all injuries resulting from physical abuse are noticeable immediately by medical or social agency personnel. Head injuries may be accompanied by hemorrhaging beneath the scalp and retinal hemorrhages or detachments in the eye. Internal injuries, such as rupture of interior organs, may result from hitting or kicking.

Child Neglect

Child neglect is a rather difficult problem with which to cope. Neglect takes on a variety of different patterns. Often neglect does not produce visible signs. The indications of child neglect usually occur over a period of time. During this time span the child is experiencing many emotionally disturbing relationships that have a negative impact on his or her growth and development. While neglect is found among all ages of children, most cases of adolescent abuse involve neglect rather than physical harm.[2]

Child neglect may take a number of different patterns. It may be neglect in the form of social isolation. The child is not permitted to socialize, play, and interact with children as is normal. Without the opportunity for social interaction while growing up, the child finds it impossible to develop positive and meaningful relationships with others in society. This often leads to many antisocial behaviors.

Neglect takes the form of failure to care for the physical needs of the child. This may be seen when the caretakers—parents or guardians—fail to provide adequate food, clothing, or hygienic measures. Lack of adequate nutrition and good hygiene can lead to chronic communicable diseases and illnesses. The child is unable to function in school owing to the presence of fatigue, colds, restlessness, or other socially unapproved patterns.

Child neglect in whatever form may be purposeful or circumstantial. It may result from the purposeful attempt to discipline the child. The parent may consider withholding food or other necessities as a means of correcting the child. Neglectful behaviors may be the result of anger, distress, and frustration of the parent generated by the child's behavior. Neglect may also stem from environmental circumstances including long-term parental illness, poverty, and marital discord. Alcoholism, overcrowding in the home, and prolonged absence of one parent are common environmental factors associated with child neglect.

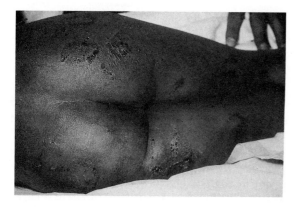

Extensive medical care and social work assistance brought this individual back to normal health. The emotional scars of the beating lasted longer than the physical wounds.

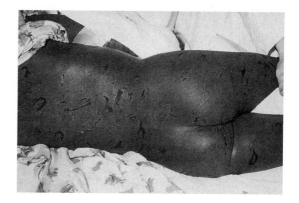

The most common kind of physical abuse of children results from beatings using belts and extension cords. These injuries are often found over several parts of the body. This boy had belt and extension cord injuries over the back and the thigh.

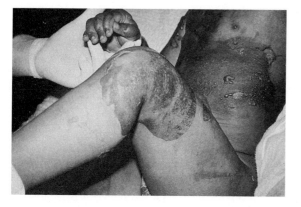

A serious type of physical abuse of children is burns. Often the abusing adult will put the child in scalding water or will place other hot substances against the child. Burns result in trauma, such as pain and infection.

The child who has been neglected will often exhibit certain behavioral indicators such as falling asleep in school, poor achievement and attendance at school, chronic hunger or fatigue, a dull apathetic appearance, socially unacceptable behavioral practices, and the use of drugs, alcohol, and tobacco. Unfortunately, child neglect goes unnoticed for long periods of time. It may not be recognized by authorities who can be helpful to the child until some physical indicators are manifested or until emotional disturbances are noticed.

Sexual Abuse

Considerable concern has been directed at the problem of sexual abuse among school age children. Victims of this type of abuse may be males or females of almost any age; however, younger adolescent females are particularly vulnerable. Sexual abuse, though occurring predominantly among adolescents, has even been reported among both male and female children of primary school age. This form of abuse is most likely initiated by a parent, guardian, or caretaker, usually a father or male relative; it is referred to by several different terms: incest, family sexual abuse, molestation, and child sexual victimization.

Sexual abuse of children by family members means using a minor child for sexual gratification of an adult or older child. Intercourse need not occur. Most cases involve genital manipulation, indecent exposure, and use of obscene language.

The magnitude of sexual abuse in the United States is uncertain. It is assumed that it is greatly underreported, leading to a lack of reliable incidence data. This underreporting of sexual abuse stems from the reluctance of most abused to follow through to prosecution. Statistics that are used in analyzing sexual abuse of children have been obtained primarily from court records. Because of the family connections, victims of sexual abuse seldom report it. This may be out of fear of retaliation by one's parents, guardians, or caretakers. Or it may not be considered unsatisfactory behavior, particularly among small children.

A basic problem associated with sexual abuse is the violation of trust that the child has had in the family. The normal processes of child development have been disrupted. Betrayal of trust, feelings of violation, and negative identity formation are noted among sexual abuse victims. Clinical studies also reveal a deep sense of low self-esteem among the abused.[3] These poor self-concepts are manifested in depression and withdrawal.

Sexual abuse causes serious psychological problems for the abused. Victims often suppress their feelings and memories of the incident. There are varying degrees of feelings of guilt, fear, anger, shame, physical pain, confusion, and depression. Often a decline in academic performance, increased involvement in substance abuse, and runaway behavior are seen in individuals who have been sexually abused.

One indication that a child is being sexually abused is expression of fear for no apparent reason. Anger and hostility may be shown toward others in daily activities. Sometimes the sexually abused child is unable to express his or her feelings adequately, and depression may be present.

Problems with sexual attitudes and behavior often follow the incidences of child sexual abuse. For victims, sexual behavior often is manifested in either a total aversion to sex or promiscuity.[4] Many individuals who have been molested sexually as children experience chronic sexual dysfunction as adults.

Unfortunately, child abuse is often a hidden problem. A very small percentage of the abused see appropriate health or social service agencies. The abused should be encouraged to openly confront the problem. Counseling needs to be provided to help break the silence concerning the abuse.

The 1984 amendments to the Federal Child Abuse Prevention and Treatment Act mandated that information about incest be disclosed to local child protective services agencies. As such, the health profession must report children who have been identified as having been molested sexually by parents, guardians, or caretakers. These reports are to be made to the local police authorities or to the child protective services agency. As a result,

health care workers, educational personnel, and social agency professionals should be trained to identify, collect, and document evidence of sexual molestation.

Emotional Abuse

This form of abuse usually involves continual degrading interactions with the individual child. Children who are constantly told that their actions are inappropriate, that they can never do something satisfactorily, or who have little feeling of success are emotionally abused. Parental behavior that is psychologically destructive to the child can be a very difficult problem.

A number of family social patterns often lead to this type of abuse. Such measures as ongoing friction in the home between the parents and the child, excessive drinking and arguing by the parents, frequent marriages and/or broken homes, and promiscuity and/or prostitution are commonly identified with emotional abuse. The child who is emotionally abused will manifest a variety of different behaviors such as hyperactivity, withdrawal, nervous skin disorders, psychosomatic disorders, and stuttering. Suicidal behavior, truancy, delinquency, and increase in substance abuse are often noted.

Causes of Child Abuse

The specific cause of child abuse or child neglect is too complex to identify. It is only possible to identify general characteristics of abusing parents. Various socioeconomic stresses affect abusing parents. Alcoholism and drug abuse are related to this problem, too. Many parents who have abused or neglected their children have a poor self-concept as well as unrealistic expectations about the development of the child. Child abuse often results in situations where parents are in conflict over child custody and visitation in cases involving divorce and separation. Very young parents are more likely to be child abusers.

Child abusers often do not have realistic expectations about the behavior of their children. They fail to understand the normal needs and developmental patterns of children at various ages. They often believe in extreme disciplinary patterns. These individuals tend to overlook the cries for help and attention that the child gives.

Other factors that have been associated with child abusers include use of substances of abuse, poverty, and unemployment. As many as three-fourths of adults who abuse children are alcohol and/or drug abusers. Though poverty doesn't cause child abuse, it does contribute to stressful situations that lead to abusive actions. The same is true of unemployment. As unemployment increases, so is the likelihood increased of there being child abuse.

Many people have no training in parenting. Specific knowledge of child development would aid all parents, but especially those prone to child abuse. Community agencies, schools, churches, and community health agencies should provide educational opportunities for parents to learn effective parenting strategies.

Child Abuse Intervention Programs

Measures that can help reduce and/or prevent child abuse are necessary. In response to that need, many community programs and agencies have been established. In addition, legal mandates relating to child abuse have been passed.

Protective and Preventive Services

A number of protective and preventive measures are available in many communities to help both the abused and the abuser. The principal agency in most communities responding to child abuse and neglect is the Child Protective Services agency. Child Protective Services are usually found in city, county, or state departments of social welfare or social services. These agencies will evaluate reports of cases of child abuse and neglect and provide necessary services. Such services include foster home care, social worker counseling with the abusers, early childhood educational programs for maltreated children, and classes in parenting.

Telephone hot lines have been established where adults can call for assistance, counseling, and help when feelings are present that could result in abuse. Often the availability of someone to talk with at times of stress can prevent an abusive action. These hot lines have also been useful for children and adolescents following abuse. These services provide someone who can be trusted at a time of trauma.

Some child abuse agencies provide the service of caring for a child at times when stressful situations may be conducive to abusive actions. When a parent is under stress due to unemployment or during a bout with alcohol, it may be best for the child to be removed from the home for a period of time.

A variety of programs and self-help activities can be found in many communities to help parents who have abused their children. One such self-help organization, known as Parents Anonymous, assists parents in solving this problem. Through the process of group dynamics and interaction, parents gain self-esteem, and social isolation is reduced. These activities help parents to overcome the problems that led to their abusive action.

An interesting program designed to assist at-risk parents with home visitor services is the Healthy Families America program. This program, launched in 1992 by the National Committee for Prevention of Child Abuse, makes use of trained, voluntary individuals to work with new parents beginning at their child's birth. Home education and support services are then provided for a period of time, some extending for the first four or five years.

This program, now operational in more than half of the states, is modeled after a program established in Hawaii in 1985 by the Hawaii Family Stress Center. The Hawaiian program is conducted within the services of the Maternal and Child Health Program of the Department of Health. New at-risk parents are visited by paraprofessionals beginning in the hospital at the time of birth. Visits continue on a weekly basis as needed for several years. The visits are voluntary; any parent can decline the services of this program.

Several risk factors have been identified for inclusion in this program. They include unemployment; single, separated, or divorced marital status; inadequate income; less than twelve years of education; history of substance abuse, psychiatric care, or marital problems; and unstable housing.

In Hawaii more than 50 percent of the new parent population is now being served by this program. After

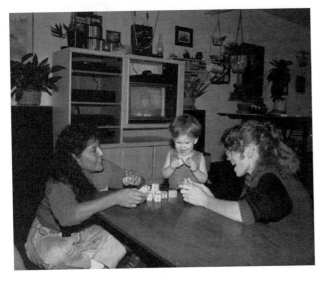

The Healthy Families America program provides voluntary in-home counseling for parents at risk for abusing their children. Counselors provide education, support, and an outlet for the inherent frustrations of parenting. Courtesy of the Healthy Families America Program. Photographer Tim L. Walker

four years of the program it was reported that no case of child abuse was reported by individuals involved in the program.[5]

It is anticipated that various combinations of state and local public agencies in cooperation with private agencies will form partnerships to work together to replicate the Hawaiian model. Pilot programs are being established with the hope of institutionalizing this model in child abuse prevention initiatives.

Legislation

All fifty states plus Washington, D.C., have mandatory reporting regulations for child abuse. Under provisions of federal legislation passed in 1974, the Child Abuse Prevention and Treatment Act, state laws regarding child abuse must cover both mental and physical injury. Legal immunity must be granted to those who report abuse and neglect. Coverage of such state legislation must include all children under the age of eighteen. The Child Abuse Prevention and Treatment Act provided funds for states to develop and implement programs to protect children. It also created the National Center on Child Abuse and Neglect, an agency within the Department of Health and

Human Services, which serves as a clearinghouse on programs relating to child abuse and neglect.

Though there are some differences in the specific legislative mandates from one state to another, most require that individuals working with children who have been abused report such incidents to appropriate authorities. School personnel, social workers, and health and medical personnel are the individuals most likely to have access to early warning signs of child abuse. In spite of concern by many professionals who wish not to become involved in these cases, it is felt that such state child abuse laws have been helpful. At the very least, they have led to increased public awareness concerning the magnitude of this problem.

Despite legislation mandating the report of suspected abuse, many instances of abuse are never recognized by school authorities, police, medical professionals, or community authorities. Many times it is not until a child is severely injured or even killed that the case comes to the attention of the legal and social authorities in a community. Many community health workers who have direct contact with families are the first to suspect or identify abuse and neglect.

Role of Schools

Because the schools play an important role in the well-being of children, school personnel must be able to identify incidences of child abuse. Educators have been slow to report child abuse except in the most severe cases. Reasons for this include fear of getting involved, reluctance to interfere in personal family matters, fear of being sued, and not knowing how and what to do.

Teachers must be aware of the pressures on young people and how to respond and assist those in need. In 1988 New York state passed legislation that requires teachers to receive two hours of in-service education regarding the identification of child abuse and how to help these children. This type of in-service training should become more widespread throughout the nation among all groups who work with children and adolescents, not just teachers.

Child abuse and sexual abuse prevention program curriculum packages are being developed throughout the nation by school districts and voluntary health agencies. Generally these curricula include in-service training to help the teachers. They need to be better informed about the various indicators of abuse and reporting procedures. Teachers also need to be encouraged to talk with students experiencing abuse and neglect.

These curriculum models also include instruction for children. Children should be taught problem-solving skills. They should be encouraged to talk with trusting adults about their feelings when in an abusive situation. Also, children must be taught how to refrain from becoming involved in circumstances that can result in child and/or sexual abuse.

In order for a curriculum package to be successful, parents need to be included. Parents must become informed about the indications of abuse. They must be made aware of the services available in the community to assist them as they are confronted with the possibility of abusing their children.

Spouse Abuse

Domestic or family violence is a very difficult problem to cope with in American society. When the matter of domestic violence or spouse abuse is considered, usually the problem involves situations where the male takes abusive action against the female. Though there are increasing reports of females abusing males, the typical pattern is for the woman to be the victim. Wife abuse occurs among all ages and is found within all social groups. Women who are most likely to be abused are very young teenage wives, those who are pregnant, and those with small children.

The extent to which spouse abuse occurs in the United States is very difficult to ascertain. It has been estimated that half of American families experience some form of violence.[6] Spouse abuse occurs at least once in two-thirds of all marriages. Half of those men who do beat their wives do so three or more times a year.[7] As many as 20 percent of the adult population may be involved in spouse abuse.[8]

In spite of the statistics, there is little doubt that spouse abuse is greatly underreported. The abused often refuse to report owing to fear, guilt, and/or shame. Embarrassment also keeps many abused individuals from reporting the incidents. Often the abused have a sense of low self-esteem and lack a support system. For some individuals the abusing situation is perceived to be normal behavior.

Spouse abuse often is referred to as the "battered wife syndrome." This syndrome usually takes one of three different forms: (1) physical abuse, (2) psychological abuse, or (3) sexual abuse. The battered wife syndrome may be the outgrowth of any intimate male-female relationship; it is not limited to legal husbands.

Physical abuse occurs when there is a physical and/or verbal dominance by the abuser over the abused. It usually involves action such as slapping, hitting, and kicking the victim. It also may involve shoving the person into something or down stairs. Physical abuse may also include the use of a dangerous weapon such as a gun, knife, or bat. This kind of abuse arouses a deep sense of fear in the abused. Often the first evidence of abuse involves bruises, fractures, and lacerations. The abused woman is hesitant to talk about the injuries. She may present some rather vague complaints and explanations as to why and how the injuries occurred.

Psychological abuse is different in that the indicators are not as readily observable as they are in cases of physical abuse. Threats made by the abuser may occur over a long period of time. This creates an atmosphere of fear. In other cases the woman may not be permitted appropriate social interaction. The male may not permit the female to socialize with certain groups, often where other males are part of the social activity. The male may isolate his wife, or lover, from her friends and relatives.

Every individual, male and female, has certain emotional needs. Abuse may occur when the abused fails to meet the emotional needs of the spouse. Psychological abuse tends to weaken the support system of the abused. This individual, usually the female, becomes more docile and is forced to depend more on the spouse. There is a destruction of the woman's self-worth and the creation of deep dependency upon the man. Independence is destroyed.

Sexual abuse of women by husbands or long-term lovers is a significant problem. Such abuse involves intercourse characterized by force, by threat of force, or by an inability of the woman to consent. Spouse abuse often is reported in the form of deviant sexual acts and marital rape, which occurs when the male forces the wife to have intercourse against her will. There have been some questions as to whether rape can occur in a husband-wife relationship. However, in recent years marital rape has had legal definition and is now punishable by law in some states.

All too often the abused female develops a "learned helplessness."[9] The woman believes that she has no power to change her life and that no one can help her. In her thinking she has lost control over her life. Guilt often develops, and she comes to blame herself for the abusive situation. A similar pattern is noted in an enforced loyalty to the aggressor; the female exaggerates her husband's good qualities.

Men who are most likely to abuse women usually have serious personal adjustment problems. They may be jealous and insecure, which leads to the various actions of social isolation and psychological abuse that are commonly seen. Males who do not trust their wives are often abusive. Men who are unable to become emotionally intimate with their wives tend to become abusive. It has been shown that many male abusers were abused themselves as children and come from families where there was spouse abuse. Further, males are at increased risk for spouse abuse when there is a high level of alcohol use. As a result, these males exhibit signs of depression and psychosis.

It is difficult for the abused female to leave the situation in which she finds herself. There are a number of risks involved in any escape attempt, not the least of which is fear and guilt. The insecurity found in most abused females adds to the difficulty of escaping the situation. Some have been killed, as well.

Assistance for Domestic Abuse

In an attempt to help the battered woman, or abused male, laws are needed and community services are necessary. Presently forty-three states as well as Washington, D.C., have laws that allow battered women to receive civil protection independent of domestic relation proceedings.[10] A victim does not have to file for divorce or separation in order to receive protection under the law.

Community shelters and protective environments for the abused female need to be available. Spouse abuse agencies should provide economic, social, legal, physical, and mental health services. When a woman is in danger of being abused, there should be a place where protection can be sought, where the abused will be understood, where help can be provided, and where the woman can reside until the conditions are acceptable for her to return to her home. It is important that a woman victim be helped as much as possible by a female advocate.

Stalking

The term *stalking* has been applied to a situation in which a person engages in a pattern of conduct that causes another individual to believe that the offender is likely to cause physical harm. Victims of domestic violence often have experienced threat, trespass, harassment, and menacing by their abuser for a period of time. Until actual injury or fatality occurs, law enforcement officers have had little legal authority upon which to act to provide protection for the victim.

Most stalking is done by men and involves spouses, ex-spouses, or boyfriends. There have been reports of the gender roles being reversed. Also there have been reports in which a female has threatened another female in a dispute over a boyfriend.

Stalking takes several forms: violation of court orders restraining one from visiting the residence of the abused, following the individual to various locations, hiding in bushes around the house, hiding in closets within the house, or causing the abused to believe the abuser will cause physical harm or mental distress.

Many law enforcement agencies feel that a need exists for legislation that will provide protection for victims of domestic violence where there is reasonable cause to believe that an individual is in potential danger. In 1990, California became the first state to pass an anti-stalking law. Since then several other states have enacted laws that prohibit a person from repeatedly following and harassing another individual. Generally, these laws make it possible to arrest and detain persons suspected of stalking an individual for the purpose of domestic violence, criminal child enticement, or theft. These laws provide civil protection in cases where there has not been recent physical assault yet menacing by stalking has occurred. Law enforcement officials can arrest an individual without a warrant where there is reasonable cause to believe that stalking has occurred. Under several of the laws the court may order an evaluation of the mental condition of the stalker.

Elder Abuse

Abuse and neglect of the elderly have become major concerns in recent years. As with child and spouse abuse, the extent of elder abuse is unknown. This is because many instances are never reported. Victims of abuse may attempt to hide the fact that they have been abused. Furthermore, many types of elder abuse behaviors are difficult to categorize.

It is estimated that between 500,000 and 2.5 million senior citizens are victims of abuse and neglect each year.[11] Possibly as many as one in ten citizens over the age of sixty-five experience some type of abuse. This type of abuse is found among all groups: racial, social, ethnic, and religious. The abusers in most instances are relatives or care givers. The victim of elder abuse is often dependent upon the abuser for physical and emotional needs. This is especially the case following the death of a spouse.

The abusers in most instances are relatives or care givers of the individual. Daughters and sons of the victims are found to be the most frequent abusers. Daughters tend to be more involved in psychological abuse and neglect, while sons are more likely to use physical abuse.[12] Often the abuser is experiencing many family problems of his or her own. It may be a period of time when the abuser is experiencing financial problems due to the demands of his or her own children. Having the added burden of an elderly relative makes for a very difficult situation that leads to both active and passive abuse.

Types of Abuse

Elder abuse takes several different forms. It may be physical abuse, neglect, psychological abuse, exploitation, and maltreatment. Often several or all of these forms may be present in a given case.

Possibly the easiest type of abuse to identify is physical abuse, which is the direct infliction of physical injury to the individual. This type of abusive action usually results in injuries, welts, sprains, fractures, and lacerations. It may take the form of beating, hitting, slapping, pushing, shaking, or other direct physical contact. All too often the elderly are unable to react, and out of helplessness appropriate medical attention and care are not obtained.

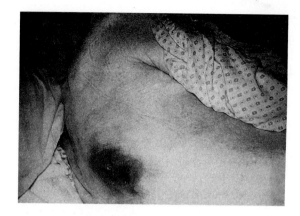

Elder abuse often takes the form of neglect. When the person is disabled and unable to move without help, serious decubitus ulcers often develop where the body is in contact with the bed for long periods of time. Such ulcers often become infected and serious related problems result.

Neglect of the elderly can take many different forms. Neglect is considered a lack of attention and/or confinement of the individual. Neglect often is not malicious but passive. Since the person may not request help and assistance or feels that to do so would inconvenience others, the needed care is unavailable. An individual who is immobile may lie in one spot long enough to cause bed sores. Failure to provide necessary treatment and services to maintain health and well-being, such as failure to give needed medication, is common among senior citizens. Active neglect is seen in situations where the care giver withholds a basic need. Withholding nutrition or fluids, medicine, personal care, or clothing and supervision are associated with this type of abuse. Individuals who are malnourished or dehydrated, have urine burns or other ulcers and sores, or have an unkempt appearance are suspect of neglect.

Situations that involve threats and produce fear create psychological abuse. Where there is a withholding of affection and where social isolation is permitted, psychological abuse occurs. Intimidation in the form of verbal abuse (shouting or scolding) and nonverbal abuse (silence, threats of abandonment or institutionalization) is commonly noted. Verbal abuse may include name calling, insults, threats, and humiliation. Individuals experiencing this type of abuse appear passive, fearful, and have a low sense of self-esteem. They are often withdrawn, passive,

Injuries to the Feet: The Result of a Fall or Abuse?

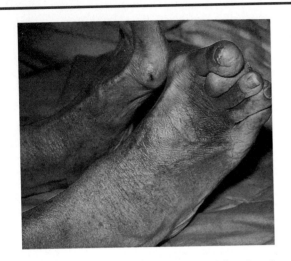

Injuries to the feet—are they the result of a fall or abuse?

Often hospital medical and social service staff are faced with contradictory stories concerning the cause of bruises and injuries of elderly individuals brought to the emergency department. All too often the explanations given do not seem appropriate for the type of injuries seen by these professionals.

The explanation given by family members who brought this individual to the municipal hospital was that the seventy-nine-year-old woman had fallen and hurt her feet. It seemed odd that the extensive injuries were on both the top and the bottom of both feet. Further examination revealed bruises on the thighs, the torso, and the arms. All indicated evidence of physical abuse.

What is, or should be, the role of the emergency room physician in such a case? The emergency room nurse? The hospital social worker? The law enforcement personnel?

Why is it necessary that medical centers develop team approaches to working with the increasing problem of elder abuse in this country?

and depressed; out of fear, they may appear to be helpless. Psychological abuse can be very devastating to the individual. Unfortunately, it is very difficult to obtain evidence against the abusers in these situations.

Exploitation is taking advantage of the resources of the elderly person. This usually involves the dishonest misappropriation of money or property. This type of abuse is seen when a senior citizen is overcharged for needed home repairs, necessary purchases, health care, or funeral costs. There are instances where the family members or caretakers will withhold pension or insurance checks and use the money for their own purposes. This kind of theft is particularly unfortunate in that the elderly person may not be able to respond. Forcing the elderly person to sign over power of attorney or forcing a change of will are other examples of exploitation. When one's possessions are missing or unknown resources are not available to cover costs of food, clothes, housing, and other necessities of life, exploitation can be suspected.

Intervention Needs

There is a growing need for intervention services to help the elderly. Those individuals whose professional responsibilities bring them into contact with the elderly, such as medical care providers, social workers, and criminal justice personnel, need to be better prepared to detect, assess, and provide treatment for elder abuse victims.[13]

There are numerous indicators of abuse. For example, when a discrepancy exists between the injury and the related history and explanation by the victim and/or others, abuse may be suspected. Other possible abuse indications are evidence of untreated injuries, multiple injuries of varying stages of healing, and the presence of injuries on areas of the body that are normally covered by clothing.

Services such as emergency shelters and therapeutic care are necessary. Counseling is important. Home help services, day-care centers, and alternative housing services can be developed in many communities to help the elderly. In addition to services for the elderly, relief

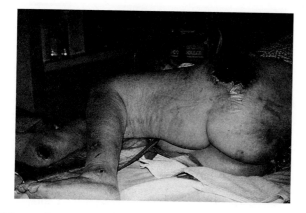

When neglect has occurred, an individual may develop decubitus ulcers over many parts of the body. This patient came to the attention of the medical staff of a hospital when the patient was brought in from a skilled nursing facility. Ulcers covered the hip and the heels, as well as other parts of the body. Infection of the wounds led to the death of this patient.

for the caretaker is essential. If such caretaker services were available, the potential abuser could obtain assistance during periods of crisis and stress.

Accompanying increased concern regarding elder abuse has come increased recognition of the need for legislation. Today forty-three states have some type of statutes for adult protection. The major provision of these laws is that they require reporting of elder abuse. However, differences exist regarding who is required to report such abuse. In most instances medical and health personnel have such obligations along with members of the clergy.

The various laws define what kinds of abuse are to be reported. Unfortunately, a type of abuse that is reportable in one state may not be reportable in another. Each state specifies to which agency a report of elder abuse is to be made; state and local departments of social services, the state attorney general's office, county probation departments, and county welfare departments are some examples.

Because of the variance from state to state, there is a need for comprehensive federal legislation relating to elder abuse. Medical personnel who work with the elderly need to be made more aware of the signs and symptoms of this kind of violence. Emergency trauma physicians, emergency nurses, and social workers are often at the forefront in identifying potential abuse cases.

The problems related to elder abuse likely will continue to increase in the years ahead with an increasing percentage of the population in the United States being over sixty-five. Historically, the rights of the elderly have received little attention. With increased concern over the rights of this population group, the incidence of elder abuse will necessitate quality care facilities, improved legislation, and better preventive measures.

Rape

An act of violence involving sex or attempted sex without the consent of the victim is rape. This action is also referred to as sexual assault, which has been defined as "nonconsensual sexual behavior, including stranger, acquaintance, and spousal assaults against either male or female victims."[14]

Incidence statistics regarding rape vary, as do those for other types of abuse. It is estimated that one in ten rapes is reported to the authorities. Further estimates have been made that as many as one in four females and one in eight males are victimized at some time in their lives.

Rape occurs in all levels of society, with most rapes being planned. Often the sexual assault takes place in the home of the victim. Sometimes the rapist forces entry, and other times the individual is known by the victim, who permits entry, not expecting the possibility of assault. Offenders typically rape more than once, but not usually the same victim.

Although most people think of the female as the typical victim, rape of males also occurs. Male rape has often been reported in the nation's prisons. It has also been reported in other locations: universities, industrial settings, and recreational areas. Usually this type of rape is committed by other males. Anal intercourse is usually the rapist's mode of entry. Male rape is often violent and conducted as a gang rape.

Rape takes a serious toll on its victims: physiologically, emotionally, and mentally. It usually has a profound and prolonged impact on the victim. The crisis resulting from sexual assault can be divided into two phases: (1) the initial experience, the confrontation, or the acute phase and (2) the long-term effect or reorganization phase. The initial crisis necessitates encouraging the victim to seek medical treatment following the assault. It

Issue—Case Study

Is It Rape or an Aggressive Affair?

Carl and Kathy have known each other for several months since meeting at a fraternity party early in the fall. They have talked several times on campus. Both are studying political science, so they have many common interests. On two or three occasions they have gone out to a movie together and stopped for a beer and pizza on the way home.

Last weekend they went to a party where Kathy met several of Carl's friends from his hometown. After the party they returned to her apartment. Since her roommate had left for the weekend, she invited Carl in to talk and watch a movie on video. As they sat on the couch and watched the movie, both began to show affection for the other.

As the time passed Carl became increasingly sexually aggressive. Despite her pleading and protests that he stop, he forced her into an act of sexual intercourse. As he left the apartment Kathy was crying and emotionally distraught.

What had happened? Had she been raped by her good friend, or was this just a case of an overaggressive relationship that happened to end in intercourse? In her mind Kathy began to feel guilty about inviting Carl into her apartment and permitting certain actions that eventually led to intercourse. What could, or should, she do now?

She was alone in the apartment with no one to talk to. A number of fears began to enter her mind. She could become pregnant since they had not used any contraception. She wanted no children at this time and had serious reservations about abortion. In addition, she had no idea how Carl felt about her other than as a friend. Then she remembered the talk she heard recently at the student union about AIDS. What if Carl was carrying HIV?

What should Kathy do? What kinds of counsel and help are available for victims of acquaintance rape on college and university campuses? Should she report this to the police authorities as a rape? What responsibilities should Carl be held accountable for in the next few hours, days, and weeks?

---

must be remembered that during this period the victim often experiences personal shock and trauma. There is a need for the medical care provider to be gentle and tactful. Some have recommended that, in the case of rape of a female, it is wise to have available the services of a female physician. It is essential that the medical examination be accomplished in private. Rape victims are usually given antibiotics during the examination to prevent sexually transmitted diseases. Pelvic examinations provide evidence that rape has taken place. However, such an examination is effective only for a short period of time, as sperm and semen will only be found for about seventy-two hours. Other physical injuries, bruises, and cuts must also be treated at this time.

Often rape occurs by an acquaintance of the victim. These occurrences take place among individuals who are known to each other as friends. They may be having a "dating" relationship. At some point in the relationship the male forces the female against her will to engage in sexual acts as part of the dating relationship. This form of rape has come to be known as *date rape* or *acquaintance*

rape. The number of date rapes being reported on college and university campuses is increasing, causing concern.

Usually the victim of date rape is acquainted with the rapist. They may have had a friendship lasting some time or may have become acquainted very recently. Studies of this type of violence indicate that as personal relationships become more involved, there is greater likelihood of rape and abuse.[15] Often this results from misunderstanding and lack of communication between the parties involved.

Acquaintance rape is most likely to take place in the room of one of the partners. Upon returning to the dormitory or apartment, the couple relaxes to music, drinks alcoholic beverages, and begins to express sexual feelings. As the sexual activity progresses, it eventually comes to a point where the male penetrates the female despite her protests. Some cases of date rape involve physical violence such as pushing, slapping, and hitting the partner as well as verbal abuse.

Unfortunately, acquaintance rape usually leads to a mixture of emotional and psychological feelings that are difficult to cope with. Often the abused will not report the rape because of feelings of guilt. Peer pressure plays a role in some situations that result in the rape. The help needed to deal with the feelings is often not available.

Although rape is a violation of one's physical person, the resulting emotional and psychological factors can require long-term care. Emotional reactions such as shock, disbelief, confusion, and fear are often found among rape victims. In an effort to help the victim overcome these problems, counseling is required.

Following the physical care, effective psychological or crisis counseling services can be most helpful. The victim should be referred to a local rape counseling service. The individual will need to express and work through the various feelings of anger, fear, hurt, and mistrust that usually follow such an assault.

Rape is a legal crime. In most states health care providers are required to report to law enforcement authorities all criminally caused injuries. In any case involving sexual assault, the medical personnel must be careful in the collection and transfer of specimens that may be used in legal documentation. Health care providers need appropriate education in helping the victim of sexual assault.

All too often the offender is never punished for the act of sexual assault. This may be the result of overburdened court schedules, improperly gathered evidence, or the failure of the victim to testify against the rapist. The importance of stricter punishment for the act of rape was noted in a summary statement of the Surgeon General's Workshop on Violence and Public Health in 1985:[16]

". . . the criminal justice system should clearly recognize sexual assault as a serious violent crime; that sanctions, including incarceration, should be imposed upon assailants commensurate with the devastating impact of the crime upon their victims; and that treatment to prevent future criminal behavior be part of sentencing wherever possible."

Suicide

Suicide is a major problem of violence, being the eighth leading cause of death in America. On one hand, we are confronted with behavior that demands our understanding, concern, and help. On the other hand, suicide is a topic about which most people in the United States would rather not talk. For many there are misunderstandings, numerous misconceptions, and even fear of the topic of suicide.

It is difficult getting an accurate indication as to how widespread the incidence of suicide is in American society. The National Center for Health Statistics reports that over thirty thousand persons a year commit suicide.[17] However, the American Association of Suicidology has estimated that approximately fifty thousand persons commit suicide annually in the United States. Both statistics may be greatly underestimated. Many suicides will never be reported as such. They will be identified as accidental death or be listed as death from some other cause. What is known is that suicide rates are increasing among all age groups and racial groups, regardless of economic status and gender.

Though suicide occurs in all population groups, it is particularly prevalent among teenagers, young adults, and the elderly. It is known that suicide is the second leading cause of death among adolescents, with as many as five thousand successful suicides a year. Suicide rates in the past fifteen years among the fifteen-to-twenty-four-age group have increased 37.5 percent. The major population involved in this rise has been white males.[18]

Concern is often expressed in a community when a series of successful or attempted suicides take place during a rather limited time period. These episodes are referred to as *suicide clusters*. Usually several individuals in the same school or locality attempt suicide in just a few weeks. Many psychiatrists, counselors, educators, and experts in mental health have studied these suicide epidemics in an attempt to learn their causes. There is no clear-cut pattern except that they tend to occur following a report of suicide. The occurrence of a cluster of successful suicides or suicide attempts causes fear and unsettledness in a community. Young people ask many questions for which answers are hard to find. Parents and adult leaders in the community often become fearful that other suicide attempts are likely to take place. Much more information is needed about these episodes, with recommendations about how all those involved, young people and adults, can cope with this very serious problem.

Suicide rates are highest among the elderly population. Though numerous reasons can be cited for this, long-term chronic illnesses and depression are commonly noted as being important causes. The death of one's spouse or close friends often results in depression, loneliness, and suicidal behavior. These difficulties often lead to a desire to bring an end to life.

For many it seems difficult to understand why a person in the prime of life should desire to take his or her life. Youth during these years experience numerous conflicts that seem to be insurmountable. Such pressures may be financial or social—the loss of an important relationship, a feeling of isolation from and by their parents, and pressures concerning academic performance and a sense of not belonging.

Attempted suicide is often a cry for help. Those working in school settings, health agencies, family care agencies, and other community settings must become aware of the various warning signs of the potential suicide. Numerous signs of potential suicidal behavior have been identified. One indication of potential suicide is that the individual tends to take actions directed toward the cessation of living. This is noticed as the individual cuts himself or herself off from some important portion of life. Often noticed is the failure to expose oneself to situations which may be painful in some way, either physically or emotionally. This may be seen in the student who is increasingly absent from classes or the employee who fails to perform at work as previously.

Another sign in a case of potential suicide is depression. Depression may have developed over the long-term, or it can have very short onset. Depression may manifest itself by feelings of sadness, tears, diminished interest in life, and feelings of failure.

Physical signs of suicidal tendency may be sleep disturbance, an unkempt appearance, and agitation. Problems with weight are often noticed among those with suicidal behavior. This may take the form of excessive or compulsive eating.

Another phenomenon that is often noticed is that the suicide victim may have spent time in putting personal affairs in order. This may take the form of paying outstanding bills or making a will. It can involve making plans and arrangements for one's funeral. It has been noted that in some instances the suicide victim says "good-bye" to certain people. It is quite common at this time for the individual to give away things that have been particularly meaningful, such as money, a prized picture, or something of personal value.

The act of suicide may include several different practices. Males tend to use more violent measures. The firearm is the chief suicide method used among males, with hanging second. Females tend to use more passive measures, such as medicines or poisons. Slitting wrists is another, more violent, procedure used by females.

There is great need in the United Sates for personnel and facilities that can provide assistance to potential suicide victims and counsel to the relatives and friends of suicide victims. Professionals involved in community health, medicine, schools, and social agencies must become aware of the many factors associated with suicide and be equipped to help those in need.

Suicide prevention and crisis intervention centers can be found in many communities throughout the United States. The first recorded effort to develop a suicide prevention program was in New York City in 1906. Today there are hundreds of prevention centers and hot lines available to those in need of these services.

These centers provide a place where the individual can get emergency help in times of suicidal crises. The basic purpose of suicide prevention centers is to stop individuals from carrying out plans to kill themselves. These centers provide twenty-four-hour calling service, which gives the individual in crisis someone to talk with. It provides opportunity to arrange professional help, medical care, or other desired assistance.

Volunteers often play an important role in a suicide prevention or crisis intervention center. This person often is the "first line of defense." A call is made and the individual on the phone, often a volunteer, will listen, talk, and refer the patient as needed. The volunteer needs to be sensitive and show understanding to the individual in crisis.

Homicide

Though homicide is the eleventh leading cause of death in the United States, it is the fourth leading cause of years of potential life lost before the age of sixty-five. Nearly twenty-one thousand individuals die at the hands of another person annually.[19] The greatest number of homicides occurs among the young, minorities, and males; the homicide rate is four times greater for men than for women.

Homicides are committed by knifings, beatings, strangulations, and firearms. Two out of every three homicides are the result of firearm use. Increased possession of weapons in American society has aggravated the problem.

Several factors are related to homicide and aggravated assaults. Drug dealing is a leading factor. Arguments over money, "turf" in the drug dealership, and other factors all too often end in shootings, stabbings, and beatings. The epidemic growth in the use of crack cocaine has resulted in a major escalation in homicides in many communities.

Alcohol is a factor in a great number of homicides. Alcohol increases the likelihood of risk-taking and provocative behavior. Inhibitions often are lessened, leading to irrational and abnormal behavior. Alcohol presence is common in the blood of a high percentage of homicide victims.

Poverty and unemployment are major risk factors for homicide, because they often lead to robbery. All too often robberies end in homicide.

Homicides also occur when people are involved in arguments and disputes. Nearly half occur where the victim and perpetrator are known or related to each other. It is estimated that less than 15 percent of all homicides occur between strangers. In the remaining third the relationship is unknown.[20]

Family conflict is the cause of many homicides, with nearly one-half occurring among spouses. Intrafamilial violence occurs among all racial and age groups. The factors that contribute to intrafamilial homicide include separation and divorce, legal issues centered around child support, and economic factors. These circumstances are often filled with anger and unhappiness toward the partner, and these feelings are eventually played out in an act of homicide.

The leading cause of death among African-American males between the ages of fifteen and twenty-four is homicide. The homicide rate is nearly ten times greater among this population group than among the non-African-American populations.[21] The homicide rate among the African-American male population is more than 90 per 100,000, while the national statistic is slightly below 9 per 100,000. Numerous socioeconomic factors have been identified that account for this. Unemployment, with accompanying stresses that lead to robbery, and alcohol and drug use are possibly the leading factors.

The Surgeon General's Task Force on Violence and Public Health addressed a number of the issues related to homicide.[22] This task force recommended specific actions that need to be implemented in communities across the nation. One recommendation stated that services should be available in communities to help both the relatives and associates of victims of homicide and aggravated assault, as well as the individuals themselves. Development of victim assistance programs was given high priority.[23]

Numerous agencies and organizations in communities throughout the country can play important roles. In addition to the health care profession and community health organizations, religious organizations, educational institutions, and criminal justice agencies can develop appropriate activities.

If any improvement in the problem of homicide and aggravated assault is to occur, efforts must take place to meet the underlying causes and risk factors associated with the problem. This will mean actions in the socioeconomic dimension as well as a serious rethinking of the need for some type of control of the weapons that are used in such assaults.

Gun Control Legislation: Yes or No?

A major controversial issue in the United States for many years has centered on gun control legislation. Should the federal government or state governments pass legislation that would limit or even ban the ownership of firearms? Particular concern is expressed about the possession of handguns.

Americans own some ninety million firearms. More than thirty thousand people are killed each year by guns. Although a number of these fatalities occur each year to individuals involved in accidents while hunting, a major percentage of these deaths occur in homicides and suicides. Over half of all homicides and suicides are committed with firearms, resulting in death to over twenty thousand individuals annually.

Thousands of innocent people are killed each year at the hand of another by the use of guns. It may be a star basketball player near his school in Illinois, the supervisor of several employees in Oklahoma, or a drug-related death in New York. Regardless of the circumstances, firearm violence results in the loss of many years of potential life productivity. It is estimated that more than 1.2 million years of potential life are lost annually owing to suicides and homicides.[24]

All too often children are the victims of firearm injuries and deaths. The report of a child taking a gun from the father's dresser drawer and accidentally shooting himself or herself is an all-too-common tragedy. It has been recommended that handguns be designed to prevent accidental discharge.[25] If safety measures were built into the manufacture of firearms, it is believed that many accidental shootings could be prohibited. Whether these measures would be effective or whether certain weapons should be totally banned is one of the major arenas of debate today.

Evidence is quite strong that in nations with bans on the possession of firearms the incidences of homicide are significantly lower. For instance, more than ten thousand homicides occur annually in the United States due to the use of firearms, while in Japan, which prohibits firearm possession, there are fewer than fifty homicides a year by firearms.[26] The same conclusion can be reached by comparing United States homicide statistics with Canada and various European nations that have firearm ban legislation.

Support for gun control legislation seems to expand after the assassination, or attempted assassination, of a leading public personality or following a mass homicide in a public setting such as a restaurant or school. This was seen in the 1960s with the assassinations of the Rev. Martin Luther King and of President John F. Kennedy and his brother Robert F. Kennedy. In the 1970s the attempted assassination of President Gerald Ford and the same action in the 1980s against President Ronald Reagan focused attention on the need for gun control legislation.

On the other hand, there is regularly strong opposition against any type of firearm control in the United States. Many people point out the constitutional right that all citizens have to own and have possession of firearms. Nationally, a leading lobby effort against gun control has been led by the National Rifle Association. This association has been instrumental in arguing against such legislation.

It has also been active in conducting educational programs to teach people proper and safe procedures for handling and storing of firearms.

Throughout the nation there are thousands of laws, federal, state, and local, that deal with the sale, use, and distribution of guns. Such laws usually deal with regulations concerning who can purchase a gun, where they can be kept or carried, and guarantees that they are safe for operation. Unfortunately, such laws have had little effect in reducing weapon use in suicides, homicides, and accidental shootings.

Declaring that there is little use for handguns other than as directed toward other humans, in 1985 the Surgeon General's Workshop on Violence and Public Health published a call for a ban on the sale, manufacture, importation, and possession of handguns.[27] The report called for criminal penalties against individuals who are in possession of any firearm where alcohol is sold or served. Alcohol consumption, firearm possession, and related interpersonal violence are very serious problems.

Near the end of 1993, after nearly seven years of debate by pro- and anti-gun control advocates, Congress passed legislation that had been highly debated, the Brady bill. This legislation mandates a five-day waiting period on the purchase of handguns. This waiting period permits a period of time in which the person wishing to purchase a handgun can be screened for criminal record or mental instability. Nearly half of the states already have some type of required waiting period for handgun purchase.

The Brady bill is a very modest attempt at solving problems of violence relating to handgun possession and use. Debate continues over the need for other legislation. Particular concern has focused upon the possession and use of semiautomatic assault weapons, particularly by teenagers. Legislation banning the possession and sale of these assault weapons is wanted by many advocates of gun control. Also, measures should be implemented to make it illegal to sell handguns to minors under eighteen years of age.

Summary

Violence has been a part of human existence since the beginning of time. Although natural occurrences have killed and maimed millions, it is interpersonal violence that must be understood and controlled by humans. Numerous agencies and organizations play important roles in providing services to the victims of violence as well as to those who commit the violence. A need exists to encourage the cooperation and integration of services of these different agencies.

Interpersonal violence includes child abuse, spouse abuse, and elder abuse. Each victim can be abused physically and emotionally. Physical abuse is probably the most easily identifiable. Neglect is less identifiable but may be just as serious. Emotional or psychological abuse often is an accumulation of years of actions and attitudes that lead to feelings of unimportance and low self-esteem for the victim.

Sexual abuse is a tragic form of violence. The incidence of child sexual abuse has increased significantly in recent years, with a majority of victims offended by relatives or acquaintances. Rape is another form of sexual abuse. Though a majority of instances of rape occur to women, male rape is increasing.

Numerous reasons can be identified for abuse. The abused, as well as the abusers, need the help of various professionals. Legislation at both the national and state levels now makes it mandatory that when there is evidence of abuse, caretakers must report it. The particular agencies to whom reports must be filed differ from one jurisdiction to another. However, all health care workers, educational personnel, social workers, religious leaders, and others involved in community work must be aware of their responsibilities.

Probably the ultimate tragedy of interpersonal violence is aggravated assault and homicide. Numerous causes for this type of violence can be identified. Though homicide occurs to all age and racial groups, it is a particular problem for young, nonwhite, minority populations. Within the African-American fifteen-to-twenty-four-year age group, homicide is the leading cause of death.

The issue of gun control in the United States has been a controversial matter for many years. There is no question that a majority of homicides and many suicides result from the use of firearms. Suicide, while not interpersonal violence in the strict sense, does result in the loss of life and accompanying loss of productive life years.

The necessity of considering violence as a community health concern was highlighted in 1985 with the Surgeon General's Workshop on Violence and Public Health. A number of recommendations for action came out of the deliberations of this workshop. Since then the necessity for including violence as an area for needed activity in health promotion and disease prevention programming and planning has been set forth in the Year 2000 Health Objectives for the Nation. A number of health objectives have been identified relating to homicide, personal abuse, suicide, and assault. A multidisciplinary approach to program development is needed in which the various factors associated with violence, such as poverty, social isolation, stress, and socioeconomic problems, are addressed.

Discussion Questions

1. Why should the matter of interpersonal violence be a program concern to the field of community health?

2. What are some of the Health Objectives for the Year 2000 that focus on interpersonal violence?

3. Discuss the differences between child physical abuse and child neglect.

4. What are some of the long-term effects of sexual abuse on children?

5. Identify some of the factors that tend to contribute to child abuse.

6. What are some community child abuse intervention programs in your community?

7. Explain the basic concept of the Healthy Families America program.

8. Discuss the various legislative provisions for reporting child abuse. What are the provisions in your particular state?

9. What are roles that the schools play in prevention of child abuse?

10. Why is it difficult to obtain accurate data on the incidence of any type of abuse: child abuse, spouse abuse, and elder abuse?

11. Discuss some of the different forms that spouse abuse takes.

12. In what ways can communities provide services to help the individual who is a victim of spouse abuse?

13. Explain the basic provisions found in antistalking laws.

14. What are some unique factors of elder abuse that do not relate to either child or spouse abuse?

15. Why do many cases of elder abuse result from actions taken by the children of the abused or care givers of the individual?

16. It is stated "rape is a legal crime." Discuss the ramifications of this statement.

17. What are several specific problems that occur as the result of acquaintance rape?

18. Identify some of the signs and indications of potential suicidal behavior.

19. What are the significance and value of suicide prevention and crisis intervention centers?

20. Why is homicide a particular problem among the young, nonwhite, minority population in the United States?

21. Discuss some of the controversy over gun control legislation.

22. Discuss the position taken by the Surgeon General's Workshop on Violence and Public Health regarding the use of handguns.

Suggested Readings

Amaro, Hortensia, and others. "Violence during Pregnancy and Substance Use." *American Journal of Public Health* 80, no. 5 (May 1990): 575–79.

American Association of Retired Persons. *Domestic Mistreatment of the Elderly—towards Prevention.* Washington, D.C.: AARP, 1988, 39 pp.

American Medical Association Council on Scientific Affairs. "Firearms Injuries and Deaths: A Critical Public Health Issue." *Public Health Reports* 104, no. 2 (March/April 1989): 111–20.

Blair, Kathryn. "The Battered Woman: Is She a Silent Victim?" *Nurse Practitioner* 11, no. 6 (June 1986): 38–47.

Centers for Disease Control. "Physical Fighting among High School Students—United States, 1990." *Morbidity and Mortality Weekly Report* 41, no. 6 (February 14, 1992): 91–94.

Centerwall, Brandon S. "Exposure to Television as a Risk Factor for Violence." *American Journal of Epidemiology* 129, no. 4 (April 1989): 643–52.

Cron, Ted. "The Surgeon General's Workshop on Violence and Public Health: Review of the Recommendations." *Public Health Review* 101, no. 1 (January/February 1986): 8–14.

Daro, Deborah, and Karen McCurdy. *Current Trends in Child Abuse Reporting and Fatalities: The Results of the 1991 Annual Fifty-State Survey.* The National Center on Child Abuse Prevention Research (April 1992).

Douglass, Richard L. *Domestic Mistreatment of the Elderly—Towards Prevention.* Washington, D.C.: American Association of Retired Persons, 1988, 39 pp.

Gold, Deborah T., and Lisa P. Gwyther. "The Prevention of Elder Abuse: An Educational Model." *Family Relations* 38 (1989): 8–14.

Gould, Madelyn S., and others. "Time-Space Clustering of Teenage Suicide." *American Journal of Epidemiology* 131, no. 1 (January 1990): 71–78.

Greenberg, Michael, and Dona Schneider. "Blue Thursday? Homicide and Suicide among Urban 15–24 Year Old Black Male Americans." *Public Health Reports* 107, no. 3 (May/June 1992): 264–68.

Guyer, Bernard, and others. "Intentional Injuries among Children and Adolescents in Massachusetts." *The New England Journal of Medicine* 321, no. 23 (December 7, 1989): 1584–89.

Herman, Judith, and others. "Long-Term Effects of Incestuous Abuse in Childhood." *American Journal of Psychiatry* 143, no. 10 (October 1986): 1293–96.

Kellerman, Arthur L., and others. "Suicide in the Home in Relation to Gun Ownership." *New England Journal of Medicine* 327, no. 7 (August 13, 1992): 467–72.

King, M. Christine, and Josephine Ryan. "Abused Women: Dispelling Myths and Encouraging Intervention." *The Nurse Practitioner* 14, no. 5 (May 1989): 47–58.

Kottmeier, Peter K. "Four Clues to Child Abuse." *Emergency Medicine* 24, no. 4 (March 15, 1992): 283–87.

Mitchell, Mark A., and Stacey Daniels. "Black-on-Black Homicide: Kansas City's Response." *Public Health Reports* 104, no. 6 (November/December 1989): 605–08.

Neergaard, Joyce A. "A Proposal for a Foster Grandmother Intervention Program to Prevent Child Abuse." *Public Health Reports* 105, no. 1 (January/February 1990): 89–93.

Nelson, Franklyn, L., and others. "Youth Suicide in California: A Comparative Study of Perceived Causes and Interventions." *Community Mental Health Journal* 24, no. 1 (Spring 1988): 31–42.

Page, Randy, and others. "Interpersonal Violence: A Priority Issue for Health Education." *Journal of Health Education* 23, no. 5 (July/August 1992): 286–92.

Payne, Thomas C. "Domestic Violence." *Michigan Medicine* 91, no. 9 (September 1992): 23–27.

Ringwalt, Chris, and Joanne Caye. "The Effect of Demographic Factors on Perceptions of Child Neglect." *Children and Youth Services Review* 11 (1989): 133–44.

Select Committee on Aging, U.S. House of Representatives, 97th Congress. *Elder Abuse: An Examination of a Health Problem.* 97–277 Committee Publication, Washington, D.C. (1981).

Shaffer, David. "Suicide: Risk Factors and the Public Health." *American Journal of Public Health* 83, no. 21 (February 1993): 171–72.

Strange, Cheri. "An Overview of Incest in Current American Society." *The Prenatal Journal* 9, no. 4 (Fall 1986).

Wintemute, Garen J., and others. "Unintentional Firearm Deaths in California." *The Journal of Trauma* 29, no. 4 (April 1989): 457–61.

Endnotes

1. Department of Health and Human Services. *Healthy People 2000: National Health Promotion and Disease Prevention Objectives.* Washington, D.C.: U.S. Government Printing Office, 1991, pp. 226–36.
2. *The Status of Children, Youth, and Families.* Washington, D.C.: U.S. Government Printing Office, 1979, p. 111.
3. Strange, Cheri, "An Overview of Incest in Current American Society." *The Prenatal Journal* 9, no. 4 (Fall 1986): 8.
4. *Ibid.,* 8.
5. National Committee for Prevention of Child Abuse, 332 South Michigan Avenue, Suite 1600, Chicago, Ill. 60604. Pamphlet.
6. Blair, Kathryn. "The Battered Woman: Is She a Silent Victim?" *Nurse Practitioner* 11, no. 6 (June 1986): 38.
7. Department of Health and Human Services. *Surgeon General's Workshop on Violence and Public Health: Report.* DHHS Publication no. HRS-D-MC 86–1 (May, 1986): 12.
8. *Ibid.,* 12.
9. Blair, "The Battered Woman," 40.
10. *Ibid.,* 44.
11. Matlaw, Jane R., and Jane B. Mayer. "Elder Abuse: Ethical and Practical Dilemmas for Social Work." *Health and Social Work* 11, no. 2 (Spring 1986): 85.
12. Mildenberger, C., and H. Wessman. "Abuse and Neglect of Elderly Persons by Family Members." *Physical Therapy* 66 (April 1986): 537.
13. Department of Health and Human Services, *Surgeon General's Workshop,* 64.
14. *Ibid.,* 69.
15. Makepeace, James M. "Courtship Violence among College Students." *Family Relations* 30 (January 1981): 97–102.
16. Department of Health and Human Services, *Surgeon General's Workshop,* 70.
17. Centers for Disease Control. Annual Summary 1984: Reported Morbidity and Mortality in the United States. *Morbidity and Mortality Weekly Report* 33, no. 54 (March 1986): 114.
18. *Ibid.,* 116.
19. Department of Health and Human Services, *Healthy People 2000,* 61.
20. Rosenberg, Mark L. "Surveillance for Suicide, Homicide, and Domestic Violence: Strengths and Weaknesses, and Issues." *Public Health Reports* 100, no. 6 (November/December 1985): 593–95.
21. Department of Health and Human Services, *Healthy People 2000,* 228.

22. Department of Health and Human Services, *Surgeon General's Workshop*, 49–54.

23. *Ibid.*

24. Centers for Disease Control, Annual Summary 1984, 120.

25. Department of Health and Human Services, *Healthy People 2000*, 284.

26. Department of Health and Human Services, *Surgeon General's Workshop*, 16.

27. *Ibid.*, 53.

You . . . and Community Health

Each person reading this book has specific health needs, problems, interests, and concerns. Your skill in coping with your individual health is dependent upon a number of variables, including economic considerations, individual values, personal knowledge, and background.

However, no one lives in a vacuum unaffected by the world and the environment. Throughout our daily activities we interact with numerous "communities." But for the most part, the focus of our concern for health is on self. We seek health care for ourselves and our families. In much of America that is accomplished through the private, fee-for-service model of health care. We do not give community health serious thought unless we cannot cope with our own health problems.

With increased urbanization, rising health care costs, and greater mobility and social concern, the fact that each of us is a part of several "communities of solution" to specific health problems necessitates a clear understanding of community health. Community health is not just providing programs for the poor or the underprivileged. Nor is it the establishment of programs funded and operated by government for the provision of health care. Community health must be viewed in terms other than curative medicine. Preventive medicine and primary health care are seen today as important foundations of the health status of our communities and individuals within those settings. Community health should include various dynamics focusing upon wellness promotion that results in good health for all.

Community health is also more than disease control and ensuring a sanitary environment as was once the case. It is no longer a discipline based solely upon the foundations created by biomedical research and development, though these are still important and necessary. Medicine and health care have long been associated with the physical sciences.

Community health is a dynamic, changing discipline that is influenced not only by the findings of biomedical research but, more important, by the social sciences. Health and wellness increasingly are recognized as having social dynamics. This means that the social sciences will play important roles in improving the health status and behavior of citizens in our communities. The dimensions of political involvement, economics, and cultural awareness as they relate to health and wellness must be understood. Nowhere is this more obvious than in the political spectrum.

As we approach the start of the twenty-first century, numerous creative approaches in community health programming and the provision of health care will be needed. It will mean development of new skills with new technology. By the year 2000, it is possible that organ transplants will be taking place with the use of connecting tubes. It will probably be possible to replace virtually every body organ. Today there is research in process attempting to develop artificial ear implants, red blood cells, and blood vessels. Work is also ongoing in the hopes of developing an implantable artificial lung and an artificial eye that are stimulated by electrodes implanted in the brain.

Today, by means of laser surgery, it is possible to replace the need to cut open a person to perform surgery. Gene therapy, a procedure of replacing defective genes with nondefective ones, could reduce most genetics-related problems. It is likely that there will be as much technological development in the next decade as in all of the past century.

Computers will increasingly be used to operate various defective body parts. The role of computer technology in the field of community health has only begun to be explored.

It can be assumed that neither a national health program nor total reliance on the private sector will be effective in solving community health problems in the future. Nations having national health insurance or health care programs have not been able to solve the same problems faced by the United States nor have they been able to control the rising costs of health care. Cost containment is every bit as much of a concern in other developed, industrial nations as it is in our country. These nations have not solved the problems of maldistribution of health care services and facilities. The poor and disadvantaged, as well as those living in rural localities, often are as poorly served as they are in the United States.

Just as one cannot expect national health programs to be totally successful, neither can it be expected that the private sector will be able to totally solve community health problems. Much of the private sector operates on the economic principle of profit and loss. It is impossible economically, and wrong morally, to suggest that the community health problems should be looked at from a profit point of view. The health, or lack thereof, of an individual or a group of persons, should not be directly affected by an individual or an organization trying to make a profit.

Another component of the private sector, the volunteer movement, cannot be expected to totally solve the nation's community health problems. Though the volunteer movement has been very effective in the health fields, it is not possible to depend on volunteers to accomplish a task so complex as the provision of health for all.

New, different, and creative models of health care provision, community health services, and programming must be at the forefront in the years ahead. Whether traditional approaches found in community health will be effective remains doubtful. It seems likely that whatever model or models become the norm, they must be based upon sociological, economical, and political dynamics.

Only as "bridges" are built will the chasm be crossed, or narrowed, between medical technology and the state of well-being for every person.[1] No single force is going to bridge the gap between existing health knowledge, skills, and technology on one hand, and the availability of adequate health care for all on the other. As has been indicated, economic and political concerns and attention to social and cultural values must be considered.

A higher degree of wellness must be the ultimate goal for all people. Community health will need to present a model, or several models, to achieve that goal. The chasm can be bridged or filled. It will take creative thinking, new models of community health programming, and concern for the fellow man, woman, boy, and girl in our communities and on our planet. Only as each of us moves and interacts within our various communities, developing an understanding and concern for the well-being of others, will effective community health be achieved. This is the future challenge for you . . . and community health.

[1]Concept of the great chasm discussed in chapter 1.

GLOSSARY

A

Abortion

Spontaneous or induced termination of a pregnancy before the fetus can survive by itself outside the womb

Acid rain

Polluted rainfall resulting when the oxides of sulfur and nitrogen react with water vapor in the atmosphere and form acids

Acquaintance rape

See date rape

Acquired immunodeficiency syndrome (AIDS)

Virus-caused illness characterized by a specific defect in the human body's natural immunity against disease

Age-related macular degeneration (AMD)

Disease in which the retina is affected resulting in visual loss among the elderly

Al-Anon

A voluntary organization for relatives of alcoholic patients

Alar

Chemical (deminozide) used by apple growers to help prevent apples from dropping from trees before they are ripe

Alcoholics Anonymous (AA)

A voluntary fellowship of recovering alcoholics who come together to help each other stay away from the use of alcohol

Almshouses

Facilities, such as jails or poorhouses, in which the mentally ill were kept in the early years of American and European history

Alzheimer's disease

Disorder of the elderly that produces memory loss and disorientation

Americans with Disabilities Act

Federal legislation that requires employers to make accommodations for employees or applicants with disabilities; included are disabled persons, people returning to work after suffering an injury, and the elderly

Angina

Reduction of the flow of blood to the heart

Anorexia nervosa

Eating disorder characterized by abnormal loss of weight and poor personal image of one's physical appearance

Anxiety disorders

Psychological disorders that include fear, distress, and a variety of phobias

APHA

American Public Health Association; professional organization of individuals employed in the various fields of community health

Arthritis

A chronic condition caused by injury or inflammation of a joint of the body

Asbestos

A mineral used in various construction activities; i.e., as a soundproofing and fireproofing agent

Azidothymidine (AZT)

An antiviral pharmaceutical that has been used experimentally with AIDS patients

AZT

See Azidothymidine

B

Bacteria

Small, single-cell microorganisms, some of which cause diseases in humans

Balloon angioplasty

Procedure used to break up atherosclerotic plaque that clogs arteries

Barbiturates

Drugs that depress the central nervous system to produce sleep or a quieting effect

Barden-LaFollette Act

1943 federal legislation that provided for vocational counseling and training for the mentally ill

Battered wife syndrome

Term used to refer to spouse abuse

BCG vaccine
Vaccine that provides protection against tuberculosis

Beers, Clifford
Author, in 1906, of *A Mind That Found Itself,* a classic on the state of affairs in mental hospitals at that time

Benign
Noncancerous or nonmalignant; localized, nonspreading, nonthreatening tumors

Beta amyloid
A protein found in plaque deposits in the brains of Alzheimer's patients; has been shown to produce degeneration of brain cells in the test tube

Black lung disease
See Pneumoconiosis

Blood alcohol concentration (BAC)
Amount of alcohol in the bloodstream

Brown lung disease
See Byssinosis

BSN (Bachelors of Nursing Degree)
The bachelor of nursing degree earned upon completion of a four-year nursing degree program

Bubonic plague
Disease transmitted to humans by fleas from infected rats; called "black death"

Bulimia
Eating disorder characterized by binging, then purging by vomiting

Byssinosis
Respiratory disease prevalent among textile workers; known as "brown lung disease"

C

Calorie
Unit used to express the energy content of food; the amount of heat required to raise the temperature of a kilogram of water (2.2 pounds) one degree centigrade

Cancer
Diseases that are the second leading cause of death in America

Cannabis sativa
The Indian hemp plant from which marijuana is derived

Carbohydrates
Group of foods, such as sugars and starches, that contain only carbon, hydrogen, and oxygen; a major source of calories in an average diet

Carbon monoxide
A colorless, odorless gas that may cause death by asphyxiation

Cardiopulmonary resuscitation (CPR)
Basic emergency life support technique involving mouth-to-mouth breathing or other ventilation technique and chest compression

Cardiovascular disease
Diseases of the circulatory system; the leading cause of death in the United States

Carpal tunnel syndrome
A painful and numbing condition of the hand caused by irritation of the median nerve that passes through the carpal tunnel in the wrist

Cataracts
A cloudiness or opacity of the lens of the eye that interferes with vision

Certificate-of-need (CON)
State laws that require state planning agency reviews and approval to spend capital expenditure monies

Cesarean section
Method of childbirth in which surgical incision is made in the abdominal and uterine walls to allow delivery of the fetus

Chemotherapy
Use of drugs in the treatment of cancer

Chernobyl
Location in the Soviet Union of a dangerous nuclear accident in 1986

Child sexual victimization
Term used to refer to sexual abuse of children and adolescents

Chiropractic medicine
Healing system based on theories of disease causation resulting from improper alignment of the vertebrae, spinal subluxations

Chlamydia
A sexually transmitted disease caused by the bacterium *Chlamydia trachomatis*

Chlorofluorocarbons (CFCs)
Chemicals containing chlorine, fluorine, and carbon used in numerous consumer products; they destroy ozone molecules

Chloroquine
An antimalarial drug

Cholesterol
Substance found in the fatty parts of animal tissue and in egg yolks that contributes to atherosclerosis

Chronic disease
Disease that is long-term and permanent

Cirrhosis
Degenerative disease of the liver characterized by the destruction of liver cells and the formation of fibrous connective tissue; often associated with alcohol consumption

Clean Air Act

The principal federal legislation directed toward improving the air quality in the United States

Cocaine

Central nervous system stimulant extracted from the leaves of the coca plant

Cohort

The grouping of individuals who are free of the disease or problem being investigated in an epidemiological study

Communicable disease

Infection that is transmitted from human to human or from animal to human

Conception

Point in time when the sperm from a male is implanted into the egg of the female

Control group

The population in an experimental study that does not receive the specific treatment under examination

Crack

Smokable form of cocaine

Cross-sectional study

A type of retrospective study often used in epidemiological research

Crude birth rate

The standard statistical datum used for stating birth rates

Crude death rate

The standard statistical datum used for stating death rates

Cumulative trauma disorders

Musculoskeletal injuries that cause damage due to wear of the musculoskeletal system at a rate faster than the body can be repaired

Curandero

Traditional healer using herbs and other modalities to cure various ailments; usually found in the Spanish-speaking countries of Central and South America

D

DAT

Drugs, Alcohol, and Tobacco

Date rape

Rape that takes place among individuals known to each other as friends

Decibels (dbs)

Unit of measurement used to indicate the loudness (intensity) of sound

Decommission

Procedure of shutting down a nuclear power plant and closing its operation

Deinstitutionalization

Removal of the mentally ill from mental hospital institutions to community care facilities

Dental caries

Tooth decay

Depression

Abnormal state of sadness or feeling of dejection

Desertification

Process of land deterioration and encroachment of the desert into previously useful and productive lands

Detoxification

Process whereby a person who is physically dependent upon a drug is gradually withdrawn from the drug

Diabetes

Disease in which the pancreas fails to produce sufficient insulin, causing an increase in blood sugar level or impairment of insulin activity

Diagnosis Related Groups (DRGs)

A prospective system of reimbursement to health providers for Medicare patients

Diastolic pressure

Blood pressure reading that indicates the arterial pressure when the heart is at rest between beats

Dioxin

Toxic chemical associated with numerous health-related problems in humans

Diphtheria

An infectious disease of the nose and throat

Doe v. Bolton

The case that the United States Supreme Court ruled on in 1973 that legalized abortion

Dracunculiasis

Parasitic disease transmitted by the guinea worm

Dram Shop Acts

Laws passed in some states which hold bartenders, servers of alcoholic beverages, and bar owners liable if they sell alcoholic beverages to an intoxicated person who later causes injury to a third person

Drug-free schools

A federal program designed to encourage cooperation within communities to work within the framework of schools to reduce and eliminate the use of drugs of abuse among school-aged young people

E

Electrocoagulation

Procedure in which malignant cells are destroyed by heat produced by electric current

Electromagnetic fields

Created in the presence of electricity, particularly electric power transmission lines; suggested as possible link to certain malignancies in humans

Elisa test

Blood test to ascertain the presence of the HIV virus that causes AIDS

Emphysema

Chronic respiratory disease resulting from the loss of normal function of the lung tissue characterized by "wheezing" and difficult breathing

Employee Assistance Programs (EAPs)

Programs supported by businesses and industries to help employees with personal problems that affect their work performance

Empowerment Education

Learning theory developed by Paulo Freire that has been useful in developing adult health education programs

Environmental Protection Agency (EPA)

The principal governmental agency charged with maintaining environmental standards

Epidemiological method

The model used in epidemiological studies that includes the interrelationships between the host, the causative agent, and the environment

Epidemiology

Study of the occurrence of disease among people

Etiology

The cause of a specific disease

Experimental group

In an epidemiological study the group that receives the treatment being studied

Export cropping

Agricultural products are exported from Third World nations to developed nations rather than being used to feed the local population

F

Fee-for-service

Concept that an individual is obliged to pay for medical services rendered by a health care provider

Fetal alcohol syndrome

Condition in which babies are born with retardation and physical abnormalities resulting from alcohol consumption of the mother during pregnancy

Fetal death

A stillbirth

Fission

Splitting of the core of an atom when it is struck by a neutron

Fluoridation

Use of fluorides to provide protection against dental caries

Fomites

Inanimate objects or material on which disease-producing agents may be transmitted

Food Guide Pyramid

A nutrition guide designed to communicate the recommendations and health messages presented in the Dietary Guidelines for Americans; published in 1992

Fungi

Parasitic, cellular organisms that lack chlorophyll

G

Galactosemia

Error of metabolism with inability to convert galactose to glucose

Gamma rays

One of the three kinds of radiation; has the ability to penetrate into the body

Genital herpes

Infectious sexually transmitted diseases caused by a herpes simplex virus and characterized by painful blisters and lesions in the genital areas of both men and women

Gerontology

Study of the aging process

Glaucoma

Increased pressure of fluid within the eye that is a leading cause of blindness

Gonorrhea

Sexually transmitted disease that affects the genitourinary tract and is spread primarily through sexual intercourse

Gout

An arthritic condition in which there is a painful swelling of the large toe

Greenhouse effect

Phenomenon in which the world's temperatures are rising owing to increased pollution in the air resulting in higher temperatures and drier world climates

Growing Healthy Curriculum Project

School health curriculum project combining the School Health Curriculum Project and the Primary Grades Curriculum Project

H

Halons

A chemical used in manufacture of fire extinguishers that can destroy ozone molecules

Health and Human Services, Department of
The federal cabinet-level department responsible for health programming

Health Belief Model
An educational learning model used by many health educators for research and for program development

Health maintenance organizations (HMOs)
An alternative system of health care where payment is made in advance on a fixed contract fee basis by a certain population

Health promotion
Term used to describe any combination of health education and related interventions designed to facilitate behavioral and environmental changes conducive to health

Hemoglobin
Substance in red blood cells that carries oxygen from the lungs to the tissues and gives blood its red color

Hepatitis
Inflammation of the liver caused by infection

Heroin
Narcotic synthesized from morphine

Hertz
Unit of measurement of sound

Hill-Burton Act
Legislation providing federal monies to construct and/or modernize health care facilities

Hispanic
Spanish-speaking population in the United States having come from Mexico, Puerto Rico, Cuba, and countries in Central and South America

Histoplasmosis
A fungal disease often marked by fever

HIV
See Human immunodeficiency virus

Homeless
Individuals who find it necessary to live on the streets and in public shelters

Homicide
Taking the life of another person; the eleventh leading cause of death in the United States

Hospital Survey and Construction Act
See Hill-Burton Act

Host
In an epidemiological study the group or individual affected by the causative agent

Human immunodeficiency virus (HIV)
The virus that is the etiologic agent of AIDS

Humectants
Food additives that help retain food texture by preventing and retarding moisture loss

Hydrocarbons
Compounds containing both hydrogen and carbon

Hypertension
High blood pressure

Hypothermia
An abnormally low body temperature

Hypothyroidism
Deficient secretion of hormones from the thyroid gland

I

Immunity
Resistance to disease and infection

Immunization
Process of providing protection against communicable diseases by use of killed or weakened strains of the causative agent to produce antibodies

Incest
Term used to refer to sexual abuse of children and adolescents; usually used when the abuser is a parent, guardian, or caretaker of the abused

Incidence rate
Numerical statistic used to express the number of cases that develop over a specific period of time

Incubation period
Period of time from the invasion into the body of a causative agent until the first signs and symptoms of the disease appear

Indian Health Service
Principal federal agency providing health care for Native Americans

Individual practice association (IPA)
One of two types of health maintenance organizations; the HMO reimburses the physician on a fee-for-service basis

Industrial hygienist
Individual that deals with environmental factors in the workplace that may cause sickness and injury

Infant mortality
Death that occurs in infants under one year of age

Influenza
A viral respiratory disease

Inpatient care
Medical care provided in the hospital

Intrauterine device (IUD)
Small plastic or metal device inserted into the uterus to prevent pregnancy

Ixodes dammini
The deer tick that is instrumental in spreading the bacterium that causes Lyme disease

J

Joints
Slang term used for marijuana cigarettes

K

Kwashiorkor
A protein deficiency disease often characterized by bloated stomachs among children

L

Lead
Chemical that causes various health problems

Leprosy
A communicable disease caused by mycobacterium leprae that affects the skin and peripheral nerves

Low infant birthweight
Weight at birth of less than 2,500 grams (5.5 pounds); popularly referred to as premature birth

LSD
Lysergic acid diethylamide, a potent hallucinogenic drug; sometimes referred to as "acid"

Lunatics
An inhumane term used to describe the mentally ill in the seventeenth and eighteenth centuries; the term was used because it was believed that the moon affected the mind

Lyme disease
Disease transmitted to humans by way of the bite of the deer tick

M

MADD
Acronym for Mothers Against Drunk Driving, a voluntary group interested in solving the problem of drunken driving

Mainlining
The practice of injecting heroin directly into the vein

Malaria
Infectious disease caused by protozoan parasites within the red blood cells and transmitted by the bite of a mosquito

Malignant
Cancerous cell growth

Malnutrition
Poor nutrition resulting in the lack of essential nutrients

Mammography
Examination procedure of the breasts for cancer

Managed health care system
A health care system in which government would regulate prices and encourage competition among health providers

Marine Health Service
The forerunner of the Public Health Service

Maternal mortality
Death of a woman from causes associated with childbirth

Measles
Infectious disease causing eruption of small red spots on the skin, referred to as rubeola

Medicaid
Federal program of health insurance for certain low-income individuals

Medical *montris*
Village health workers as they are referred to in Indonesia

Medicare
Federal program of health insurance for the elderly

Mescaline
A hallucinogenic drug sometimes known as peyote

Metastasis
Separation of malignant cells that spread to other parts of the body

Metazoa
Animal organisms that can infect humans

Mumps
Contagious viral disease with inflammation and swelling of the parotid and other salivary glands, fever, and pain

N

Narcotics
Drugs that have a depressant effect on the central nervous system

Neonatal death
Infant death that occurs within the first twenty-eight days after birth

Nicotine
A central nervous system stimulant that is present in the leaf of tobacco

Nitrogen oxides
Colorless, odorless gas making up most of the atmosphere and found in all living things

Norepinephrine
Neurotransmitter that is important in normal brain functioning that governs emotions

Norplant contraceptive
A subdermal implant contraceptive that provides protection against pregnancy over a relatively long period of time

Notifiable disease
Diseases that are required to be reported to the federal government

Nurse-midwives
Nurses with special training in the care and delivery of the pregnant woman

Nurse-practitioner
A health professional with specialty training beyond that of a registered nurse

Nursing home
The principal health care facility providing long-term care for the elderly

O

Occupational health nurse
A nurse who has specific training, experience, and skills unique to problems found in the industrial setting

Occupational physician
Medical doctor who services the medical needs in the occupational setting

Occupational Safety and Health Act
Federal legislation that established the Occupational Safety and Health Administration and the National Institute of Occupational Safety and Health

Official health organization
Health agency that receives a majority of its funding from tax sources

Omnibus Budget Reconciliation Act
Federal legislation that created the "block grant" program

Onchocerciasis
A filarial disease caused by *Onchocerca,* a filarial parasitic worm; popularly known as "river blindness"

Oncogenesis
Process by which a normal cell is changed to an abnormal cell

Oncology
The study of and treatment of cancer

Opiates
Drugs that are derived from opium, such as codeine, morphine, and heroin

Optometrist
A nonmedical doctor trained in the diagnosis of refractive errors of the eyes

Oral rehydration therapy (ORT)
An inexpensive, effective measure used to orally rehydrate patients; procedure is particularly useful where children have suffered dehydration from diarrhea

Organic mental disorders
Psychological disorders that are the result of physiological factors

OSHA
Term used to identify the Occupational Safety and Health Administration

Osteoarthritis
An arthritic disease that occurs as a result of injury or overuse of a joint

Osteopathic medicine
The diagnosis and treatment of diseases with particular attention to impairments of the musculoskeletal system

Osteoporosis
Loss of bone or thinning of bones that can result in pain and disability

Osteosarcoma
A rare bone cancer

Otitis media
An inflammation of the middle ear

Outpatient care
Medical care provided in such a manner that the patient does not need to be hospitalized

Ozone
Photochemical oxidant formed when atomic oxygen combines with oxygen already in the atmosphere that irritates the lungs, eyes, and throat, damages plants, and causes rubber to crack and decompose

Ozone layer
Ozone gas in the stratosphere ten to twenty-five miles above the earth

P

Particulate matter
Airborne particles of solid or liquid substances; soot, dirt, dust, fly ash

Pediatric AIDS
AIDS cases among infants and children

Pellagra
Dietary deficiency disease

Pelvic inflammatory disease (PID)
Severe inflammation of the upper part of the female reproductive system and the abdominal cavity

Pertussis
Whooping cough

Peyote
See Mescaline

Phenylketonuria
Metabolic disorder caused by the absence of the enzyme phenylalanine hydroxylase

Philanthropic foundations
Nonprofit funding foundations that support a broad range of social, education, and health services

Physician's assistant
An individual with one to two years of specialty training who can provide primary health care under the supervision of a physician

Plaque
Fatty deposits that form on the inner layer of the arterial walls

Pneumoconiosis
Respiratory disease that results from exposure to various dusts, principally found among coal miners; known as "black lung disease"

Pneumonia
Inflammation of the lungs caused by bacteria, viruses, chemical irritants, and allergens

Podiatrist
An allied health professional who provides care and treatment of problems of the feet

Polychlorinated biphenyls (PCB)
Chemical compounds found in industrial products and wastes that may accumulate in animal tissue and cause birth defects and liver damage

Postpartum
That which occurs after childbirth; after the delivery

PRECEDE Model
An educational learning model used by many health-educators for research and program development

Preferred provider organization
A system of health delivery designed to reduce the costs by developing a prearranged negotiated fee service

Prevalence rate
Statistical data that indicates the number of persons with a given problem at a particular point in time

Pro-choice
Term used to describe those who favor abortion

Prohibition
Period of time in the 1920s when it was illegal to manufacture and market alcoholic beverages

Pro-life
Term used by those who are opposed to abortion

Promotores del salud
Village health workers as they are referred to in Latin America

Proprietary for-profit hospital
Privately owned health care facility established and operated by a profit-making corporation

Prospective payment system
Provision of health care at a predetermined rate based on a particular diagnosis. See Diagnosis Related Groups (DRGs)

Prospective study
A type of epidemiological study that examines a given factor over a long-term period of time

Psychiatrist
A medical doctor whose specialty includes the diagnosis and treatment of emotional disturbances and mental disorders

Psychologist
An individual who studies the nonmedical science of human behavior

Public Health Service
Governmental agency that is part of the Department of Health and Human Services; principally responsible for maintaining and protecting the health of the American public

PVOs
Term used in international health work to designate those organizations in the private sector; private voluntary organizations, nongovernmental agencies

R

Radioactivity
The release of radiation

Radon
An odorless, colorless, tasteless, natural radioactive gas that is produced naturally in the ground; the product of underground uranium decay

Rape
An act of violence involving sex or attempted sex without the consent of the victim

Recommended Dietary Allowances (RDAs)
Standards of adequate nutritional intake published by the Food and Nutrition Board of the National Research Council

Reefers
Slang term used for marijuana cigarettes

Registered care technician
Semi-skilled bedside technician recommended by the American Medical Association to help fill the gap created by the shortage of registered nurses

Respite care
Type of care for the elderly that provides periodic relief for the family; adult day-care centers

Retrospective study
In epidemiological study an observational technique in which the specific population group is examined for a particular factor under investigation

Rheumatoid arthritis
An arthritic condition in which there is an inflammation of a joint

Roe v. Wade
The legal case upon which the United States Supreme Court ruled that abortion was legal

Roentgens
Basic unit of measurement of radiation

Role delineation project
A project designed to identify competencies of those individuals who are health educators

Rubella

Infectious disease causing eruption of small red spots on the skin; referred to as German measles; of shorter duration than rubeola

Rubeola

See Measles

S

Saccharin

Artificial sweetening substance used as a substitute for sugar

SADD

Acronym of Students Against Drunk Driving, a voluntary group of adolescents interested in assuring that they will not drive intoxicated or ride with others who have been drinking

Safety engineer

Worker involved in dealing with potential hazards in the workplace

Salmonella

Most common cause of foodborne disease in the United States

Sanitarian

An individual employed by health departments to conduct environmental inspections and carry out sanitation measures as required by rules and regulations of the local and state health department

Sanitary landfill

Site where solid wastes are buried in layers under dirt as a means of waste disposal and land reclamation

Schistosomiasis

Parasitic disease carried by snails that reside in slow-moving or stagnant water

Scurvy

A dietary deficiency disease resulting from inadequate ascorbic acid

Sedative

A drug that produces a calming effect, relaxes muscles, and relieves feelings of tension, anxiety, and irritability

Senile dementia

Results from narrowing of blood vessels that supply the brain with oxygen

Sickle-cell anemia

An inherited disorder of the red blood cells in which the normal flow of blood is blocked; this condition is found principally among the African-American population and those individuals from the Mediterranean region

Sidestream smoke

The smoke that affects the person in proximity to the individual who is smoking

Silicosis

Respiratory disease prevalent among workers exposed to silica

Smallpox

Acute, contagious disease (caused by a virus) that is characterized by fever, headache, abdominal pain, and lesions of the skin; has been eradicated since the early 1980s

Smokeless tobacco

Use of tobacco as snuff or chewing tobacco

Social Security

Social retirement insurance program for the elderly established by the federal government in 1935

Sodium

Salt

Somatoform disorders

Psychological disorders characterized by unfounded or unsubstantiated physical complaints when there is no observed or identifiable cause for the individual's symptoms

Stimulant

Drug that increases central nervous system function

Stroke

Impairment of the blood supply to the brain

Sudden infant death syndrome (SIDS)

Condition in which a child dies unexpectedly from unknown causes, usually while asleep in bed

Suicide

The taking of one's own life

Superfund

Federally authorized fund to provide support for cleaning up toxic waste sources

Synanon

First therapeutic community program for drug addicts founded in 1959

Syphilis

Sexually transmitted disease that is spread by person-to-person contact

Systolic pressure

Force exerted on the arteries when the heart beats

T

Temperance Movement

A movement that started in the early 1800s that called for total abstinence from the use of alcohol; a leading organization in the movement to bring about Prohibition in the 1920s

Temperature inversion

Meterological condition in which cooler air becomes trapped under a warmer layer of air and the cooler layer becomes heavily polluted

Tetanus
  Acute infectious disease caused by the toxin of *Clostridium tetani:* lockjaw

Tetrahydrocannabinol (THC)
  Active ingredient in marijuana that causes the euphoric effects

Thalidomide
  Tranquilizing drug taken by many pregnant women during the late 1950s that caused severe birth defects

Therapeutic community
  Residential programs providing drug abuse treatment

Toxemia
  Condition in which toxic substances are in the blood cells; caused by bacteria

Toxic wastes
  Hazardous chemicals such as dioxin, PCB, PBB, vinyl chloride, mercury, lead, and arsenic

Tuberculosis
  Respiratory disease caused by the tubercle bacillus

Tumor
  Abnormal, nonfunctional cell mass that grows independent of surrounding structures

Typhus
  Acute infectious disease usually prevalent in unsanitary localities

U

Understanding AIDS
  Brochure mailed to every household by the United States Surgeon General regarding AIDS in 1988

V

Vaccine
  Preparations of weakened or killed pathogens that stimulate antibody formation without causing observable signs of the disease

Vector
  An organism that transmits a disease-producing microorganism

Veterans Administration
  Operates a network of medical centers and clinics for former members of the military

Vinyl chloride
  Toxic chemical that can cause respiratory distress in humans

Virus
  Microscopic infectious organism that is parasitic and depends on nutrients inside cells for metabolic and reproductive survival

Voluntary health organizations
  Nonprofit organizations whose programming involves much use of voluntary time and financial support from nongovernmental sources

W

WIC
  A federally funded nutritional program for women, infants, and children

Women's Health Initiative
  A long-term federal government initiative established in 1993 designed to provide information and to enhance women's health

World Health Assembly
  The governing body of the World Health Organization

World Health Organization (WHO)
  International health organization with headquarters in Geneva, Switzerland

Y

Yellow fever
  An acute viral disease that affects the liver and is transmitted by certain mosquitoes

Z

Zoonosis
  Animal diseases that can be transmitted to humans

CREDITS

Chapter 13
Page 255: © Michael J. Okoniewski/The Image Works; **p. 257, 258:** AP/Wide World Photos; **p. 263:** © James L. Shaffer; **p. 264:** © Jack Spratt/The Image Works; **p. 265:** © Tony Freeman/PhotoEdit

Chapter 14
Page 273 left: Photo provided by the National Cancer Institute, Bethesda, MD.; **p. 273 right:** Courtesy of the American Cancer Society; **p. 274:** © Michael Siluk; **p. 278 both:** Erie County General Health District; **p. 279:** © Michael Siluk; **p. 280:** © Erika Stone/Peter Arnold, Inc.; **p. 285:** Photo provided by the National Cancer Institute, Bethesda, MD.

Chapter 15
Page 294: National Library of Medicine; **p. 302 top & bottom left:** Courtesy of the National Institute of Mental Health; **p. 302 right:** © Michael Siluk; **p. 305:** © Michael Siluk

Chapter 16
Page 310: Keep Toledo/Lucas County Beautiful Program; **p. 313:** Provided by the W. K. Kellogg Foundation, Battle Creek, Michigan; **p. 314:** Ohio Department of Education; **p. 316:** © Michael Newman/PhotoEdit; **p. 317, 318:** Courtesy of the American Cancer Society; **p. 323:** © Brian J. Miller; **p. 325:** Courtesy of the Ohio Environmental Protection Agency, Northwest District Office; **p. 326:** © Brian J. Miller

Chapter 17
Page 337: © A. Perlstein/Photo Researchers, Inc; **p. 338:** Provided by the W. K. Kellogg Foundation, Battle Creek, Michigan; **p. 339:** © Dean Miller; **p. 341 top:** Ohio Department of Education; **p. 341 bottom:** © James L. Shaffer

Chapter 18
Page 354: © Donna Jernigan; **p. 355:** Photo provided by the National Cancer Institute, Bethesda, MD.; **p. 356:** © Donna Jernigan; **p. 360 left & top right:** Courtesy of the Indian Health Service; **p. 360 bottom right:** © Michael Siluk; **p. 361 both:** Courtesy of the Indian Health Service

Chapter 19
Page 371: © Ron Byers; **p. 377 left:** © Dean Miller; **p. 377 right:** © James L. Ballard; **p. 379:** AP/Wide World Photos; **p. 382:** © Jean-Claude Lejeune

Chapter 20
Page 390: Courtesy of the National Institute of Aging; **p. 393:** Defiance Ohio Health Department; **p. 396:** Courtesy of the National Institute of Aging; **p. 400:** © Lynn Ritter; **p. 402:** Provided by the W. K. Kellogg Foundation, Battle Creek, Michigan; **p. 403 top:** © Julie O'Neil; **p. 403 bottom:** © Lynn Ritter

Chapter 21
Page 411: © Bill Bachman/PhotoEdit; **p. 414:** AP/Wide World Photos; **p. 420 both:** Courtesy of the American Cancer Society; **p. 429:** © Dean Miller

Chapter 22
Page 437: UPI/Bettmann Newsphotos; **p. 443:** © James L. Shaffer; **p. 446:** American Red Cross; **p. 447:** Courtesy of the American Cancer Society

Chapter 23
Page 459 all: Courtesy of Julie Coyle; **p. 462:** Courtesy of Healthy Families America/Photographer Tim L. Walker; **p. 465, 466, 467:** Courtesy of Julie Coyle

INDEX